Communicating About Health

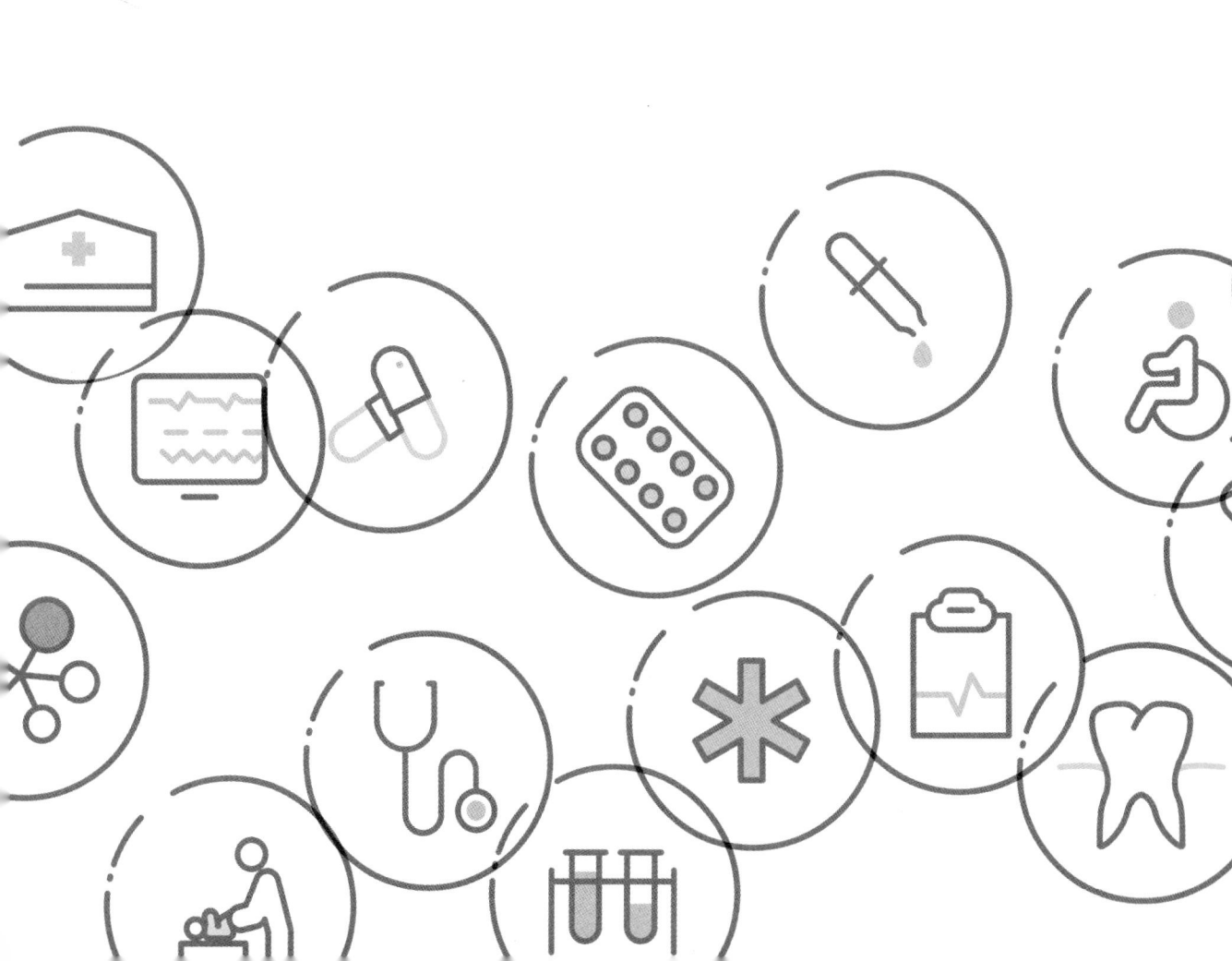

Communicating About Health

Current Issues and Perspectives

SIXTH EDITION

Athena du Pré
University of West Florida

WITH

Barbara Cook Overton
Louisiana State University

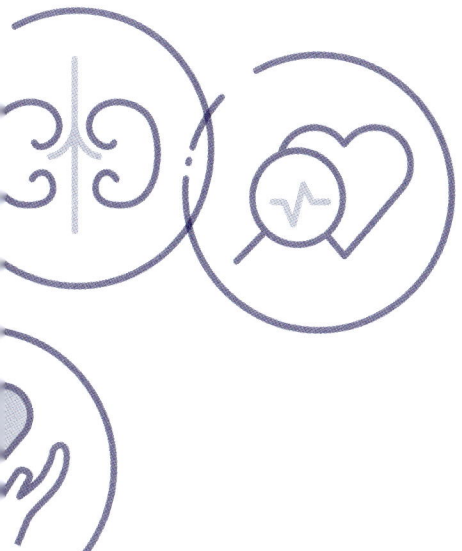

New York   Oxford
Oxford University Press

Oxford University Press is a department of the University of Oxford.
It furthers the University's objective of excellence in research, scholarship,
and education by publishing worldwide. Oxford is a registered trade mark of
Oxford University Press in the UK and certain other countries.

Published in the United States of America by Oxford University Press
198 Madison Avenue, New York, NY 10016, United States of America.

© 2021, 2017, 2014, 2010 by Oxford University Press
© 2005 by McGraw-Hill
© 2000 by Mayfield Publishing Company

> For titles covered by Section 112 of the US Higher Education
> Opportunity Act, please visit www.oup.com/us/he for the latest
> information about pricing and alternate formats.

All rights reserved. No part of this publication may be reproduced, stored in
a retrieval system, or transmitted, in any form or by any means, without the
prior permission in writing of Oxford University Press, or as expressly permitted
by law, by license, or under terms agreed with the appropriate reproduction
rights organization. Inquiries concerning reproduction outside the scope of the
above should be sent to the Rights Department, Oxford University Press,
at the address above.

You must not circulate this work in any other form
and you must impose this same condition on any acquirer.

Library of Congress Cataloging-in-Publication Data
Names: DuPré, Athena, author. | Overton, Barbara Cook, author.
Title: Communicating about health : current issues and perspectives /
   Athena du Pré, University of West Florida with Barbara Cook Overton,
   Louisiana State University.
Description: Sixth edition. | New York : Oxford University Press, [2021] |
   Includes bibliographical references and indexes. | Summary: "Our goal in
   this edition of Communicating About Health: Current Issues and
   Perspectives is to provide a manageable way of understanding the complex
   array of factors (both new and longstanding) that affect health. Along
   the way, we share the latest research and give voice to the stories of
   many different people. We believe you will find this to be an
   insightful, rich, and thorough overview of health communication. Our
   wish is that readers come away with a sophisticated knowledge of current
   issues, a real-life appreciation of the human side of health care and
   advocacy, and practical strategies for communicating more
   effectively and ethically about health"—Provided by publisher.
Identifiers: LCCN 2020002319 (print) | LCCN 2020002320 (ebook) | ISBN
   9780190924362 (paperback) | ISBN 9780190924379 (epub) | ISBN
   9780197525531 (ebook)
Subjects: LCSH: Communication in medicine. | Medical personnel and patient.
   | Health education. | Health promotion.
Classification: LCC R118 .D87 2021 (print) | LCC R118 (ebook) | DDC
   610.69/6—dc23
LC record available at https://lccn.loc.gov/2020002319
LC ebook record available at https://lccn.loc.gov/2020002320

Printing number: 9 8 7 6 5 4 3 2 1

Printed by LSC Communications, Inc.
United States of America

Brief Contents

Preface xv

PART I Establishing a Context for Health Communication 1

CHAPTER 1   Introduction 2
CHAPTER 2   The Landscape for Health Communication 20

PART II The Roles of Patients and Professional Caregivers 39

CHAPTER 3   Patient–Caregiver Communication 40
CHAPTER 4   Patient Perspectives 63
CHAPTER 5   Care Provider Perspectives 79

PART III Sociocultural Issues 103

CHAPTER 6   Diversity in Health Care 104
CHAPTER 7   Cultural Conceptions of Health and Illness 131

PART IV Coping and Health Resources 157

CHAPTER 8   Social Support, Family Caregiving, and End of Life 158
CHAPTER 9   eHealth, mHealth, and Telehealth 187

PART V Communication in Health Organizations 215

CHAPTER 10 Health Care Administration, Human Resources, Marketing, and PR 216

PART VI Media, Public Policy, and Health Promotion 237

CHAPTER 11 Health Images in the Media 238
CHAPTER 12 Public Health and Crisis Communication 268
CHAPTER 13 Planning Health Promotion Campaigns 295
CHAPTER 14 Designing and Implementing Health Campaigns 319

References 345
Credits 399
Author Index 401
Subject Index 415

Contents

Preface xv

PART I Establishing a Context for Health Communication 1

CHAPTER 1 Introduction 2

The Importance of Health Communication 2

BOX 1.1 Career Opportunities: Profiles of More Than 125 Health-Related Jobs 3

A Systems-Level Approach 5

Philosophy of This Book 6

BOX 1.2 Learn While You Make a Difference 7

What Is Health? 7

What Is Health Communication? 8

BOX 1.3 Perspectives: True Stories About Health Communication Experiences 8

    Defining Communication 8
        COLLABORATIVE SENSE-MAKING 9
        MULTIPLE LEVELS OF MEANING 9
        CONTEXT AND CULTURE 9
    Defining Health Communication 10

BOX 1.4 Theoretical Foundations: The Basis for Health Communication 10

    The History of Health Communication 11

BOX 1.5 Resources: Health Communication Organizations and Resources 11

Health Care Models 12
    Biomedical 12
    Biopsychosocial 13
    Sociocultural 13

BOX 1.6 Perspectives: A Memorable Hospital Experience 14

Communication's Influence on Health 15

BOX 1.7 Ethical Considerations: An Essential Component of Health Communication 16

BOX 1.8 Perspectives: Down, but Not Out 17

Summary 18
Glossary 18
Discussion Questions 19

CHAPTER 2 The Landscape for Health Communication 20

Current Issues in Health Care 20
    Early and Preventive Care 21
    Access and Health Disparities 21
    Navigating a Complex System 22
        COMMUNICATION SKILL BUILDERS: NAVIGATING THE HEALTH CARE SYSTEM 23

Health Communication in a Changing World 23
    Global Health 24
    Changing Populations 24
        AGING 24
        RACIAL AND CULTURAL DIVERSITY 24
    Communication Technology 25

Communication in Managed Care 25
    Conventional Insurance 26
    Health Maintenance Organizations 27
    Preferred Provider Organizations 27
    High-Deductible Health Plans 28
    Pros and Cons of Managed Care 28
        ADVANTAGES 28
        DISADVANTAGES 29

Health Care Reform 30
    Universal Coverage 30

BOX 2.1 Selecting a Managed Care Plan 31
        PROS AND CONS OF UNIVERSAL COVERAGE 31
    Single- and Multi-Payer Systems 32
        SINGLE-PAYER 32
        MULTI-PAYER 33
    The Affordable Care Act 34

BOX 2.2 Ethical Considerations: Classroom Debate on Health Care Reform 35

Summary 35
Glossary 36
Discussion Questions 37

PART II The Roles of Patients and Professional Caregivers 39

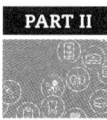

CHAPTER 3 Patient–Caregiver Communication 40

BOX 3.1 Career Opportunities: Health Communication Research 41

Medical Talk and Power Differentials 42
- Knowledge and Power 42

BOX 3.2 Ethical Considerations: The Truth, the Whole Truth . . . or Not? 43
- Who Talks and Who Listens 44
- Sensitive Subjects 44
- Patronizing Behavior 45
- Transgressions 45
- Why Do We Do It? 46

Collaborative Communication 47
- Reasons for a Shift 48
- Model of Collaborative Interpretation 48
- Focus on Quality of Life 49
- Shared Decision Making 50

Communication Skill Builders 51
- Motivational Interviewing 51
- Dialogue 53
  - NONVERBAL ENCOURAGEMENT 53
  - VERBAL ENCOURAGEMENT 54

BOX 3.3 Perspectives: A Mother's Experience at the Dentist 55
- Narrative Medicine 56

BOX 3.4 Theoretical Foundations: Integrative Health Model 59

BOX 3.5 Communication Tips for Patients 60

Summary 61
Glossary 61
Discussion Questions 62

CHAPTER 4 Patient Perspectives 63

Patient Socialization 63

BOX 4.1 Perspectives: The Agony of Uncertainty 64

Voice of Lifeworld 65
- Feelings Versus Evidence 65
- Specific Versus Diffuse 66
- Bridging the Gap 67
- Communication Skill Builders: Talking to a Care Provider 67

Health and Identity 68
- Identity and Facework 68
- Identity and Chronic Health Concerns 69
- Communication Challenges 69
- Communication Skill Builders: Responding to Identity Threats 70

Satisfaction 70

BOX 4.2 Ethical Considerations: Does Satisfaction Reflect Quality? 72

Cooperation and Consent 72

BOX 4.3 Career Opportunities: Patient Advocacy 72
- Reasons for Noncooperation 73
- Care Providers' Investment 73
- Informed Consent 74

BOX 4.4 Ethical Considerations: Patients' Right to Informed Consent 76

Summary 77
Glossary 78
Discussion Questions 78

CHAPTER 5 Care Provider Perspectives 79

BOX 5.1 Career Opportunities: Care Providers 80

Care Provider Preparation 80
- Historical Perspective 80
- The Role of Communication 81
- Socialization 81
  - VOICE OF MEDICINE 82
  - HIDDEN CURRICULUM 82
  - ISOLATION 82
  - IDENTITY IN LIMBO 83
  - PRIVILEGES 83
  - LOSS OF EMPATHY 84
  - IMPLICATIONS 84
- Communication Training and Integrated Approaches 84
  - INTERPROFESSIONAL EDUCATION 84
  - PROBLEM-BASED LEARNING 84
  - BIOPSYCHOSOCIAL FOCUS 85

Systems-Level Influences on Care Providers 85
- Organizational Culture 85
- Time Constraints 86

Psychological Influences on Caregivers 87
- Emotional Preparedness 87
- Mindfulness 88

Confidence 88
Satisfaction 89

Stress and Burnout 89

BOX 5.2 Perspectives: Blowing the Whistle on an Impaired Physician 90

Causes 90
CONFLICT 90

BOX 5.3 Communication Skill Builder: Dealing with Difficult Patients 91

EMOTIONS 91
WORKLOAD 92

Healthy Strategies 92

Medical Mistakes 93

"Doctor Amputates Wrong Leg" 93
Why Mistakes Happen 93
What Happens After a Mistake? 94
Communication Skill Builder: Managing Medical Mistakes 95
FROM THE BEGINNING 96
IF AN ERROR DOES OCCUR 96

Interprofessional Teamwork 97

Advantages 98
Difficulties and Drawbacks 99
Communication Skill Builder: Working in Teams 99

Summary 100
Glossary 100
Discussion Questions 101

 **PART III** Sociocultural Issues 103

 **CHAPTER 6** Diversity in Health Care 104

Intersectionality Theory 104

Socioeconomic Status 105

Health Literacy 108

Skill Builders for Public Health Care Professionals 109
Skill Builders for Health Care Providers 110
Skill Builders for Patients 110

Gender Identity and Sexual Orientation 110

Race and Ethnicity 112

Distrust 113
High Risk, Low Knowledge 113
Limited Access 113

BOX 6.1 Ethical Considerations: Who Gets What Care? 114

Stereotypes 115
Intercultural Health Communication 115

BOX 6.2 Genetic Profiling: A View Into Your Health Future 116

Language Differences 117

BOX 6.3 Perspectives: Language Barriers in a Health Care Emergency 118

Disabilities 120

BOX 6.4 Career Opportunities: Diversity Awareness 120

What It Means to Have a Disability 120
Communication Dilemmas 121

BOX 6.5 Perspectives: My Disability Doesn't Show 122

Communication Skill Builder: Interacting with People Who Have Disabilities 122

Age 123

Children 123
PARENTS' ROLE IN CHILDREN'S CARE 124
COMMUNICATION SKILL BUILDER: TALKING WITH CHILDREN ABOUT ILLNESS 124

Older Adults 124
COMMUNICATION ACCOMMODATION THEORY 125
COMMUNICATION PATTERNS 127
COMMUNICATION TECHNOLOGY AND OLDER ADULTS 127

Summary 128
Glossary 129
Discussion Questions 130

 **CHAPTER 7** Cultural Conceptions of Health and Illness 131

Culture and Health Communication 132

The Challenge of Multiculturalism 132
CULTURAL ADAPTABILITY IN HEALTH CARE 133

Cultural Conceptions of Health 134

Health as Organic 134
Health as Harmonic Balance 135
PHYSICAL, EMOTIONAL, AND SPIRITUAL 135
HARMONY WITH NATURE 136
HOT AND COLD 136
ENERGY 136

Making Sense of Health Experiences 137

BOX 7.1 Theoretical Foundations: Theory of Health as Expanded Consciousness 137

Health Condition as Social Asset 139
Health Condition as Social Liability 139
  DISEASE AS CURSE 139
  STIGMA 140
  THE MORALITY OF PREVENTION 141
  VICTIM ROLE 141

Social Roles and Health 141
  Sex, Gender, and Health 142
    FEMALE IDENTITY AND HEALTH 142
    MALE IDENTITY AND HEALTH 143
  Family Roles and Health Communication 143

BOX 7.2 Perspectives: Thai Customs and a Son's Duty 144

Illness and Coping Metaphors 145
  "Fight for Your Life" 145
  "Strive for Peace and Flexibility" 146

Sick Roles and Healer Roles 146
  Mechanics and Machines 147
  Parents and Children 147
  Spiritualists and Believers 148

BOX 7.3 Ethical Considerations: Physician as Parent or Partner? 148
  Providers and Consumers 149
  Partners 150

BOX 7.4 Perspectives: Partners in Care 151

Holistic Care 151
  Terminology 152
  Popularity 152
  Advantages 152

BOX 7.5 Holistic Medicine at a Glance 153
  Drawbacks 153

BOX 7.6 Career Opportunities: Holistic Medicine 154

Summary 155
Glossary 155
Discussion Questions 156

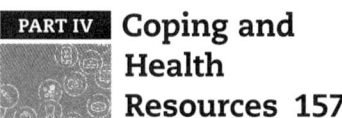

PART IV Coping and Health Resources 157

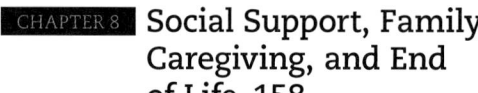

CHAPTER 8 Social Support, Family Caregiving, and End of Life 158

Conceptual Overview 159
  Theoretical Perspectives 159

BOX 8.1 When Communication Ability Is Compromised 161
  Coping 161
  Sense of Control 162
  Dialectics 163
  Crisis 163
  Normalcy 164

Coping and Communication 165
  Action-Facilitating Support 165
  Nurturing Support 166
    COMMUNICATION SKILL BUILDER: SUPPORTIVE LISTENING 166

BOX 8.2 Theory of Problematic Integration 167
    COMMUNICATION SKILL BUILDER: ALLOWING EMOTIONAL EXPRESSION 168
    SOCIAL NETWORKS 169

When Social Support Goes Wrong 169
  Friends Disappear 169
  Hurtful Jests 170
  Too Much Support 171
  A Note of Encouragement 171

Animal Companions 172

Transformative Experiences 172

Friends and Family as Caregivers 174

BOX 8.3 Organ Donations: The Nicholas Effect 174
  Stress and Burnout 176
  Caring for Caregivers 176

BOX 8.4 Perspectives: A Long Goodbye to Grandmother 177

End-of-Life Experiences 178
  Life at All Costs 178
  Death with Dignity 179
  Communication Skill Builder: Coping With Death 181

Advance-Care Directives 181

Communication Skill Builder: Delivering Bad News 182

BOX 8.5 Ethical Considerations: Do People Have a Right to Die? 182

BOX 8.6 Career Opportunities: Social Services and Mental Health 184

Summary 184
Glossary 185
Discussion Questions 186

CHAPTER 9 eHealth, mHealth, and Telehealth 187

Health Information Haves and Have Nots 189
- ePatients 189
- Digital Divide 189
  - SOCIODEMOGRAPHICS 189
  - VISION CHALLENGES 190
  - CONFIDENCE 190

Why and When Do People Seek Ehealth Information? 190
- Information Sufficiency Threshold 191
- Health Information Acquisition Model 191
- Theory of Motivated Information Management 191
- Integrative Model of Online Health Information Seeking 192
- Unified Theory of Acceptance and Use of Technology 193

Is eHealth Information Useful to Everyday People? 194
- Advantages 194
  - RICH ARRAY OF INFORMATION 194
  - SOURCE OF PRACTICAL ADVICE 194
  - SOCIAL SUPPORT 194
- Disadvantages 195
  - UNRELIABLE INFORMATION 195
  - CONFLICTING INFORMATION 196
  - OVERWHELMING AMOUNTS OF INFORMATION 196
  - PRIVACY CONCERNS 196
- Communication Skill Builder: Using the Internet Effectively 196

Is eHealth Information Useful to Care Providers? 197

Impact of eHealth 198

mHealth 200
- Health Apps 201

BOX 9.1 Ethical Considerations: The Pros and Cons of Telemedicine 202

- Texting for Health 203
- Disadvantages 204

Telehealth 204
- Telemedicine 204
- Patient Portals 205
- Telemonitoring 206
- Potential Advantages of Telehealth for Consumers 206
  - PATIENT-CENTERED COMMUNICATION 206
  - ACCESS TO SERVICES 207
  - COST SAVINGS 207

- Potential Advantages of Telehealth for Health Professionals 207
  - EFFICIENCY 207
  - TEAMWORK 208
  - ACCESSIBLE INFORMATION 208
- Potential Disadvantages of Telehealth 208
  - SCHEDULING CHALLENGES 208
  - WORKFLOW DISRUPTIONS 208
  - COST 208
  - COMPENSATION QUESTIONS 208
  - LIABILITY 209
  - THREATS TO PRIVACY 209
  - UNORGANIZED INFORMATION IN ELECTRONIC MEDICAL RECORDS 209
  - COMPROMISED QUALITY OF CARE 210
  - EFFECTS ON PATIENT–PROVIDER COMMUNICATION AND THERAPEUTIC RELATIONSHIPS 210

BOX 9.2 Career Opportunities: Health Information Technology 211

Summary 211
Glossary 213
Discussion Questions 213

PART V Communication in Health Organizations 215

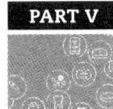

CHAPTER 10 Health Care Administration, Human Resources, Marketing, and PR 216

BOX 10.1 Career Opportunities: Health Communication Specialists 217

Health Care Administration 217
- Enhancing Health Care Experiences 218

BOX 10.2 Journals in the Field 219

- Communication Skill Builder: Servant Leadership and Empowerment 219
  - INVERT THE PYRAMID 219
  - BUILD RELATIONSHIPS BY LISTENING 220
  - PUSH DECISION MAKING TO THE LOWEST LEVEL POSSIBLE 221
  - HOLD PEOPLE ACCOUNTABLE 222
  - CELEBRATE SUCCESSES 222

Human Resources 223
- Theoretical Foundations 223

BOX 10.3 Staffing Shortages in Health Care 224

Communication Skill Builder: Building Great Teams 225
    HIRE CAREFULLY 226
    TEACH THE CULTURE AND VALUES 226
    CONTINUALLY RECRUIT INTERNAL TALENT 226

Marketing and Public Relations 227
    Foundations for Theory and Practice 228
        FOCUS ON RELATIONSHIPS 228
        INTEGRATE 229
        DEVELOP REPUTATION, NOT ONLY IMAGE 229
    Communication Skill Builder: Two-Way Communication and Social Media 230

Crisis Management 231

Service Excellence 232

Summary 233

Glossary 234

Discussion Questions 234

PART VI Media, Public Policy, and Health Promotion 237

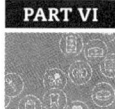

CHAPTER 11 Health Images in the Media 238

Theoretical Foundations 239
    Third-Person Effect 240
    Cultivation Theory 240
    Social Learning Theory 240
    Social Comparison Theory 241

Advertising 241
    Nutrition and Obesity 241
        EFFECTS ON CHILDREN 241
        EFFECTS ON ADULTS 242
        ACTIVITY LEVELS 243
    Alcohol 243
    Tobacco and Nicotine 245
    Pharmaceutical Advertisements 245

BOX 11.1 Perspectives: Viagra Ads Promise Male Transformation 246
        ADVANTAGES OF DTC ADVERTISING 247
        DISADVANTAGES OF DTC ADVERTISING 248
        COMMUNICATION SKILL BUILDER: EVALUATING MEDICAL CLAIMS 249

News Coverage 249
    "New Study Suggests that Vaccines Don't Cause Autism" 249
    Accuracy and Fairness 250
    Sensationalism 250
    Advantages of Health News 251
    Communication Skill Builder: Presenting Health News 251

BOX 11.2 Perspectives: Barbie: Feminist Icon or Woman as Sex Object? 252

Media and Body Image 253
    Health Effects 254

BOX 11.3 Perspectives: Boys' Toys on Steroids 255
    Beauty Sells . . . Sometimes 256

Entertainment 256
    Portrayals of Health Care Situations 256
    Portrayals of Health-Related Conditions 257
        MENTAL ILLNESS 257
        DISABILITIES 258
    Portrayals of Health-Related Behaviors 258
        SEX 258
        VIOLENCE 260
    Entertainment and Commercialism 261
        ENTERTAINOMERCIALS 261
        PRODUCT PLACEMENT 261
    Entertainment-Education Programming 262

BOX 11.4 Ethical Considerations: Is the Entertainment Industry Responsible for Health Images? 263
    Impact of Persuasive Entertainment 264

Media Literacy 264

Summary 265

Glossary 266

Discussion Questions 267

CHAPTER 12 Public Health and Crisis Communication 268

What Is Public Health? 268

BOX 12.1 Career Opportunities: Public Health 269

Risk and Crisis Communication 270
    Managing Perceptions 271

BOX 12.2 Parents Grapple with Vaccine Information 272
    How Scared Is Scared Enough? 273
    In the Heat of the Moment 274

BOX 12.3 Risk Management/Communication Framework 275

Crisis Communication Models and Guidelines 276
    World Health Organization's Guidelines on Communicating Risk 276
    The IDEA Model 277
    The Crisis and Emergency Risk Communication (CERC) Model 278

Social Media and Crisis Communication 278

Case Studies: A Global Perspective 279

BOX 12.4 Typhoid Mary and TB Andy 280
    Ebola 281
        COMMUNICATION WITH THE WORRIED WELL 281
        COMMUNICATION IN THE MIDST OF TRAUMA 282
        AIDS 283
        SARS 285
    Avian Flu 286

BOX 12.5 Ethical Considerations: Who Should Be Protected? 287
    Zika 288
    The Opioid Epidemic 289

BOX 12.6 Lessons for Public Health and Crisis Communication 291

Summary 292
Glossary 293
Discussion Questions 294

CHAPTER 13 Planning Health Promotion Campaigns 295

BOX 13.1 Career Opportunities: Health Promotion and Education 297

Background on Health Campaigns 297
    Motivating Factors 297
    Exemplary Campaigns 298
        GET TO KNOW THE AUDIENCE 298
        INVEST IN COMMUNICATION INFRASTRUCTURES 298

BOX 13.2 Storytelling Connects Underserved Women and Care Providers 299
        MAKE HEALTHY OPTIONS ACCESSIBLE 300
        TAKE A MULTIMEDIA APPROACH 300
        SET CLEAR GOALS AND MEASURE YOUR SUCCESS 300

Step 1: Defining the Situation and Potential Benefits 301
    Benefits 301
    Current Situation 301
    Diverse Motivations 302

Step 2: Analyzing and Segmenting the Audience 302
    Data Collection 302
        ETHICAL COMMITMENTS 303
        DATA-GATHERING OPTIONS 303
    Choosing a Target Audience 305
        THEORETICAL FOUNDATIONS 305
        REACHING UNDERINFORMED AUDIENCES 306
    Segmenting the Audience 306
    Audience as a Person 307
    Young Audiences 308
    Sensation-Seekers 308

BOX 13.3 Ethical Considerations: The Politics of Prevention—Who Should Pay? 310

Step 3: Establishing Campaign Goals and Objectives 311

Step 4: Selecting Channels of Communication 312
    Channel Characteristics 312
    Message Impact 313
        AROUSAL 313
        INVOLVEMENT 313
    Multichannel Campaigns 315

Summary 316
Glossary 317
Discussion Questions 318

CHAPTER 14 Designing and Implementing Health Campaigns 319

Theories of Behavior Change 321
    Health Belief Model 321
    Social Cognitive Theory 322
    Theory of Reasoned Action 323
    Transtheoretical Model 324
    Wrapping It Up 325

Critical-Cultural Perspective 326

BOX 14.1 Ethical Considerations: Three Issues for Health Promoters to Keep in Mind 327

Step 5: Designing Campaign Messages 329
    Choosing a Voice and/or Spokesperson 330

BOX 14.2 Career Opportunities: Health Campaign Design and Management 331
    Designing the Message 331

THEORETICAL FOUNDATIONS: MESSAGE FRAMING 332
COMMUNITY EXPECTATIONS 334

BOX 14.3 Theoretical Foundations: What Does Science Say About Peer Pressure? 334

NARRATIVE MESSAGES 336
LOGICAL APPEALS 337
EMOTIONAL APPEALS 337
NOVEL AND SHOCKING MESSAGES 339

BOX 14.4 S-mething Is Missing 339

Step 6: Piloting and Implementing the Campaign 340

Step 7: Evaluating and Maintaining the Campaign 341

Evaluation 341
Maintenance 342

Summary 342

Glossary 343

Discussion Questions 344

References 345

Credits 399

Author Index 401

Subject Index 415

Preface

A great deal has changed since the first edition of *Communicating About Health* was published 20 years ago. Our watches and telephones have become important sources of health communication. Vaping has emerged as a health threat, as have vaccination denial and the emergence of a number of lethal viruses. Health care reform has transformed how services are offered and allowed tens of millions of previously uninsured people to have coverage. And the list goes on.

Yet many fundamentals of health communication are as (or more) important than ever. Communication skills remain crucial for sharing information, offering comfort, and negotiating health options. The world population is increasingly diverse, opening people's eyes to new ideas about health and healing. Lingering social inequities mean that a person's health can still largely be predicted by their race and socioeconomic status. Information, access to care, and health literacy remain challenges, especially in the context of complicated health care systems and a mind-boggling amount of health information available online.

Our goal in this edition of *Communicating About Health: Current Issues and Perspectives* is to provide a manageable way of understanding the complex array of factors (both new and long-standing) that affect health. Along the way, we share the latest research and give voice to the stories of many different people. We believe you will find this to be an insightful, rich, and thorough overview of health communication. Our wish is that readers come away with a sophisticated knowledge of current issues, a real-life appreciation of the human side of health care and advocacy, and practical strategies for communicating more effectively and ethically about health.

Our Approach

Because health care is so dynamic and complex, it's difficult to keep up with everything. We often feel we are doing well to stay up to date in any one sector. That's understandable. But it is also the greatest weakness in the system, and it can be a fatal flaw. We miss opportunities for innovative teamwork. Our efforts are often duplicative and contradictory. And we often don't see the larger patterns at work. As the great systems theorist Peter Senge (2006) observes, *"Structures of which we are unaware hold us prisoner"* (p. 93).

In health care, this often equates to mistakes and duplications, expensive care that might have been avoided, well-intentioned campaigns that don't work, and administrative oversight that is cumbersome and distracting rather than smooth, supportive, and integrated. Effective communication isn't a nicety. It's good medicine, and it's good business.

Communicating About Health is readable enough to serve as an introduction to the field. But as feedback from experienced health professionals bears out, this is not a skim-the-surface book. It offers deep insights that are helpful even for experienced practitioners and researchers. By the book's end, readers should be able to speak knowledgeably, not just about one aspect of health care, but about how the many pieces fit together and influence each other.

Intended Audience

This book is designed primarily for people pursuing careers in the health industry and those with a research interest in health communication. This includes care providers, health care administrators, marketing and public relations professionals, media planners and producers, public health promoters, human resources personnel, researchers, educators, and others.

It may seem that such a diverse audience could not be served by the same text, and to some extent that is true. By all means, read other works as well. Specialized texts have a great deal to offer. But our advice is to read this book first or alongside the others. It provides something that specific-interest books cannot—a revealing overview of how various professions, cultures, and current concerns converge. We believe that, where health is concerned, understanding the big picture is as important as mastering a particular skill set. Your success will be enhanced if you are able to speak authoritatively about current issues in the health care field overall. (And truth be told, we're counting on you to address some of the ongoing challenges in health care.)

Strengths of the Book

Communicating About Health has several advantages:

- **Up-to-Date Coverage** The book describes how managed care, health care reform, mobile technology, social media, and other factors are changing the nature of health communication. Readers are exposed to innovations unimagined just a few years ago and encouraged to consider the pros and cons in terms of health communication.
- **Diversity in Health Care** Readers are exposed to culturally diverse ways of thinking about health and healing. Topics include gender identity, age, socioeconomic status, race, and more. The book looks at health care through the eyes of care providers, patients, administrators, health promoters, and others who contribute to the process.
- **Communication Skill Builders** *Communicating About Health* is a useful guide for people interested in improving their health-related communication skills. It includes suggestions for encouraging patient participation, providing social support, listening, developing cultural competence, working in teams, designing health promotion campaigns, and more.
- **Critical Thinking and Discussion** Throughout the book, *Perspectives* features, *Ethical Considerations* boxes, photo captions, and discussion questions challenge students to weigh the merits of various communication options and apply what they are learning to their own lives.
- **Instructional Resources** An instructor's manual, available both in print and online at www.oup.com/he/dupre-6e, features a sample syllabus, daily lesson plans, learning activities, handouts, test questions, and more. Corresponding PowerPoint presentations are designed to stimulate student engagement either in person or online.

Communicating About Health is much more than a literature review. It explores the diverse perspectives of people involved in health communication and shows how they blend and negotiate their ideas to create communication episodes. The book integrates research, theories, current issues, and real-life examples. This blend of information enables students to understand the implications of various communication phenomena. At the same time, readers learn how they can contribute to health communication in a positive way as professionals, patients, and researchers.

Features in the New Edition

This edition features a more streamlined format that maintains the readability and real-life examples that have made previous editions so popular. Each chapter now ends with a glossary of terms, an easy-reference summary in outline form, and updated discussion questions. Here is an overview of new coverage:

- **Chapter 1 (Introduction)** includes updated examples and research along with new coverage of the World Health Organization's perspective on health in the context of everyday life.
- **Chapter 2 (The Landscape for Health Communication)** has been significantly updated with insights and tips about navigating the health care maze. The chapter also includes new information about health disparities and health care reform, including an explanation of concepts such as managed care, multi-payer systems, Medicare for All, and the Affordable Care Act.
- **Chapter 3 (Patient–Caregiver Communication)** includes updated information about the impact of patient–provider communication on health, diagnoses, satisfaction, and pain. New sections offer strategies for discussing sensitive subjects and engaging in shared decision making.
- **Chapter 4 (Patient Perspectives)** has been reorganized to focus more on patient satisfaction and identity work. New segments provide patients tips for talking to care providers and responding to face-threatening health concerns.
- **Chapter 5 (Care Provider Perspectives)** features new information about interprofessional education and teamwork. It also includes updated information about diverse career opportunities in patient care.
- **Chapter 6 (Diversity in Health Care)** includes new and expanded coverage of gender identity and sexual orientation, ethnicity and race, and the link between health and socioeconomic status. Additional skill builder tips and examples have been added to provide diverse perspectives.
- **Chapter 7 (Cultural Conceptions of Health and Illness)** presents new coverage of a

culture-centered approach to health communication as well as the effects of social stigma and cultural adaptability.
- **Chapter 8** (**Social Support, Family Caregiving, and End of Life**) features expanded coverage of the dialectical push and pull people feel when managing health concerns as well as new research about adapting to a "new normal" after a serious health event.
- **Chapter 9** (**eHealth, mHealth, and Telehealth**) has been updated to reflect current issues and cutting-edge research in eHealth. Special attention has been given to emerging mobile technologies, wearable devices, and health apps. Providers' experiences and perspectives relevant to eHealth and telehealth are included.
- **Chapter 10** (**Health Care Administration, Human Resources, Marketing, and PR**) presents new and updated examples of communication specialists in health care and the work they do. Coverage of staffing shortages is updated along with communication skill builders related to leadership, human resources, and public relations.
- **Chapter 11** (**Health Images in the Media**) presents new research on the ways media can inform our reading of certain health issues and behaviors, such as binge drinking, vaping, and sexual assault. Social media's effect on health is addressed, and an expanded discussion of direct-to-consumer pharmaceutical advertisements explores media's impact on provider–patient relationships.
- **Chapter 12** (**Public Health and Crisis Communication**) has been revised with a renewed focus on crisis and risk communication models from the CDC and the World Health Organization. Social media's role in crisis communication is explored and recommendations are offered. Case studies have been updated to reflect current research on HIV/AIDS, Zika, and the opioid epidemic.
- **Chapter 13** (**Planning Health Promotion Campaigns**) has been updated to reflect new research and trends in health promotion campaigns. Special attention has been given to campaigns addressing vaping and methamphetamine abuse, as well as those using social media. An expanded discussion on message tailoring explores multiple ways messages can be designed for diverse audiences.
- **Chapter 14** (**Designing and Implementing Health Campaigns**) presents research on health promotion campaigns that extend the utility of the health belief model and transtheoretical model. Updated examples highlight the latest research on source credibility, narrative messages, gain- and loss-frames, and affect appeals.

Overview of the Book

Part I: Establishing a Context for Health Communication

The first two chapters provide an introduction to health communication. Chapter 1 establishes the nature and definition of health communication, current issues, and important reasons to study health communication. Chapter 1 also provides tips for making the most of features such as *Ethical Considerations*, *Theoretical Foundations*, and *Career Opportunities* boxes that appear throughout the book.

Chapter 2 explores how health communication is evolving within the context of social and public issues. Understanding these issues allows for deeper appreciation of topics described in the rest of the book. The chapter culminates with a look at health care reform measures, helping students better understand how policy debates and topics in the news affect them personally.

Part II: The Roles of Patients and Professional Caregivers

Part II focuses on interpersonal communication between patients and health care providers. Chapter 3 describes patient–provider communication in terms of who talks, who listens, and how medical decisions are made. It features a broader array of providers than in the past, thanks to emerging research about nurses, pharmacists, paramedics, physical therapists, technicians, and others. The chapter features a discussion of narrative medicine and real-life examples of patient–provider communication.

Chapter 4 examines health communication through patients' eyes, considering what motivates patients, what they typically like and do not like about health care, and how people express themselves in health encounters. This edition looks closely at how communication is influenced by the nature of illness, patient disposition, and threats to personal identity. It includes information about communication skills training for patients and updated information about patient narratives and self-advocacy.

In Chapter 5, readers view health from the perspective of professional care providers. This edition explores the philosophy behind caregiver training programs and how that has changed through the years. As in Chapter 3, coverage includes a broader array of professionals than in the past. This chapter features coverage of mindfulness and other strategies to help care providers remain emotionally resilient. It also presents tips for communicating with difficult patients, communicating when time is limited, and disclosing medical mistakes. It concludes with a unit on multidisciplinary teamwork. Information is provided on more than 30 careers in medicine, dentistry, nursing, and allied health.

Part III: Sociocultural Issues

Chapter 6 focuses on diversity among patients and health professionals. It begins with a feature on intersectionality theory and includes expanded coverage of nuanced gender identities. The chapter presents information and strategies for communicating effectively with people who differ in terms of social status, gender, race, language, ability, and age. The section on health literacy is substantially updated. Case studies describe the experiences of a Spanish-speaking woman in an English-speaking hospital and a college student coping with a physical disability.

Chapter 7 describes social and cultural conceptions of health and healing. It presents a model of cultural competence and exposes readers to ideas about health around the world, including conceptualizations of health as a balance between the physical and spiritual, between elements of "hot" and "cold," between different types of life energy, and more. Coverage of holistic medicine appears in this chapter, as do diverse expectations about the roles of patients and caregivers. The chapter includes a feature about the theory of health as expanded consciousness and many examples illustrating diverse perspectives.

Part IV: Coping and Health Resources

Part IV focuses on the array of resources we may use to maintain and regain health, and when that is not possible, to cope at the end of life.

Chapter 8 illustrates the importance of social support and provides tips for supportive communication. This edition features updated coverage about the role of communication in family caregiving and end-of-life experiences. The chapter also examines instances of social support "gone wrong"—episodes in which people's efforts to help actually hurt, and how we can avoid making the same mistakes. Another section within the chapter explores the notion of animals as supportive companions. The chapter includes sections on transformative health care experiences and organ donation decisions.

Chapter 9 presents updated information about eHealth, mHealth, and telehealth. It presents evidence that, around the world, more people now have mobile technology than have electricity in their homes. We explore how health communication specialists are trying to make the most of this new information resource to benefit diverse patent populations around the world. The chapter addresses such questions as *Why and under what circumstances do people seek electronic health information? Is eHealth information mostly helpful or counterproductive?* and *How does eHealth communication compare with face-to-face interactions?* Readers will learn more about the emergence of virtual hospitals, mobile devices, and health apps, and will debate the pros and cons of telehealth in terms of health communication. Information about medical information and technology careers is presented.

Part V: Communication in Health Organizations

Chapter 10 presents new examples of roles that communication specialists play in health. The chapter is loaded with theories and expert tips related to health care administration, public relations, being a servant leader, promoting a shared vision, working in teams, and rewriting the rules by which health care organizations operate. The chapter culminates with tips for service excellence from some of the best medical centers in the world. Coverage includes theories and related stories from professionals in the field.

Part VI: Media, Public Policy, and Health Promotion

Chapter 11 provides the latest information about health images in advertising, news, and entertainment. It features new coverage about body image and social media, as well as media influence on obesity, alcohol and nicotine use, sex, and violence. The chapter also includes a section on the international impact of entertainment-education and information about careers in health journalism. It includes tips for reporting health news, using interactive media to present health information, and developing media literacy.

In Chapter 12, readers explore the real-life lessons of health communication professionals involved with Ebola, AIDS, SARS, avian flu, Zika, the opioid epidemic, and other health threats. The chapter presents advice for preventing and minimizing crises, responding in the heat of the moment, and managing public fears and information needs. The emphasis is on collaborative communication that is timely, data based, and culturally sensitive.

Chapters 13 and 14 guide readers through the creation and evaluation of public health campaigns. Both chapters include real-life campaign exemplars and sample PSAs, as well as expanded coverage of campaign design resources and message framing. An updated section discusses the lessons of the critical-cultural approach as we contemplate the ethics of persuading people in diverse cultures to reexamine health-related behaviors. These chapters showcase careers in health promotion and health campaign design.

Acknowledgments

A great number of people have contributed to the creation of this text. Our first thanks go to editor Karon Bowers, assistant editor Alyssa Quinones, production editor Marianne Paul, and copyeditor James Fraleigh whose wonderful work has and will influence this edition, and other colleagues at Oxford University Press for their remarkable guidance, enthusiasm, and good humor. We are also grateful to the following reviewers who suggested ideas for this edition:

- Jen Anderson, *Bellevue College*
- Stewart Auyash, *Ithaca College*
- Deborah R. Bassett, *University of West Florida*
- Emily Cripe, *Kutztown University of Pennsylvania*
- Steven Giles, *Wake Forest University*
- Geoffrey D. Klinger, *DePauw University*
- Diana Karol Nagy, *University of Florida*
- Brian Rogers, *University of Wisconsin Whitewater*
- Jayne L. Violette, *University of South Carolina Beaufort*

We continue to be grateful, as well, to those who have edited previous editions, including Toni Magyar, Mark Haynes, Peter Labella, Josh Hawkins, Nanette Giles, and Holly Allen; and to those who have reviewed previous editions, including Mariaelena Bartesaghi, Maria Brann, Salome Brooks, Mary L. Brown, Tricia Burke, Rebecca Cline, Brooke Hildebrand Clubbs, Ellen R. Cohn, Joy Cypher, Crystal Daugherty, Michael Dennis, Rebecca de Souza, Patrick J. Dillon, Elizabeth Edgecomb, Jessica Elton, June Flora, Randa Garden, Jo Anna Grant, Laurie A. Grosik, Stephen Haas, Amy Hedman, Stephen Hines, Vernon F. Humphrey, Kate Joeckel, Haywood Joiner, Virginia McDermott, JJ McIntyre, Katherine Miller, Chris R. Morse, Cheri Niedzwiecki, Jill O'Brien, Christine Parkhurst, Donna Pawlowski, Loretta L. Pecchioni, Elizabeth Petrun, Rajiv N. Rimal, Christina Sabee, Juliann C. Scholl, Pam Secklin, Jiunn-Jye Sheu, Christine Skubisz, Daniel Steinberg, Richard L. Street, Jr., Claire F. Sullivan, Sharlene Thompson, Teresa Thompson, Monique Mitchell Turner, Julie E. Volkman, Kandi Walker, Ken Watkins, Elaine Wittenberg-Lyles, Catherine Woells, Debra L. Worthington, Kevin Wright, Jill Yamasaki, Gust A. Yep, and Alan Zemel.

We would also like to thank colleagues and students who have contributed ideas, narratives, and feedback, most notably Annina Dahlstrom, Beth McPherson, Josh Newby, Chris Elkins, Alejandra Ryan Escobar, Patricia Barlow, Jennifer Terry, Susanne Fillmore, Dawn Murray, Praewa Tanuthep, Beverly Davis Willi, Jennifer Seneca, Lori Juneau, Stefanie Howell, Melanie Barnes, Amy Jenkins, Bridget King, Micah Nickens, Samantha Olivier, Gwynné Williams, Brittany Jay, Dustin Saulmon, Vickie Payne, Chris Thomas, Nicole Yeakos, Drew Bryson, and Evelyn Briere.

We also owe heartfelt thanks to our partners Grant Brown and Clayton Overton, whose support, inspiration, and patience are astonishing and much appreciated.

About the Authors

Athena du Pré is a Distinguished University Professor who teaches in the Department of Communication at the University of West Florida. She is also co-author of *Essential Communication* and the latest editions of *Understanding Human Communication*.

Barbara Cook Overton has a doctorate degree in health communication from Louisiana State University and is the author of *Unintended Consequences of Electronic Medical Records: An Emergency Room Ethnography*.

Establishing a Context for Health Communication

PART I

It's an exciting time to study health communication. To contribute in meaningful ways, we must be up to date, well informed, and aware of the big picture. This section lays the groundwork for that. You can read the rest of the book in any order you like, but begin with this section. In Chapters 1 and 2, you will learn about philosophical perspectives and recent events that have led us to the current moment. Understanding that journey makes it easier to envision the future—and ways that you can make a difference in it.

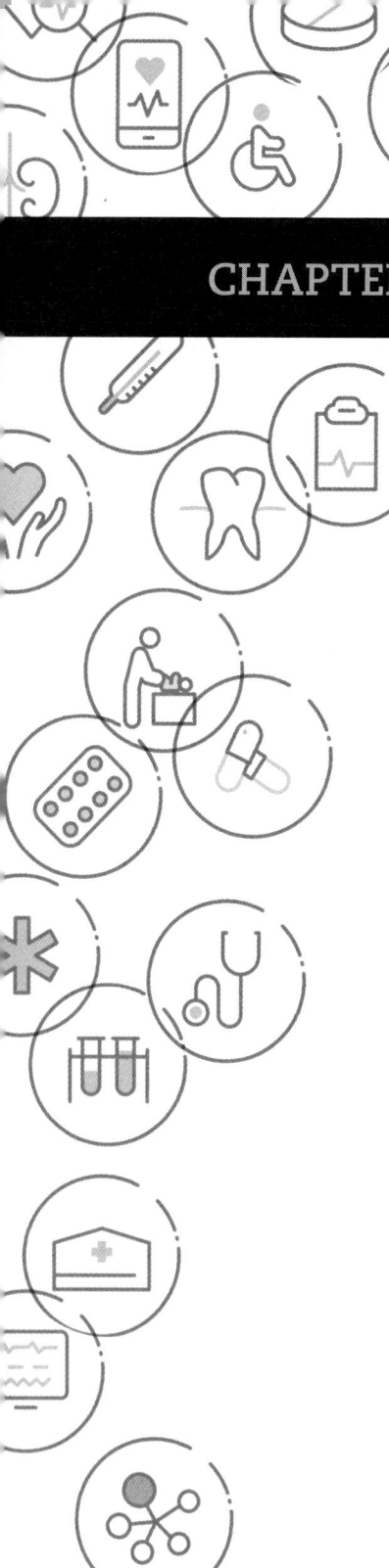

CHAPTER 1

Introduction

In 2020, a new virus spread around the world, sickening or killing at least 2 million people. As the crisis escalated, communication was a powerful tool for persuading people to engage in protective behavior. But the message was mixed. On the same day the World Health Organization declared a global health emergency, the United States president announced that the virus was "under control" and a week later said the "risk was low." Within weeks, hospitals in hardest hit areas were overwhelmed. As officials prepared tents and auditoriums to serve as makeshift hospitals, some government leaders issued stay-at-home orders to reduce the risk of contagion, while others encouraged people to continue shopping and going to work and school.

Pandemics present a powerful reminder how important (and challenging) health-related communication can be. But health communication doesn't occur only during a crisis. It's part of our everyday lives. We communicate about health with friends, family members, coworkers, and health professionals. Our ideas about health are influenced by the internet, movies, public service and announcements, and more.

In this chapter, we consider what health and health communication are all about. We examine philosophical perspectives of health and healing. Then we focus on how and why people communicate as they do about health. The chapter concludes with key reasons to study health communication, including particularly promising career growth. (See Box 1.1 for a list of health-related careers featured throughout the book.)

The Importance of Health Communication

While Lisa Suennen was a hospital patient, she felt "at times comforted and at other moments abandoned." Some care providers were thoughtful, attentive, and helpful. However, others failed to listen to her, explain procedures, or communicate well with one another (Suennen, 2015). Some nurses told her they were too busy to respond when she rang the bell for help, diagnostic tests weren't ordered on time, and her insurance claim was denied after paperwork was mishandled.

BOX 1.1 Career Opportunities

Profiles of More Than 125 Health-Related Jobs

Career boxes throughout the book showcase careers related to health and health care. Here are some of the jobs profiled in each chapter.

CHAPTER 3 Research/Education
- Consultant
- Professor
- Researcher

CHAPTER 4 Patient Advocacy
- Case manager
- Patient advocate
- Patient care coordinator
- Patient navigator
- Social worker

CHAPTER 5 Care Providers
- Clinical laboratory assistant
- Dental assistant
- Dental hygienist
- Dentist
- Doctor of osteopathic medicine
- Emergency medical technician
- Hospitalist
- Licensed practical nurse
- Medical doctor
- Medical records technician
- Nurse practitioner
- Occupational health/safety technician
- Occupational therapist
- Pharmacist
- Pharmacy technician
- Physical therapist
- Physician assistant
- Psychiatric technician or aide
- Psychiatrist
- Psychologist
- Radiology technologist
- Recreational therapist
- Registered nurse
- Respiratory therapist
- Speech-language therapist
- Surgeon
- Surgical technologist

CHAPTER 6 Diversity
- Diversity officer
- Equal Employment Opportunity (EEO) officer
- Health care interpreter

CHAPTER 7 Holistic Medicine
- Acupuncturist
- Chiropractor
- Holistic nurse
- Massage therapist
- Midwife
- Naturopathic physician
- Nutritionist/dietician
- Reiki practitioner
- Yoga instructor

CHAPTER 8 Mental Health
- Home health aide
- Hospice/palliative care provider
- Mental health counselor
- Psychologist
- Senior citizen services providers
- Social service manager
- Social worker

CHAPTER 9 Medical Technology
- Computer and information systems manager
- Health information administrator or technician
- Software developer

CHAPTER 10 Health Care Administration
- Chief financial officer
- Chief operating officer
- Departmental director
- Director of human resources
- Health information manager
- Medical director
- Medical office manager
- Nursing director
- President or CEO
- Strategic planning director

Health Care Human Resources
- Compensation and benefits manager
- Customer service representative
- Human resource manager
- Recruiter
- Training and development specialist

Health Care Marketing and Public Relations
- Advertising designer
- Community services director
- In-house communication director
- Marketing professional
- Pharmaceutical sales representative
- Physician marketing coordinator
- Public relations professional
- Strategic planning manager

CHAPTER 11 Health Journalism
- Health news editor/reporter
- Health publication editor
- Journal or magazine editor
- Media relations specialist
- Nonprofit organization publicity manager

CHAPTER 12 Public Health
- Business or billing manager
- Communication specialist
- Emergency management director
- Environmentalist
- Epidemiologist
- Fundraiser
- Health campaign designer
- Health department administrator
- Health educator
- Health inspector
- Health researcher
- Media relations professional
- Nonprofit organization director
- Nurse
- Nutritionist/dietician
- Patient advocate or navigator
- Physician
- Public policy advisor
- Risk/crisis communication specialist
- Social worker

CHAPTER 13 Health Promotion and Education
- Community health educator
- Corporate wellness director
- Fitness instructor
- Health campaign designer/manager
- Health information publication designer
- Hospital-based health educator
- Patient advocate or patient navigator
- School-based health educator

CHAPTER 14 Health Campaigns
- Communication director
- Director of nonprofit organization
- Media relations specialist
- Professor/educator
- Public relations specialist
- Publication designer

During a health care experience, communication is more than a nicety. It can enhance healing via a two-way exchange of information, comfort, stress reduction, trust, and mutually satisfying solutions (Street, Makoul, Arora, & Epstein, 2009). By contrast, ineffective health communication often leads to increased anxiety, errors, mistrust, and poor decisions. For these reasons, dissatisfying interactions are linked to adverse health outcomes and to burnout among health care professionals (e.g., Clayton, Iacob, Reblin, & Ellington, 2019; Kodjebacheva, Estrada, & Parker, 2017). And the effects go both ways. Burnout tends to lead to worse communication, causing an even steeper downward spiral (Clayton et al., 2019).

Interpersonal interactions are only part of the picture. They occur in the context of culture, economics, environmental conditions, and public policy. As you will see throughout the book, communication is often the vehicle through which these factors are realized and negotiated. A great deal is at stake. As health communication scholar Gary Kreps (2005) observes, "many of the people who are most at risk for poor health outcomes from cancer and other serious health problems are members of underserved populations" (p. S68). In the United States, people of low socioeconomic status are five times more likely to be in poor health than affluent individuals are (Khullar & Chokski, 2018, para. 5).

There is no "us" and "them" when it comes to health. About 1 in 4 people in the United States has a chronic health condition such as heart disease, mental illness, depression, or diabetes ("National Health Council," 2014). Medical costs escalate when these conditions are not well managed. There is also a price to pay in terms of pain, stress, and lost productivity. People with chronic illnesses are six times more likely than others to miss work regularly (Fouad et al., 2017). Experts say we could save trillions of dollars (and untold suffering) worldwide by helping people prevent and manage long-term health concerns ("Heart Disease," 2015; National Alliance on Mental Illness, 2019; "National Diabetes," 2017; Rapaport, 2018).

The good news is that along with challenges come new possibilities. The future may belong to those who not only improve health care but fundamentally *reimagine* the way it is provided. "Health in 2040 will be a world apart from what we have now," predict analysts (Batra, Betts, & Davis, 2019, para. 4).

For one thing, technology is changing the health information available to everyday citizens. To return to our opening example, Suennen might realize in the future that her heart is malfunctioning even before she feels symptoms or visits a doctor. Wearable devices such as smartphones can now monitor people's health and alert them to seek care when needed. This has already saved a number of lives (Smith, 2018). And the trend is growing. Before long, it may be possible to equip your bathroom mirror and other features of daily life to monitor key health indicators (Batra et al., 2019). At another level, the days of one-way communication from health experts to health care consumers are giving way to more collaborative models in which patients can more easily ask questions and share health data with care providers, even when they cannot be with them in person. We talk more about the impact of health information technology in Chapter 9.

Another change involves the way that health care services are provided. Clinics and hospitals aren't going away, but additional services are emerging that embed health care more into everyday life. For example, many neighborhood pharmacies now function as "health hubs" that offer vaccinations and nutrition counseling and monitor people's blood pressure, diabetes, cholesterol, and more. Considering that the United States spends 90% of its health care money on chronic conditions, affordable and convenient care is crucial to moderating costs ("Health and Economic," 2019).

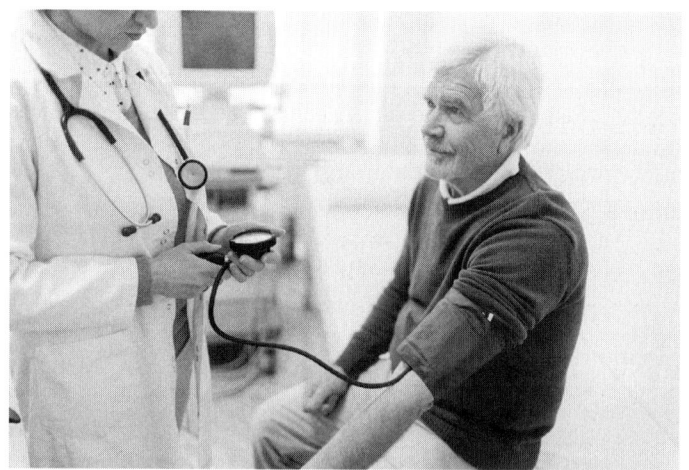

Some neighborhood pharmacies now serve as "health hubs" where people can have their blood pressure and other health indicators monitored without a trip to the doctor's office.

Have you ever asked a pharmacist for advice or assistance? If so, were you satisfied with the interaction? Why or why not?

Of course, these new resources are only helpful if you can readily use them. In Chapter 2 we talk about the cost of receiving care, and in Chapter 6 about literacy challenges that make it difficult for many people to understand and use health communication.

A Systems-Level Approach

No facet of health occurs in isolation. Recognizing that, we explore health communication from a systems perspective in this book. Health care is a *system* in that it consists of interrelated elements that influence and rely on one another to function as a cohesive whole (von Bertalanffy, 1968). Your family is a system, as are your university, your workplace, and the larger industries and cultures that influence you.

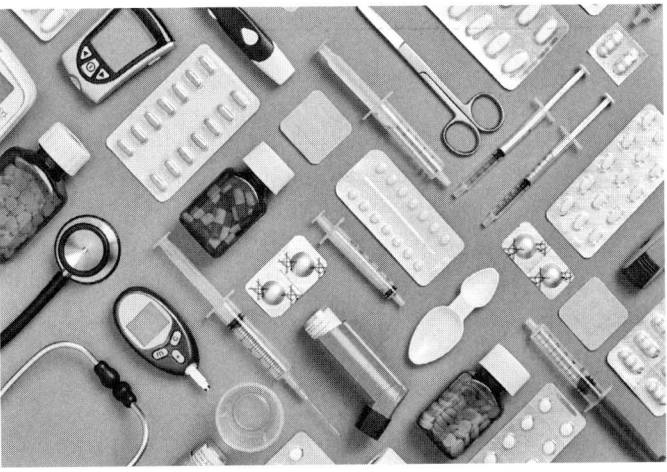

Much like a living organism, components of the health care system are interdependent and resistant to radical change. However, small changes can be pivotal.

If you could make one change to the health care system, what would it be and why?

Health care is an overarching system composed of many subsystems, such as clinics, pharmaceutical firms, nonprofit organizations, hospitals, community groups, and more. The implications of a systems approach, as we will apply it, are captured well by management theorist Peter Senge (2006). Here are four tenets of systems theory as he explains them that will help you develop a sophisticated understanding of health communication.

The structure of a system influences the people within it. As Senge (2006) observes, "when placed in the same system, people, however different, tend to produce similar results" (p. 42). That's not to say that people have no choice about their behavior. But it reminds us of the larger reality—that our choices are strongly influenced by the relationships, structures, and norms in which we find ourselves. To return to the example that opens this chapter, the care providers who communicated poorly with Suennen may have been careless or indifferent. On the other hand, they may have been stressed, burned out, or struggling to keep up in understaffed units.

Superficial "fixes" seldom lead to long-term success. Senge (2006) points out that "the easy way out usually leads back in" (p. 60) and very often "today's problems come from yesterday's solutions" (p. 58). For example, it seems reasonable on the surface to reward care providers when patients experience extraordinary gains in good health. However, that practice presents a disincentive to take on patients with complex and high-risk conditions. As a result, people in the greatest need may have difficulty finding someone to care for them—not because care providers are unconcerned but because the system discourages it. In systems theory, the law of unintended consequences points out that even well-intentioned solutions may have undesirable effects. To avoid simplistic assumptions that may cause more problems than they solve, look below the surface. Former health care executive Robert Hugin (2018) makes the case, saying that "to produce the right solutions, we must ask the tough questions, and not grasp at quick fixes just because they seem popular or convenient" (para. 6).

Systems resist radical change. A central tenet of systems theory involves homeostasis, a system's tendency to favor balance and stability. This quality makes systems resistant to radical or fast changes, especially if they challenge well-established ways of thinking or behaving. Senge (2006) warns that, based on the very nature of a system, "the harder you push, the harder the system pushes back" (p. 58). You have probably noticed this if you have tried to drastically change your diet or lifestyle, or if you have witnessed grand initiatives at work that tend to be abandoned and forgotten in favor of the next big initiative (which is likely to meet the same fate). However much we may wish for sudden, sweeping changes in health care, truly long-term solutions are likely to be achieved gradually.

Seemingly small changes can produce powerful results. The good news is that the interdependent nature of systems makes them highly sensitive to slow, small changes. A key leverage point can have powerful results. For example, the health care system isn't likely to become simpler any time soon, but in Chapter 2 we discuss how health care navigators in some areas are helping patients understand and navigate the system more effectively. Another example involves efforts to promote community wellness. Health campaigns designed by outsiders are often ineffective at changing a target audience's attitudes and behaviors. However, when professionals work *with* members of a particular culture to identify their health-related goals and culturally acceptable options, the outcomes may be more successful (Dutta & de Souza, 2008; D. B. Friedman, Hooker, Wilcox, Burroughs, & Rheaume, 2012).

All in all, Senge (2006) points out, "systems thinking is both more challenging *and* more promising than our normal ways of dealing with problems" (p. 63). Improving health communication is not as simple as saying "Do better!" By the same token, blaming individuals seldom gets us far. But a sophisticated understanding of the underlying factors at play can help reveal leverage points with lasting impact.

Philosophy of This Book

This book is based on two main convictions. One is that the best health communication strategies are effective, sustainable, and respectful to the people involved. The other is that we are best equipped to understand (and to improve) the system when we understand health communication from a wide range of perspectives—cultural, physical, interpersonal, social, organizational, and political.

Here are some examples of what can go wrong when people focus on one area of communication but neglect others:

- Patients are well treated, but their families feel distraught and uninformed.
- A campaign director unfamiliar with cultural ideas about health creates messages that are unappealing or offensive to the target audience.
- A marketing/public relations director who does not understand the dynamics of patient–caregiver communication is unable to help shape and promote services that meet stakeholders' needs.
- A team member uninformed about health care administration and current issues misses out on leadership opportunities.
- Care providers who do not communicate effectively with each other confuse patients and their loved ones with contradictory information.
- Health communication researchers focus only on individual actions rather than recognizing the social and organizational constraints that may limit people's options.
- A high-tech means of sharing health information benefits people who are already well informed but increases the gap between information haves and have-nots.

After establishing the context for current issues in health communication in Part I, the book is organized roughly from micro- to macrolevel perspectives. We focus on interpersonal connections between patients and professional caregivers in Part II, and then broaden the scope in Part III to consider the influence of diversity and culture. Part IV explores health care resources, including social support and technology. In Part V, we consider the ways that people in health care organizations use communication to lead, inspire, and support team members, and to partner with the community. The book concludes in Part VI with coverage of health communication in the media, public health, and health care campaigns. In real life, of course, we encounter these factors simultaneously rather than one by one. Keep the interplay between them in mind.

Here are some ways to get the most from this book:

- *Don't overlook boxes and sidebars.* Key terms and theories appear in boxes as well as in the main text.
- *Engage in critical thinking.* Questions throughout the book prompt you to reflect on your viewpoints and experiences. Critical thinking, the ability to link abstract ideas to actual practices, is one of the most useful ways to put what you learn to good use.
- *Apply what you learn.* Throughout the book, *Communication Skill Builder* sections present practical tips for communicating effectively about health. Experts suggest strategies for communicating with a diverse range of people, presenting our concerns as patients, being effective leaders, using social media, designing health campaigns, and more. (See Box 1.2 for ideas about how you can put your skills to work in a service-learning project or internship.)

BOX 1.2

Learn While You Make a Difference

Whether it's a service-learning project, an internship, or a volunteer effort, there are many ways that you can gain experience and learn about health care while you make a difference in people's lives. It helps to establish learning objectives and goals at the beginning and to reflect on what you have learned and accomplished when the project is complete. Here are a few ideas.

Work with a Nonprofit Organization
- Help with strategic planning
- Create a media packet and marketing plan
- Publicize an event or program
- Provide assistance with training
- Recruit volunteers
- Help with an event already scheduled
- Conduct surveys
- Host a health fair booth
- Help develop a crisis management plan
- Stage a mock crisis for practice

Plan, Publicize, and Host an Event
- Fundraiser
- Awards banquet
- Celebration
- Cleanup or spruce-up activity
- Image-building outreach activity
- Health-enhancing event

Advocate
- Focus on a particular need, risk, or group of people
- Research the issue
- Partner with people in need; honor their agenda
- Identify needed resources and/or policies
- Educate the public
- Meet with policy-makers and community leaders
- Host strategy sessions
- Create coalitions and long-term plans

Educate People
- Host a public lecture
- Organize a symposium
- Hold a mini-conference
- Present communication workshops
- Write articles and PSAs for the media

Raise Money
- Host a fundraising event
- Collect contributions
- Recruit sponsors and partners
- Sell items of value
- Host a chance drawing

Health Campaigns
- Conduct market research
- Create a campaign or assist with one
- Promote healthy behaviors
- Raise awareness of risks
- Assess campaign exposure
- Evaluate outcomes

What Is Health?

It sounds like an easy question. We know when we are healthy and when we are sick. At least that's how it feels most of the time. But sometimes we are not even sure ourselves. There is space in the middle. And depending on our personal and cultural perspectives, our very idea of being *healthy* can differ from other people's definitions.

The World Health Organization (WHO) defines **health** as "a state of complete physical, mental and social well-being and not merely the absence of disease or infirmity" (WHO, 1948, p. 1). This definition, unchanged for more than 70 years, reminds us that *healthy* is not the opposite of *sick*. Health often involves a sense of harmony and equilibrium between many aspects of life. It may call into play our feelings, physical abilities, and relationships with others.

Layered onto the WHO's definition of health is the observation that a person's environment influences the degree to which they are able to function effectively in everyday life (WHO, 2002). WHO's International

Classification for Functioning, Disability and Health (known commonly as the ICF) distinguishes between *capacity* (what a person is able to do in a general sense) and *performance* (the person's ability to function in particular environments). To illustrate, imagine that you have trouble seeing clearly at a distance. Your performance as a student may suffer if you can't read what a professor posts on a PowerPoint. However, if someone assists you in taking notes, or if you can simultaneously view the PowerPoint on your laptop, you may perform as well as people whose eyesight (capacity) differs from yours. Social support, as well as self-concept and other factors, also influence how people perform.

This idea is familiar to Tanya Khvitsko (2018), who uses prosthetic legs. Khvitsko says that most of the time she doesn't feel "disabled." She performs much like anyone else, or even better. She explains:

> I live a normal life. I went to school. I am married with a baby on the way. I've ran a marathon. I socialize with friends. I have a full time job . . . Yes, I have to adapt to things. But I am not disabled, because I don't feel disabled. Instead, I feel like I am more abled, because I have more challenges to accomplish on a daily basis. (para. 4)

But there are occasions when Khvitsko feels disabled—not because of her own capacities but because of the way people treat her. She says that, when people focus on her legs, ask personal questions they wouldn't ask others, or cheer her on during races simply because she uses prosthetic limbs, she feels "extremely disabled" (para. 5).

Based on this contextual understanding of health, a person might experience better health because their capacity changes or because their environment does. We'll talk more about this interface throughout the book.

What Is Health Communication?

Health communication is shaped by many influences, including personal goals, skills, cultural values, situational factors, and consideration of other people's feelings. The definitions presented in this section emphasize the interdependence of these factors. As communicators, we influence, and are simultaneously influenced by, the people and circumstances around us. We rely on others to help us meet goals and make sense of life events. Sometimes the most important thing we do is simply be present for others.

Defining Communication

Communication is anything but simple. Imagine a scenario in which a person says to you, "I'm pregnant." If we believe that meaning lies only in the words we use, this is a simple two-word parcel of information. As we know, however, communication involves a lot more than that. Even in the case of relatively simple interactions, people negotiate a myriad of potential meanings and implications.

The **transactional model of communication** proposes that people collaborate to construct meaning in a process of ongoing, reciprocal influence (Barnlund, 1970). If you were asked to comment on the "I'm pregnant" statement, you would probably want answers to a number of questions first, such as *Who said it? Under what circumstances? Did the speaker look and sound happy, sad, fearful, or some other way? Is the person who made this statement my wife? My teenage daughter? My cashier in the grocery store?* The transactional communication model reminds us that communication is a sophisticated process. It does not happen within people, but between them, in the midst of many factors

---

BOX 1.3 PERSPECTIVES

True Stories About Health Communication Experiences

In *Perspectives* boxes throughout the book you will read about the real-life experiences of people involved with health communication. These accounts represent the viewpoints of patients, loved ones, caregivers, executives, social activists, health campaign managers, and others. They provide insight about how people of different races, cultures, ages, languages, abilities, sexual orientations, and educational levels experience health communication.

that influence how they behave and what sense they make of the situation and each other. To clarify, let's take a closer look at three key aspects of transactional communication: collaboration, multiple levels of meaning, and the importance of context and culture.

COLLABORATIVE SENSE-MAKING

A central tenet of transactional communication is that meaning does not lie in discrete units of information or in any one person. Rather, it emerges within experiences that participants collaboratively create.

If a friend tells you she is pregnant, you are likely to notice her nonverbal cues, do a quick mental inventory of her situation and prior comments, and experience feelings of your own. Your reaction to the news may show on your face even before the words are completely out of her mouth. In such a situation, your friend may pick up on your reaction and reframe the announcement and even how she feels about it. Ultimately, whether an exchange takes on the key of celebrating, comforting, or any number of other options depends on how the people involved co-construct it.

One implication of transactional communication is that participants do not take turns being senders or receivers. Instead, they simultaneously send and receive messages all the time. Even a blank expression is likely to be considered feedback, suggesting that the listener is bored, uninterested, or so on. Thus, the transactional model highlights the importance, not only of words, but also of ever-present nonverbal cues.

As you will see in Chapter 3, many people criticize the traditional model of patient–caregiver communication in which patients are mostly silent and health professionals do most of the talking. Such a dynamic is likely to result in misunderstandings and in a power differential that limits patients' opportunities to help shape their own care. From a transactional perspective, the blame does not lie solely with health professionals, however. Patients are often observed to be quiet and submissive. Whether they realize it or not, they may contribute to the very dynamic they dislike.

MULTIPLE LEVELS OF MEANING

Transactional communication is consistent with a **relational approach**, which proposes that meaning is interpreted at both a content and a relational level

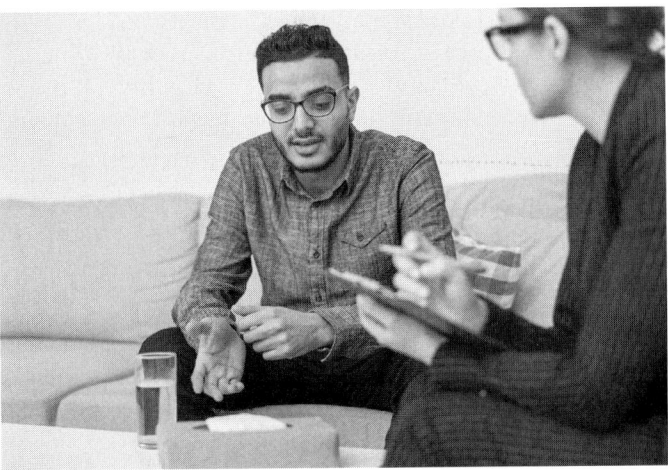

Have you ever felt like the underdog in a health care encounter? If so, what contributed to this feeling? Is there anything you or other people might have done differently?

(L. E. Rogers & Escudero, 2004; Watzlawick, Beavin, & Jackson, 1967). At a content level, meaning is considered to be mostly denotative—that is, subject to literal interpretation. "I'm pregnant" is a simple statement of fact.

At a relational level, participants consider the implications of communication in terms of their relative status and feelings about each other. Relational messages are often conveyed implicitly, as by considering *how* something is said, *who* says it and *when*, and what they *do not* say. Although relational cues may be subtle, they often convey powerful implications regarding the expectations, emotions, power, and status of the participants. For example, in Chapter 8 we discuss the conundrum that individuals often over-assist people with physical limitations. Although their intentions are good, the relational-level implications may be that "you are needy and incapable" and "you are different from me and from other people." In reality, people with physical challenges often say they prefer to be treated just like anyone else (e.g., Nemeth, 2000). In a similar way, a person may feel gratified by a health professional who treats him as an equal but put off by one who insinuates that he is ignorant or irresponsible about his health. (Bear in the mind that, as a collaborator in the process, the person's response will help to shape the ultimate meaning and tone of that encounter.)

CONTEXT AND CULTURE

The anthropologist Clifford Geertz (1973) famously observed that people are suspended in "webs of significance" (p. 5). In other words, none of us exists as an island. We are influenced by larger environments and contexts such as past experiences, the neighborhoods in which we live, the cultures with which we identify, and so on. Each of these is likely to influence what we consider acceptable and how we interpret what happens around us.

In Chapter 2, we consider how health care has evolved over time and the effects of recent reform efforts. On the surface, these happenings may seem irrelevant to the way we communicate about health as individuals. However, they probably influence us more than we realize. For example, a health professional might wish to spend an hour with each patient but be prohibited from doing so by organizational rules and structures. Patients who criticize the professional for being "hurried and inattentive" may miss the reality that the system is more to blame than the individual.

From a transactional perspective, cultural mores are woven into the sense-making endeavors of everyday communication. Cultural expectations influence how we behave as patients (Chapter 4), how society regards health concerns such as mental illness and obesity (Chapters 6 and 7), and so on. You might know someone who does not seek care for depression because, in the culture in which she was raised, mental illness is considered shameful.

In summary, the transactional perspective reminds us that communication episodes are collaborative and unique accomplishments. The people involved interactively shape the meanings that emerge at both a content and relational level, and they do so within many layers of context. Awareness of this perspective may help you appreciate the sophisticated nature of health communication phenomena you read about in this book and avoid drawing simplistic conclusions about them. That being said, don't expect every communication study that is described to be transactional in nature. Researchers sometimes single out or isolate particular aspects of health communication for study, and rightfully so. With an understanding of transactional communication, perhaps you can appreciate these as components of a larger process as you continue to learn and put the pieces together.

Defining Health Communication

Gary Kreps and Barbara Thornton (1992) define **health communication** as "the way we seek, process, and share health information" (p. 2). We search out and pass along messages and mingle what we hear and see with our own ideas and experiences. In this way, we are actively involved in health communication,

---

BOX 1.4 THEORETICAL FOUNDATIONS

The Basis for Health Communication

He who loves practice without theory is like the sailor who boards the ship without a rudder and compass and never knows where he may cast.

—**LEONARDO DA VINCI**

As we explore the field of health communication, theories connect the dots, just as constellations reveal patterns in the stars. Good theories make sense of diverse information and help us to get our bearings. They help us know, in advance, where we are headed and what paths are available to us. *Theoretical Foundations* segments (sometimes in the text, sometimes in boxes of their own) showcase theories relevant to health communication. These theories address such issues as:

- What is health?
- How do we make sense of health crises?
- What behaviors enhance and compromise coping efforts?
- How do interpersonal relationships influence health?
- How does multiculturalism influence health and health care?
- How can health care organizations stimulate teamwork and innovation?
- In what ways do media messages influence our health?
- How do people respond to public health campaigns?
- What factors influence people to become more knowledgeable and proactive about their own health?

not just passive recipients of information. A great deal of health communication involves professional care providers such as doctors, nurses, pharmacists, aides, therapists, counselors, and technicians. But we serve as caregivers for friends and loved ones as well. Chapter 8 demonstrates the value of social support when we are ill, healthy, and even (perhaps especially) when we cope with death and dying.

The History of Health Communication

Health communication emerged as a defined area of study in the late 1960s. Interest was spurred most notably by researchers and practitioners in psychology, medicine, sociology, and persuasion who recognized that communication is central to the process of health and healing (Kreps, Query, & Bonaguro, 2008, p. 5). Health communication has also flourished as a component of communication, business, nursing, public health, and allied health programs, to name just a few.

One lesson that has emerged is that communication is not separate from health care, but is therapeutic in itself. It is also the vehicle through which people learn about health and reach agreement about what is wrong and what could be better. This involves individual health as well as organizational structures and public policy.

Health communication scholars have also brought attention to social factors. It is common to think about health in terms of personal choices—a good diet, an active lifestyle, regular checkups, and good information. But the evidence is clear (see Chapters 6 and 14) that these options are not available to everyone in the same measure. Improving the health of a community requires that we consider social equity, community resources, access to care, and the environment.

Health communication is often persuasive in nature. Communication—be it through news stories, PSAs, entertainment programming, or conversations with health professionals or loved ones—has an impact on whether we smoke, exercise, drink and drive, get enough sleep, take part in health screenings, and so on. Persuasive communication is a powerful tool. How, and under what circumstances, should we use it to influence people's behavior? What persuasive appeals are most effective? Which are unethical? We examine answers to these questions and others in Part VI.

Today, health communication research is a thriving field. Notable publications include the journal *Health Communication*, first published in 1989 and still led by founding editor Teresa L. Thompson of the University of Dayton, as well as *Qualitative Health Research*, the *Journal of Health Communication, Communication & Medicine, The Routledge Handbook of Health Communication* (T. L. Thompson, Parrott, & Nussbaum, 2011), the *Encyclopedia of Health Communication* (T. L. Thompson, 2014), and many others.

As you probably realize by now, health communication is quite diverse. It unites interdisciplinary practitioners and scholars and covers a gamut of issues ranging from interpersonal communication, to culture, media, public health, education, and more. It involves the work of scholars around the world—from Europe to Australia and New Zealand, Asia, Canada, the United Kingdom, and the Americas (Thompson et al., 2011).

The following section introduces three approaches to health care that are fundamental to how and why people communicate as they do.

BOX 1.5 RESOURCES

Health Communication Organizations and Resources

This book is designed to give you a rich and current overview of health communication. We will visit a number of locations (social settings, doctors' offices, boardrooms, movie theatres, and more) and look at health through different people's eyes. Our hope is that, as you explore each perspective, your appreciation of the nuances that influence health and health communication will increase. Along the way you will probably want to know more than can be fit into one book. To get you started, here is a list of organizations and websites you might wish to investigate for more information about health communication:

- American College of Health Care Administrators: http://www.achca.org
- American College of Health Care Executives: http://www.healthmanagementcareers.org

continued

> continued
>
> - American Communication Association: www.americancomm.org
> - American Public Health Association: www.apha.org
> - American Society for Healthcare Human Resource Administration: http://www.ashhra.org
> - Association for Education in Journalism & Mass Communication: www.aejmc.org
> - Centers for Disease Control and Prevention: http://www.cdc.gov
> - Central States Communication Association: www.csca-net.org
> - Coalition for Healthcare Communication: www.cohealthcom.org
> - Eastern Communication Association: www.ecasite.org
> - European Association for Communication in Healthcare: www.each.eu
> - European Public Health Association: www.eupha.org
> - Health Care Public Relations Association: https://www.hcpra.org
> - International Communication Association (Health Communication Division): https://www.icahdq.org/group/health
> - International Union for Health Promotion and Education: www.iuhpe.org
> - National Cancer Institute: http://www.cancer.gov
> - National Center for Health Marketing: www.cdc.gov/healthmarketing
> - National Communication Association (Health Communication Division): www.natcom.org
> - National Institute of Health: www.nih.gov
> - National Prevention Information Network: https://npin.cdc.gov
> - Public Relations Society of America, Health Academy: healthacademy.prsa.org/index.html
> - South Asian Public Health Forum: www.saphf.org
> - Southern States Communication Association: www.ssca.net
> - U.S. Department of Human Services Health Communication Activities: www.health.gov/communication
> - Western States Communication Association: www.westcomm.org
> - World Federation of Public Health Associations: www.wfpha.org
> - World Health Organization: www.who.int/en

Health Care Models

What causes ill health? If your answer is germs, you have probably been influenced by the biomedical model, which is not surprising, considering that it has been the primary basis of conventional Western medicine for the last 100 years. But if you believe that illness is caused by a variety of factors—such as people's frame of mind, their values, and the communities in which they live—your views more closely reflect a biopsychosocial or sociocultural model. Following is a description of each model and its impact on health communication.

Biomedical

The **biomedical model** is based on the premise that ill health is a physical phenomenon that can be explained, identified, and treated through physical means. Biomedicine is well suited to a culture familiar with engines and computers. "Repairing a body, in this view, is analogous to fixing a machine," wrote Charles Longino (1997, p. 14). Physicians are like scientists or mechanics. They collect information about a problem, try to identify the source of it, and fix it.

The focus is often reductionist. That is, in accordance with the scientific method, health professionals try to isolate key variables by bracketing out extraneous information. A medical interview may sound a lot like this: *When did the symptoms start? . . . Does it hurt when I do this? . . . On a scale of 1 to 10, how bad is the pain? . . . Have you had a fever?* Health communication influenced by the biomedical model is typically focused and specific. Health professionals' questions require only brief answers, such as *two weeks ago* and *yes*.

Biomedical talk tends to have its own vocabulary, which can be puzzling and intimidating to patients.

A mother summoned to the hospital after her son had been injured remembers:

> When I walked into the trauma center, they told me Justin had suffered severe trauma to his brain, a subarachnoid hemorrhage in the sylvian fissure and right posterior fossa, frontal lobe contusions, diffuse axonal shearing injuries, and a non-displaced vertical fracture of the C6 vertebra. What I heard was "brain damage, broken neck."

Although Justin's condition was critical, he eventually recovered. His mother says she feels lucky about the outcome, but she will never forget the terror of being confronted with medical jargon that frightened and confused her, rather than actually helping her understand what was wrong.

At its best, the biomedical approach is efficient and definitive. Medical tests and observations may yield evidence that can be logically analyzed and treated with well-established methods. One criticism of the model, however, is that it marginalizes patients' feelings and social experiences, sometimes to the extent of treating people as impersonal collections of parts or symptoms. People are often dissatisfied when care providers don't listen to their concerns surrounding an illness, and they may mistrust diagnoses if they feel that the providers don't fully understand their problems.

Biopsychosocial

The **biopsychosocial perspective** takes into account people's physical conditions (biology), their thoughts and beliefs (psychology), and their social expectations. It's consistent with WHO's definition of health and the ICF model we discussed previously. From a biopsychosocial perspective, health experiences are not solely physical phenomena but are also influenced by people's feelings, their ideas about health, and the events of their lives.

The biopsychosocial perspective emphasizes that no one approach works well with everyone. For example, some family caregivers welcome loved ones' help, whereas others find it disruptive. A caregiver interviewed by Elaine Wittenberg-Lyles and colleagues put it this way: "After not having anybody for a while and then having somebody here all the time kind of makes

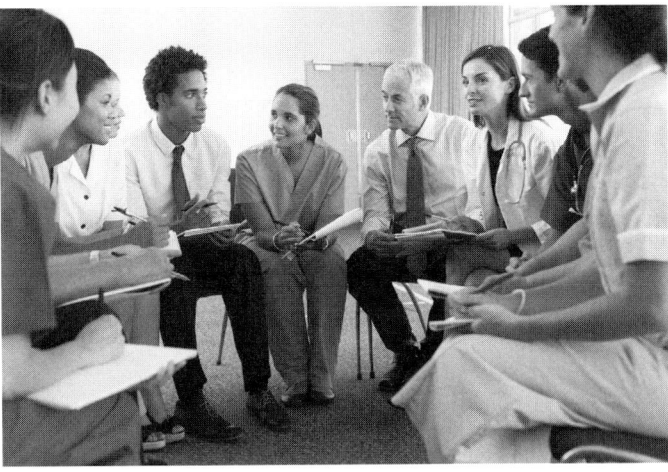

Think beyond the boundaries of conventional care to design a team ideally suited to help you stay healthy.

Who would you want on your team? By what means would you prefer to communicate with these people? How do you think your health would be affected?

me—adds to my stress" (p. 906). The researchers observe that more social support is not always better. A more important consideration is how well it meets the recipient's preferences and psychological needs (Wittenberg-Lyles, Washington, Demiris, Oliver, & Shaunfield, 2014).

There is evidence to support the biopsychosocial premise that people's thoughts and emotions have an influence on their overall health and coping ability. Researchers have long known that emotional stress tends to elevate people's heart rates and blood pressure. They are now finding that excessive stress reduces the body's resistance to disease (e.g., Lovell, Moss, & Wetherell, 2011). On the bright side, health is sometimes enhanced by good humor, a positive attitude, and social support (e.g., Gallagher, Phillips, Ferraro, Drayson, & Carroll, 2008).

Sociocultural

From a **sociocultural perspective**, health reflects a complex array of factors involving personal choice, social dynamics, and culture. Social variables include wealth, poverty, prejudice, access to health services, and living conditions, to name a few. Culture is embodied in shared values, traditions, and rituals.

The sociocultural perspective rejects the notion, on the one hand, that health is purely personal, and on the other hand, that people are simply products of

BOX 1.6 PERSPECTIVES

A Memorable Hospital Experience

In my short 27 years I have visited hospitals in four states, and only one stands out in my memory: St. Jude Children's Research Hospital in Memphis, Tennessee. My family spent nearly two years of our lives walking in and out of the doors of St. Jude while my sister was being treated for leukemia.

Walking into the administrative office the first day we arrived was like being in Grandma's house seated by a warm, open fireplace. During those first hours of our shock and fear over my sister's diagnosis, the hospital staff worked quickly on her paperwork without making us feel the least bit rushed. The warmth and tone of their voices was like that of a family member. We were assured we could always reach them—if not at work, at home! They were our new family.

The doctors at St. Jude stopped and spoke with families and patients and answered any questions they were asked. The doctors were not the only gems in the hospital, though. I remember two very special nurses, Jackie and Mary. One night my parents and I went to eat and were late getting back (it was shrimp night!). We found Mary, who had gotten off work 1½ hours earlier, reading to my sister. Jackie assisted my sister with manicuring her nails, even though it was not part of her technical duties. The nurses at St. Jude stepped out of their textbook roles to accommodate the needs of their patients.

Members of the housekeeping and dietary staff were always helpful, too. When my sister thought she had an appetite for a hamburger or macaroni and cheese, they always did their best to get some up to her before she realized she did not want anything at all.

The last person I recall from the support staff was Mrs. Fran, our social worker. She was a dream, not just a friend you could talk to but one you could count on to take care of the little things you naturally forget in situations such as ours. When my sister died, Mrs. Fran was there for my family and made all the arrangements to get us back home to Louisiana.

There were many difficulties in dealing with the death of a loved one, and my sister was only 15. However, my parents and I feel an incredible debt to St. Jude. We have founded a fundraising chapter for St. Jude in Baton Rouge and I hope to pursue a career to help caregivers, families, and the public understand the importance of interpersonal communication skills in hospitals and other health care centers.

—GWYNNÉ WILLIAMS

---

their environment. Instead, it recognizes that these factors are mutually reflexive. Therefore, focusing on only one factor is typically counterproductive.

As an example, the popular Drug Abuse Resistance Education (DARE) program has been largely ineffective at changing schoolchildren's long-term attitudes and behavior concerning illegal drugs (Birkeland, Murphy-Graham, & Weiss, 2005). After studying the data, Nicole Stephens and colleagues concluded that DARE's impact is limited because it has focused almost exclusively on drug use as a matter of personal choice. The larger reality, they found, is that some young people live in environments in which drug use is prevalent, highly encouraged by their peers, and considered normal. Those youth "may find it harder to resist drug use by simply 'saying no,'" the researchers assert. "Instead, a different set of intervention strategies—for example, decreasing students' exposure to situations where drug use is likely—may be more useful or effective" (Stephens, Markus, & Fryberg, 2012, p. 729).

Ultimately, no medical model is comprehensive enough to cover all facets of health. The best option may be awareness that health can be approached in different ways and the versatility to use dimensions of these models appropriately. The biopsychosocial and sociocultural models are appealing for their thoroughness and personal concern (see Boxes 1.6 and 1.8). However, implementing a holistic approach is no easy task, and sometimes a biomedical solution is enough. In Chapters 3 through 5, we explore patterns and techniques of patient-provider communication. In Chapters 6 and 7, we investigate the link between health and sociocultural factors such as social status, race, gender, age, and ability. Then we return to the idea in Chapter 14, where we consider how a critical-cultural perspective can help health promoters give voice to marginalized groups and allow them to challenge and perhaps transform inequitable social structures.

Communication's Influence on Health

Health communication is integral to individuals, organizations, and society overall. It is necessary to meet medical goals, enhance personal well-being, save time and money, and make the most of health information. Following are six reasons to study health communication. Each of these is addressed more fully in the chapters that follow.

First, *communication is crucial to the success of health care encounters*. Without it, caregivers cannot hear patients' concerns, make diagnoses, share their recommendations, or follow up on treatment outcomes. "Health communication is the singularly most important tool health professionals have to provide health care to their clients," wrote Kreps and Thornton (1992, p. 2) and it continues to be true. Patients who take an active role in medical encounters are more likely than others to be satisfied with their care (Ashraf et al., 2013).

Interpersonal communication is crucial, considering that about 32 million people in the United States (roughly 1 in 7 adults) are unable to read more than a simple children's storybook (U.S. Department of Education, 2015). Added to that figure are people who, although they can read, have language differences and physical challenges that make it difficult to understand and use health information. All of these fall within the category of health literacy. People with health literacy challenges are usually less knowledgeable about health issues than others, and they may miss appointments, avoid medical care because they are embarrassed or frustrated, prepare incorrectly for surgery and other procedures, misinterpret the instructions for medications, and more. Experts estimate that health literacy challenges result in avoidable medical costs totaling more than $106 billion a year in the United States (Vernon, Trujillo, Rosenbaum, & DeBuono, 2007), and the loss in productivity and quality of life is immeasurable. Effective communication can offset the tragic and costly consequences of low literacy.

Second, *wise use of mass media and social media can help people learn about health and minimize the influence of unhealthy and unrealistic media portrayals*. Media consumers—especially those who rely on newspapers, magazines, and computers—are likely to be well informed about health issues and to take an active role in maintaining their own health (Koch-Weser, Bradshaw, Gualtieri, & Gallagher, 2010; Rains, 2008a). However, the media is also filled with glamorous images of people engaging in unhealthy behaviors, making media literacy especially important. In Chapter 9, we survey innovative ways that health promoters are making use of online and mobile communication. In Chapters 11, 13, and 14 we explore health images in the media, media literacy, and how to create effective health campaigns.

Third, *communication is an important source of personal confidence and coping ability*. Health professionals are less likely to experience burnout and less likely to leave the profession if they are satisfied

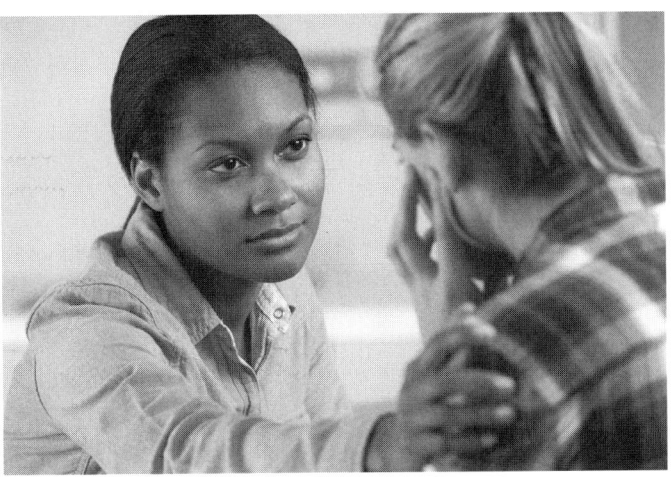

Health communication includes conversations with friends and loved ones in everyday life.

How is your physical and emotional health influenced by communication with people you know?

(Dyrbye et al., 2013). Likewise, patients cope best when they feel comfortable talking about delicate subjects such as pain and death. And people involved in support groups often cope better and even live longer than similar persons who are not members (Chapter 8). In short, good communication is conducive to good health.

Fourth, *effective communication saves time and money*. Caregivers who listen attentively and communicate a sense of caring and warmth are less likely than others to be sued for malpractice (Dym, 2008). Likewise, patients who communicate clearly with their care providers have the best chance of having their concerns immediately addressed, which is likely to improve their health and save time and money.

Fifth, *communication helps health care organizations operate effectively*. Communication skills are useful in recruiting employees, establishing innovative teams, creating efficient systems, and sustaining service excellence (Chapter 10). Studies show that supervisors' communication skills are one of the most important determinants of employees' satisfaction and their intention to stay on the job. Organizational leaders can also use communication to assess market needs and respond to patient preferences.

Sixth, *health communication may be important to you because of career opportunities*. The health industry already employs about 18 million people in the United States, and that number is expected to reach 20 million within a few years ("Healthcare Workers," 2017; U.S. Bureau of Labor Statistics, 2019). The number of jobs in health care is growing faster than in any other industry (U.S. BLS, 2019). Communication skills are central to jobs in clinical care, public relations, marketing, health care administration, human resources, education, community outreach, crisis management, patient advocacy, and more.

Reasons for the notable job growth are threefold: (1) Baby boomers are retiring, which diminishes the current pool of professionals in health care; (2) health needs are simultaneously escalating as the average age of the population increases; and (3) health care reform has added about 20 million Americans to health insurance rosters, qualifying them to receive medical care. Labor analysts predict a particularly high demand for nurses, allied health professionals, health educators, public health specialists, and health care administrators. Communication skills are a valuable asset in these and every other aspect of the health industry.

BOX 1.7 Ethical Considerations

An Essential Component of Health Communication

> "Our customers routinely bare their bodies, as well as their souls, within our organizations. I can think of no other enterprise in our society where so much is placed in the hands of others."
>
> **LARRY SANDERS, CHAIR OF THE AMERICAN COLLEGE OF HEALTH CARE EXECUTIVES**

Sanders (2003) advises those who provide and study health care, "One of the most significant ways we can demonstrate how much we care about those we serve is to visibly display our personal commitment to operating with extraordinary integrity, ethics and morality each and every day" (p. 46).

It is imperative that people involved with health care understand the ethical implications of their actions and conduct themselves with honor and integrity. They must also be aware of the perceptions of others. If people perceive—rightly or wrongly—that health-related professionals are unethical, they may experience stress, avoid medical care, lie to health care providers, or withhold information to protect themselves.

Many of the ethical dilemmas that people in health care face are essentially matters of communication. They involve honesty, privacy, power, social stigmas, media images, advertising, and persuasive messages about health. In most cases, there is more than one option, but no simple solution. What seems right in one situation may be wrong in another. Personal preference and culture, among other factors, shape what people want and expect. Even so, there is value in thinking through the implications and exploring diverse reactions with others.

Ethical Considerations boxes present ethical dilemmas as well as discussion questions and additional resources. We encourage you to discuss and debate

continued

these issues, eliciting diverse views. Do not be afraid to change your mind or to argue both sides of an issue. It is usually easier to behave ethically if you have thought the issues through *before* you find yourself in a real-life dilemma. Following are some questions you might ask yourself as you consider your options concerning ethical challenges posed in this book and elsewhere.

- Is this option legal?
- Is it honest? Is deception or omission of the truth involved?
- Who will be hurt? Who will be helped?
- Will the decision benefit me personally but hurt others?
- Are the results worth the hardship involved?
- Is it culturally acceptable?
- Will my decision compromise people's privacy or trust?
- Will my decision be demeaning or degrading to anyone?
- Is it fair? Will my action unfairly discriminate against anyone?
- Is the action appropriate for the situation?
- Have I considered all the options?
- How would I wish to be treated in the same situation?
- How would I feel if my decision or action were published in tomorrow's newspaper?

BOX 1.8 PERSPECTIVES

Down, but Not Out

As a high school baseball pitcher, it was devastating to hurt my shoulder just three weeks from the playoffs. My doctor helped to lighten the mood a bit by saying, "You're a great kid and I like you, but I hate seeing you here in my office. That means something's wrong." I always felt comfortable with him because he knew how to connect with me and assure me that whatever the problem was, he would get it fixed and get me back out on the field.

As it turned out, I didn't need surgery, but I did need physical therapy five days a week. The therapists were really great. They were very strict when it came to my rehab and throwing program. "Absolutely no throwing if you feel any pain whatsoever. You got it?" one therapist said to me. They treated me like royalty, even though I wasn't, and made sure I was doing the right things to get healthy again. With the urgency to get back in the game quickly, they placed me on a fast-paced, demanding rehabilitation regimen. They made sure I received the appropriate amount of work every day, and they repeatedly asked me how my shoulder was coming along.

I can't say enough about how helpful and flexible they were with me. It was tough for me to come in during office hours, so they sacrificed their own time to come in early and stay late for me. Not once did they complain. They always had smiles on their faces and always seemed positive and excited to be helping me.

After two weeks of the well-conditioned rehab they put me through, I felt completely pain free and ready to pitch again. "Now if you ever need to come in again for any therapy or some shoulder exercises, you just come on in. Don't hesitate. We'll be here," the head physical therapist told me.

"Yes ma'am, I appreciate everything you all have done for me," I replied.

I am thankful to have had those professionals who gave me their best effort and went to the absolute maximum to ensure that I was taken care of and treated properly. I can never repay them for what they did for me.

—DREW

Drew went on to earn titles as Pitcher of the Year in Alabama, All-County Pitcher of the Year, and Most Valuable Pitcher of the Year, in addition to pitching for his college team.

Summary

Importance of Health Communication
- Effective communication can enhance healing.
- Ineffective health communication can cause anxiety, errors, mistrust, and poor decisions.
- If some members of a population are underserved, the suffering, costs, and lost productivity affect everyone.

Systems-Level Approach
- Health care is an overarching system composed of many subsystems.
- The structure of a system influences the people within it.
- Superficial "fixes" seldom lead to long-term success.
- Systems resist radical change.
- Seemingly small changes can produce powerful results.

What Is Health?
- The World Health Organization (WHO) defines health in terms of overall physical, mental, and social well-being within the context of daily life.

What Is Health Communication?
- The transactional communication perspective holds that meaning is collaboratively created by people as they simultaneously send and receive messages.
- Relational messages are often conveyed implicitly, as by considering how something is said, who says it and when, and what they do not say.
- Health communication emerged as a defined area of study in the late 1960s.
- Healthy options are not equally available to everyone. Issues of social equity, community resources, access to care, and environment are involved.
- Health communication includes a focus on interpersonal communication, culture, media, public health, education, and more.

Health Care Models
- From a biomedical perspective, care providers are like scientists or mechanics who collect information about a problem, try to identify the source of it, and fix it.
- From a biopsychosocial perspective, health experiences are not solely physical phenomena but are also influenced by people's feelings, their ideas about health, and the events of their lives.
- Sociocultural influences on health include wealth, poverty, prejudice, access to health services, living conditions, shared values, traditions, and rituals.

Communication's Influence on Health
- Communication is crucial to the success of health care encounters.
- At their best, mass media and social media can help people learn about healthy options and resources.
- Communication can be an important source of personal confidence and coping ability.
- Effective communication saves time and money.
- Communication can help health care organizations operate effectively.
- Health communication is relevant to many career opportunities.

Glossary

biomedical model The premise that ill health is a physical phenomenon that can be explained, identified, and treated through physical means. *See page 12.*

biopsychosocial perspective An approach that takes into account people's physical conditions (biology), their thoughts and beliefs (psychology), and their social expectations. *See page 13.*

health Defined by the World Health Organization (WHO) as "a state of complete physical, mental and social well-being and not merely the absence of disease or infirmity." *See page 7.*

health communication The way we seek, process, and share health information. *See page 10.*

relational approach The perspective that meaning is interpreted at both a content (literal) level and a relational level that implies the relative status of communication partners and their feelings about each other. *See page 9.*

sociocultural perspective The view that health reflects a complex array of factors involving personal choice, social variables (e.g., income, prejudice, access to health services, living conditions), and culture (shared values, traditions, and rituals). *See page 13.*

transactional model of communication The theory that people collaborate to construct meaning in a process of ongoing, reciprocal influence. *See page 8.*

Discussion Questions

1. Imagine that you have been given responsibility for your family members' health. You can hire any collection of professionals you like, but you should not limit your thinking to traditional aspects of health care. What factors would you consider in terms of each person's health? Who would you involve in making sure that your family members stay as healthy as possible?

2. Spend a few minutes writing about a health care encounter you have experienced as a patient, loved one, or health professional. Identify at least three content-level and three relational-level messages in the encounter. How were the relational-level messages conveyed? What role did culture and prior experiences play in the encounter? Were you mostly satisfied with communication during this encounter? Why or why not?

3. What do you think of the case studies about St. Jude Hospital (Box 1.6) and the baseball player's physical rehabilitation (Box 1.8)? Have your experiences been mostly similar to these or different? How?

4. Divide a sheet of paper into three columns. Label them "biomedical," "biopsychosocial," and "sociocultural." Under each heading, list aspects of your health well described by that perspective. Reflect on how these factors influence the way you think about and communicate about your health.

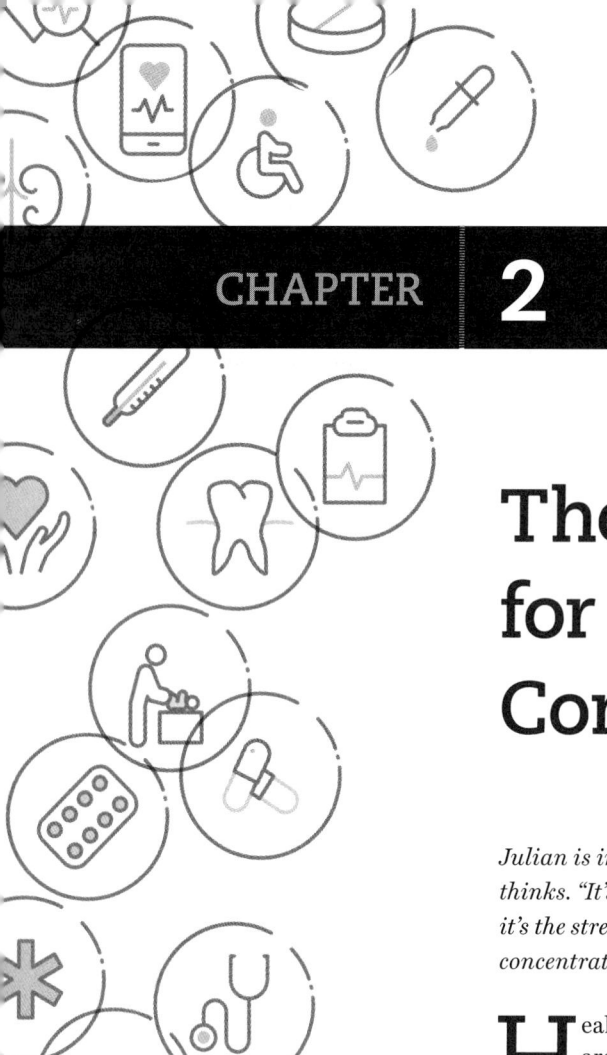

CHAPTER 2

The Landscape for Health Communication

Julian is in class one day when he begins to feel queasy. "That's weird," he thinks. "It's probably that late-night pizza catching up with me. Or maybe it's the stress of final exams in a few weeks." He rubs his stomach and tries to concentrate on the class.

Health issues, both large and small, arise nearly daily in our lives. They are often resolved with a good night's sleep or an internet search. At other times, they require that we navigate the health care system. Either way, one thing is certain: We will all be involved in health care in one way or another—as patients, loved ones, community members, professionals, researchers, and/or policy-makers. This chapter provides a foundation for understanding some of the most pressing issues in health care.

As you may remember from Chapter 1, one tenet of transactional communication is that we are influenced by the larger contexts and systems in which we live. Therefore, before we launch an in-depth exploration of health communication issues, it's important to understand the landscape in which they occur. We will delve further into many of these issues throughout the book.

Current Issues in Health Care

When Julian's stomach is still bothering him several days later, his friends urge him to see a doctor. Julian knows it's good advice. If this is something serious, he'd like to stop it before it gets worse. On the other hand, he has a number of reservations: He would hate to miss school or work right now. The last time he tried to get a doctor's appointment, he had to wait a week and then sit in the waiting room for more than an hour. He's not sure he can afford to pay for a doctor's visit. And even if he had the time and money, he doesn't quite know whom to call.

Julian's internal dialogue reflects many of the important issues in health care and health communication today—early care and prevention, access, and challenges navigating the system.

Early and Preventive Care

It is healthier, and ultimately less costly, to prevent illnesses and injuries than to treat them once they become serious. If Julian has appendicitis, for example, early care might prevent surgery, permanent damage to his health, and even death. This is true of many health concerns. As mentioned in Chapter 1, when conditions such as diabetes, cancer, obesity, and asthma are not well managed, they typically cause serious complications that are costly and difficult to treat (CDC, 2019).

The value of early and preventive care is evident in countries that make it a priority. Japan spends an average of $4,600 per citizen on health care annually, whereas the United States spends about $8,100 (World Health Organization [WHO], 2018a). Japan invests its much smaller budget heavily in prevention, regular care, and early detection of disease. Partly as a result, Japanese citizens live an average of five years longer than Americans and outperform the United States on many other health indicators as well (Organisation for Economic Co-Operation and Development, 2019a, 2019b, 2019c).

Clearly, it's in everyone's best interest to keep people healthy, but providing early and preventive care is not simple. It requires a different orientation and infrastructure than reactive care, and it relies on the concerted efforts of everyday citizens and a diverse array of professionals. A large part of the effort involves communication. As we will discuss in Chapters 12 through 14, public health involves mass-mediated messages, face-to-face communication, crisis management, and more. And since prevention usually involves ongoing attention to a complex array of factors, the most effective efforts involve multidisciplinary teams and everyday people. In Chapter 5, we talk about the rewards and challenges of a team approach.

Access and Health Disparities

Experts can predict roughly how long a person will live based on where the person lives and how much money they make. For example, a baby born and raised in Africa will die an average of 16 years sooner than a child born at the same time in Europe (WHO, 2017).

In the United States, women in the top 1% income bracket live an average of 10 years longer than women in the bottom 1% (Chetty, 2016). And the wealth–longevity differential is even larger for American men, at 15 years.

"There is no biological or genetic reason for these alarming differences in health and life opportunity," says an analyst for the World Health Organization (2011, para. 1). Instead, one culprit is the different care and information people receive. For example, some observers say there are "two Americas" (Commonwealth Fund, 2013). One is populated by residents of states such as Massachusetts, Hawaii, Washington, Minnesota, and Connecticut that lead the nation in percentage of insured residents and access to affordable care. The other "America" includes states such as Texas, Mississippi, Oklahoma, Arkansas, and Nevada, where barriers to care are far higher (Commonwealth Fund, 2019). On average, even low-income residents of "first America" are healthier and live longer than middle-class residents of "second America."

One barrier to care involves health insurance. As you might predict, people without insurance tend to forgo regular checkups and health screenings. They are likely to seek care only when they are seriously ill or injured, and they may be unable to afford prescription medication and other treatments such as counseling and physical therapy (Kaiser Family Foundation, 2019). Even among those who are insured in the United States, about 3 in 10 have a hard time paying for premiums and copays (Kaiser Family Foundation, 2019). Later in the chapter, we will explore health care reform measures that impact who can afford health insurance and what it covers.

Another challenge is to provide culturally sensitive care to members of underserved populations. When polled, 9 out of 10 personnel at community health centers in the United States say that the most needed improvement is better communication with diverse patients to assist them in identifying and meeting personal health goals (Broderick & Haque, 2015). "You must appeal to patients with relevant, personalized communications," agrees health care strategist Brent Walker (2017, para. 6). Instead of assuming that everyone feels the same, care providers might pose questions such as *What are your main goals and priorities? What questions do you have about your health? What factors help you stick with health-related goals?* and *What factors make it difficult?*

Better access to health care and information can be cost saving and life enhancing. There are no simple solutions, but a range of communication modalities play a factor, including direct patient–caregiver communication (Chapter 3), awareness of diverse needs and cultural assumptions (Chapters 6 and 7), system-level processes and resources (Chapter 10), and the use of communication technology (Chapter 9).

Navigating a Complex System

When Julian visits with a general practitioner, the doctor tells him, "You may be experiencing a virus or the effects of stress. But to be on the safe side, I'd like you to see to a gastroenterologist for some tests." Julian's head is swimming with questions such as What is a gastroenterologist? What sort of tests? *and* How long will I have to wait for that appointment? *The doctor seems to be in a hurry to conclude the visit, though, so Julian simply says thanks and leaves, feeling a bit adrift.*

Julian isn't alone in feeling that he has entered an environment that can be difficult to navigate. In a recent study of 1,500 people affected by chronic illnesses, two-thirds said they have felt "anxious, confused, or helpless" about the process of seeking and receiving care (Schneider, Abrams, Shah, Lewis, & Shah, 2018). The most common frustrations involve communication: unclear instructions, contradictory information from different providers, hard-to-understand insurance policies, and a sense that health professionals don't communicate well with one another (Roche et al., 2016; Schneider et al., 2018).

"We show up and expect that Doctor A talked to Doctor B and that they're all on the same page. In reality, that's not happening," observes nurse Sana Goldberg (quoted by Lefferts, 2018, p. 33). Consequently, patients often feel that they have to be their own case managers, scheduling and coordinating care with little knowledge of how the health system works (Roche et al., 2016, p. e976). The results include added stress, treatment delays and oversights, communication gaps, adverse patient outcomes, and additional emergency department visits and hospitalizations (Kern, 2018).

The fault lies not so much with individuals as with the health care system overall. Providers often work for different organizations, with duties and time constraints that prevent them from also acting as

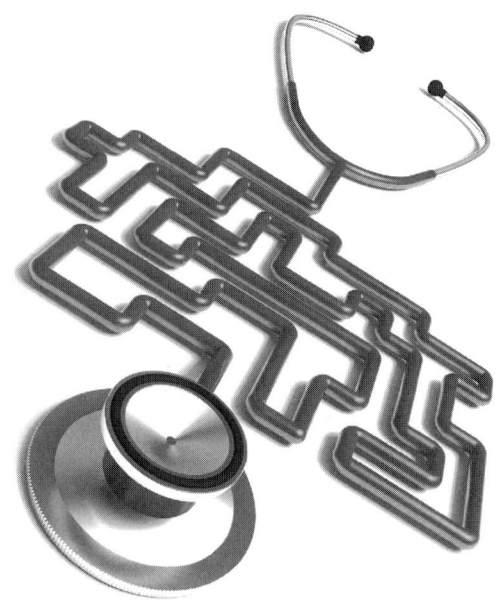

The health care system can feel like a maze, especially when a serious illness requires treatment by providers in many different organizations. In some markets, health care navigators help chart the way for patients and their loved ones.

Have you ever wished you could enlist the services of a health care navigator? If so, what type of assistance would have been most helpful?

full-blown case managers. As some analysts put it, the U.S. health system (and many others) suffers from a "lack of scaffolding" (Roche et al., 2016, p. e977). The building blocks may be there but a coherent structure to organize and synchronize them is lacking.

On the bright side, some large medical organizations and communities have had success pairing patients with health care navigators. In Queensland, Australia, the government funds about 400 nurse navigators who don't work for any one medical center, but who know them all well (Hudson et al., 2019). Here are a few services the navigators provide:

- They advocate for patients, answer questions, and provide emotional support and information.
- Because navigators often have an inside track when it comes to scheduling, they can sometimes arrange appointments with a range of specialists on the same day to spare patients excessive travel and disruptions.
- Navigators review diagnostic and treatment information with patients, all the while looking for red

flags (inconsistencies, missing test results, duplications, or oversights) that others might miss.
- Navigators help patients draft questions and summaries to share with care providers.
- They also organize team meetings at which health professionals gather to discuss specific patients.

In Queensland, navigators' contributions help patients and providers alike. One person recalls what happened when she showed her pediatrician a personal health care synopsis her navigator had created for her. The doctor said, "That's fantastic and amazing, it's all there for me" (Hudson et al., 2019, p. 115). Studies show that well-trained health care navigators, even when they don't have medical backgrounds, are able to reduce health care costs and improve patient access, satisfaction, and health outcomes (Catania, Bagnasco, Zanini, Aleo, & Sasso, 2016; Rocque et al., 2017; Sharmeen Shommu et al., 2016).

The challenge, particularly in the United States, has been funding. When care spans the boundaries of multiple organizations, who foots the bill? So far, there's no clear answer.

COMMUNICATION SKILL BUILDERS: NAVIGATING THE HEALTH CARE SYSTEM

Here are a few communication approaches that may be helpful if you or a loved one experiences a serious, long-term health concern.

- *Develop a strong relationship with a principal care provider (PCP).* Choose the health professional most likely to manage your overall care and with whom you have a good relationship. Keep your PCP well informed about your health status and share their name and contact information with everyone involved in your care, including specialists, emergency department personnel, and so on. Insist that all records and test results be shared with your PCP (Brookhardt-Murray, 2005).
- *Recruit a personal health care quarterback.* In addition to a PCP, choose someone you love and trust (perhaps a good friend or family member) to help you. Leslie Michelson, author of the book *The Patient's Playbook*, calls this person a "health care quarterback" (Michelson, 2015). A good quarterback can provide emotional support, talk through medical decisions with you, help you manage appointments, look up information, and so on.
- *Maintain a roster of key players.* Even if no specific health care team is assigned to you (it usually isn't), develop your own list of players and their contact information. You might include physicians, nurses, social workers, scheduling personnel, health insurance professionals, and others who can provide assistance and answer questions.
- *Keep and share clear records of your medications, health care visits, allergies, and test results.* Bring this information to all visits. It may help prevent oversights, duplications, and mistakes.
- *Listen to your body.* In the midst of an ongoing health concern, it can be difficult to know what is serious and what isn't. Experienced patient and blogger William Bilicic (n.d.) offers this advice: "I know you might be scared and think you are overreacting, but you are probably not. Trust me, if you feel like something is off, then something is off and you need to get it looked at" (para. 5).
- *Network.* Support groups and online communities can be valuable guides as you make your way through unfamiliar territory. For example, Rhiannon, a blogger who copes with depression and posttraumatic stress, says that people who have similar challenges have provided her with practical advice and emotional support when she has felt lost in the system (Rhiannon, 2018).

So far, we have looked at three current issues in health care: early care and prevention, access, and the challenge of navigating an often-fragmented system. In each case, communication can be an important tool to make connections, reduce uncertainty, share information, and provide emotional support. In the next section, we broaden the scope to consider more macro-level influences on health communication.

Health Communication in a Changing World

When Julian looks up "pain near the belly button," he notices a news story about an illness that has killed or sickened people in several countries. He notes with relief that his symptoms are nothing like theirs, but it reminds him to take precautions before his study-abroad experience in a few months.

Changes in the world around us have profound influences on health. Here we examine three of those changes in terms of global issues, population shifts, and technological advances.

Global Health

Travel, immigration, and the international exchange of food and products mean that diseases are continually carried across national borders. The Coronavirus provided a striking example of how quickly a disease can spread. In March 2020, the number of cases outside mainland China doubled every few days, escalating from 10,000 to 1 million by April 2, and then doubling to 2 million by mid-April.

The AIDS epidemic has been even more deadly and long lasting. Thanks to aggressive health promotion efforts, new cases are not emerging as quickly as in years past, but the situation remains critical. Tens of millions are still infected, and about 40% of them are not receiving treatment that might reduce symptoms and extend their lives (WHO, 2018c).

Other global issues related to health include climate change, reluctance to vaccinate, addiction, pollution, and a growing number of drug-resistant illnesses (WHO, 2019a). In Chapter 12 we focus on international communication and the intercultural competence necessary to deal effectively with global health concerns.

Changing Populations

Improving health and well-being ranks third on the United Nation's "17 Goals to Change Our World," behind reducing poverty and hunger (United Nations, 2019). One challenge is to respond effectively to population shifts. Here we explore how changes in the population affect health and the way we communicate about it.

AGING

By the year 2050, the percentage of people worldwide who are 60 or older will be twice what it was in 2015 (WHO, 2018b). That's good news in many respects. Older adults have a great deal to offer their families and communities, and living longer provides "the chance to pursue new activities such as further education, a new career or pursuing a long neglected passion," point out analysts for the WHO. Yet, they add, "the extent of these opportunities and contributions depends heavily on one factor: health" (WHO, 2018b, para. 4).

Although many older adults are healthy, they are more likely than others to have chronic health concerns, which will increase the need for medical care, assisted living facilities, social services, and home care. We will explore facets of health communication with older adults (Chapter 6) and the joys and challenges of providing at-home care for loved ones (Chapter 8).

RACIAL AND CULTURAL DIVERSITY

If there is a theme for the years ahead, it may be multiculturalism. In the United States, people of Hispanic, Asian, and Native American descent together are expected to comprise the majority of the population within the next 25 years (Vespa, Armstrong, & Medina, 2018). Diversity is also rising in other parts of the world, mostly because a record number of people are now being forced from their homelands by war and other hardships (WHO, 2019b).

A more culturally integrated world presents an unprecedented richness of diversity. The challenge will be to address the health needs that arise. Immigrants and refugees are at higher-than-average risk for depression and anxiety, inadequate health care, and the effects of poverty (WHO, 2019c). And experts predict that Americans of color will still have disproportionately fewer educational and professional opportunities than White Americans do.

An ongoing dilemma is that people who are most in need of health care are often least likely to be well informed about health issues and to utilize health services. It's not yet clear whether technology will help bridge literacy gaps—by presenting information in clear, visual terms and in multiple languages—or whether people already at a disadvantage will fall further behind because they do not have equal access to information-rich resources such as the internet.

Complicating the issue even further, diversity among health care workers is not expected to keep pace with the overall population. In the United States, for example, although Black and Latinx individuals comprise about 31% of the population, they make up only 15% of physicians and 20% of registered nurses (U.S. Bureau of Labor Statistics, 2019; U.S. Census Bureau, 2018). As a result, patients are likely to be treated by caregivers who differ markedly from them in terms of knowledge, needs, and cultural beliefs. This is regrettable because, as physician Dhruv Khullar (2018) puts it,

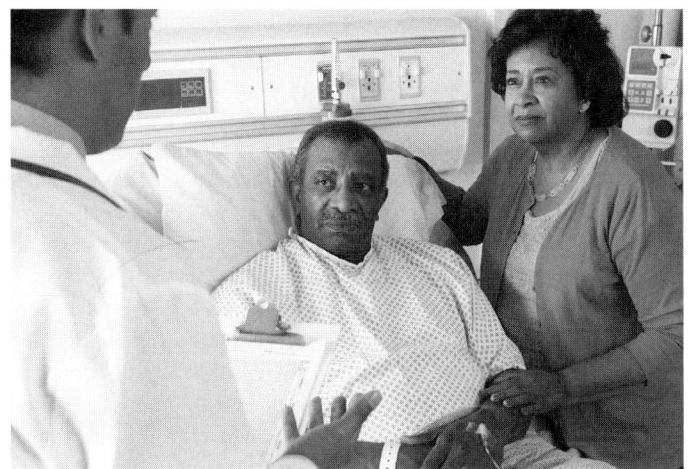

Care providers in the United States do not yet reflect diversity in the overall population, which can lead to misunderstandings and missed cues.

What techniques would you recommend to people of different cultural backgrounds to help them bridge the gap during health care encounters?

more diverse health professionals "could help us move toward a system in which the lived experience of minority groups is better understood and validated, and the barriers they face more readily identified and addressed" (para. 16). In Chapters 6 and 9 and elsewhere in the book, we explore facets of health communication related to age, culture, and other forms of diversity.

Communication Technology

When Julian visits a gastroenterologist, she confirms that his appendix is enlarged. She prescribes antibiotics and asks Julian to check in with her daily via email so they can closely monitor his symptoms. "If you don't feel better in the next few days, call the phone number on this card," the doctor says. "A nurse is available around the clock to answer questions and make arrangements for emergency care, if necessary. Or, if you prefer, use our online chat service to communicate with a member of our care team any time."

As Julian's experience illustrates, new options in technology are expanding the opportunities for health communication. Nearly 1 in 3 Americans has communicated online with a physician, mostly via email (Jiang & Street, 2017). As you might predict, people ages 18 to 34 are more receptive than older individuals to the idea of instant-messaging their doctors and following/friending them on social media (American Osteopathic Association, 2018). Older adults are taking advantage of different technology. Among those surveyed, more than half of Americans in their fifties and sixties said they have established online patient portals that they use mostly to review medical test results, request prescription refills, and schedule appointments (Clark, Singer, Solway, Kirch, & Malani, 2018).

In addition, new mobile apps allow people to measure and record health indicators such as heart rate and blood sugar, and if they wish, to share that data with health professionals. Another promising eHealth option involves multimedia storytelling in which people are not only consumers of information but are actively (and interactively) involved in sharing health-related narratives that they create themselves (Cozma, 2009). The process can be rich, therapeutic, and informative. At the same time, it sometimes diverts attention from scientific information, which is typically more complex and less emotionally immediate than personal stories (Cozma). We explore issues related to telemedicine, eHealth, and media storytelling in Chapter 9.

In closing this section, although it may seem that the average person is not directly affected by global changes, that is far from the case. They influence the type of care providers people are likely to see, what services are available, and what role individuals play in maintaining their own health. People who work in the health industry are likely to experience the stress and promise of change, the opportunity to use new technology, and the need to communicate effectively with a variety of people and include them as partners in their own care.

In the next two sections, we take a closer look at two efforts to make health care more affordable, less wasteful, and more accessible—managed care and health care reform.

Communication in Managed Care

Let's back up a bit in Julian's story.... Before he called a doctor, he phoned his parents to check on his insurance status, remembering that his older sister was not insured her last year in college because, like him, she was a part-time student. Julian's parents assure him that the rules have changed since then and he is indeed covered on their health insurance policy. On that encouraging note, they tell him how to access a website that lists care providers included on their plan.

Julian's conversation with his parents reflects elements of managed care as well as health care reform (which we will talk about later in the chapter).

Managed care organizations coordinate the costs and delivery of health services. Whereas health decisions were once made almost entirely by health care professionals and patients, managed care organizations now recruit patients, match them up with care providers and facilities, and monitor expenses. As such, managed care represents the influence of people (or entities) other than patients and caregivers. By managing resources such as money, labor, technology, and facilities, people in managed care organizations seek to make health care more efficient and affordable. Since managed care took root in the 1980s, it has expanded to include 99% of U.S. residents with employer-sponsored health plans (Henry J. Kaiser, 2018). To understand the variety of managed care organizations, let's fast-forward a year or so and pretend that Julian is choosing between health insurance options, which he is likely to do when he gets a full-time job. Here is a description of his managed care health insurance options and the implications of each in terms of health communication.

Conventional Insurance

At one point, nearly everyone who had health insurance in the United States had conventional (also known as *indemnity*) insurance. Now, less 1% of employee-sponsored plans meet this description (Henry J. Kaiser, 2018), but let's imagine that Julian's employer is one of the few that do.

As a conventional insurance subscriber, Julian will pay a set monthly amount (**insurance premium**) and the first $1,000 or so of his annual medical expenses (his **deductible**). If his expenses exceed this deductible, insurance will pay most of the remaining costs (usually about 80%) and he will pay the rest. To prevent him from going into overwhelming debt, there is an upper limit, called a **catastrophic cap**, on the amount of out-of-pocket money he will be required to pay each year. Beyond that limit, insurance will pay 100%.

On the downside, premiums for conventional insurance are usually higher than in other plans. However, subscribers have more freedom to choose their own doctors and other providers. From a communication perspective, this means Julian will have the chance to choose care providers with whom he feels most comfortable.

Conventional insurance is classified as **fee-for-service** because providers are paid (reimbursed) for specific care they provide. In other words, doctors, hospitals, physical therapists, and so on, make money only if people use their services. One implication is that care providers may overprescribe tests and treatments. Another is that wellness is not highly rewarded in the fee-for-service model. Traditionally, conventional insurance policies have not covered routine checkups.

Conventional insurance represents a **third-party payer** system because, as you can see, there are three parties involved—the provider, the patient, and the payer (insurance company). Over time, the balance of power between these parties has shifted. For example, insurance companies used to pay hospitals based on the costs they incurred while providing care. Beginning in the early 1980s, however, the U.S. government and insurance companies began establishing flat-rate reimbursement amounts for inpatient hospital procedures. Because the rates were classified within general types of care (e.g., cardiac, oncology), they came to be known as **diagnosis-related groups** (**DRGs**). This is known as a **prospective payment structure** because reimbursement is established in advance rather than after care has been provided. This payment structure has made communication between care providers and funding agencies particularly important. If they are not on the same page in terms of what care a patient needs, it is unlikely that the provider will receive full payment.

DRGs are meant to reward hospitals for cutting costs and expediting care. They probably have, to some extent. A hospital whose expenses fall below the reimbursement rate can keep the difference as profit. A few other things have happened as well. For one, hospital stays (which are more expensive to provide than outpatient treatment) have become dramatically shorter and available only to people with serious illnesses and injuries. Some hospitals have also begun to limit or discontinue procedures with low reimbursement rates.

DRGs are not only a factor in traditional insurance, but also in managed care. Let's consider Julian's options in that arena. The averages presented here are based on the Henry J. Kaiser Family Foundation's 2018 employee health benefits survey.

Health Maintenance Organizations

A **health maintenance organization** (**HMO**) is designed to be more or less a one-stop shop for members' health needs. An HMO hires physicians and other care providers, who work directly for the HMO. Their salaries are covered by the premiums that members pay each month.

If Julian chooses an HMO, he will pay a monthly premium and a **copay** (a cost per visit) every time he visits a doctor.[1] This includes checkups and preventive care visits. Most HMOs do not have deductibles, but about a third of them do.

Knowing that he will probably never pay more than a $25 copay to visit a general practitioner, Julian might be more willing to have annual checkups and to seek care for minor health concerns than if he had conventional insurance. This is meant to save money in the long run, both for members and for HMOs.

Among managed care options, HMOs present the smallest set of provider options. Julian may only see care providers who work for the HMO, and he may not always have a choice about whom he sees among them.

As an HMO member, Julian cannot see specialists unless such care is recommended by a provider (usually a primary care physician) in the HMO. This is designed to avoid unnecessary visits and costs, but the approval process and limitations can be frustrating.

You guessed it: HMOs are not third-party payer systems. In their case, it's as if the insurance company and the medical center have merged into one. And they are not based on fee-for-service. Instead, HMOs are capitated systems. **Capitation** involves the payment of an established (capitated) amount paid in the form of premiums (plus minor copays), no matter what care is provided. It's the job of HMOs to manage both the budget and the care.

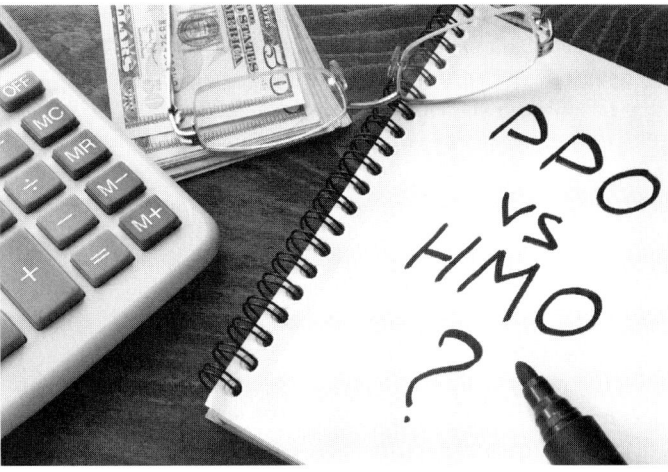

Managed care health plans differ in terms of premium costs, provider options, deductibles, and more.

As a health care consumer, are you most interested in an HMO, PPO, or high-deductible health plan? What are the pros and cons of each?

Some people (including many care providers) worry that combining the insurance company with the medical center presents a conflict of interest. We'll talk more about that shortly. First, let's continue the tour of managed care options.

Preferred Provider Organizations

A **preferred provider organization** (**PPO**), also in the managed care family, works a little differently. If Julian joins a PPO, his premium will probably be about the same as if he joined an HMO, but he will have an annual deductible, and his copay will vary by procedure.

Here's how it works. Rather than hiring care providers outright, as HMOs do, PPOs contract with independent care providers. The PPO agrees to put the provider on a "preferred" list if the provider offers services at agreed-on discount rates to the PPO's members. Julian's copay will be a percentage of this discounted fee. This means he will pay different amounts for different services. It also means he can choose any care providers he wishes, with one caveat: As the name implies, providers on the "preferred" list cost less than those who are not. There are often higher copays and/or separate deductibles for providers not on the list. But unlike HMO members, Julian will receive *some* financial coverage no matter which caregivers he chooses.

If Julian requires a lot of care or if he sees non-preferred providers, he is likely to pay more as a

---

[1] For now, let's leave prescription drugs, outpatient surgery, and hospital care out of the mix. With managed care, separate copays and deductibles usually apply to those services.

PPO member than as an HMO member. But he will have more freedom of choice in a PPO, which can be a bonus in terms of relationship building. He may also encounter less conflict of interest because (1) PPO providers do not work directly for the managed care organization, so they may be spared some of the pressure to cut costs and speed up patient visits, and (2) they operate on a fee-for-service basis that gives them more incentive to prescribe (rather than avoid) tests and treatment. These advantages may be why the majority of people with employee health plans choose PPOs (49% compared to 16% in HMOs).

High-Deductible Health Plans

Perhaps Julian is in excellent health and almost never seeks medical care. He may wonder, "Why should I pay high premiums when I never meet the deductible anyway? My money goes in, but it doesn't come out—at least it doesn't come to me." And if he is really thinking long-term, he might also wonder, "Rather than paying high premiums, why can't I save that money for the future, when my medical bills are likely to be higher?"

These are the basic concepts behind **high-deductible health plans** (**HDHPs**). Members pay relatively low monthly premiums. In exchange, their deductibles are nearly double that of other plans, and the catastrophic cap is higher. The smaller up-front costs make HDHPs appealing to people on limited budgets. Nearly 1 in 3 employed Americans is now enrolled in a high-deductible plan.

HDHP members may qualify to invest in tax-deferred **health savings accounts** (**HSA**) that they can use to pay for current and future medical expenses. This is meant to encourage people to control their own health costs.

Unfortunately, this is also the downside of HDHPs. Some people buy into them because they can afford the lower premiums only to find that they cannot afford the out-of-pocket costs that lie ahead. Reports abound of people who are insured but still cannot afford to buy prescription drugs or see a doctor. Even if Julian has not needed much medical care in years past, one accident or major illness can wreck his finances.

Managed care also affects hospitals, medical centers, treatment and diagnostic centers, and other organizations. Their budgets and decisions are heavily influenced by budget constraints, paperwork, and capitation, as you will see in the following synopsis of the pros and cons of managed care.

Pros and Cons of Managed Care

Overall, there are upsides and downsides to managed care. Following are a few considerations both ways. One note before we begin: In the parlance of health care, *insurers* include both conventional insurance companies and managed care organizations. However, as you have seen, 99% of insurance policies are now managed care memberships. So when people talk about "insurers" these days, they mostly mean managed care organizations.

ADVANTAGES

Following are some factors in favor of managed care.

PREDICTIVE BUDGETING The beauty of capitation is that it offers predictable, steady income based on members' contributions. Although the budget under managed care is typically smaller than before, advance planning is more feasible. "Capitation gave us the flexibility to use our budget with creativity limited only by our imaginations and habits," recall physicians Joseph Dorsey and Donald Berwick (2008, p. A9) of Harvard Pilgrim Health Care. They invested in innovative and patient-friendly services such as reminder calls, after-hours phone access, extended clinic hours, time-saving technology, and more. As a result, in the early days of managed care, their patient/members made half as many visits to emergency departments as the state average.

INCENTIVE TO REDUCE COSTS Managed care rewards health care organizations for streamlining processes and eliminating wasteful practices. As you may remember, with capitation and DRGs, only organizations that operate in a cost-effective way make money.

MORE AFFORDABLE CARE A related benefit is that managed care is designed to make health care more affordable. In a global sense, the system is oriented toward making the most of every health care dollar. At an individual level, patients pay set or reduced fees, even if they need a lot of care. This can be especially valuable to people with chronic illnesses who benefit from regular treatment.

WELLNESS The expectation early on was that managed care organizations would invest in disease prevention and education because, with capitation, well patients would cost them less than sick or injured ones. (As you will soon see, this potential has not been well realized so far.)

ADMINISTRATIVE ASSISTANCE AND TEAMWORK Individual health professionals may also benefit from managed care. One physician says that managed care gave him his life back. He does not make as much money as before, but as an HMO employee he doesn't have as many administrative responsibilities. He is only on call one day a week, and he can schedule days off—all luxuries he did not have as a physician entrepreneur.

CAREER JUMP START Managed care organizations can also offer the advantages of a ready-made caseload. Signing on as an HMO employee or a preferred provider means built-in advertising among hundreds or thousands of available patients.

DISADVANTAGES

Unfortunately, as the system has evolved, the disadvantages of managed care have become numerous. It may help as you read the following list of drawbacks to keep in mind that *something* had to be done. It is conceivable that we would be in even worse shape without the managed care revolution. But clearly, we still have a long way to go.

COSTS CONTINUE TO RISE One disappointment is that, overall, the goal of cutting costs has not been realized. Managed care may have slowed spiraling costs to some extent, but premiums have climbed steadily. Since the 1990s, health insurance premiums have risen an average of 55%, with employees of small businesses being hardest hit (Economic Research Initiative on the Uninsured, 2005; Henry J. Kaiser, 2017).

Some spokespersons for managed care say that premium hikes are necessary because health expenses are rising and the population is getting older. However, critics accuse managed care organizations of making large profits while patients and providers lose money (Center for Consumer Information, 2011).

PREVENTION STILL NOT A PRIORITY It is sometimes said that the United States does not have a health care system, it has an illness care system. Managed care was supposed to change that by shifting the focus to cost-saving prevention. That has not happened on the scale many people had hoped. This is mostly because prevention efforts cost in the short run but save in the long run. "The managed care plans don't think it's worthwhile to invest in prevention programs when people change their plans frequently, trying to get lower costs," said a managed care executive on an anonymous survey ("Health Economics," 2003, p. 56). In other words, managed care organizations are, predictably enough, often reluctant to invest in the long-term health of short-term members.

INCENTIVE TO LIMIT CARE Critics are also troubled that managed care organizations sometimes pressure providers to limit care and speed up patient visits. Journalists coined the phrase "death by HMO" to refer to instances in which people's health was hurt or destroyed when decision makers in managed care organizations refused to authorize expensive treatments or delayed approval until it was too late. Some 9 out of 10 physicians surveyed said that patients' health has been negatively impacted by the approval process, sometimes leading to death, hospitalization, or permanent damage to their health (American Medical Association, 2019).

Some people worry that these incentives will interfere with care providers' professional judgment. It's common for HMOs to withhold a portion of physicians' pay, to be awarded only if the treatment they prescribe comes in under budget and only if they see a specified (usually large) number of patients per day.

LIMITED CHOICES As mentioned, patients in managed care lose some of the ability to choose or switch caregivers. Even with PPOs, there is a strong financial incentive to see providers on the short list. To receive full benefits, members are limited to providers who participate in their care plans, and they may be forced to switch providers if they change employers or if their employers change managed care affiliations. Such disruptions may compromise the quality of patient–caregiver relationships. Some people are more worried than others. Less than half (44%) of older adults surveyed said they would switch doctors to save money (Tu, 2005). However, people ages 18 to 34 felt differently. A large majority (70%) of them would choose a lower-priced plan, even if it required them to change doctors (Tu).

RED TAPE OVERLOAD Last, a great deal of energy in managed care is diverted to bureaucracy. Many caregivers say that it's nearly impossible to do their jobs well and meet the increased demand for paperwork. Physicians rank "too much paperwork" as one of the top three reasons for burnout in the field (Peckham, 2013).

Of a similar mind, Bhupinder Singh, a New York general practitioner, told the *New York Times*:

Thirty percent of my hospital admissions are being denied. There's a 45-day limit on the appeal. You don't bill in time, you lose everything. You're discussing this with a managed care rep on the phone and you think: "You're sitting there, I'm sitting here. How do you know anything about this patient?" (quoted by Jauhar, 2008, p. 5)

Nearly 1 in 3 physicians surveyed say they have staff who work on nothing but filing pre-authorization paperwork (American Medical Association, 2019). See Figure 2.1 for more.

The extra paperwork translates to less time with patients. An extensive study of hospital nurses revealed that the nurses spent less than one-fifth of their time (just shy of 2 hours per 10-hour shift) providing direct patient care (Hendrich, Chow, Skierczynski, & Lu, 2008). They spent the most time (nearly 4 hours per shift) doing required paperwork. The rest was spent communicating with other care team members, getting supplies, moving between rooms, and so on.

All in all, the managed care landscape is unsatisfying and even frightening. It has changed significantly from the early days when, as physicians Dorsey and Berwick (2008) recall, "neither of us can recall a single instance of being told by management to withhold from a patient any care that we thought, based on evidence, could help" (p. A9). Dorsey and Berwick's initial optimism has turned to disillusionment. Now, they charge, managed care has been "hijacked by insurance companies" such that physicians are "handcuffed" to procedures and limitations meant to save money today rather than provide high-quality care that will pay off in the long run (p. A9).

For some questions to ask as you consider various managed care plans, see Box 2.1.

Health Care Reform

If health equaled wealth, U.S. citizens would live longer than anyone else. The United States spends eight times the worldwide average, per capita, on health care. However, 44 countries have longer life expectancies (World Population Review, 2019). This surprises many people who assume that the U.S. health care system is the best in the world. Actually, it ranks 29th compared to other nations (Fullman et al., 2018). That's mostly because some people in the United States receive no or little care while others receive a disproportionate share of the pie. As you will see, that imbalance adversely affects health and drives up costs for everyone.

This section explores issues related to health care policy and reform. It should help you communicate knowledgeably about concepts that you are likely to hear about in the news—such as the *universal coverage*, *Medicare for all*, *individual mandates*, and the *Affordable Care Act*. The goal isn't to convince you of any particular viewpoint. Instead, pros and cons are provided for each, and your challenge (now and in the future) is to consider what is most important from your perspective.

Universal Coverage

Imagine knowing that, from the moment you are born until you die, you can get health care any time you need it. **Universal coverage** means that all citizens (and, in some countries, all temporary residents and visitors as well) are assured of health care. Italy is an example. A few years ago, when the Vidrines (an American family) were visiting Rome, one of them got food poisoning. Local residents escorted the family to the emergency room of a Roman hospital. "They immediately gave Joshua a stretcher," recalls Andrea Vidrine of her son's care. "He had two rounds of antibiotics, several liters of IV fluids, an ultrasound, and three blood tests, and he spent a night in the ER." There was no charge for the visit.

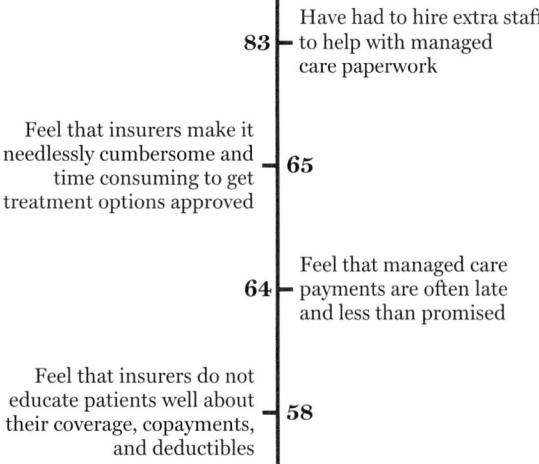

FIGURE 2.1 The majority of Texas physicians surveyed about managed care felt the system wastes money and time.

BOX 2.1

Selecting a Managed Care Plan

Here are some questions to ask when reviewing health insurance plans.

1. What are my monthly premiums, and, if applicable, what portion of the premium will my employer pay?
2. Will I have copays? If so, how much are they?
3. Is there an annual deductible? If so, how much is it? (If you are considering a family plan, ask if this amount applies to each person's care or to the family overall.)
4. Does the deductible apply to preventive care visits?
5. Do separate deductibles or copays apply to preventive care, prescription drugs, outpatient surgery, hospital stays, or visits to nonpreferred providers?
6. Is there an annual catastrophic cap (an out-of-pocket limit) on expenses? If so, what is it? What expenses count toward this amount?
7. How many (and which) physicians and specialists are on the plan or the preferred provider list? (It's a good idea to call a few of these before you sign on, to see if they are accepting new patients and to gauge how long people typically wait to get an appointment. Just because a provider appears on the list doesn't mean they have time for more patients.)
8. Are there conditions or treatments not covered by this plan? (Managed care has not been particularly good about funding care for mental health and some other concerns. Ask in advance what's covered and what's not.)
9. Is it required that I establish a primary care physician? If so, who are my options? If an HMO, will I be able to see the same physician every time, or will I be required to see whoever is available?
10. To what extent will the plan restrict the prescription drugs I am able to buy with benefits? (Every plan has formularies, which are lists of approved drugs that the plan covers. Some plans have long lists, and some have short ones. Particularly if you know which drugs you prefer or need to take, it is wise to ask in advance if they are covered.)
11. Which hospitals are included in this plan? If more than one, can I choose from among them?

As you may notice in Table 2.1, nearly all of the top 40 health systems offer universal coverage to some extent. The status of universal care in the United States is uncertain. We'll talk more about that in a moment.

PROS AND CONS OF UNIVERSAL COVERAGE

To enter the debate about health care reform, it's important to understand the pros and cons of universal coverage. Here are the basics.

Some people oppose universal coverage on the grounds that individuals should take personal responsibility for their own health and health care expenses. Some of the arguments from that perspective are (Amadeo, 2019):

- If health care is available to all, healthy people may end up paying disproportionately for unhealthy ones.
- People guaranteed of care might be lax about maintaining their own health.
- Offering care to all citizens might overwhelm the health system and lead to longer wait times.

On the other side of the issue, proponents of universal coverage hold that health care should be available to everyone who needs it. Here are their arguments ("Should All," 2019):

- Neglecting the health of some people hurts all people because contagious diseases left untreated are likely to spread, and medical care for diseases in advanced stages is more expensive than preventive care would have been.
- Universal coverage reduces the risk of personal financial disaster if someone experiences a health crisis.
- Providing care for everyone may lead to healthier citizens and a more prosperous and productive society.
- Funding for universal coverage may ultimately bolster the health care system in terms of resources, jobs, and services.

TABLE 2.1 Ranking of World Health Systems

RANKING AMONG WORLD HEALTH SYSTEMS		TYPE OF HEALTH COVERAGE
1	Iceland	Universal
2	Norway	Universal
3	Netherlands	Universal
4	Luxembourg	Universal
5	Australia	Universal
6	Finland	Universal
7	Switzerland	Universal
8	Sweden	Universal
9	Italy	Universal
10	Andorra	Universal
11	Ireland	Universal
12	Japan	Universal
13	Austria	Universal
14	Canada	Universal
15	Belgium	Universal
16	New Zealand	Universal
17	Denmark	Universal
18	Germany	Universal
19	Spain	Universal
20	France	Universal
21	Slovenia	Universal
22	Singapore	Universal
23	United Kingdom	Universal
24	Greece	Universal
25	South Korea	Universal
26	Cyprus	Universal
27	Malta	Universal
28	Czech Republic	Universal
29	United States	Uncertain Future
30	Croatia	Universal
31	Estonia	Nearly Universal
32	Portugal	Universal
33	Lebanon	Nearly Universal
34	Taiwan	Universal
35	Israel	Universal
36	Slovakia	Universal
37	Bermuda	Not Universal
38	Puerto Rico	Universal
39	Poland	Universal
40	Hungary	Universal

Source: Fullman, N., Yearwood, J., Abay, S. M., Abbafati, C., Abd-Allah, F., Abdela, J., . . . & Lozano, R. (2018). Measuring performance on the Healthcare Access and Quality Index for 195 countries and territories and selected subnational locations: A systematic analysis from the Global Burden of Disease Study 2016. The Lancet, 391(10136), 2236–2271.

Funding for universal coverage typically involves single-payer and/or multi-payer systems. We consider those options next.

Single- and Multi-Payer Systems

You've probably seen headlines such as "Candidate Supports Medicare for All" and "The Future of Our Multi-Payer System." In this section we consider what those terms mean and the relative advantages and disadvantages of each.

SINGLE-PAYER

As the name suggests, in a **single-payer** system, one source pays the bills for all essential health care. It's as if everyone uses one main insurance company—which may be a government agency or a privately run national health insurance plan. In this way, everyone is guaranteed essential services (universal coverage). Most single-payer systems are funded by tax dollars that people contribute throughout their lives.

An example of a single-payer system is Medicare, which was begun in the United States in 1965 principally to provide health insurance for individuals age 65 and older. Before its enactment, about half of Americans of retirement age had no insurance coverage at a time in their lives when they were likely to need more care than ever (Davis, Schoen, & Bandeali, 2015). Medicare now defrays health care costs for 98% of older Americans (Davis et al., 2015). It is funded via income tax and employer contributions. The system isn't all inclusive. About 8 in 10 people on Medicare buy supplemental insurance to help with out-of-pocket expenses (Cubanksi, 2018). But the program has been successful enough to inspire the rallying cry "Medicare for all" among people who support a single-payer option.

Here are some advantages of a single-payer system.

- Because people pay into the same system throughout their lives, the dividends they contribute when they are healthy offset the costs they incur when they are not.
- In single-payer systems, people are able to receive health benefits without incurring significant debt at the time of service.
- System administrators know they will care for the same people all of their lives, so they have a vested interest in maintaining their health.
- Single-payer systems typically offer more continuity, lower administrative costs, and less paperwork because the same benefits are available to all people, compared to the myriad of coverage options available through private insurance companies (Hsiao, Knight, Kappel, & Done, 2011).

Keep these points in mind as you consider the relative advantages of a multi-payer system.

MULTI-PAYER

In **multi-payer** systems, health insurance is provided by a variety of sources, usually including both private companies and government programs. The United States is primarily a multi-payer system. Ask your friends who provides their insurance coverage and are you are likely to hear about a range of different companies.

Unlike the single-payer model, multi-payer systems are typically funded by a mixture of individual contributions and tax dollars. Here are some components of the multi-payer system in the United States:

- People who can afford health insurance buy it on their own or through their employers.
- Some employers (usually large companies) contribute a portion of employees' premium costs and decide which coverage options are available to them.
- Public "safety net" programs—such as state-based Medicaid and children's health insurance programs—provide coverage for people who qualify. (Qualifying criteria differ by state.)

Although these are the main options, they don't cover everyone. An estimated 2.5 million people in the United States fall into a "coverage gap," meaning that they don't qualify for public assistance yet they can't afford health insurance (Garfield & Orgera, 2019).

Multi-payer systems may or may not involve universal coverage. For most of its history, the United States has been a multi-payer system without universal coverage. People have had the option to purchase health insurance or not. One challenge is that, if people only enroll in insurance when they expect to have high medical bills, insurance treasuries are lower and premiums rise to cover the costs. Consequently, fewer people can afford insurance, which leads to even steeper rates, and so on. By 2013, some 44 million people in the United States had no health insurance and didn't qualify for government-sponsored plans ("Key Facts," 2018).

One option for universal coverage in a multi-payer system is an **individual mandate**, which is a rule that people who don't qualify for public assistance must purchase health insurance. Individual mandates are usually accompanied by subsidized premiums for people with low incomes. Those in favor of individual mandates argue that it's fair to expect everyone to pay into the system based on what they can afford. Those who oppose individual mandates maintain that the government should not require anyone to make a purchase that they don't want or can't afford.

Multi-payer systems present several advantages:

- The overall tax burden is usually lower than in single-payer systems, since individuals typically pay out of pocket in multi-payer systems.
- Multi-payer systems typically involve more marketplace competition than in single-payer systems. This may stimulate more innovation, a wider array of coverage options, and more competitive salaries to attract workers.
- Some people consider it a plus that there is less government involvement in multi-payer systems.

Although we have presented these as two distinct options, a combination of single- and multi-payer options is possible. Some people in the United States advocate for a single-payer system to provide prevention and essential health services to all citizens *and* a supplementary multi-payer option for people who would like to buy additional insurance and customizable options.

Now that you are familiar with the options, let's consider them in the context of actual health care reform efforts.

The Affordable Care Act

Health care debates in in the United States occur against the backdrop of one of the most sweeping health care reform efforts in the nation's history, the Affordable Care Act (ACA) of 2010. The provisions of the ACA are likely to change over time, but knowing about them will give you a leg up as a voter and a participant in public discourse.

The first thing to know about the ACA is that it initiated universal coverage in the United States for the first time by implementing an individual mandate requiring U.S. citizens to either submit proof of insurance with their annual income tax returns or pay a fine. To help accomplish this, the ACA established a *health insurance marketplace*, essentially a central database of insurance plans and options along with tax credits for low-income citizens and information about public assistance programs. The ACA also implemented a number of insurance company reforms and tax credits for states (to help fund Medicaid), employers (to reward them for offering employees health benefits), and health care organizations (designed to encourage efficiency and quality care).

In addition to the individual mandate and insurance marketplace, here are the main provisions of the ACA:

- *Coverage of the "essential 10."* The ACA stipulated that, at a minimum, health insurance policies must cover services in 10 essential categories: emergency care, outpatient care, inpatient hospitalization, maternity and newborn care, mental health services, prescription drugs, rehabilitation for injury and disease recovery, lab work, pediatric care, and preventive care.
- *Parental coverage until age 26.* Under the ACA, insurance companies were required to allow policyholders' children up to age 26 to be included on their parents' plans. (In reference to our earlier example, this is why Julian was eligible to be covered by his parents' insurance plan although his sister, a few years earlier, was not.)
- *Free prevention and wellness exams.* The ACA entitled people to receive immunizations, annual checkups, and 15 to 26 types of health screening without paying copays or deductibles.
- *Ban on preexisting-condition clauses.* Prior to the ACA, it was common practice for insurance companies to refuse coverage or elevate premiums for people with preexisting conditions. The ACA outlawed these practices as well as lifetime and annual spending limits on coverage.

Under the ACA, about 20 million previously uninsured Americans had gained coverage by the year 2016 ("Key Facts," 2018). But the ACA's future is still uncertain. In 2017, President Donald Trump reduced the individual mandate fine to $0, which essentially ended the expectation of universal coverage in the United States, at least for the time being. That year, about 700,000 people in the United States returned to the ranks of the uninsured ("Key Facts," 2018).

The most heated debates about the ACA have revolved around the issue of whether people should be required by law to have health insurance. Related debates center around the cost of health care and usefulness of health insurance. In the United States, about 1 in 4 people under age 65 who have insurance say they still cannot afford to pay the deductibles required to actually receive care (Commonwealth Fund, 2015). Although these people are protected from catastrophic medical bills, the care that might keep their illnesses from worsening

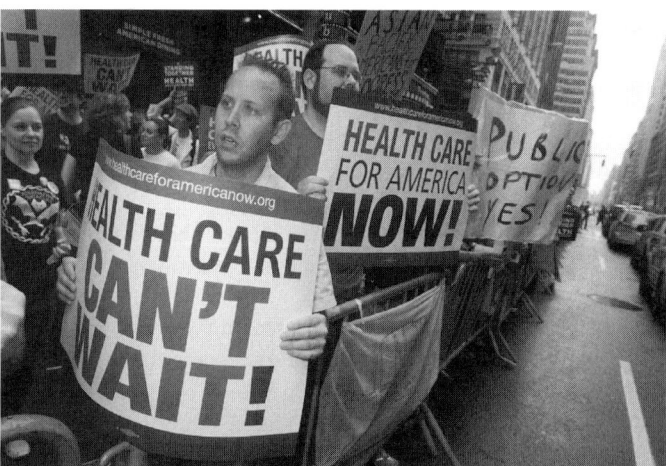

Public discourse over health care reform has been passionate in recent years. Joining the debate means becoming familiar with the vocabulary and issues involved in universal coverage and other reform elements.

Which aspects of health care are you most passionate about—communication with care providers, access and affordability, public health, technology-mediated health information, or another issue?

> **BOX 2.2 Ethical Considerations**
>
> ## Classroom Debate on Health Care Reform
>
> You have been exposed to numerous options for health care reform. Look up recent events and changes and develop your own viewpoints. Then hold a series of classroom debates. Here are some topics you might address: (1) in favor of universal coverage and against it; (2) arguments for a single-payer model, a multi-payer system, or a combination of the two; (3) for or against individual mandates; (4) for or against the Affordable Care Act.
>
> Appoint team captains or have the instructor moderate. One group at a time should present its arguments, with time after each argument for questions and challenges. (Make sure talking time is divided fairly among the participants.)
>
> As the debate progresses, people may change their minds. If so, they should get up and move to the group that best represents their viewpoints.

may still be out of reach. And the "coverage gap" we discussed earlier continues to leave many in a quandary.

As we have said, health care reform is not a static issue. Stay tuned to the news and political debates to stay abreast of what is happening, and exercise your right to take part. We are living in a historic time. The future of health care is being crafted now, and it is safe to say that you will be involved in it, one way or another. Hopefully what you have learned here will make you a more active participant in the process, whatever role you play.

Summary

Current Issues in Health Care

- Chronic conditions not well managed are costly and difficult to treat.
- Preventive care is relatively inexpensive and relies on communication and teamwork.
- Income predicts lifespan, partly because of the the different health care and information people receive.
- Effective communication is needed to serve members of underserved populations.

Navigating a Complex System

- Communication breakdowns cause added costs, stress, delays and oversights, adverse patient outcomes, and extra care.
- Patient navigators can help people understand information and manage the health care system.

Health Communication in a Changing World

- The average age worldwide is increasing substantially, leading to high demand for health care services.
- Ethnic and racial diversity increase the need for culturally sensitive health communication.
- Diversity among health care workers is not keeping pace with that of the overall population.

Communication in Managed Care

- Managed care organizations recruit patients, match them with care providers, and monitor expenses.
- Members of health maintenance organizations (HMOs) pay monthly premiums and copays for health care visits. They only see care providers approved by the HMO.
- Members of preferred provider organizations (PPOs) pay less if they visit care providers on "preferred" lists, but they receive some benefits no matter who they see.
- High-deductible health plans (HDHPs) offer relatively low monthly premiums but high deductibles and high catastrophic caps.
- Potential advantages of managed care include predictive budgeting, incentive to reduce costs (at least theoretically), focus on wellness, administrative assistance, and career jump starts.
- Disadvantages of managed care include rising costs, lower emphasis on prevention than was hoped, incentives to limit care, limited choices, and excessive red tape.

Health Care Reform

- U.S. health care ranks 29th in the world, mostly because some people receive no or little care.
- Critics of universal coverage argue that healthy people may pay for unhealthy ones, people may be lax about maintaining their health, and the health system may be overtaxed.
- Arguments in favor of universal coverage are that untreated diseases may spread to others and escalate costs; patients won't face financial hardship if they become sick; a healthy society is more prosperous; and more resources, jobs, and health services may result.
- Arguments in favor of single-payer systems are that people pay throughout their lives, there are no high charges at the time of service, there is an incentive to maintain public health, and administrative demands are lessened.
- Arguments in favor of multi-payer systems include lower overall tax burden, more marketplace competition, and less government involvement.

Provisions of the Affordable Care Act of 2010

- Evoked individual mandate
- Established national health insurance marketplace
- Required insurance companies to cover 10 essential health care services
- Guaranteed coverage on parents' insurance until age 26
- Offered free prevention and wellness exams
- Banned preexisting condition clauses
- Required insurance companies to pay promised benefits without a price cap

(Some of these provisions are still in effect. Others may not be.)

Glossary

capitation A set fee paid to cover a person's health needs, regardless of the care actually required. *See page 27.*

catastrophic cap An upper limit on the amount of out-of-pocket expense an insurance subscriber is required to pay each year. *See page 26.*

copay The portion of a health care bill the patient is required to pay when services are rendered. *See page 27.*

deductible The amount of out-of-pocket medical expense an insured individual is required to pay before receiving financial assistance from the insurer. For example, you might pay the first $500 of your emergency room bill, and insurance will pay 80% of the remaining cost. *See page 27.*

diagnosis-related groups (DRGs) Flat-rate reimbursement amounts for specified inpatient hospital procedures (e.g., a certain amount paid for an appendectomy, established in advance rather than based on actual costs incurred by the health provider). *See page 26.*

fee-for-service The practice of paying a care provider for specific care provided, as opposed to a capitated amount paid in advance regardless of services rendered. *See page 26.*

health maintenance organization (HMO) A managed care organization that offers enrollees a variety of health services for a set monthly fee and copays. Caregivers are usually employed directly by the HMO and provide services only to HMO members. *See page 27.*

health savings account (HSA): A tax-exempt savings plan in which people can set aside money to pay future medical bills. U.S. taxpayers qualify for HSAs if they are part of high-deductible health plans. Money saved can be used over many years. *See page 28.*

high-deductible health plan (HDHP) A managed care plan with lower-than-normal premiums but higher-than-normal deductibles and out-of-pocket spending caps. Most HDHPs qualify members to establish tax-exempt health savings accounts. *See page 28.*

individual mandate A rule requiring everyone to have health insurance. *See page 30.*

insurance premium A membership fee paid by subscribers in a conventional insurance or managed care plan. Often deducted from one's paycheck. *See page 29.*

managed care organizations A health care system in which income, resources, and health services are supervised by a managing body such as a health maintenance organization or preferred provider organization. Patients pay the organization a set fee each month to receive health services. *See page 26.*

multi-payer A system in which health insurance is provided by a variety of sources, usually including both private companies and government programs. May involve universal coverage or not. Typically funded by a mixture of individual contributions and tax dollars. *See page 33.*

preferred provider organization (PPO) A managed care organization that pays independent caregivers a discounted fee for each service they provide to PPO members. Patients may visit providers not on the preferred list, but they pay higher fees to do so. *See page 27.*

prospective payment structure A system in which reimbursements are established in advance rather than after care has been provided. *See page 26.*

single-payer A system of universal coverage in which one source (a government agency or a privately run national health insurance plan) pays the bills for everyone's health care. Usually funded by tax dollars. *See page 32.*

third-party payer A benefits provider (usually an insurance company) that is separate from the patient and the care provider. Common with traditional indemnity insurance but less common in managed care. *See page 26.*

universal coverage The provision that all citizens (and, in some countries, all temporary residents and visitors as well) are assured of health care. *See page 30.*

Discussion Questions

1. Have you ever been frustrated trying to navigate the health care system? If so, how? What might you suggest to improve the system for patients?
2. Do you think managed care is mostly good or mostly detrimental? Why? What pros and cons are most important to you? If you were able to change managed care for the better, what might you do?
3. Are you in favor of universal coverage or not? Why?
4. Which do you consider more appealing, a single-payer or a multi-payer system? Why?
5. Do you support or oppose the idea of an individual mandate? Why? What role, if any, do you think employers should play in defining and paying for employees' health insurance?
6. Which provisions of the Affordable Care Act do you support? Which do you oppose? Why?

PART II

The Roles of Patients and Professional Caregivers

It is fitting that we begin our in-depth exploration of health communication at the most personal level—those moments when we connect with another person to offer comfort and care, or, as patients, open ourselves to receive what another can do to help us. There is something remarkable about the patient–provider relationship that makes it far more than a business transaction. In this section we will explore common patterns of patient–provider communication—from brusque, rushed encounters that may leave us feeling exposed and disappointed, to moments of true connection and compassion that, whether or not they heal our bodies, comfort our souls. In Chapter 3, we explore the communication patterns that characterize patient–provider communication—who talks, who listens, what stories are shared, and so on. Then, in Chapters 4 and 5, we immerse ourselves, first, in what it means to be a patient, and next, in what it feels like to be a professional care provider, including the hopes, fears, joys, and frustrations of both roles. Hopefully, you will finish the section with an enhanced respect and appreciation for everyone involved.

Each patient ought to feel somewhat the better after the physician's visit, irrespective of the nature of the illness.

—**WARFIELD THEOBALD LONGCOPE**

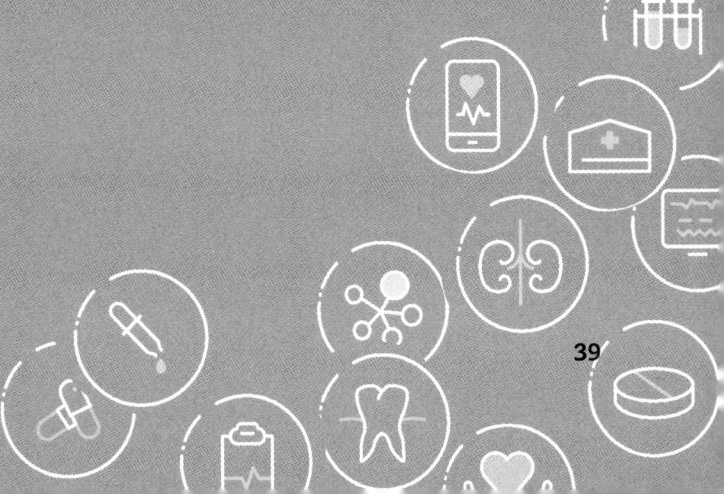

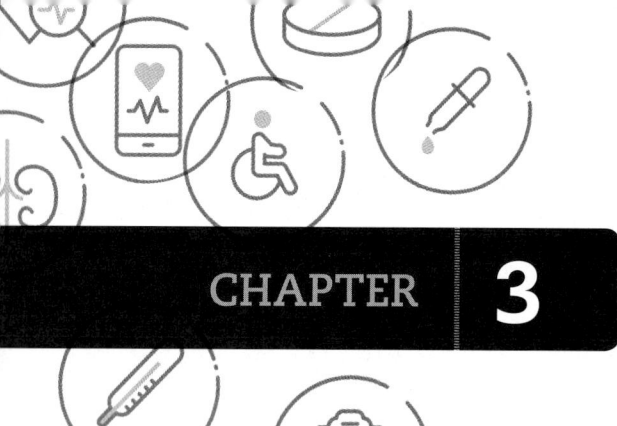

CHAPTER 3

Patient–Caregiver Communication

Ben noticed a lump in his breast just after his fifty-eighth birthday. Embarrassed about the problem, he avoided mentioning it to his wife for several months, thinking it would probably go away on its own. When she learned about it, his wife encouraged, then begged Ben to see a doctor. In the next few months other family members joined her entreaties. Finally, Ben made a doctor's appointment. On the day of the appointment the family was anxious to hear what the doctor said. Imagine their surprise when Ben returned and said the visit went "just fine," but he didn't tell the doctor about the lump. When the shocked family asked why, Ben shrugged and said, "He didn't ask me."

This true story illustrates some of the complex factors that affect patient–caregiver communication. Although it may sound foolish not to tell a physician about our health concerns, research suggests that episodes like Ben's occur quite frequently. As you will see, there are numerous reasons for this pattern. In this case, Ben felt that the doctor did not encourage him or even give him a chance to share the information. Health professionals may see the matter differently, wondering why patients seem to play guessing games with them rather than coming to the point.

This chapter examines what happens during medical transactions—who talks, who listens, and how people behave. Effective patient–provider communication is important for a number of reasons:

- Communication can help people feel valued, supported, and understood, which can reduce stress and improve well-being (Jacobsen, Bouchard, Emed, Lepage, & Cook, 2015; Jiang, 2017; Li, Matthews, Dossaji, & Fullam, 2017).
- Open communication can help patients and care providers reach accurate diagnoses and negotiate treatment options (Rosti, 2017).
- Satisfied and well-informed patients are more likely to stick with treatment plans and to engage in follow-up care (Eriksson, 2015).
- Patients tend to perceive less pain when they feel valued and empowered by health providers (Ruben, Meterko, & Bokhour, 2018) and when they

have realistic expectations about pain (Adams & Field, 2001).
- Patients who have good relationships with their care providers are less likely to file malpractice suits if things don't go as planned (Dym, 2008; Watson, 2014).
- Care providers who feel good about their communication with patients are typically more satisfied and less likely than others to experience burnout (Clayton, Iacob, Reblin, & Ellington, in press; Li et al., 2017).

Considering these factors and others, Richard Street and colleagues conclude that there is a link between patient–provider communication and health outcomes (Street, Makoul, Arora, & Epstein, 2009).

Because patient–provider communication is so important, you may be tempted to blame one party or another if it seems ineffective or insensitive. A student asked to sum up health communication literature once declared, "What I get is that doctors are mean and patients are dumb." Although few people might be so blunt, experts and students alike are often guilty of similar assumptions.

Resist the urge to draw simplistic conclusions. Keep in mind that patients and caregivers work together to shape their communication patterns. As we discussed in Chapter 1, communication is a transactional process, meaning that communicators exert mutual influence on each other such that the approach one participant takes suggests how the other should respond (Rawlins, 1989, 1992; Watzlawick, Beavin, & Jackson, 1967). For instance, if a health professional acts like a parent, the patient is encouraged to behave in the complementary role of a child (and the other way around). Patients sometimes become frustrated with their care providers' parent-like behavior, unmindful that they may have encouraged it by adopting meek and submissive roles themselves (R. Adams, Price, Tucker, Nguyen, & Wilson, 2012). Stephen Bochner (1983) famously urged us not to consider patients and caregivers as adversaries but as "reasonable people of good will, trying to exchange views with other reasonable people of equally good will" (p. 128) in circumstances that are sometimes very challenging.

The chapter is divided into three sections. The first describes a lopsided power dynamic that has traditionally characterized medical encounters. The second contrasts that pattern with a more collaborative model of patient–provider communication that is gaining favor. The third section presents communication skill builders involving motivational interviewing, dialogue, narrative medicine, and tips for patients.

Before we begin, here are a few notes about what appears in this chapter and what doesn't. First, content is guided in large part by published research, the majority of which focuses on physician communication. However, the field is gradually broadening to include more research about nurses, pharmacists, paramedics, physical therapists, technicians, and others. Therefore, you will see references to communication with a broader range of caregivers than in years past. Second, you will also notice that this chapter focuses on interactions with professional care providers. This excludes the more than 40 million family caregivers who care for ill or injured loved ones at home in the United States (Stepler, 2015). Since the challenges and rewards of family caregivers deserve special attention, we will focus on them separately, in Chapter 8.

BOX 3.1 Career Opportunities

Health Communication Research

Consultant
Professor
Researcher

Career Resources and Job Listings
- Association of American Medical Colleges: www.aamc.org
- *Chronicle of Higher Education*: chronicle.com
- European Association for Communication in Health Care: www.each.eu
- International Communication Association: www.icahdq.org
- National Communication Association: www.natcom.org
- Society of Behavioral Medicine: www.sbm.org
- Society of Teachers of Family Medicine: www.stfm.org
- U.S. Bureau of Labor Statistics: www.bls.gov

Medical Talk and Power Differentials

When a psychiatrist responds to friendly emails from a child she counsels regularly, some of her colleagues say she should keep a greater distance. Elsewhere, a fellow psychiatrist grapples with how to respond when a patient who is mentally ill refuses to undergo testing for a serious disease that can be treated if doctors can confirm that he has it.

These real-life scenarios were shared by participants in a Swedish study of ethical considerations that psychiatrists regularly encounter[1] (Pelto-Piri, Engström, & Engström, 2013). Both situations concern issues of power. In the first, the physician's colleagues believe she is too involved with her young patient. She feels otherwise—that being "happy and friendly" is natural and that it supports a sense of shared power between her and the patient. In the second scenario, the psychiatrist grapples with whether to give the patient power (by complying with his wishes) or to exert power on his behalf by insisting that he be tested.

In some ways, it makes sense to give health professionals power. They have the benefit of advanced education, access to technology, and high social status. Moreover, the very definition of patienthood suggests someone who requires assistance. As a consequence, we often speak in terms of *doctor's orders*, *patient compliance*, and the like. This language suggests that health professionals have authority that patients do not.

However, patients are in the driver's seat in many ways. For the most part, health professionals cannot treat them without their permission, nor can they require patients to follow medical advice. They cannot even require people to show up for exams. All the same, patients may not perceive that they have much choice in these matters. In this section, we look at traditional communication patterns in patient–provider communication in terms of who does

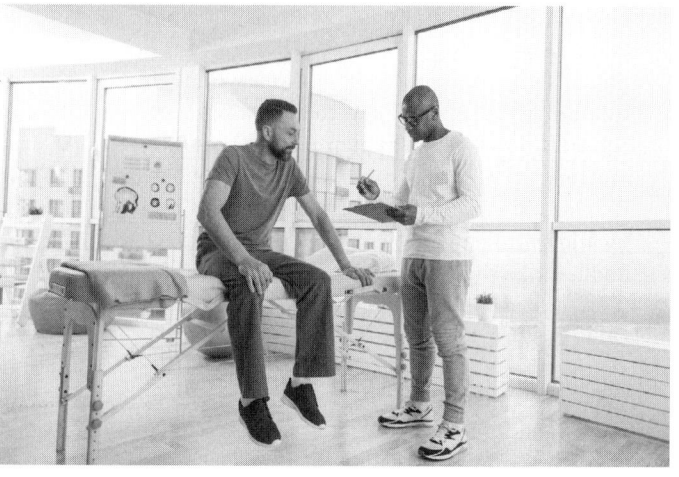

Some care providers get to know their patients well and engage with them largely as peers. Others maintain a distance.

In what circumstances, if any, do you think health professionals should engage in friendly chats with patients? When, if ever, should they maintain interpersonal distance? Why?

most of the talking, listening, questioning, and topic selection.

Knowledge and Power

One aspect of caregiver-centered communication involves unequal access to information. For many decades, doctors felt it was unkind to "confuse" patients with medical details or to "burden" them with making medical decisions (Katz, 1984). "It was not until 1979 that a majority of physicians reported disclosing cancer diagnoses to their patients," say Bryan Sisk et al. (2016, para. 1).

Therapeutic privilege is the prerogative sometimes granted to physicians to withhold information from patients if they feel that disclosing the information would do more harm than good (Katz, 1984). The odds are that most care providers have patients' best interests at heart. But traditionally, they have withheld information for some of the following reasons (Sisk, Frankel, Kodish, & Isaacson, 2016):

- At different points in history, physicians have been encouraged to keep patients in the dark to maintain their dependence on the medical establishment.
- Doctors have sometimes been told to omit details that would make them or the medical profession look bad.

---

[1] In these examples, pronouns have been assigned randomly to the participants solely for the purpose of talking about them. The article is not specific about their gender.

- Some doctors have worried that people will be so afraid of possible side effects (however unlikely) that they will refuse treatment if made aware of them.
- Care providers might worry that bad news will hamper a patient's ability to cope.
- It can be gut-wrenching to share bad news. As the famous physician William Osler reflected, "It is a hard matter . . . to tell a patient that he [or she] is past all hope" (quoted by Sisk et al., para. 6).

A move toward full disclosure became significant beginning in the 1980s and 1990s. For one thing, as everyday people gained access to health information online, they became less satisfied receiving limited information from care providers. For another, the public became less trusting of medical professionals as atrocities such as the Tuskegee Syphilis Study (Chapter 4) and the unauthorized use of Henrietta Lacks's cancer cells (Chapter 4) came to light (Sisk et al., 2016).

Some people still feel there are times when health professionals should withhold information from patients. Others feel that patients should be guaranteed complete disclosure and the power to make their own decisions. (See Box 3.2 for an ethical consideration of the factors involved.)

BOX 3.2 Ethical Considerations

The Truth, the Whole Truth . . . Or Not?

Although Anna (age 68) is seriously ill, she feels relatively well and her spirits seem high. She often remarks to those around her that she is feeling much better and she is eager to talk of future plans. However, it's obvious to her care providers and to her family that she will not live more than a few months. The family has asked Anna's physician not to tell her she is dying. They argue that she probably knows she is nearing the end of life but her behavior implies a request that people not bring up the issue. They feel that Anna's current happiness matters most at this point, and they are reluctant to impose bad news on her, particularly when there is nothing that can be done about it.

The current American Medical Association code of ethics states that physicians should only withhold information about a patient's condition or treatment when disclosing that information would present such distress that it would harm the patient's health (Wynia, 2004). As with many ethical principles, that can be a difficult call to make. It's not easy to gauge how patients will respond. And even when people seem distressed, they often say they are glad to know the truth so that they can make informed decisions, and if necessary, get their affairs in order and say goodbye to loved ones (Yang et al., 2018).

Cultural preferences also play a role. In Japan, for instance, although people typically want to know the truth about their own health, they often insist that physicians shield family members from distressing diagnoses—afraid of destroying their loved one's hope and fearful that talking about adverse outcomes might lead to their occurrence (Kakai, 2002). In other cultures, the expectation may be that adults can handle difficult truths, but that pediatric patients should be protected from them (Rosenberg, Starks, Unguru, Fuedtner, & Diekema, 2017).

What Do You Think?

1. If you were Anna's physician, would you tell her that she does not have long to live? Why or why not?
2. If physicians withhold information, should they go so far as to lie if patients ask outright about their prognosis?
3. How do you respond to the argument that physicians can never be sure about patients' odds of recovery, so it's sometimes better to withhold information that might diminish their hope?
4. What if you were a physician and a patient told you, "If this condition is terminal, don't tell me"? Would you withhold information even if it meant making treatment decisions on the patient's behalf?
5. What if patients do not say "Don't tell me" outright, but their actions seem to suggest that they don't want to know if the news is bad? Would you tell them?
6. Is it ever permissible to give a patient's family information without telling the patient? If so, under what circumstances?
7. If you were the patient, are there any circumstances in which you would wish information to be withheld from you?

Who Talks and Who Listens

An asymmetrical pattern in which physicians do most of the talking has long been common. For example, when Tessie October and colleagues (2018) studied consultations between health care teams and parents of children in critical care units, they found that the health professionals were almost always first to speak (setting the tone and agenda for the conversations), and they spoke, on average, nearly three times as much as the parents, often presenting complex medical jargon without explanation. The researchers call these "monologue heavy" exchanges "missed opportunities" to involve families in decisions about their children's care (October, Dizon, & Roter, 2018, para. 18).

Sometimes, providers' word choices influence how patients respond. Close study reveals that patients give more detailed responses when care providers ask open-ended questions (such as *What can I do for you today?*) than when they ask yes-or-no questions (*So you're sick, huh?*) or comment on a patient's symptoms (*You're having body aches.*) (Heritage & Robinson, 2006). Closed-ended questions and comments may give patients the impression that health professionals do not want details or that they already know them. This may be lost on providers who assume that patients will speak up if they have concerns, regardless of how the conversation begins.

The tenets of transactional communication remind us that health communication is a collaborative enterprise. Therefore, it may not surprise you that patients often support an unequal balance of power in their own ways. For example, they typically yield the floor to doctors. In one study, patients went silent 94% of the time when physicians began talking, and the patients rarely finished what they had been saying before the interruption (Li, Krysko, Desroches, & Deagle, 2004).

An inequitable pattern of talking and listening may occur because health professionals feel rushed and because they have been trained to zero in on specific causes of illness. This makes sense from a certain perspective, but it may be counterproductive considering that patients may consider it extremely risky (or even rude) to disclose embarrassing or distressing information in the first few seconds of the conversation. They are more likely to build up to their main concerns slowly. This means that a care provider who focuses on a patient's initial statement may miss the real issue or learn about it belatedly.

The term **doorknob disclosure** describes a pattern in which patients blurt out their main concerns at the last instant of a visit, as when the care provider is at the door ready to leave. For example, a patient who initially says she is suffering from fatigue or a sore throat may blurt out that depression is actually her biggest problem. The care provider in such a situation can focus on that concern another time or, as more often happens, launch another medical interview with the patient. (Think about this the next time you wonder why the wait is so long in a doctor's office.) All in all, it may be worthwhile for care providers to earn patients' trust and to take the time to establish a clear agenda at the beginning of medical encounters. For their part, patients can try to be forthcoming sooner. Later in the chapter, we'll consider some tips to help with both of these goals.

Sensitive Subjects

"It comes to the point where they have to ask you, 'Are you having sex?' Some of them [clinicians] don't feel comfortable asking those questions because they're like, 'It's a kid here. I'm asking this kid.' And it's kind of weird for them."

This statement, by a teenager girl in David Córdova and associates' (2018, p. 1180) study, highlights how difficult it can be for patients and care providers to speak frankly with one another.

Evidence suggests that patients usually want to talk about the hard stuff if their care providers seem nonjudgmental and will keep the information private. But patients are unlikely to bring up the issues themselves (Córdova et al., 2018). Said one teenager, "I just want them [clinicians] to ask me. And if they ask me, I'm gonna be honest. . . . I really want to discuss it, but I'm not gonna say anything until you ask" (Córdova et al., 2018, p. 1181). Sex is a touchy subject. Substance abuse is another, especially among young people. By age 18, about 60% of American youth have tried alcohol and 12% have tried illicit drugs (Drug Facts, 2018; Underage Drinking, 2017). Nevertheless, about half of young adults surveyed said that care providers do not bring up issues of substance abuse with them (Blevins, Anderson, Caviness, Herman, & Stein, 2019).

Open communication can also be complicated by language barriers. Hispanic women interviewed for one study described a discouraging cycle in which they struggled to express themselves in English, which seemed to frustrate their doctors, which in turn made the women feel even more tongue tied (Julliard et al., 2008). Especially when the women's concerns involved sensitive issues such as genital health, domestic violence, or sexual orientation, they were most likely to stay silent about them, even though they wanted their doctors to know. Most of the women said they could overcome their hesitancy when doctors seemed compassionate and interested and when they used skilled interpreters as needed.

Although regrettable, it's easy to see why sensitive subjects are often glossed over or ignored. Health professionals are not immune to the embarrassment and discomfort that patients feel. Added to that, care providers may worry that they are not well qualified to discuss emotional topics (Lumma-Sellenthin, 2009; McBride, 2012). Medical school professor Lenore Buckley (2008) remembers a student struggling to comfort a patient with HIV who wasn't sure life was worth living after he lost his job and his family. The student told Buckley, "I just don't feel that I know enough to offer him any advice. I can't imagine how difficult this is for him" (p. xii). Buckley reflects that the student did not lack empathy. Instead, he feared, as anyone might, that saying the wrong thing might make the patient feel worse.

Patronizing Behavior

Especially hurtful are incidents in which health professionals **patronize** patients (treat them as if they are inferior) by withholding information, speaking down to them, and shrugging off their feelings as childish or inconsequential. For example, blogger Emma Maathuis (2018) recalls feeling slighted while undergoing surgery on her foot. "The doctor wasn't particularly rude but was dismissive and it felt like he didn't care," she says (para. 2). He didn't introduce himself when he entered the room and injected anesthetic into Maathuis's foot. Then he left for 20 minutes without explanation. During the surgery, the physician spoke only to the nurse, not to the patient, describing his raucous weekend. When the procedure was complete, he left without addressing the patient. Maathuis, a social worker, filed a complaint and refused to see that doctor again, but she wonders how many other patients feel distressed and alienated by similar behavior.

Some behavior is clearly patronizing. But much of it involves a judgment call. For example, is it patronizing when a nursing home staff member talks to an older adult in a high, singsong voice using simple words? When researchers Mary Lee Hummert and Debra Mazloff (2001) asked older adults to view a video simulation of such an encounter, some participants felt the staff member was condescending. One said that she treated the older woman "like she was a 4-year-old," and several observed that the staff member did most of the talking and did not listen (Hummert & Mazloff, 2001, p. 174). However, some others in the focus group thought the staff member was being kind or that she inadvertently sounded patronizing, although she probably meant well (Hummert & Mazloff, 2001).

Transgressions

Health care encounters often involve touch, personal disclosures, and physical exposure usually reserved for intimate relationships. Usually, everyone involved recognizes the boundary between intimacy (a unique sense of closeness, interdependence, and trust) and detached concern (the effort to understand another person, but with restricted emotional involvement). However, patients and caregivers sometimes breach those expectations. Farber et al. (1997) call actions that cross the line between intimacy and professionalism **transgressions**, from the Latin phrase meaning "to step across."

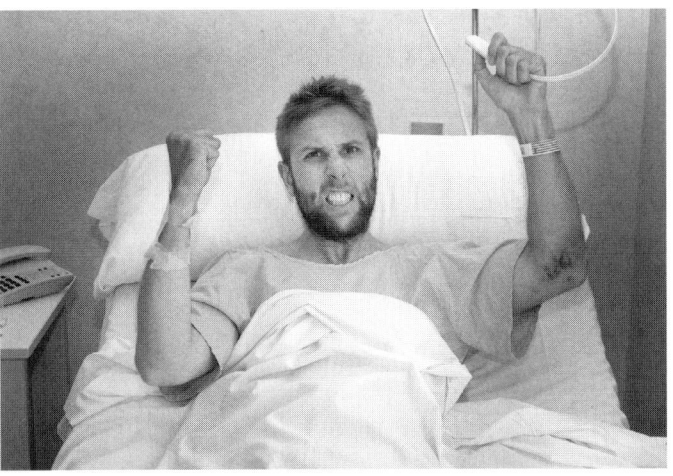

Patients and health professionals commit transgressions if they become verbally or physically abusive, insulting, or overly flirtatious.

What would you do if you felt uncomfortable in a health care encounter?

Transgressions frequently have painful and confusing results. Feelings of heartache, disappointment, guilt, and loss of reputation may result. Patients, typically in positions of lesser power, may feel violated or forced into behaving against their wishes (Brüggemann, Wijma, & Swahnberg, 2012). Professionals may feel harassed or embarrassed and may face legal action and loss of professional privileges.

Sexual contact is an obvious transgression, but other behavior can be inappropriate as well. Doctors say that patients sometimes transgress by demanding more time than they can give, asking for money or favors, being overly flirtatious or seductive, giving frequent or expensive gifts, being verbally abusive, bringing or threatening to bring weapons, making bigoted remarks, and shouting. Nurses and others are sometimes harassed by patients who touch them inappropriately or make suggestive comments. Care providers may transgress by making sexual advances, asking unnecessary personal questions, insulting patients, or sharing confidential information with others.

Researchers propose that transgressions may result from patients' vulnerability, their need for assurance, and the trust they place in their care providers. Providers, too, may experience strong feelings (either positive or negative) in relation to patients, feelings that may be heightened by a sense of isolation from family and friends.

Following are some steps for addressing transgressions based on work by Pateet, Fremonta, and Miovic (2011), Farber, Novack, and O'Brien (1997), and R. Zook (1997).

- Take stock of personal needs and social expectations that may motivate a transgression (e.g., loneliness or need for approval).
- Establish clear boundaries for touch and talk, perhaps by creating and distributing a list of prohibited behaviors.
- Be careful not to send ambiguous or mixed messages.
- Seek the counsel of support groups, friends, and colleagues.
- Enlist the help of mental health professionals if it seems warranted.
- Have others present during potentially problematic transactions.
- Acknowledge transgression attempts and discuss them in a calm way with the other person.
- If inappropriate behavior does not stop, let the other person know you intend to take formal action. If it still does not stop, contact a supervisor or the local medical society.

Why Do We Do It?

Patterns such as those just described point to power inequities between patients and health professionals. Power is not inherently negative. It can be used to help others, as when care providers use their influence to advocate on patients' behalf. However, you may feel frustrated by examples that suggest an unfair or abusive use of power. The reality is that patients do not usually like a lopsided power dynamic, but neither do most health professionals. So, if neither side typically likes it, why do we engage in it?

Our reason is that we may not feel we have a choice. We may underestimate our options, concluding that "I have to take control because many patients either don't speak up or they talk too much," or "The nurse practitioner didn't give me a chance to say much."

A second reason reflects the power of social expectations. Accepted rules of politeness and professionalism may guide our actions, even if we do not particularly like them. Traditionally, society has expected doctors to be dominant and patients to be submissive. Changing such deeply ingrained ideas is usually a slow and cautious process. Indeed, professionals who want patients to be forthcoming may find some are still uncomfortable doing so. Kathryn Greene's (2009) **disclosure decision-making model** (**DD-MM**) proposes that many patients do not simply say what is on their minds. Instead, they weigh three key factors first:

- *What outcomes can I predict if I share this information?* Patients are most likely to share information if they believe they will not be judged negatively because of it, if the information seems relevant, and if they think it will lead to better care. However, if they do not feel ready to hear what might result, they may still remain silent.
- *How is the other person likely to respond?* Patients who trust their care providers and feel they can predict how they will respond usually feel safer disclosing private information.
- *Can I share this information effectively?* Even if the information is important, patients who worry that they will sound stupid or awkward sharing it might shy away from doing so.

As this list suggests, trust is important, particularly when sharing serious or embarrassing concerns that people are unlikely to know about otherwise (Greene, 2009; Greene et al., 2012).

Third, as mentioned, institutional routines and rules influence how people behave. Open communication is discouraged when patients and professionals feel rushed, lack privacy, and/or do not have a chance to interact regularly. Health professionals are sometimes "ruled by the tyranny of the urgent," in the words of nursing professor Kenneth Walsh and colleagues (2009, p. 176). When faced with overwhelming workloads or strict time limitations, care providers may limit communication, act in brusque ways, and fail to listen.

Fourth, health professionals who wish to share power may find themselves in an ethical bind. As the examples that open this section illustrate, it's not always easy to decide when to be assertive and when to be accepting. A course in Turkey was useful in helping nursing students manage that tricky balance. The students studied communication techniques related to both empathy and assertiveness and then coached each other during experiential activities (Ünal, 2012). A majority of the students finished the course significantly more assertive and more self-aware than when they began, suggesting that they were better prepared both to empower patients and to express their own viewpoints.

It should also be said that, although asymmetrical power has long been the norm, many care providers are quite responsive and patient centered. Blogger Caitlin McCall (2018) describes the communication she shares with a therapist who has helped her overcome hardship and feel healthy again:

> I love my therapist. In the, we're best friends but she just doesn't know it kind of way. We've talked about her daughter, if lululemon is worth the money, and our obsession with Meghan Markle. She made the consci[ous] effort to journey with me. We mourned over things I lost, fought for hope, and celebrated small victories. Our togetherness removed my isolation and confusion. (para. 8)

Everyone's idea of ideal patient–provider communication is different, but McCall's story points to the comfort that can come from a mutual sense of trust. In the following section, we explore a trend toward more equal footing between patients and professionals.

Collaborative Communication

Dr. Price has just confirmed that Victor, a teenage boy in her care, has type 2 diabetes. Significantly overweight, Victor has often been teased at school, although he is a good student. Dr. Price must decide how to share the life-changing news that Victor will need immediate and long-term treatment for diabetes (Edgar, Satterfield, & Whaley, 2005).

Health professionals regularly experience pivotal points such as this. One option is to present the information in an authoritarian way, with strict instructions about what Victor must do to protect his health. Another is to involve him as an active and well-informed participant in the process. **Collaborative medical communication** involves participants' proactive desire to treat each other as peers who openly discuss health options and make mutually satisfying decisions (Balint & Shelton, 1996; Laine & Davidoff, 1996). Whereas traditional communication often supports a power differential, collaborative communication signals an explicit desire to be partners. This approach is neither entirely patient centered nor provider centered. Instead, participants work together. To illustrate, let's return to Dr. Price and Victor, as Timothy Edgar and colleagues (2005) tell the story.

Rather than use medical terminology that most people do not understand, Dr. Price helps Victor understand his condition by comparing it to a logjam on a river. "Picture for a minute your bloodstream as a river and the sugar as logs," she says (p. 99). If workers downstream do not get the logs out of the river, they cause a logjam. In your case, she explains to Victor, your pancreas does its job by getting sugar into your blood, but the receptor sites "downstream" do not absorb it effectively. Because of that, she points out, Victor probably feels hungry and tired a lot, but eating the wrong things just makes him feel worse (Edgar et al., 2005). During a conversation in which Dr. Price shares information and invites Victor and his family to ask questions, he comes to realize that he will feel better once he puts fewer logs (less starch and carbohydrates) into his system and starts an exercise program to help "open" the receptor sites that will turn the sugar into energy he can use. At the end of the visit, Dr. Price gives Victor a blank notepad on which

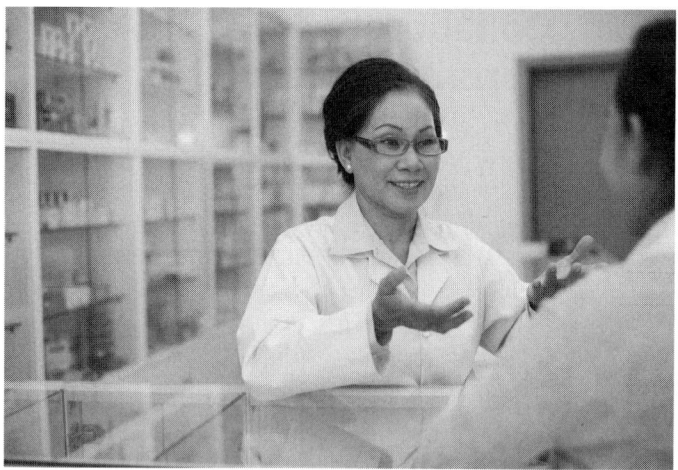

Health professionals who listen well, share information with patients, and invite their input embody a collaborative communication style.

Describe one of your favorite health professionals and why their communication style appeals to you.

he can write questions as they occur to him before their next visit (Edgar et al., 2005).

Health care interactions in which the participants function as collaborators—rather than boss and subordinate—are becoming more popular. We consider why next.

Reasons for a Shift

There are two main motivations behind the shift toward more collaborative patient–provider communication: knowledge and outcomes.

First, if knowledge is power, everyday people have more of it. Health is the subject of apps, websites, television channels, magazines, books, news programs, advertisements, and extensive online databases. As the public becomes more educated about health matters, many people are no longer content answering closed-ended questions and following orders. They wish to discuss options and participate in decision making. This can be challenging. Self-educated patients sometimes frustrate health professionals, especially when they interpret the patients' assertiveness as disrespect and feel they must "de-educate" patients about unreliable information. A patient in Alex Broom's (2008) study overheard his physician call him "difficult and overinformed" after he asked the doctor about information he had learned online (p. 101). However, many professionals feel that well-educated and active patients are a bonus. Says Gail Weiss (2008), "It's the rare physician who doesn't acknowledge that now, more than ever, physicians learn from their patients" (para. 3).

Second, many people realize that, although provider-dominated communication seems efficient in the short run, it is often counterproductive. Patients who perceive their physicians to be domineering talk less than others and are less likely to share important information with them (Schmid Mast, Hall, & Roter, 2008). In contrast, patients who perceive their care providers to be caring are more at ease than other patients and share their feelings more easily (Schmid Mast et al., 2008). People who are actively involved in medical encounters are also likely to remember more than others about treatment recommendations (Dillon, 2012).

When patients are forthcoming about their concerns, health professionals have an easier time understanding what is wrong. It's no wonder that both patients and care providers appreciate these encounters. Physicians, nurses, and genetic counselors (particularly female care providers) who feel they are highly engaged with patients usually consider their work more meaningful and are less likely to burn out than other providers (Clayton et al., in press; Geller, Bernhardt, Carrese, Rushton, & Kolodner, 2008).

All in all, provider-centered communication is not a thing of the past, and collaborative communication is not entirely new. Some health professionals have always been careful to empower and listen to patients. But we have a better understanding now of the benefits and techniques involved. Next, we consider a theory of collaborative engagement and explore some practical ways to encourage partnerships between patients and providers.

Model of Collaborative Interpretation

Michelle, a 15-year-old caring for her 5-month-old daughter, seeks emergency care for excessive menstrual bleeding. Although Michelle was hospitalized two weeks earlier for asthma and she suspects that the asthma and her current problem are the result of stress, she does not mention either the hospitalization or the stress to her doctors.

This true story, described by Amanda Young and Linda Flower (2002), illustrates what they call a *rhetoric of passivity*, based on participants' assumptions that patients should go along with what care providers say and do. Back in the emergency department, the medical student caring for Michelle asks leading and closed-ended questions that do not encourage her to share her concerns. For her part, Michelle makes only brief replies and is not assertive about sharing what is on her mind. Consequently, Young and Flower report:

> Michelle leaves the hospital with a referral to see a gynecologist with no discussion of what she thinks is causing her problem—a list of stressors that would boggle the mind of a middle-class adult, let alone a 15-year-old single mother in the inner city. (p. 82)

Young and Flower (2002) propose an alternative model of communication based on a *rhetoric of agency* that recognizes patients as co-agents in health encounters. Their **model of collaborative interpretation (CI)** proposes that health communication is most effective when patients actualize the roles of decision makers and problem solvers and when health professionals function as counselors or friends who work alongside patients to help them achieve shared goals. This rhetorical shift relies on the mutual efforts of everyone involved. It cannot work if patients are unwilling to share their stories or to take an active role in health care transactions. Nor will it work if care providers embody a paternalist notion that they know what is best for patients. With the CI model, patients and professionals, together, establish shared goals and work collaboratively to pursue them.

Importantly, the CI model does not privilege either patients or professionals. Instead, as Young and Flower (2002) describe it, the goal is "an experience that validates the expertise of both patient and provider and that dignifies the patient's needs" (p. 89). Such a model can be difficult to create, especially since it is a new idea for many people. As a guide, Young and Flower describe communicative acts that support collaborative interpretations. They include the following:

- Draw on each other's expertise by asking for details about past experiences with the health concern;
- Consider how the patient feels the health concern influences their lifestyle and physical, mental, and emotional health;
- Explicitly discuss both parties' interpretations of the health concern;
- Encourage both parties to share their goals and expectations; and
- Develop a mutual sense of control by identifying strategies that you both feel are beneficial, practical, and acceptable.

Now let's take a closer look at research about the collaborative model.

Focus on Quality of Life

In an issue of *Health Communication* devoted to "The Patient as a Central Construct," Robert Kaplan (1997, p. 75) forecast a move away from the "find it—fix it" biomedical model to an "outcomes model" that emphasizes long-term quality of life. Such a model focuses on the importance of everyday health and fulfillment. Oncologist Jamie Van Roen believes in this. She says:

> The first thing I do to try to make the relationship real is teach them [patients] to complain. I tell them I don't know what it's like to be the patient, to have cancer. It's a matter of control. Patients often feel like they have lost control of everything. I try to give it back. (quoted by Magee & D'Antonio, 2003, p. 202)

A quality-of life model requires a wide-angle focus that extends beyond organic indications of illness. It may involve a range of care providers—such as nutritionists, exercise physiologists, and counselors—and a focus on the complex features that bear on an individual's health.

Collaborative care involves listening and partnering. In the book *On Call: A Doctor's Days and Nights in Residency,* Emily Transue (2004) describes her first conversation with a patent she knew to have terminal cancer. Aware that he had been experiencing depression, Transue asked the man, "How are your spirits?" and he replied, "As good as you could expect them to be, I guess. . . . Not that I don't have my moments." Rather than brushing his words aside, Transue said, "Tell me about the moments" (p. 13). The patient shared with her that he sometimes considered taking his own life, but he stuck around to have more time with his beloved dog. Transue says that such details helped her understand the man's health and quality of life in context better and provide the care he needed. Together, she says, they learned about dying and all the steps along the way.

Patient-centered care has been shown to enhance satisfaction, help overcome racial and ethnic discrimination, lower costs, and improve medical outcomes (Benjamin et al., 2015; Epstein, Fiscella, Lesser, & Stange, 2010; "Patient Centered," 2015). As a result, some funding agencies and health care advocates have begun to measure providers' proficiency at it. They earn highest marks if they engage in rapport-building behaviors, are nonverbally attentive, encourage patients to tell their stories, ask follow-up questions, are tactful and respectful, present information clearly, and show empathy and support (van Zanten, Boulet, & McKinley, 2007).

All the same, there are several reasons that care providers may be reluctant to engage fully in collaborative communication (Légaré & Witteman, 2013):

- They may feel that the treatment is so straightforward as not to require collaboration. (Patients may or may not share this sense of routine.)
- They may worry that negotiating the decision will take too long or be distressing.
- They may be unaware of the collaborative communication approach or unsure how to go about it.
- They feel that there aren't many good treatment options to choose from.

Paramedics in one study say that it's fairly easy to communicate about facts and procedures, but it's often difficult to talk about uncertain outcomes, especially when there is no easy solution to a patient's problem or when the prognosis is poor (Nordby & Nøhr, 2011). For that reason, they say, they sometimes keep a bit of distance so they don't "put a foot in it" or invite requests they will be unable to fulfill. At the same time, the paramedics describe episodes in which patients are deeply grateful for personal attention. For example, one paramedic was able to arrange for a patient in the final stages of cancer to go straight into a hospital room rather than wait in the hospital reception area first. The paramedic said of the experience:

> We tried to make everything as comfortable as we could, and when we were finished, I said, "I cannot say have a good recovery, but I hope we have contributed to making this journey as pain free as possible for you." The patient had tears in his eyes, and said that if there were angels on earth, then they had to be us. (Nordby & Nøhr, 2011, p. 220)

In the spirit of productive collaboration, three New Zealand nursing scholars propose that participants approach health encounters as "puzzles" rather than as "problems." As they describe it, puzzling involves people with different but equally valid perspectives "thinking aloud" about what they would like to achieve and why (Walsh, Jordan, & Apolloni, 2009). In contrast to a "problem" orientation ("Here's what I think we should do . . . ") that presupposes clear answers and certainty, a puzzle approach involves people as partners in setting goals and choosing options in a context that they acknowledge to be ambiguous.

Shared Decision Making

When people's "life stories" are disrupted by serious illness, physicians Peter Anderson and Rabi Hanna consider it their job to help them to "re-imagine the next chapters." They take a team approach inspired by the vision of geese flying in a V. Sometimes one member or another is in the lead, but always, they strive to be part of a cohesive team in which no one is left out, even the patient.

Anderson and Hanna, who work with patients at Cleveland Clinic, use face-to-face interactions and computer-mediated "virtual visits" to collaborate with patients and other care providers (Anderson & Hanna, 2019). The idea, they say, is that well-informed people who work together are likely to produce the best results. All team members have access to full medical information, meeting summaries, and personal items such as family photos that help them feel personally connected to one another (Anderson & Hanna, 2019, p. 4). Anderson and Hanna say it's one of the best ways they know to provide expert, integrated care.

Shared decision making is consistent with a collaborative, quality-of-life approach. Patients who are actively involved in decisions about their care are often better informed, more engaged with their care providers, more confident in their decisions, and more likely than others to engage in follow-up care (Arnetz, Zhdanova, & Arnetz, 2016; Zikmund-Fisher et al., 2010; Zisman-Ilani et al., 2019).

Care providers might set the stage for shared decision making with questions such as *"What have you tried so far?"* (Barnes, 2018, p. 136). Beyond that, they might take stock of how they present recommendations. Tanya Stivers and associates (2018) identified common approaches, ranging from provider-centered to patient-centered:

- *Pronouncements* state what the care provider plans to do, without encouraging input from the patient. For example, a physician might say, *"I'm going to start you on Sudafed."*
- *Proposals* ostensibly treat the patient as a decision maker, but only in response to a specific plan of action, as when a care provider says, *"Why don't we try Allegra?"*
- *Assertions* do not include a clear directive, but instead state a benefit, as in *"Advil would help with your pain."*
- *Suggestions* propose a possible plan of action but imply (or state outright) that the choice lies with the patient, as in, *"You could try Claritin."*
- *Offers* display that the care provider is receptive to the patient's wishes. They might sound like this: *"Would you like some samples?"*

As you can probably tell, pronouncements assert the most professional authority, whereas offers give patients the most decision-making power. That is not to say that patients always want or need full authority to make decisions. Depending on the situation, they may feel adrift without caregivers' input. For the most part, patients usually appreciate when care providers offer them information, support, resources, and perspectives so they can make decisions *together* (Palmer-Wackerly, Krieger, & Rhodes, 2017).

Communication Skill Builders

Collaborative communication can be rewarding for everyone involved, but it is not always easy. Here are three communication approaches that may be useful in initiating and taking part in medical dialogues: motivational interviewing, dialogue, and narrative medicine.

Motivational Interviewing

We may as well admit it: Most of us *know* about healthy behaviors, but we don't always do them. We are aware that we should work out more, eat less fast food, drink more water, get more sleep, and so forth. But sometimes other options seem more appealing or important. Even when we have the healthiest of intentions, once the day starts, a hamburger is a quick meal on the way to school, it seems too hot or too cold to jog, and so on. A whole range of factors seems to keep us from doing what we intended. Theorist Brenda Dervin calls these *gaps*.

Dervin and colleagues propose that life is an enterprise in sense making (Dervin, 1999; Dervin & Frenette, 2001). They use the terms *nouning* and *verbing* to illustrate the point. **Nouning** implies that things are static and predictable. From this perspective, we decide to drink more water, and we do, as simple as that. But more often, life feels more like **verbing**, a process in which we continually make sense of changing circumstances because new information becomes available to us, our perspective changes, circumstances transform, or the like. As this occurs, gaps emerge in what we believe and in the actions available to us.

To employ a simple example, perhaps you are determined to drink more water today, but the vending machine is out or a friend surprises you with a latte. Now there is an unforeseen gap. To visualize what Dervin and colleagues call *gappiness,* imagine walking down a sidewalk, fairly certain about where you are going, and then finding that a significant section

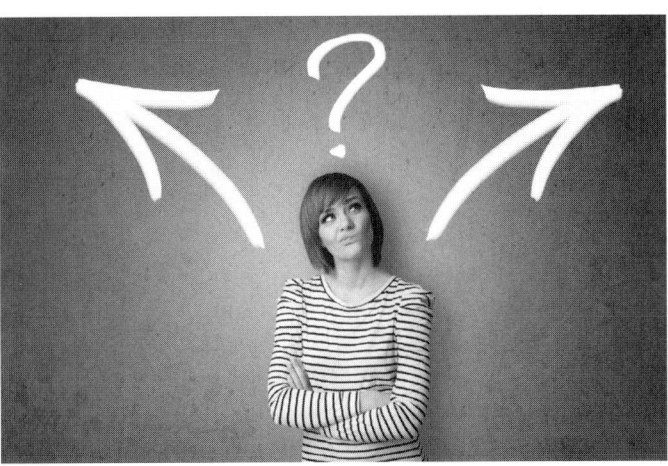

Motivational interviewing helps people weigh the relative pros and cons of decisions, with respect for the reality that health-related choices involve a good deal of ambivalence.

What would you like to do (or stop doing) to improve your health? What factors make it easy to follow through with your intentions? What factors make it difficult?

of the pavement ahead of you is missing. It may be an easy matter to bridge the gap, or it may not. But if you are to keep going in the original direction, you must bridge it in some way. In our example, bridging might mean finding a different vending machine or refusing the latte. If you foresaw the gap, perhaps you planned ahead and brought a bottle of water with you. Conversely, you might abandon the gappy path for now and resolve to try again tomorrow. This is a simple example. As you might imagine, it is often a lot more complicated. The main point is that life is inherently gappy. We continually adjust our goals and behaviors in light of changing circumstances. It is no wonder health professionals want to throw up their hands sometimes. Health (a noun) *is* really important. Yet for a wide range of reasons, people's actions (the verbs) do not always support that ideal.

This leads us to a communication approach that recognizes the verbing side of life—**motivational interviewing (MI)**. Stephen Rollnick and William Miller (1995) conceptualized MI as a client-centered process in which an interviewer (e.g., a health professional, counselor, or friend) helps a interviewee "explore and resolve ambivalence" about a decision, all the while respecting the interviewee's "autonomy and freedom of choice" (paras. 3 and 4, respectively). Let's break that definition down into key points:

- The interviewer does not play a coercive or prescriptive role. They do not tell the interviewee what to do.
- Although the interviewer may be knowledgeable about options, they do not presume to know what is best for the other person.
- The interviewer respects that, because people weigh a variety of factors when making decisions, they almost always experience mixed feelings (ambivalence).
- The interviewer's job is respectfully and nonjudgmentally to ask questions about the interviewee's feelings, to help clarify those feelings, and to support them in making choices (resolving the ambivalence).

In one study, nurses used MI to help people experiencing cancer-related pain examine their feelings about various treatment options (Fahey et al., 2008). From a distance it may seem that a person in pain would naturally seek pain relievers, but as you probably know from personal experience (even considering a headache or sore muscle), the decision is more complicated than that. For one thing, there is no one right way to respond to pain. We might consider it weak to seek relief, or we may be afraid that we will mute our body's natural warning signs. We might fear that we will become addicted to painkillers, that they will make us groggy, and so on. MI practitioners respect this natural ambivalence and try to help people sort through it on their own terms. MI is a true partnership.

Following are some common techniques and assumptions of MI, illustrated with questions adapted from Miller & Rollnick (1995) and Fahey and colleagues' (2008) work with people experiencing pain and from Gerry Welch and colleagues' (2006) work with diabetes patients.

- *Set a respectful tone.* Explain the basic ideas of MI, and express a sincere commitment to listen to and learn from the other person.
- *Let the decision maker set the agenda.* Identify what is important to the interviewee by asking questions such as *Are you happy with the way things are? What is going well? Is there anything that could be better? Do you have concerns about pain?* or *Why do you think you have pain?*
- *Gauge the decision maker's interest.* Change is self-motivated. If the issue is not important to the decision maker, it's probably not fruitful to focus on it. You might ask: *On a scale of 1 to 10, how important is it to you to reduce this pain?*
- *Explore ambivalence.* People almost always have mixed feelings about change. To invite discussion of these factors, you might ask, *It sounds like eating sweets makes you feel unwell, yet you crave them. Is that how it feels? . . . What would change in your life if you had less pain? . . . What factors might prevent you from eating a healthy diet?*
- *Listen.* Let the interviewee do most of the talking.
- *Elicit–provide–elicit.* Ask a question, reflect your understanding of the answer, and then ask questions to get a deeper understanding of the issue, as in: *I hear you saying that you would enjoy being around loved ones more if you were in less pain, but you're worried that you might become addicted to the medication. Why does that worry you?*
- *Identify multiple options (including doing nothing) and weigh their merits.* Some questions to ask include, *What options are you aware of? . . . What are the advantages of your current*

diet? What are the disadvantages? ... What are the advantages of changing your diet? What are the disadvantages?

- *Partner; don't persuade.* If you would like to suggest options or information, make sure they do not sound like prescriptions. For example, you might say: *If you'd like, I'll tell you a bit more about . . .* or *Here are a few things that work for some people . . .*
- *Roll with resistance.* Avoid arguing or convincing. Instead, try to understand thoroughly the decision maker's reluctance to change: *It sounds like you're interested in biofeedback, but you're not confident that it will work.*
- *Gauge the decision maker's sense of confidence and self-efficacy.* You might ask: *On a 1-to-10 scale, how confident are you that you can manage the pain by . . . ?* Keep in mind that confidence, in this case, is not simply a matter of positive attitude. Someone may be unconfident that she can engage in speech therapy twice a week because she doesn't have reliable transportation.
- *Focus on small, incremental changes.* Often, we are not confident that we can make drastic changes, but small ones seem doable. Focus on baby steps: *You indicated that your pain level is usually an 8 out of 10. What do you think it would take to get it down to a 6?*
- *Collaborate and empower.* Emphasize that you are partners in the process and that you will work together and adjust the strategy as you go: *I hear you saying that you would like to try sugar-free snacks. Would you like to try that for two weeks, then come back and we'll see how it's going? . . . What can I or other people do to help you reach your goal?*

This is but a brief overview of MI. Research supports its efficacy at helping people overcome their reluctance to have their adolescent children vaccinated for human papillomavirus (HPV) (Reno et al., 2018), cope with and continue dialysis (McCarley, 2009), quit smoking (Bock et al., 2008), lose weight (Riiser et al., 2014), seek help when considering suicide (Britton, Williams, & Conner, 2008), and more.

Dialogue

A **dialogue** is a conversation in which both people participate fully and equitably, each influencing the encounter in ways that make it a unique creation (Geist & Dreyer, 1993). When conversational partners engage in dialogue, they do not simply adopt ready-made roles; they create them to suit their own situations and preferences.

John Suchwalko remembers a doctor's visit that changed his life and that illustrates a patient's perspective on dialogic communication. "My blood pressure was off the charts, but I didn't feel anything," Suchwalko says (quoted by Magee & D'Antonio, 2003, p. 49). He was also overweight, seldom exercised, was a smoker, and had high cholesterol. It's easy to imagine that a physician might convey disapproval. But Suchwalko's doctor, George Hanna, didn't. As Suchwalko describes it:

> *The thing that impressed me about Dr. Hanna was that he didn't come down on me real hard. I didn't feel like I had been sent to the vice principal's office and he was wagging a finger in my face saying, "You better do this" or "You better do that." Instead he came across like he was a very knowledgeable friend. . . . From then on, I was on a diet, I started walking every day, and I came into his office every two weeks. He would talk to me, encourage me, keep me going. That helped a lot.* (p. 49)

Following are some other techniques for encouraging dialogue in health encounters. Although patients as well as care providers may use these, the majority of the literature is addressed to providers, recognizing perhaps that patients are traditionally more likely to follow health professionals' cues than the other way around.

NONVERBAL ENCOURAGEMENT

> *A couple was dismayed when a doctor spent the entire meeting with them standing with his hand on the doorknob while they were seated. "For them, it implied that he was rushed and did not care much about them," relates Dan Small (2019), who later interviewed the couple. "Although the level of clinical information provided by the clinician met the expected standard of care, the couple went away feeling unfulfilled"* (p. 517).

A hand on the doorknob is hard to miss. But even far more subtle nonverbal cues can be powerful. Researchers have noted several ways that care providers can nonverbally encourage patients to take a more active role in medical encounters.

- *Act interested.* Patients respond well when providers make frequent eye contact, display an attentive posture, and use a caring tone of voice (He, Sun, & Stetler, 2018; Nicolai, Demmel, & Farsch, 2010).
- *Touch (cautiously).* People may interpret touch in a number of ways. Subjected to physical contact and proximity usually reserved for intimate relationships, some patients may feel defensive or violated. However, patients undergoing stressful procedures often say they are comforted when a trusted nurse touches them or holds their hand (Bundgaard, Sørensen, & Nielsen, 2011).
- *Allow silence.* Physician Frederic Platt, the author of numerous books and articles on patient-provider communication, says that asking the right questions is only half the challenge. The rest is waiting for the answers. "Pausing long enough to allow the patient to find that answer is hard," Platt acknowledges. "Nature and doctors abhor a vacuum; we rush to fill the silences. It works better if we can trust the silence to do its work" (Platt, 1995, p. 13).
- *Adapt to the other person.* Communication scholars call it convergence when conversational partners display the same or similar nonverbal cues (Coupland, Coupland, & Giles, 1991). Convergence is typically experienced as a sense of alignment between people. In one study, staff members were most successful at recruiting people to be part of clinical trials when they adopted similar eye contact, touch, and vocal qualities as the people with whom they were interacting (Morgan, Occa, Mouton, & Potter, 2017).

VERBAL ENCOURAGEMENT

The challenge has sometimes been to get patients to open up and share concerns. Suchman et al. (1997) lament lost opportunities for sharing emotions, asserting that "the feeling of being understood by another person is intrinsically therapeutic" (p. 678). However, many patients feel inhibited, fearing that it is inappropriate for them to share feelings. Some providers have overcome patients' inhibitions by using open-ended questions, treating people as equals, encouraging self-disclosure, coaching patients, and using humor. Here are a few tips.

- *Start on a friendly note.* Patients are most likely to feel rapport with a care provider when they smile, shake hands, and engage them in a polite greeting and introduction (Koermer & Kilbane, 2008; Norling, 2005).
- *Listen and encourage.* People experience health on many levels. Listen for what Ashley Hesson and colleagues (2012) call a patient's three stories: a *physical story* that involves bodily symptoms, a *personal story* that situates the person's experiences within a personal and psychosocial context, and an *emotional story* that describes how they feel about the health issue and its effects.
- *Ask "what else?"* Invite the patient to talk about their concerns, listen attentively, and then ask *"What else is on my your mind?"* several times (Branch & Malik, 1993). Only then should you collaboratively establish an agenda for the encounter—which may not include all concerns, but should focus on the most important of them.
- *Avoid abrupt topic shifts.* If you suddenly change the subject, patients may wonder if they have offended you or if you have really been listening. To reduce misunderstandings, strive for smooth transitions, such as "I appreciate your sharing these things; we're going to have to shift gears now and I'll ask you some different types of questions about your symptoms" (suggested by Smith & Hoppe, 1991, p. 464).
- *Pay attention to distress markers.* Remember that patients often stutter and stammer when they are working up to important disclosures. Don't change the subject before you know what's on their minds. Your reassurance may help them speak openly.
- *Ask for the patient's feedback.* Most people will not interrupt you to let you know they cannot follow your advice. You must ask, as in, *"How do you feel about this option?"* and *"Is there anything that would make this hard for you to do?"*
- *Reassure patients.* People have many goals for a health encounter—to be reassured, forgiven, comforted, cured. Words mean a lot *("You needn't feel embarrassed about this." "It's not your fault." "I understand." "You're in pain, aren't you?")* (Harres, 2008). Patients typically consider that providers who are open and reassuring understand them better than those who seem controlling (Silvester, Patterson, Koczwara, & Ferguson, 2007).

- *Consider using humor.* The use of mild, respectful humor seems to be a particularly effective means of minimizing status differences between patients and caregivers (du Pré, 1998; McCreaddie & Payne, 2012) and helping family caregivers relieve stress (Bethea, Travis, & Pecchioni, 2000). Conversational humor can help participants speak candidly without seeming like "bad patients" and can help people in health care situations develop a sense of immediacy and friendliness (Scholl, 2007).

For an example of especially pleasing patient–provider communication, read the mother's story in Box 3.3.

BOX 3.3 PERSPECTIVES

A Mother's Experience at the Dentist

When I first took Kathryn to the dentist, she was very apprehensive. She had never been before due to lack of dental insurance and money, and she only went to the doctor when she was really sick, which was once every 2 years or so. Most illnesses we handled at home, and the idea of preventive care was foreign to her. I knew she needed to go. I knew she wasn't brushing as good as she should, and I also knew that sometimes she lied to me about brushing at all. I couldn't watch her every minute.

When I remarried last year, we were finally fortunate enough to have dental insurance, only we found out there was a 1-year waiting period for anything other than cleanings. So I waited.

Finally, the year was up, and in July I took Kathryn to the dentist for the first time in her life. I tried in advance to make her understand that it was all right to be scared, but that did not mean that it was all right to whine, cry, and generally throw a fit. I told her again and again that I would never take her to anyone I didn't trust or anyone I thought would harm or hurt her unnecessarily.

On a Saturday morning we drove 40 miles to the dental center. Right away, the staff tried to make Kathryn feel at home. The receptionist greeted me and Kathryn by name and asked Kathryn if she was tired from getting up so early on a Saturday. But as I filled out the forms, Kathryn hid behind me, and she spent a lot of time trying to hug me and kiss my cheek. She always does this when she is nervous.

I found I was nervous as well. Not only could I not ease Kathryn's fears, but I found myself feeling like I was a bad parent for not bringing her to the dentist until she was 8. I wasn't sure, as nice as the receptionist was, if she would understand things like no money and no insurance. So we didn't talk about the fact that Kathryn should have been to the dentist years ago; we just talked about easy things, like the nice weather and my wedding pictures.

Soon it was time for Kathryn to go back. After taking X-rays the hygienist led us back to an examination room and found me a small stool to sit on so that I could stay in the same room. She was very friendly and made me feel comfortable. She was also nice to Kathryn and didn't put us down for not coming in sooner.

The cleaning was a little nerve racking, since it was a bit uncomfortable, and Kathryn has a wonderful gag reflex. But the hygienist never seemed to get upset, and she even talked to Kathryn as though she understood, asking her questions like "It's a little scary at first, isn't it?" and "Are you okay? We can wait a minute if you want to, but if we go ahead, we'll be done sooner." It was great that she was so understanding.

By this time, Kathryn was less apprehensive about me leaving the room for a few minutes. The dentist and I walked to the other end of the hall, where he explained that Kathryn had a lot of cavities. He recommended a series of four brief appointments to help Kathryn become more at ease as they repaired her teeth. He made me feel at ease, telling me what a pretty girl Kathryn was. Then he got serious and let me know he understood my concerns about not bringing her in sooner, but not to worry. The cavities were not severe, they were all in baby teeth, and although there were several, they would be easy to fix.

I collected Kathryn and stopped by the front desk, where the receptionist pulled out a surprise box and let Kathryn pick out what she wanted. The next visits

continued

continued

were not as bad as Kathryn thought they would be. Every time she was a little happier and not so apprehensive about what would happen. Once she had been through the routine, she knew what to expect, and that helped. She said she liked everyone at the dentist's office. Once I brought a newspaper article I had written about Kathryn's school with her picture in it. The staff insisted on reading the whole thing and remarked what a good writer I was and how pretty Kathryn was. They also insisted on seeing my wedding pictures. It wasn't just something to be nice; they really wanted to see them.

I feel good taking Kathryn there because I know, no matter what, we will get the best treatment. Not only that, but we have established friendships with these people that will last. They truly believe they are there to serve, and they show that in everything they do. Just ask Kathryn. She'll tell you.

—DONNA

Narrative Medicine

Anne had seen a lot of doctors over the years, but Dr. Falchuk was different. He smiled and said to her, "I want to hear your story in your own words." He showed no signs of being rushed or impatient. In fact, Anne recalls, "his calm made it seem as if he had all the time in the world" (Groopman, 2007, p. 12).

Dr. Falchuk's kind attention came at a good time, because Anne was nearing death. Although she was eating 3,000 calories a day, she was unable to keep food down and she had become critically underweight. The problem had persisted for 15 years, and although Anne was only in her thirties, her body's systems were crashing. Of the 30 or so doctors she had consulted before Dr. Falchuk, none had asked to hear her whole story, as he did. Instead, most doctors had asked only brief, closed-ended questions. Their subsequent diagnoses ranged from depression to bulimia, to irritable bowel syndrome, and more. Some felt that the illness was "all in her head." Most urged her to eat a high-carbohydrate diet of cereals and breads to gain weight. But her health kept deteriorating.

After listening carefully to Anne's story from beginning to end, Falchuk was the first to identify her disease correctly. He suspected—and confirmed—that she had celiac disease, a severe allergy to the gluten found in many grain products (notably the same products that other doctors were urging Anne to eat). Falchuk's diagnosis and the subsequent diet change saved Anne's life. When Groopman (2007) interviewed Falchuk about the episode, he denied doing anything extraordinary. Listening to patients' stories *should* be a doctor's first priority, Falchuk said, avowing that "once you remove yourself from the patient's story, you are no longer truly a doctor" (quoted by Groopman, p. 2007).

Narrative medicine is an approach championed most notably by physician and medical school

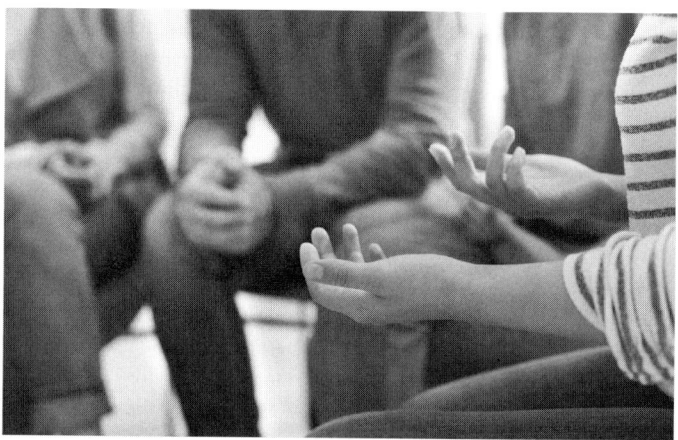

Storytelling is a natural way of explaining experiences and sharing information. Narrative medicine embraces stories as rich opportunities to share and connect.

Consider a health concern you have now or have experienced in the past. What story would you tell about it to a willing listener?

professor Rita Charon. It involves respect for people's stories and the awareness that storytelling unites both the teller and the listener in a unique and shared experience with profound implications for life and for healing (Charon, 2006). Charon proposes that narrative medicine is both an ideal and a method. It involves a commitment to deep and sincere listening, a belief in the power of stories to heal and to reveal what needs healing, and the courage to, as Charon puts it, "inhabit" another person's point of view for a while.

Charon (2009b) presents narrative medicine as a means of bridging the "chasms and divisions and discontinuities" of health care and the experience of being ill (p. 197). The disconnect may have blinded Anne's previous caregivers to the true problem. Falchuk was different from them in that he attentively listened to her. In doing so, he was able to identify what the others had missed. Charon shares his belief that medicine, at its best, bridges the gaps between people. Genuine engagement, she says, requires the courage to face raw and uncomfortable emotions. But it also offers revelations and connections beyond imagining. Here are a few of the key principles involved.

Narrative medicine embraces the idea that storytelling is a natural way of making sense of the world. Any time people gather, even for a few moments, they tell stories. One person tells another what it was like to undergo surgery, have a baby, go on a blind date, or so on. Communication scholar William Rawlins (2009) proclaims, from personal experience and many years researching the topic, that "making stories with friends is good for the heart and the soul" (p. 168). This is especially true when we are trying to make sense of a serious occurrence such as a health event that interrupts the storyline we imagined for ourselves. "Sickness summons stories," writes narrative theorist Lynn Harter (2009, p. 141).

Moreover, people tell stories for some very compelling reasons. At a surface level, narratives are informative. They tell people of specific goings-on and perhaps prepare them to take part in similar circumstances. But at an even deeper level, narratives shape interpretations and viewpoints—some would say that they shape reality. In Charon's words, through the events of life and our stories about them "we become who we are, discover who we are, accept who we are, rage or pleasure toward who we are" (2009a, p. 120).

Narrative medicine involves compassionate engagement and a respect for the uniqueness and wholeness of each individual. Here is a powerful example told by Charon:

> *My first gesture after hearing out a woman with muscular dystrophy and impending respiratory failure was to sit as close to the patient as I could, thigh to thigh, my hands in my lap, trying to inhabit her climate of panicky despair so as not to leave her alone in it. And so we were on a search together right from the beginning.* (2009a, p. 123)

Charon begins conversations with new patients by saying, "I will be your doctor, so I must learn a great deal about your body and your health and life. Please tell me what you think I should know about your situation" (2009a, p. 122). Then she listens, without writing or typing or any other activity that might distract.

Far from being a waste of time, Charon says that listening without interrupting has enabled her to learn things that might have taken years to discover otherwise. "Having hastened the development of genuine listening and learning about the patient, I found myself able to do things that mattered right from the beginning" (2009a, p. 122). But the process is not only for her benefit. Telling one's story has a value even more inherent. "The patient's body talks with the patient's self, in an odd and powerful way, while I, the witness, listen," Charon says, observing that we often come to understand and integrate facets of ourselves through storytelling (p. 122).

Narrative medicine embraces the idea that health professionals are not, and cannot be, all knowing and all powerful. Indeed, many would argue that the expectation that they should be omnipotent and infallible fosters a sense of distance and authority that is at odds with true engagement. From the perspective of narrative medicine, even when there is nothing a professional can do to cure a patient, the act of being present with that person is therapeutic and affirming. As Charon puts it, "one knows, one feels, one responds, and one *joins with* the one who suffers" (2006, p. 12).

Harter (2009) tells of a physician who includes in patient charts notes about what and whom they love and what they dream of doing. In the chart of Anna, a young woman with bone cancer, he included her prom and graduation photos, two life events he knew were important to her. Later, in a poignant meeting in which he had to tell Anna that her cancer had spread to her lungs, he asked, "What other chapters in your life do you want to write, Anna? How can I help you write those?" (quoted by Harter, 2009, p. 141). Rather than talking, he listened.

Narratives are important to health communication in several ways. As mentioned, patients naturally speak in narrative form, describing their concerns within a sequence of events that they consider relevant. Narratives often address a sophisticated array of factors simultaneously, and they may be a means of conveying what we would not otherwise blurt out. Timothy Halkowski (2006) observed that patients often present a "sequence of noticings" that involve emerging indications of a potential health problem and what the patient did about them at each step. These narrative details may seem superfluous to caregivers, who may wonder, as one doctor puts it, why patients don't just come to the point and "bottom-line it." But for patients, Halkowski says, these narratives allow them to manage the dilemma of simultaneously impressing care providers that their concerns are legitimate while avoiding being typified as melodramatic or overly self-concerned. The patient is able to present a number of indicators that are demonstrated as being relevant to the current concern, underscoring its status as real rather than imagined. Patients can also share useful information about what has or has not worked so far. This sequential narrative, Halkowski says, gives patients a mechanism for presenting their concerns in an informative and identity-supporting way.

This leads to another reason that narratives are important: They are loaded with information. A sensitive listener can detect cues to a person's hopes, fears, doubts, future intentions, and more. Particularly since patients are often nonassertive about expressing these feelings, caregivers may find that narratives offer valuable insights. Subtle cues may be the only indications that a person is dissatisfied, in despair, reluctant to cooperate, overly anxious to please, or so on. All of these feelings can be directly relevant to the success of medical care.

Janice Brown and Julia Addington-Hall (2007) identified four types of narratives in the stories told by people with motor neuron disease (MND), a neurological disorder that gradually diminishes people's ability to move and speak. Most people with MND die in 3 to 5 years.

- *Sustaining narratives* emphasize hope and positive thinking. For example, one mother of two young children said she was grateful for what she could still do, even though her ability to walk and talk were ebbing. "I mean, I still feel I could be a lot worse off. I mean I know everything's hard work, but there's no pain in it" (p. 204).
- *Enduring narratives* describe a process of stoically living through one's suffering, ambivalent about whether it would be better to live or to die. One man in the study, who could no longer move his hands or arms, said, "They say there's not much they can do about it, you have just got to take it" (p. 205). He said he had instructed caregivers not to resuscitate him if he had a heart attack because dying would be better than "sitting here like this" (p. 205).
- In *preserving narratives*, people describe illness as something to be conquered, with varying levels of confidence in their ability to do so. One participant in the study had turned to holistic therapies in addition to pharmaceutical prescriptions, changed his diet, and eliminated chemicals from his home. "I am just willing to try anything," he said (p. 205).
- *Fracturing narratives* describe fear, loss, denial, and threats to self-concept. Said one woman with MND: "I try and remain optimistic and fear that if the day comes when I have to fully embrace this illness, possibly because of increasing symptoms, then I will totally fall apart. I am trying to postpone that moment" (p. 206).

The researchers reflect that caregivers can better understand people by listening to their narratives and appreciating that those narratives are likely to evolve over time.

Finally, there is something more to narratives—something less easily measured, but unquestionably powerful in the act of bearing witness to another person's story. As Richard Zaner (2009) expresses it, there is, in narrative, something between people "that does not belong exclusively to either person" (p. 170) but lives in the "terrain where wonder holds sway" (p. 170). Within that terrain, says Charon (2006), caregivers connect with others through a sense of genuine curiosity and concern, and they learn a great deal about themselves in the process.

If the move toward patient empowerment continues, narratives are likely to become more influential components of patient–caregiver communication. Geist and Gates (1996) describe the process as "movement from biology to biography" (p. 221). When caregivers listen and ask open-ended questions, they can learn a great deal, not only about patients' physical conditions, but also about their expectations and values (Eggly, 2002). How relevant are such factors to personal health? Very relevant, according to the integrative health theory (Box 3.4), which proposes that health is not an isolated condition, but an alignment between multiple factors.

In this section, we have focused a great deal on what caregivers can do to encourage effective communication. See Box 3.5 for communication tips designed specifically for patients.

BOX 3.4 THEORETICAL FOUNDATIONS

Integrative Health Model

Health cannot accurately be reduced to a failure of body, identity, or behavior, say the creators of integrative health theory (Lambert et al., 1997). Instead, **integrative health theory** proposes that health is the alignment between interpretive accounts (assumptions and explanations), performance (activities and behaviors), and self-image (understanding of one's own identity).

Ideally, alignment is stable and enduring (the person is healthy), but a change in any one force can upset the alignment. Lambert and colleagues (1997) present the example of a man who feels healthy despite undiagnosed high blood pressure. However, once his condition is diagnosed and he begins taking medication for it, the man experiences a side effect (impotence). His interpretive account—that, as a healthy male and husband (his self-image), he should have a sexual relationship with his wife—is threatened by his inability to engage in sexual intercourse (performance). In short, "the impotence is a resistance that destabilizes his healthy alignment," write Lambert and associates. "When he realizes he is impotent, he no longer feels healthy" (p. 34).

Lambert and colleagues (1997) use the term *resistance* to describe factors that threaten alignment. The effects of resistance are not predictable or universal. The man in the previous example might respond by altering his self-image, redefining his ideas about being a good husband, or resuming sexual activity by ceasing the medication (Lambert et al.).

People may have a difficult time adjusting to resistance factors that seem small to others. By the same token, over time, people sometimes achieve alignment that others would not think possible. Marianne Brady and David Cella (1995) described the resiliency with which some cancer patients ultimately adapt to their illness: "Many even say they are strengthened by the experience and note an improved outlook on life, enhanced interpersonal relationships and a deepened sense of personal strength" (para. 13). Although their physical abilities may be compromised by the disease, these people apparently adjust other factors to achieve a new (even an improved) sense of alignment.

The integrative health model presents several implications for health communication. For one, it sets aside the centuries-old question of whether health is fundamentally a matter of mind or body. By rejecting reductionist notions, it provides an inclusive definition of health that relies more on alignment between factors than isolation of any one element. From this perspective, a health examination would not be focused on identifying the "cause" of a health concern but in considering how it is situated within broader contexts.

Another implication is that restoring alignment may be simple or complex. Sometimes there is primarily one form of resistance. Lambert and coauthors (1997) give the example of an appendectomy that restores a young woman to full health. In her case, alignment is disrupted but quickly restored. In other situations, however, focusing on one resistance point may not help (or may even worsen) overall alignment. For example, amputating a limb may remove physical danger but plunge the patient into personal crisis. Considering this, the biomedical model may be appropriate for some medical encounters but woefully insufficient for others.

A third implication is that outcomes are neither static nor definitive. Lambert and colleagues (1997) write, "It is never known in advance which accommodations will be successful, nor is it known whether accommodations will themselves lead to the emergence of new resistances" (p. 35). Even when alignment is present, there is no guarantee it will stay that way. In fact, it almost certainly will be challenged. Because of

continued

continued

this, health is viewed more productively as a process, as a temporal emergence, than as an outcome.

Finally, in the midst of this complexity, Lambert and colleagues (1997) argue that there is one constant: *The patient is always central in the process.* As an individual involved in the ongoing work of balancing identity and performance, a "patient is at the center of the aligned elements" and is "also the one doing the work of interactive stabilization" (p. 31).

What Do You Think?

1. In what ways do your daily activities support your self-image? How would you feel if you lost the ability to perform these activities?
2. Think of the last time you felt unhealthy. What resistance factors were involved? Was alignment restored? If so, how?

BOX 3.5

Communication Tips for Patients

Here are some suggestions from the experts.

- *Take stock.* Consider Rita Charon's question: "Please tell me what you think I should know about your situation." You need not memorize or rehearse an answer, but do give some thought to what you want caregivers to know, as well as your goals for the visit and your concerns at a physical, emotional, and social level.
- *Create a one-page health history.* In an easy-to-read format, present information about your health (medications, illnesses, hospitalizations, allergies, surgeries) and any diseases diagnosed in your immediate family. Bring a copy to all doctor visits and hospital stays.
- *Write down and rank-order your concerns.* Care providers like a list—*if* it helps them get a succinct overview of all your concerns and *if* the list identifies what you consider most important. (Keep in mind that you may not have time to go through all the items on the list in one visit. Bring an extra copy to share and to include in your chart.)
- *Prepare for the standard questions.* Be ready with answers to such questions as, *What does it feel like? When? Where? For how long?*
- *Choose health care providers carefully.* Find professionals who are well respected by their peers and who listen well and make you feel comfortable. Your feelings are as legitimate as your medications and health history. Find someone who pays attention to both.
- *Don't overlook valuable resources.* There are probably more people available to help you than you realize. For example, pharmacists can offer advice about prescription and nonprescription medications, address concerns, and serve as ongoing advisors and guides (Gade, 2007). Likewise, dieticians, athletic trainers, and others can help with health-related behaviors.
- *Know what treatment you are supposed to get, and make sure your caregivers know it, too.* As we will discuss in Chapter 5, medical mistakes happen. Tell care providers why you are at the clinic or hospital, and make sure everyone agrees. This might prevent a wrong-side surgery or medication error.
- *Help set the agenda.* Be as clear as possible when making an appointment so that the caregiver knows your concerns and expectations. ("*I'm experiencing sharp abdominal pains*" or "*I'd like an overall physical and a chance to ask some questions.*")
- *Don't abuse the clock.* The reality is that care providers must budget their time. Most are willing to listen when they appreciate that what you are saying is relevant to your concern. For your part, speak freely, but emphasize the relevance of what you want to share and avoid going off on tangents.
- *Take an active role.* Doctors usually understand patients' goals more clearly and share more information when patients ask questions and state their concerns, preferences, and opinions (Cegala, Street, & Clinch, 2007).
- *Acknowledge reservations.* If something prevents you from speaking frankly, let the care provider know ("*I'm embarrassed*" or "*I'm afraid I have cancer*" or "*I can't afford that*").
- *Be assertive.* If your questions have not been answered, or if you do not agree with the advice given, state your feelings in a clear and respectful way. Walking away dissatisfied helps no one.

Summary

Importance of Patient–Provider Communication

- Good communication (open, trusting, clear, and thorough) can help participants in medical encounters arrive at accurate diagnoses, mutually acceptable treatment plans, clear expectations, a shared sense of support and solidarity, and proactive strategies for health maintenance.
- Effective communication also promotes well-being by easing patients' anxiety and pain.

Medical Talk and Power Differentials

- The traditional power difference between patients and caregivers is manifested in conversations in which patients tend to acquiesce and professionals to dominate.
- Unwittingly or not, patients often collaborate in the lopsided nature of these medical conversations by speaking hesitantly and abandoning topics when interrupted. They may do this because it seems polite, culturally appropriate, or in keeping with institutional routines.
- Patients tend to save embarrassing and distressing information until they feel comfortable divulging it. They aren't alone in their discomfort. Care providers may be embarrassed and may feel unqualified to address emotional issues.

Patronizing Behavior and Transgressions

- Patients may feel patronized (treated as if they are inferior) when providers seem to ignore them.
- Transgressions frequently have painful and confusing results. Experts suggest that participants in health care encounters take stock of their needs and emotions, set clear boundaries, avoid sending mixed messages, seek the counsel of friends and colleagues, have others present, and address unwanted behavior with the person involved, and when warranted, with authorities.

Collaborative Communication

- Collaborative communication is neither caregiver centered nor patient centered, but instead is dedicated to active partnerships.
- Many caregivers, far from being anxious to abuse the power granted them, are frustrated by the barriers it creates. They attempt to empower patients through the use of encouraging words and nonverbal gestures.
- The model of collaborative interpretation (CI) distinguishes between the rhetoric of passivity and the rhetoric of agency, suggesting that patients and care providers develop mutual trust and work together as partners.
- Shared decision making is consistent with a collaborative, quality-of-life approach.

Communication Skill Builders

- In motivational interviewing, the interviewer issues no orders or commands and makes no judgments. Instead, the interviewer asks questions to help the other person explore the advantages and disadvantages of various options.
- When conversational partners engage in dialogue, they do not simply adopt ready-made roles. They create them to suit their own situations and preferences.
- Narratives reveal how people view the world, how they see themselves in relation to others, and what events are most significant to them. Information of this sort can give caregivers valuable insight and can provide a therapeutic way for them to authentically engage with patients.
- Patients may respond to illness in many ways—from relief to terror—and may experience changes in their personal identity as a result of illness. Integrative health theory describes the importance of alignment and resistance in maintaining good health.

Glossary

collaborative medical communication An approach in which communication partners treat each other as peers who openly discuss health options and make mutually satisfying decisions. *See page 47.*

disclosure decision-making model (DD-MM) The perspective that patients consider answers to the following questions before disclosing sensitive information: *What outcomes can I predict if I share this information? How is the other person likely to respond?* and *Can I share this information effectively? See page 46.*

dialogue A conversation in which conversational partners participate fully and equitably, each influencing the encounter in ways that make it a unique creation. *See page 53.*

doorknob disclosure A pattern in which patients blurt out their main concerns at the last instant of a visit. *See page 44.*

integrative health theory The proposition that health is the alignment between interpretive accounts (assumptions and explanations), performance (activities and behaviors), and self-image (understanding of one's own identity). *See page 59.*

model of collaborative interpretation (CI) The theory that health communication is most effective when patients actualize a rhetoric of agency by taking part in decision making and problem solving and when health professionals function as counselors or friends who work alongside patients to help them achieve shared goals. *See page 49.*

motivational interviewing (MI) A client-centered process in which an interviewer (e.g., a health professional, counselor, or friend) helps an interviewee explore and resolve ambivalence about a decision, all the while respecting the interviewee's freedom of choice. *See page 49.*

narrative medicine An approach that involves respect for people's stories and the awareness that storytelling unites both the teller and the listener in a unique and shared experience with profound implications for life and healing. *See page 56.*

nouning The assumption that people's behavioral patterns are static and predictable. *See page 51.*

patronize Treating someone as if they are inferior, as by withholding information, speaking down to them, or dismissing their feelings as childish or inconsequential. *See page 45.*

therapeutic privilege The prerogative sometimes granted to physicians to withhold information from patients if they feel that disclosing the information would do more harm than good. *See page 42.*

transgressions Inappropriate actions that cross the line between intimacy and professionalism. *See page 45.*

verbing The notion that behavior is a process in which we continually adapt in light of changing circumstances and perspectives. *See page 51.*

Discussion Questions

1. Traditionally, health professionals have had more control over medical conversations than patients have had. What factors contribute to the prevalence of provider-centered communication? Describe some of the communication patterns involved. How do patients' behaviors contribute to these dynamics? How do care providers' behaviors contribute?

2. What is therapeutic privilege? What guidelines would you suggest for using this privilege?

3. What actions by patients and care providers might qualify as transgressions? What are some methods for handling transgression attempts? Provide a few examples.

4. How could patients and care providers lessen the likelihood of doorknob disclosures?

5. According to the disclosure decision-making model, what three considerations affect whether people disclose nonvisible health concerns to someone else?

6. Compare a "rhetoric of passivity" with a "rhetoric of agency." What are some communication strategies caregivers and patients can use to accomplish collaborative interpretation? Apply these to an example of your own.

7. Compare the assumptions of physician-centered and collaborative communication. How is the care provider's role different in each model? How is the patient's role different? What are some of the reasons that many people are shifting from provider-centered to collaborative communication?

8. What are the assumptions and techniques of motivational interviewing? Would you enjoy being part of such an interview? Why or why not?

9. Think of a health concern you have experienced personally. When asked about it, what does your narrative include? What elements of the narrative are most important in terms of your feelings about it and its importance in your life? Now analyze the experience in terms of integrative health theory. In what ways did you experience *alignment? Resistance?*

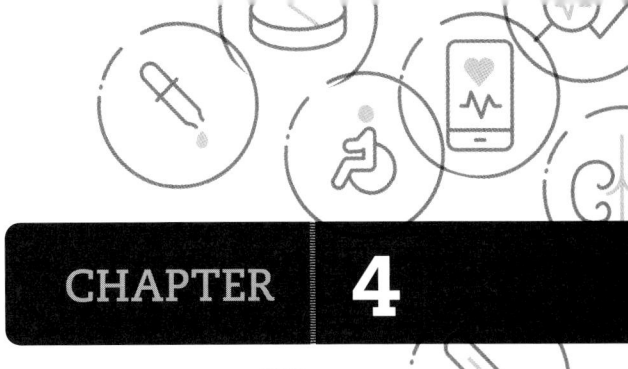

CHAPTER 4

Patient Perspectives

I remember, as a child, the distinct smell of the doctor's office. It's different than any other odor, and it leaves a lasting impression. The smell of rubbing alcohol, the smell of medicines, and the smell of antibacterial soap on the doctor's hands. As a child, you don't know what to make of it.

These musings by a college student evoke vivid images of patienthood. Whatever else we remember of childhood, most of us will never forget the sensory alert of waiting anxiously to be seen by a doctor.

Being a patient can be a frightening experience, even as an adult. Uncertainty is guaranteed, and pain is a strong possibility. At the same time, though, there is the promise of relief, a cure, or a reassuring health assessment. (See Box 4.1 for a true story about one patient's experience managing uncertainty.)

In this chapter we look at health care situations through patients' eyes. We investigate the informal socialization process that helps people learn how to behave in that role, how health shapes and reflects our personal identity, what patients generally like and dislike, and what motivates people to follow (and, just as often, to ignore) medical advice.

As we explore these topics, bear in mind that, although there are facets of patienthood (such as embarrassment, anxiety, hope, and gratitude) that we are all likely to experience at some point, the experience of being a patient is highly personal and cultural. Examples throughout this chapter highlight some of that diversity, and Chapters 6 and 7 are devoted to diverse perspectives, including the intersection of health and culture, race, gender, age, and many other factors.

Patient Socialization

Being a patient often means suspending the rules of everyday interaction. For example, the touch and physical exposure usually reserved for intimate relationships occurs under bright lights in the company of strangers. In emergencies or intense circumstances such as childbirth, modesty may not be on anyone's mind. During routine exams, however, participants tend to display in subtle ways that the body-as-examined is more an object than

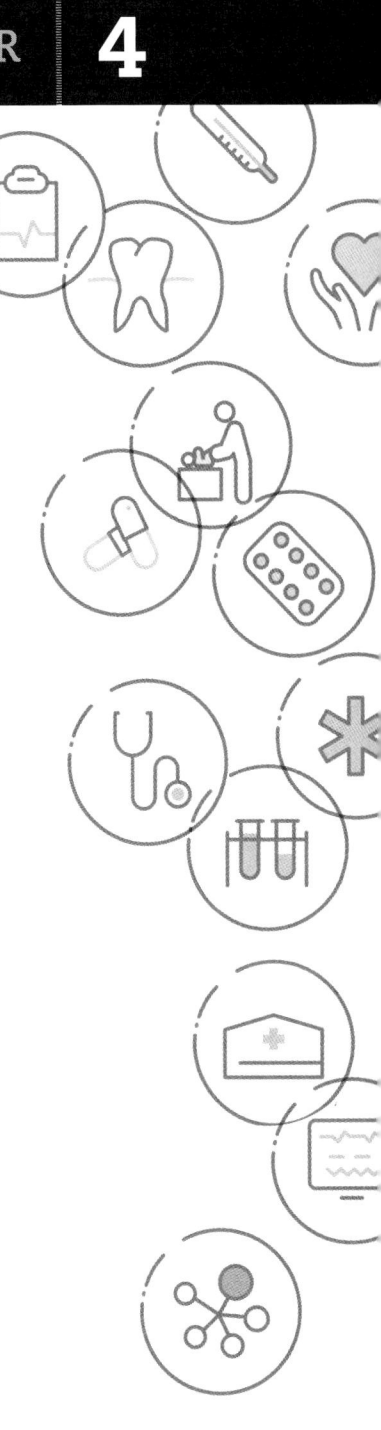

BOX 4.1 PERSPECTIVES

The Agony of Uncertainty

It all began one day when I was in eighth-grade physical education class. As the class began to warm up and stretch, I noticed a knot on my knee. A month passed and the knot did not go away. In fact it grew from the size of a pencil eraser to the size of a quarter. My mother made an appointment with our family doctor, and I began to panic. I personally gave myself one year to live.

During my appointment the doctor asked questions like, "Have you fallen down recently?" I was so distraught I felt like screaming, "I did not come in here for a bump and scrape!" But I just said no.

After ordering X-rays, the doctor said he could not tell if the knot was a cyst or a tumor and referred us to a bone and joint specialist. I was beyond scared. I was only 13 and had never had anything worse than the flu. I had so many questions, but there wasn't much chance to ask them. Every question I asked got a brief response, when what I really wanted was a full explanation and, above all, reassurance. The conversation went something like this:

> **DOCTOR:** It looks like you have a cyst or a tumor. I'm going to refer you to a specialist.
> **ME:** What does that mean?
> **DOCTOR:** It means he will look at your knee and figure out what is going on.
> **ME:** Is it serious?
> **DOCTOR:** That's what he'll be able to determine.
> **ME:** Well, OK.

I wasn't sure about the difference between a cyst and a tumor, and both sounded horrible. I was afraid the doctor would laugh if I said I was afraid of having cancer. Or had he just told me I *did* have cancer? I left not knowing, and I had to wait a month to see the specialist.

On the day of the appointment with the specialist, Dr. Benze, we waited 2½ hours to see him. However, his personality and gentle manner made up for the wait. Dr. Benze compassionately and carefully told me the lump (now the size of a small orange) was a tumor. When I began to cry, he explained that not all tumors are cancerous. He arranged to surgically remove the tumor in two days, and he promised to tell me everything about the surgery in advance and to share the lab results with me as soon as he received them.

On the day before surgery my mother and I visited the hospital to make arrangements. The admitting attendant was detached and unfriendly, but the nurses and doctors were wonderful. They tried to make me feel comfortable and relaxed. An outpatient nurse sat down with us and described in detail what would happen before, during, and after the surgery. I felt comfortable asking every question I did not feel safe asking the first doctor.

Suffice it to say that the surgery went well. The tumor was not cancerous, and I have had no more tumors. Overall, the experience was a positive one. The worst part was leaving the first doctor's office with so many fears and questions I never got to voice. Although the surgery was frightening, I felt better once people started telling me what was going on.

—SARAH

What Do You Think?

1. Do you think the first doctor could have communicated more effectively with Sarah? If so, how?
2. Do you think Sarah could have communicated more effectively? If so, how?
3. Sometimes doctors feel they will alarm or confuse patients (especially young patients) by giving them medical details. Do you agree?
4. How can patients help ensure that they get the information they want?

---

an intimate landscape. Christian Heath (2006) observed that patients typically lower their eyelids, turn their heads aside, and gaze into the middle distance during potentially embarrassing or painful examinations. At the same time, health professionals typically avoid direct eye contact, focusing instead on particular parts of the patient's body. This "body work," as Heath calls it, is a sophisticated, collaborative performance in which participants display that what might otherwise seem to be an intimate or callous infringement is—by mutual consensus—an acceptable, clinically approved interaction with its own rules of appropriateness.

Verbal interactions can be equally as challenging. Although patients are unlikely to agree with everything their care providers say, they may fear that speaking up will make them seem difficult or disrespectful (Frosch, May, Rendle, Tietbohl, & Elwyn, 2012). Most patients who disagree with their doctors either stay quiet or hint at their disagreement by asking questions or talking about their preferences. In one study, only 1 in 7 patients said that they tell their doctors outright when they disagree with them (Adams, Elwyn, Légaré, & Frosch, 2012). It's easy to imagine the misunderstandings that occur as a result.

Considering the challenges, how do people learn to embody a patient role? Unlike health professionals, patients are usually in medical situations only briefly and occasionally. Moreover, whereas providers-in-training are usually required to observe experienced professionals, everyday people seldom get to observe other patients. Thus, socialization into the role of patient requires a good deal of guesswork and experimentation. People apply their everyday knowledge to the role and generally display all the hesitancy you might expect. This section describes the Voice of Lifeworld, the typical power difference between patients and professionals, and the dilemmas people face when they disagree with their caregivers.

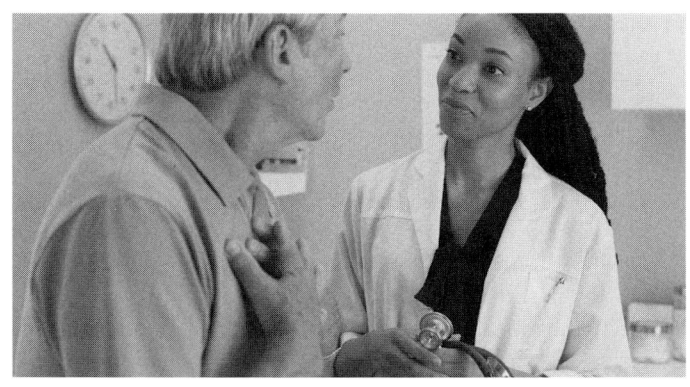

A great deal rides on how effectively patients communicate with care providers. However, there is typically little instruction on how to do that well.

Have you ever found yourself reluctant or unable to tell a care provider what you wanted to say? If so, what factors might make it easier for you to communicate openly?

Voice of Lifeworld

When 25-year-old Jessica Tar told her dentist that her tongue had been hurting, she didn't expect it to be anything serious. But when tests revealed cancer, the prescribed treatment was nearly as frightening as the diagnosis. Doctors would have to remove a portion of her tongue. As an aspiring singer and actress, Tar was devastated to realize that her speech might be affected. "I was crying that day like I had never cried before," she remembers ("Jessica's Story," n.d.).

We follow Tar's experiences in this section, in which we explore the role of communication in making sense of health care experiences. Patients typically speak with what Elliot Mishler (1984) calls the **Voice of Lifeworld**, which is primarily concerned with health and illness as they relate to everyday experiences. Whereas a health professional may understand back pain in terms of specific discs and muscles, from a lifeworld perspective, the main issue may be that the pain interferes with a person's ability to pick up a child or perform tasks at work. When asked what is wrong, patients typically describe sensations and events, as in, "I get a horrible pain behind my eyes when I try to read the newspaper. It really scares me."

In contrast to the Voice of Medicine—which is primarily oriented to evidence, measurement, and precision—the Voice of Lifeworld is more oriented to feelings and contexts. From this perspective, it's natural that Tar was worried, not only about her physical condition, but about how treatment would affect her daily life and her career.

Feelings Versus Evidence

Patients typically gauge whether they are sick or healthy based on personal experience, comparisons with others, and gut instinct (Mishler, 1981, 1984). Health professionals, however, are typically taught to rely on empirical verification. Therefore, they may put more faith in their own observations and in diagnostic tests than in patients' descriptions of what is wrong.

Put another way, as a general principle, patients typically trust feelings, whereas health professionals trust evidence. This disconnect can lead patients to feel that they are not being

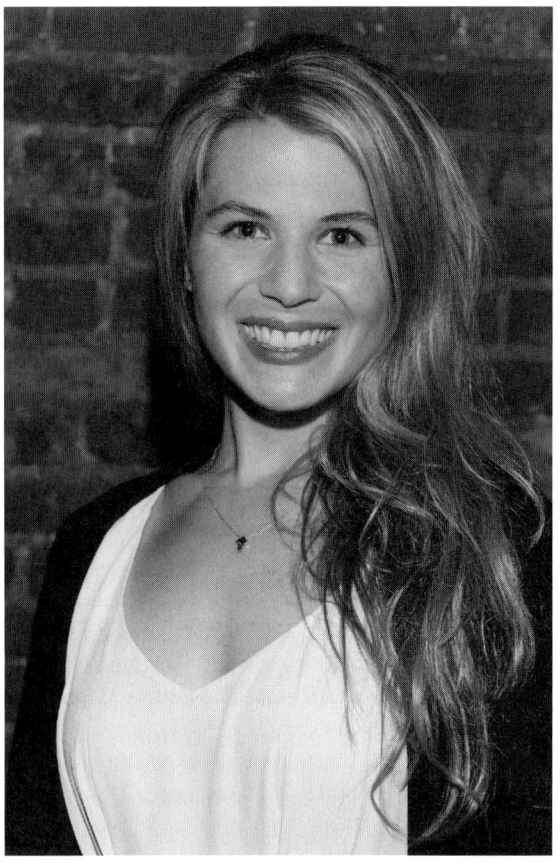

Actress Jessica Tar's ambitions were threatened when doctors had to remove a small portion of her tongue because of a tumor. Oral surgeon Jatin Shah took her lifeworld concerns seriously and worked with her to devise a treatment plan that saved her life and helped her resume life as usual.

Describe a time when a care provider paid attention to your feelings. How did that affect your satisfaction with the encounter? Your feelings about your condition?

heard and that health professionals are unsympathetic to their feelings (Cousin, Mast, Roter, & Hall, 2012).

Health professionals may have many reasons for diverting talk away from lifeworld issues. They may consider them irrelevant to the patient's medical condition or outside of their control. Or, as we discussed in Chapter 3, they may be uncomfortable discussing issues because they lack experience with them or they have not been trained to engage in those types of conversations. "Under these circumstances doctors typically interject questions, interrupt, or otherwise change the topic, to return to the voice of medicine," says medical theorist Howard Waitzkin (1991, p. 25).

Although the contrast between the Voice of Lifeworld and the Voice of Medicine can lead to misunderstandings, it's possible to bridge the gap. Tar was treated by oral surgeon Jatin Shah, who reviewed laboratory reports about her condition but realized that Tar's emotional health was as important as her physical recovery. In the midst of her distress, Dr. Shah asked her, "Other than the cancer you have, what is bothering you?" ("Jessica's Story," n.d.).

Specific Versus Diffuse

One result of disparate philosophies is that health professionals are often precise, whereas patients are diffuse. To illustrate, a care provider may hear "pain behind the eyes" and want to know exactly where, how strong, how long. Patients, however, may be concerned with surrounding issues (*Will I die? Can I still be a good parent? Am I going blind? Do I have a tumor? What have I done to deserve this?*). Although both mean well, health professionals may be frustrated when patients "go on and on," and patients may feel rebuffed when caregivers seem uninterested in their stories.

Patients also tend to be diffuse in their perception of what gives rise to illness. Unlike conventional medicine practitioners, who typically strive to find specific causes, patients often perceive that an illness has multiple origins, common among them stress and relationship issues. Consequently, scientific specificity may seem sorely deficient in explaining illnesses as patients perceive them. People may leave exams wondering if their care providers really understood their problems at all.

Patients may also have numerous goals that take precedence over purely physical healing. They may wish to vent emotions, confess, or be reassured, forgiven, or comforted during a medical visit. These goals may pose a challenge to some professionals' efforts to set aside what they consider extraneous factors and focus on measurable ones.

All in all, patients tend to interpret illnesses in the broad context of everyday life, whereas many professionals are taught to reduce diseases to their simplest, most measurable parts. As we saw in Chapter 3, however, some patients and health professionals adopt a collaborative approach that integrates medical and lifeworld voices. Working together, Tar and Dr. Shah determined to preserve her verbal abilities and self-image as much as possible, without compromising her chances of physical recovery. The surgery was successful in removing the cancer, and after months of therapy to help her eat, talk, and swallow effectively, Tar found her voice again. She has since become a mother of two and a professional actor. (You can catch her as Christine Benash in *The Meat Puppet* and as a nurse in *Alien vs. Zombies.*) Tar says she feels lucky to have found a collaborator in Dr. Shah, who listened to her and was "invested in my life" ("Jessica's Story," n.d.).

Bridging the Gap

> An American physician is put on the spot when a Russian family in his care complains that physical therapy sessions in the United States are briefer and more superficial than those in their homeland. The physician might spring to the defense of American health care. Instead, he says, "Maybe it's not as good, but that's all we can afford. You know?" (Lo, 2010, p. 491).

In this real-life episode, the doctor bridges the gap between his experiences and his patients' by acknowledging that, indeed, theirs may be a better model. The physician later reflected that his nondefensive response seemed to help the family accept the different care model and cooperate in making the most of it (Lo, 2010).

This is one example of how patients and caregivers might meet in the middle. The trend toward preventive care might also narrow the divide between medical and lifeworld voices. Prevention is, by nature, a diffuse topic involving an array of risk factors and lifestyle decisions. Furthermore, talking about prevention is usually not as emotionally intense as talking about existing illness. Some speculate that a third voice will emerge that feels natural to both patients and professionals.

Communication Skill Builders: Talking to a Care Provider

> A middle-aged woman whose previous doctors had written off her symptoms to menopause helped her new doctor see beyond that stereotype by saying: "I know I'm in menopause, and all five doctors have told me that's the cause of my problems. And two told me that I'm crazy. And, frankly, I am a little crazy. . . . But I think this is something else, that what I'm feeling is more than just menopause" (Groopman, 2007, p. 56).

Physician Jerome Groopman shares this story in his book *How Doctors Think* (2007) as an example of how patients can, as he puts it, "help doctors think." In this case, the woman's doctor listened, and she was right. She had a rare tumor that, if left untreated, might have threatened her life.

People who are confident about their communication skills are usually more satisfied than others with the health care they receive (Chou, Wang, Finney Rutten, Moser, & Hesse, 2010). Even proficient communicators, however, may find themselves out of their depth conversing about health-related topics. Here are some tips from the experts:

- *Try the PACE method.* The acronym stands for *present information, ask questions, check your understanding,* and *express any concerns*. Patients coached to use PACE often share more information with doctors without extending the length of exams (Harrington, Norling, Witte, Taylor, & Andrews, 2007).
- *Accept medical uncertainty.* Patients may find comfort in believing that health professionals know exactly what is wrong with them, but that degree of certainty is not always possible. Sometimes the underlying causes of an illness are revealed only gradually with persistent investigation over time. Jumping to conclusions can blind both professionals and patients to the real or multiple causes of an illness. Groopman (2007) encourages patients not to criticize care providers for uncertainty or pressure them into acting more certain than they feel.
- *Ask questions.* Care providers are subject to cognitive errors and limitations, just like everyone else. Groopman (2007) admits, "Sometimes I come to the end of my thinking and am not sure what to do next" (p. 264). He encourages patients to stimulate health professionals' thinking and communication by asking such questions as, *What else could this be? What's the worst-case scenario? What should I expect next? Is it possible I have more than one problem?* and *Is there any evidence that doesn't fit?*

In the next two sections we look at factors that contribute to patient satisfaction and patient–caregiver cooperation.

Health and Identity

"The old story goes, 'When life gives you lemons, make lemonade.' But what do you do when life gives you cancer?" So begins a video by Stephen Sutton (2014), a teenage boy with incurable, advanced-stage cancer. His next words are, *"This is not a sob story. This is Stephen's story."*

Stephen's story attracted worldwide attention when, soon after his diagnosis, he uploaded to Facebook a bucket list of 46 experiences he wished to enjoy. In the 4 years before his death, Sutton accomplished nearly everything on his list and then some. He set out to raise 10,000 pounds for teens with cancer, and eventually raised 469 times that much (the equivalent of more than $7 million in the United States). He organized charity events, spoke to audiences about his life journey, recruited more than 500 people to help him set a Guinness World Record, and more. Even since Sutton's death, people have continued to raise millions in his name.

Sutton's story is not an ideal or typical illness experience. There *is* no ideal or typical experience. Although people with long-term illnesses tend to experience recognizable phases of identity management, the way they cope and define themselves is as unique as people themselves.

Identity and Facework

To understand the effects of health concerns on personal identity, consider for a moment who you are. A few words might come to mind: student, son,

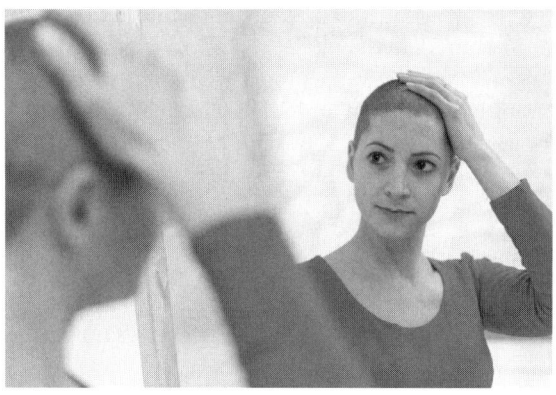

It can be difficult to reconcile one's sense of self with the physical effects of some illnesses and treatments.

Have you ever felt that an illness or injury changed the way that others regarded you, even temporarily? If so, how?

daughter, parent, athlete, kind, smart, energetic, and the like. To the extent that you and the people around you agree on these roles and descriptions, they make up your identity. **Personal identity** is a relatively enduring set of characteristics that define a person.

At first consideration, having an identity may seem easy. You simply are who you are. However, the deeper reality is that you work hard to "be" who you are. Sociologist Erving Goffman (1971a, 1971b) used the word face to describe the *self* we present to others and facework to describe the verbal and nonverbal ways that we maintain that image and collaborate in supporting (or challenging) the images of others. Like other people, you are no doubt invested in maintaining the qualities and talents that make you unique.

Communication is the primary means by which people negotiate their identities. Health concerns can make this challenging. What if your appearance or your ability to talk changed substantially? What if people began treating you differently, as in speaking loudly and slowly to you or avoiding eye contact with you? Even minor illnesses and injuries can interfere with your ability to "be" who you are.

Facework is not a simple process. Blended into your personal identity is a collection of **social identities**, characterized by perceived membership in societal groups such as "teenagers," "Asian Americans," and "retired persons" (Harwood & Sparks, 2003). Based on the groups with which you identify, you may expect yourself (and others like you) to think and behave in particular ways. For example, you may be surprised when a youthful friend reveals that she has a serious heart condition, and you may thereafter view her as "older" than her peers (Kundrat & Nussbaum, 2003). Dilemmas are also presented for people with conditions such as inflammatory bowel disease that are highly personal (Defenbaugh, 2013) and for those undergoing treatments such as chemotherapy that cause visible changes in their appearance. A woman in one study who lost her hair during cancer treatments describes looking in the mirror and alternating between two reactions: *"The reflection is not me . . . It's me . . . It's not me"* (quoted by Koszalinski & Williams, 2012, p. 119).

Sometimes, people's health status is part of their identity. Jake Harwood and Lisa Sparks (2003) call this a **tertiary identity**—a label that defines simultaneously the illness and a person's alignment toward it. For example, a participant in a leadership retreat introduced herself as, among other things, a "breast cancer survivor." The group responded with applause and hugs. Surviving cancer was treated as courageous and admirable, and group members felt a sense of intimacy that she had shared this news with them. Harwood and Sparks propose that a number of tertiary identities are available to people with the same health conditions. For example, the woman in this example might have said, "I'm a cancer victim" rather than a "survivor." It is likely that the group's reaction (and their image of her) would have been somewhat different. Perhaps even more importantly, different wording might reflect something important about the way she viewed her *own* circumstances.

If the effects of a health concern are short lived, you may not experience a serious threat to your identity. However, long-term conditions can change how you see yourself and how others treat you.

Identity and Chronic Health Concerns

Shelly's life has not been the same since she was diagnosed with and treated for cancer in her sinuses. The process has altered her appearance and left her physically frail and unable to conceive a child. Although doctors may consider her relatively "healthy" as a result of the treatment, she lives a different reality.

This true story from Laura Ellingson and Kristian Borofka's (2018) study of long-term cancer survivors illustrates tenets of the **managing meanings of embodied experiences** (**MMEE**) theory, which proposes that health is interwoven with aspects of *being* (who we are), *doing* (how we behave), and *directed becoming* (what we want to become) (Field-Springer & Margavio Striley, 2018). From this perspective, health is not a label or status, but a lived experience that involves self-image, physical ability, social identity, relational status, and more.

Communication is central to MMEE. For example, Shelly's account of life as a long-term survivor involves aspects of *being* ("I feel like such a burden" and "I feel sometimes worthless"), *doing* ("There are things I can't do anymore. I mean, we were very athletically active [before the illness] . . ."), and *directed becoming* as she wonders whether she will ever be interested in sex again and if her husband will leave her (Ellingson & Borofka, 2018, p. 5).

Individuals' reactions to a health crisis may be surprising, even to themselves. Kathy Charmaz has studied the way that people with long-term illnesses seek to reconcile their previous identities with the changed circumstances in which they find themselves. She has identified four stages common to the process:

- First, people typically take on a **supernormal identity**, determined not to let the illness stop them from being better than ever.
- The next stage is usually a sense of **restored self**, in which people are not quite as optimistic but typically deny that the illness has changed them.
- The third stage is **contingent personal identity**, in which people admit that they may not be able to do everything they could previously do and they begin to confront the consequences of a changed identity.
- The final stage, **salvaged self**, represents the development of a transformed identity that integrates former aspects of self with current limitations (Charmaz, 1987). When people are diagnosed with identity-threatening illnesses, their health status may become part of their identity as well.

Communication needs differ at every stage, and reflect some common dilemmas.

Communication Challenges

People with conditions that are chronic or hard to define may have a difficult time navigating those issues with professionals. In some cases, the challenge is to establish what is most important. For example, a patient with depression may feel that other concerns are brushed aside as psychosomatic even when they are legitimate. After studying low-income patients experiencing depression and chronic health problems, Renée Gillespie (2001) concluded that many of them "resented feeling as though they had to prove or stress how sick they 'really' were" to doctors (p. 109). Their frustration was compounded by the fear that doctors would consider them "neurotic" if they became emotional about their health concerns and frustration.

Another challenge is keeping people with chronic conditions well informed and involved in their care

(Wright Nunes et al., 2011). Some health organizations pair these patients with nurses who communicate with them regularly, help monitor their health, and support them in making healthy lifestyle choices. Patients often say that the nurses are able to spend more time with them than doctors can, and they are well qualified to monitor their health, even when nothing out of the ordinary is worrying them (Mahomed, St. John, & Patterson, 2012). Said one patient: "[The nurse] really listens to you, which is important. . . . She gives you good quality time" (Mahomed et al., p. 2544).

Communication Skill Builders: Responding to Identity Threats

Following are a few communication strategies for loved ones and health professionals that arise from awareness that a health crisis can be experienced as an identity challenge:

- *Listen*. People use narratives to convey, establish, and negotiate their identities. Listening is often the best thing you can do.
- *Look below the surface*. People who seem to be upbeat and "taking it well" may be hiding deeper feelings or harboring unrealistic expectations.
- *Expect varied reactions*. Sometimes people are determined to "beat" an illness, as if it's an enemy. At other times, they may feel their condition is degrading or unfair. Or they might feel relieved that it's not worse or simply glad to know what's going on.
- *Honor the importance of multiple perspectives*. When physical treatment goals are at odds with identity goals, as they often are, communicate openly and collaboratively about the differences. Honor the importance of multiple perspectives.
- *Be careful about the words you use*. Survivor supports a different identity than *victim*, and so on. Also pay attention to the words other people use. These may present openings for conversation, as in, "*You refer to yourself as 'a crip' since the accident. Do you feel that people treat you that way?*"

Stephen Sutton, whose story began this section, ultimately said that his goal was to show people "what it's like to have something go wrong with your life but not to be defined by it" (Sutton, 2014). Not everyone goes through every stage or spends the same amount of time in each stage. However, Charmaz's model illustrates that people actively work to manage their identity when illness or injury threatens the "self" they normally project.

In the next two sections we look at factors that contribute to patient satisfaction and patient–provider cooperation.

Satisfaction

A physician committed to empowering patients was initially at a loss when an immigrant patient wanted him to simply tell her what to do, even after he laid out the pros and cons of various treatment options. Then he arrived at a solution: He said to the patient, "I'm going to tell you what I would advise for my own mother. . . . But in America we don't make you do things. So now you have to adjust to the fact that we don't make you do things."

This encounter, described by Ming-Cheng Miriam Lo (2010, p. 491), reflects a blend of perspectives that satisfied both participants. It underscores that communication is at the heart of satisfying interactions. And the stakes are high. Satisfied patients are more likely than others to trust care providers, engage in follow-up care, and follow treatment advice (Fico & Lagoe, 2018). Patient satisfaction is often a good reflection of quality. In hospitals where patients are highly satisfied, health outcomes are better and hospital stays shorter (Tsai, Orav, & Jha, 2015). That benefits everyone involved *and* the budget.

Patient satisfaction is more closely linked to providers' communication than to their technical skills (Tarrant, Windridge, Boulton, Baker, & Freeman, 2003). This may be because it's difficult to judge technical skills and because people tend to assume that health professionals are technically competent. It may also reflect how important communication skills are to diagnosis and treatment.

First, let's consider what *not* to do in terms of communication. A sense of being undervalued or overlooked is particularly displeasing to patients. The following communication approaches tend to give a bad impression:

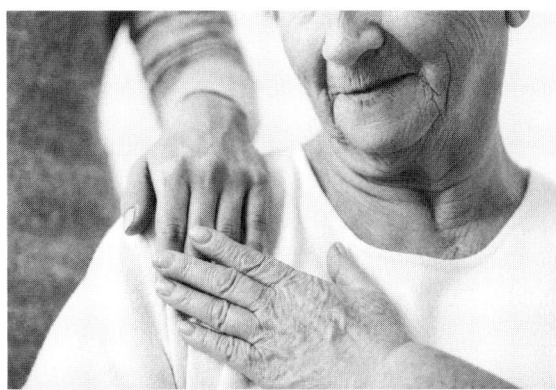

The term *patient* connotes a person in ill health who seeks the services of a care provider. Some theorists suggest that the terms *health citizen*, *health decision maker*, and *health client* are preferable because they acknowledge that people are involved in health care all the time, not just when they seek professional assistance.

Do you feel the term patient *is accurate when describing well people seeking to maintain their own health? Brainstorm some other terms we might use. Which is your favorite?*

- *Lack of explanation.* People are frustrated when they experience long waits and excessive red tape without knowing why (Bleustein, Valaitis, & Jones, 2010; Fenton, Jerant, Bertakis, & Franks, 2012). An apology or explanation can ease that frustration considerably.
- *Curt, discourteous, or disrespectful communication.* Patients say they resent it when caregivers neglect to introduce themselves or when they ignore them, seem disinterested, or talk down to them. Some patients also prefer not to be addressed by first name (Milika & Trorey, 2008).
- *Invasions of privacy.* Patients say they feel dishonored when staff members allow them to be physically exposed to others and when others can read or overhear their private information. Physician John Egerton (2007) had a rule for the front-office staff: "Avoid mentioning the patient's name and diagnosis in the same sentence" (Milika & Trorey, 2008, para. 6.) For instance, never say, "John Smith has prostatitis again" or "Helen Will has head lice" (para. 6). Naturally, caregivers must discuss patients and their conditions, but they should do so in private.

- *Feeling rushed and bewildered.* Patients resent it when professionals use words they don't understand and when they seem to be in a hurry. These two often go hand in hand. One care provider interviewed said she tends to use medical jargon to save time, even when she knows patients will not understand it (Dahm, 2012, p. 684). Patients in the same study said they pick up on the urgency and tend to stay quiet about their questions. As one patient put it: "There is just a whole line of people . . . You don't wanna keep the doctor up in saying 'oh what does this mean?'" (p. 685). Ironically, the resulting misunderstandings can take more time than a clear explanation would have.

On the bright side, the following communication approaches are known to *enhance* patient satisfaction:

- *Expressions of empathy.* Nothing beats a sense of being heard and respected. Patients want to know they can speak freely and that their doctors will not turn against them if they seek second opinions (Jadad & Rizo, 2003).
- *Information.* Patients appreciate feeling well informed about their conditions and treatment (Jangland, Gunningberg, & Carlsson, 2009). Some also say they would appreciate it if physicians were more forthcoming about the costs of various options (Brick, Scherr, & Ubel, 2019).
- *A sense of control.* Although people appreciate doctors' advice, only about 20% of patients want their caregivers to make decisions without them (Deloitte, 2008). This applies to everyday decisions as well as major treatment options. One hospital patient said he appreciates it when nurses who bathe him wash body areas he cannot reach and then ask, "Would you like to do the rest for yourself?" (quoted in Milika & Trorey, 2008, p. 2713).

Researchers Alejandro Jadad and Carlos Rizo (2003) conclude that, "in most cases it would not take fancy technology, extra time, or increased costs to satisfy what patients 'want.' It would take only an assertive patient and a confident healthcare provider who is willing to listen" (para. 6). See Box 4.2 for ethical considerations involved in judging a health care experience.

BOX 4.2   Ethical Consideration

Does Satisfaction Reflect Quality?

In a *New York Times* editorial, oncology nurse Theresa Brown (2012) proposes that a focus on patient satisfaction might diminish the quality of medical care. She worries that health professionals might cut back on painful, but important, procedures and overinvest in pleasing amenities that do not improve health outcomes. "Evaluating hospital care in terms of its ability to offer positive experiences could easily put pressure on the system to do things it can't, at the expense of what it should," says Brown (para. 11).

What Do You Think?

1. Would you be more likely to rate medical care more favorably if it's pleasant? Why or why not?
2. Do you think it is more effective to rate health care centers on the basis of health outcomes or on patient satisfaction? Why?
3. What do you say to those who feel that ratings based on health outcomes will penalize health care centers and professionals who take on high-risk and end-of-life cases?
4. In your opinion, what's the best way to rate the effectiveness of health care?

Cooperation and Consent

Tiger Woods limped up the sloping hill of Torrey Pines golf course in 2008. He made the final shot to finish one stroke ahead of his nearest competitor after a grueling playoff in a golf tournament that included 91 holes. Woods won the tournament, thrilling fans but confounding his doctors, who had urged him not to play because of a knee injury.

In this respect Tiger Woods is not so different from the majority of us. Although we are unlikely to challenge our doctors' advice in person, only about 50% of us follow medical advice completely or most of the time (Hall, Tangka, Sabatino, Thompson, Graubard, & Breen, 2018; Neiman et al., 2017).

As Michael Burgoon and Judee Burgoon (1990) observe, it's curious that we do not follow medical advice more closely, considering that we pay for the advice, presumably stand to benefit from it, and typically revere the expertise of medical professionals. In this next section we explore some of the reasons why we may not follow through. Then we examine health professionals' stake in treatment outcomes and policies concerning informed consent. (See Box 4.3 for more resources about related careers.)

BOX 4.3   Career Opportunities

Patient Advocacy

Case manager
Patient advocate
Patient care coordinator or consultant
Patient navigator
Social worker

Career Resources and Job Listings

- Patient Advocate Foundation: www.patientadvocate.org
- National Patient Advocate Foundation: www.npaf.org
- Patient Navigator Outreach and Chronic Disease Prevention Demonstration Program: http://bhpr.hrsa.gov/nursing/grants/patientnavigator.html
- National Association of Social Workers: www.socialworkers.org
- Council on Social Work Education: www.cswe.org
- Case Management Society of America: www.cmsa.org
- National Organization for Human Services: www.nationalhumanservices.org
- U.S. Bureau of Labor Statistics Occupational Outlook Handbook: www.bls.gov/ooh

Reasons for Noncooperation

If patients don't follow medical advice, it doesn't necessarily mean they are lazy or indifferent about their health. A number of more legitimate concerns may affect their decisions.

For one, medical recommendations may be impossible or impractical to carry out. A person may be unable to afford prescribed medications or may be physically incapable of performing suggested routines. For example, people who miss dialysis treatments often report that no one is available to drive them to and from appointments (Gordon, Leon, & Sehgal, 2003). Likewise, people with low incomes may have little choice concerning their exposure to "avoidable" health threats. As Gillespie (2001) describes it:

> Low-income families live in older homes filled with lifetimes of dust and molding timber. They breathe the air polluted by factories that never cease production and by the cars of daily downtown professionals who sleep in clean, suburban air each night. Often depressed, they are more likely to smoke and less likely to eat well. Many sleep on the floor, knowing that the asthma this triggers could kill them, but afraid that a stray bullet shot through the window will do so sooner. (p. 114)

In other situations, recommended regimens may be so foreign to people that they cannot easily integrate them into their lifestyles. For instance, it may seem inconceivable to remove red meat completely from one's diet. Or, like Tiger Woods, people may feel that some goals and obligations are too important to miss, even if it means risking a personal illness or injury.

Second, people may not agree with health professionals' assessments or treatment recommendations. Research suggests that people are likely to distrust diagnoses and ignore medical advice if they are not able to describe their concerns during medical visits (Zhong, Nie, Xie, & Liu, 2019). People may also deny diagnoses that threaten their self-image. It may be difficult to admit obesity, hearing loss, depression, sexually transmitted infections, and the like.

Third, people may stop medical routines prematurely if they perceive that they have no effect or if their symptoms cease (Hamdidouche et al., 2017). For example, it's difficult to convince people to continue treatment for conditions such as high blood pressure because they cannot directly perceive that the medicine has a positive effect.

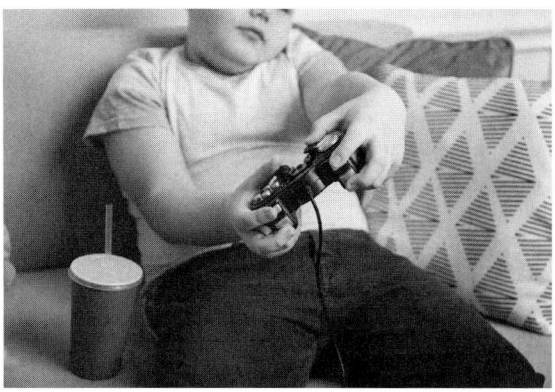

A variety of factors sometimes make unhealthy choices appealing.

When are you tempted to do things you know to be unhealthy? Why?

Finally, patients may stop taking medication if they experience unpleasant side effects (Emilsson, Gustafsson, Ohnstrom, & Marteinsdottir, 2017) or if they don't believe it will help (Makarem, Smith, Mudambi, & Hunt, 2014). Under those circumstances, they may try other methods or conclude that the cure is worse than the disease.

These factors are exacerbated when care providers do not encourage patients to express their concerns and reservations at the time they give medical advice. Evidence suggests that many people leave their doctors' offices knowing they cannot or will not follow through with the advice given, but they do not feel free to say so. Doctors who assume that patients should follow orders regardless of their circumstances may be discouraged when treatment outcomes are less than optimal. And, if people do not feel comfortable talking with a care provider, they may not fess up later that they did not follow their advice.

Care Providers' Investment

It may be tempting to assume that, if patients do not follow medical advice, they have only themselves to blame. But health professionals may be blamed as well. Lack of patient–provider cooperation often results in harmful health outcomes. Nonadherence is linked to diabetes treatment failures (Mizobe & Fukuda, 2016), increased hospitalization for heart failure (Gilotra et al., 2017), and asthma-related complications and deaths (Papi et al., 2018), to name just a few. These are not just patients' problems.

Care providers' careers may be damaged by excessive treatment failures. With capitation and restricted reimbursements, health care organizations lose money on patients who do not improve as expected. Consequently, hospitals may refuse to grant physicians privileges if their treatment outcomes are below par, and medical groups may deny them employment for the same reason. Health professionals' reputations among patients may suffer as well. Physician Wesley Sugai says he does not treat patients who chronically ignore medical advice without explanation:

> As a rural solo pediatrician, I have neither the time nor the desire to try to convince parents about the importance of childhood immunizations, follow-up with specialists, or medications.... I tell parents that I have to be able to trust them to carry out the treatment plan, just as they must trust me to prescribe the proper therapy. If neither of us trusts the other, then the patient-doctor relationship is nonexistent and we must go our separate ways. (Sugai, 2008, p. 14)

Sugai says that he does work with patients who are up front about reservations or limitations that affect their health behaviors. All in all, it's important for everyone that patients who cannot follow treatment advice or who do not agree with it feel comfortable admitting that and negotiating more suitable options.

Public health is at stake as well. Good communication and healthy behaviors can avert epidemics and reduce the incidence of avoidable illnesses and injuries. In the United States, the cost of preventable hospitalizations is about $25 billion per year, equal to nearly 10% of total health costs (United Health Foundation, 2015). Analyst Bill Clements (1996) advises, "Make no mistake about it: Bad communication costs you money" (para. 3).

Considering these factors, how far should health professionals go to gain patients' cooperation? Some medical centers are implementing ways to stay in touch with patients between visits and treat them as partners in decision making. As the next section illustrates, over time, public policy has changed concerning patients' role in medical decisions.

Informed Consent

For centuries, physicians considered it wise to tell patients only as much as they could understand (in the doctors' opinion) and nothing that might dissuade them from following medical advice (Chapter 3). For example, if a doctor judged that the potential advantages of a drug outweighed its possible side effects, the doctor might not tell the patient about side effects, for fear the patient would not take the drug (J. Katz, 1995). Likewise, although doctors have always been required to get patients' permission before they operated on them, they have not been required to tell patients about the risks involved.

In most cases physicians were presumably following their best judgment. In some cases, however, patients were subjected to risks, even to deadly medical experiments and exploitation, without their knowledge. At particular risk have been members of some racial and ethnics groups and financially impoverished members of society. One example is the **Tuskegee Syphilis Study** conducted in Alabama (Box 4.4). Another famous case involves Henrietta Lacks, an African American mother of five who died of cervical cancer in 1951. But "not all of Henrietta Lacks died that day," explains her family ("The Lacks Family," 2012, para. 1). Lacks's cancer cells had the unprecedented ability to live and multiply in a laboratory environment. Without

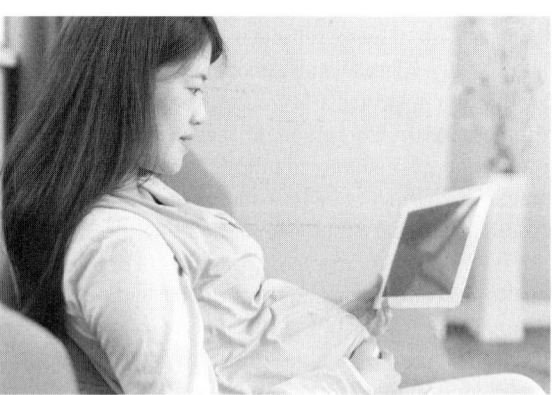

Videos about treatment options can help people become well informed about risks and benefits before they decide whether to consent to treatment.

Have you ever said yes to treatments when you were unsure about potential side effects? If so, what factors led you to say yes?

Lacks's consent, medical researchers kept some of her cells, multiplied and cloned them, and shared them with colleagues worldwide. To date, scientists have grown 50 million metric tons of Lacks's cells (known by the code name HeLa) and have used them as the basis for some of the most transformational medical breakthroughs in history, including a vaccine for polio, and treatments for cancer, herpes, leukemia, Parkinson's disease, AIDS, and more (Margonelli, 2010; Silver, 2013). The Lacks family was not informed about the use of her cells for more than 20 years, and they have never received proceeds from the sale of her organic material (worth tens of millions of dollars and counting). The upshot is that the Lacks family is still unable to "afford access to the health care advances their mother's cells made possible" (Henrietta Lacks Foundation, 2015, para. 3).

Public outrage over the Tuskegee Syphilis Study and others like it led the U.S. government to pass informed-consent laws. **Informed consent** means that patients must (a) be made fully aware of known treatment risks, benefits, and options; (b) be deemed capable of understanding such information and making a responsible judgment; and (c) be aware that they may refuse to participate or may cease treatment at any time (Ashley & O'Rourke, 1997). When patients are children or are otherwise unable to make decisions, close family members may be allowed to consent on their behalf.

Informed-consent requirements are designed to allow patients enough information so that they can make knowledgeable judgments about their own care. Some theorists believe that health care should go even further toward including patients in treatment decisions. As early as 1973, medical analyst Harold Walker predicted that doctors would become less authoritarian and more persuasive. The difference is subtle but important. From an authoritarian perspective, patients are expected to *comply* with doctors' orders. From a persuasive perspective, however, patients take an active role in decision making. They *cooperate* in the process as informed and influential participants.

If people are included in decision making as patients, it may be possible to overcome or accommodate many of the factors that have kept them from following medical advice. The health professional who is aware of a patient's financial and physical limitations, cultural reservations, denial, or discouragement is better able to negotiate acceptable options with them. At the very least, patients and caregivers can establish outright what each is willing to do. This may ultimately be less frustrating than allowing their differences to go unspoken.

Informed consent is a victory for patient empowerment. However, the terms are sometimes hard to apply, even when people try hard to do so. For example, a long list of complications (many of them extremely unlikely) might result from a simple procedure. It may be impractical or impossible to list every possible outcome. However, physicians may be accused of negligence if an unlikely outcome results and the patient was not warned about it in advance. Language differences also present challenges. It is sometimes difficult to understand medical and legal terminology. In focus groups, Spanish speakers in the United States with literacy challenges said that consent and privacy forms that had been translated into Spanish were too long and wordy, the fine print aroused their suspicious, and they felt rushed to comply without fully understanding the forms or discussing them with family members (Cortés, Drainoni, Henault, & Paasche-Orlow, 2010). (We talk more about health literacy challenges in Chapter 6.)

On the bright side, when they are available, multimedia presentations about medical procedures often increase understanding prior to informed consent. Melissa Wanzer and colleagues invited the parents and guardians of children who were recommended for endoscopies to view a four-minute video about hospital procedures and an interactive presentation about informed consent, including optional voice-over and a true-false quiz they could take as many times as they liked at their own pace. Compared to parents and guardians who simply reviewed informed consent forms with a physician, those who took part in the multimedia presentation understood more about the procedure and were subsequently less anxious about it and more satisfied with the care their children received (Wanzer et al., 2010).

Partly because complete disclosure is so difficult to define, the courts have been reluctant to hold physicians responsible for informed-consent violations except in clear-cut cases. See Box 4.4 for ethical implications concerning informed consent.

BOX 4.4 Ethical Considerations

Patients' Right to Informed Consent

During the infamous Tuskegee Syphilis Study, which began in 1932, some 600 African American men were enrolled without their knowledge in a medical experiment. They were patients of the Public Health Service in Macon County, Alabama, and the experiment was conducted by the U.S. government through the Tuskegee Institute in Alabama.

Although medical researchers knew that 399 of the men had syphilis, the men were not told. Doctors simply told all the men they had "bad blood" and provided them with medicine, meals, and burial expenses. However, the medicine was not really medicine at all. It was a harmless but ineffectual placebo.

The study was designed to help medical researchers learn more about the effects of syphilis among African Americans. Syphilis is a sexually transmitted disease that affects the bones, liver, heart, and central nervous system. In advanced stages, it can cause open sores, heart damage, tumors, blindness, mental illness, and death. When the study was begun, there was no effective treatment for syphilis. However, by 1940, penicillin was known to be effective at treating and even curing it.

The syphilis patients in the Tuskegee experiment were not given penicillin. Instead, researchers continued to watch the disease progress until the experiment was called off in 1972, some 40 years after it began.

When details of the Tuskegee study were made public, there was an angry outcry. Some likened it to the Nazis' medical experiments on Jewish prisoners during World War II. The courts eventually ordered the federal government to pay the men and their families a total of $10 million for the injury and indignity they had suffered. Twenty-five years after the end of the experiment, President Bill Clinton publicly apologized for the government's behavior.

Now, before patients are given medical treatment (experimental or otherwise), they must be fully informed, give consent, and be aware that they can cease treatment at any time. It is hoped that informed consent will prevent atrocities such as the Tuskegee Syphilis Study. But informed consent is sometimes hard to apply. Jauhar (2008) describes the ethical challenges of informed consent in some instances:

[An] issue I continue to struggle with today is how to balance patient autonomy with the physician's obligation to do the best for his patient. As a doctor, when do you let your patient make a bad decision: When, if ever, do you draw the line? What if a decision could cost your patient's life? How hard do you push him to change his mind? At the same time, it's his life. Who are you to tell him how to live? (p. 233)

Jauhar (2008) describes a particularly difficult case when a hospital patient, Mr. Smith, began to cough up blood and have trouble breathing. His condition quickly deteriorated, and doctors knew they would have to act quickly to save his life. Their only hope was to insert a temporary breathing tube. But the patient adamantly refused. In his mind, being intubated seemed a worse fate than death. Mr. Smith's fear seemed irrational, yet he was coherent and capable of communicating—thus he was capable of giving (or refusing) informed consent. As the doctor responsible for Mr. Smith's care, Jauhar faced a dilemma. He could honor the patient's wishes and allow him to die, or he could overrule the patient and insert the breathing tube by force. What would you have done?

Jauhar chose to insert the breathing tube, although the staff had to restrain Mr. Smith physically to do it. During the procedure Jauhar worried that the patient would hate him for disobeying his wishes. "'If you live through this,' I whispered to Mr. Smith, 'I hope you can forgive me'" (Jauhar, 2008, pp. 236–237). Two weeks later, as Mr. Smith neared recovery, Jauhar stopped by his room and told the patient he was responsible for the decision. The patient considered his response for a moment. "I've been through a lot," he finally said, his voice still hoarse from two weeks of intubation. . . . "But thank you" (p. 237). This is an extreme case, but it illustrates some of the ethical dilemmas involved in informed consent.

What Do You Think?

1. Do you agree with Jauhar's decision? Why or why not? What would you have done in his place?

continued

2. Sometimes medical information is difficult to understand fully. How should we establish if the consenting person is informed enough to give consent?
3. Some people, such as those with terminal illnesses, are willing (even anxious) to try untested therapies. Researchers may not know what results to expect, and they may even anticipate negative outcomes. Who should decide whether the patient undergoes untested therapies? Should public money be used in these cases?
4. In medical research, is it ever justified to deceive people (as in giving placebos) to make sure they are not just responding to the power of suggestion? If so, under what conditions?
5. Sometimes it is in the best interest of society or health care workers to know if a person has a contagious disease (such as AIDS). If the person doesn't consent to a test for that disease, do you think it should be permissible to perform the test without the person's knowledge? (A vial of blood may be used for a variety of tests without the patient knowing it.)
6. On what grounds, if any, should health professionals judge whether a patient is emotionally capable of making a life-or-death judgment about emergency treatment?

Summary

Patient Socialization

- In contrast to the well-established ways in which caregivers are socialized, people learn how to be patients mostly through life experience and watching others.
- Patients often communicate in hesitant and nonassertive ways because they are uncertain what is expected of them and afraid to seem rude or ignorant.

Voice of Lifeworld

- Although a professional may conceive of health as a biological phenomenon to be identified by its physical manifestations, patients are more likely to interpret illnesses in light of their effects on everyday activities.
- The Voice of Lifeworld is concerned with feelings and events.

Health and Identity

- Patients' communication and their willingness to self-advocate are influenced by a variety of factors, including the nature of their illnesses, their personalities, and their communication skills.
- Illness can affect people's very identity. Evidence suggests that people work to maintain their identities, even when illness changes their patterns of behavior.

Patient Satisfaction

- Patient satisfaction is often based more on how caregivers listen and empathize than on patients' perception of their technical competency.
- People typically prefer care providers who seem interested, caring, and sympathetic.
- They also appreciate having a sense of control and being treated with dignity.

Cooperation and Consent

- People's adherence to medical advice is surprisingly low for a range of reasons, including limited money and resources, mistrust of the diagnosis or treatment plan, a sense that the illness is cured, and a perception that the treatment is worse than the disease.
- Although patients may have good reasons for not following medical advice, the results can be disastrous for them, for health professionals, and for the public.
- Many health advocates urge patients and professionals to be more explicit about negotiating treatment options that are practical and acceptable.
- Ethical principles and U.S. laws stipulate that patients be well informed about health choices and allowed to decide for themselves what care they will and will not receive.
- Informed-consent laws protect people from atrocities such as the Tuskegee Syphilis Study, but some cases fall within a gray zone in which it is difficult to determine when patients are too distraught or fearful to make informed choices.

Glossary

contingent personal identity A stage of identity management in which a person with a serious illness admits that they may not be able to do everything they could do previously and begins to confront the consequences of a changed identity. *See page 69.*

informed consent The requirement that patients must (a) be made fully aware of known treatment risks, benefits, and options; (b) be deemed capable of understanding such information and making a responsible judgment; and (c) be aware that they may refuse to participate or may cease treatment at any time. *See page 75.*

managing meanings of embodied experiences (MMEE) The theory that health is interwoven with aspects of *being* (who a person is), *doing* (how that person behaves), and *directed becoming* (what that person wants to become). *See page 69.*

personal identity A relatively enduring set of characteristics that define a person. *See page 69.*

restored self A stage of identity management in which a person with a serious illness is less optimistic than in the supernormal stage but typically denies that the illness has changed them. *See page 69.*

salvaged self A stage of identity management in which a person with a serious illness develops a transformed identity that integrates former aspects of self with current limitations. *See page 69.*

social identities Characterizations associated with membership in different societal groups such as "teenagers," "Asian Americans," or "retired persons." *See page 68.*

supernormal identity A stage of identity management in which a person with a serious illness is determined not to let the illness stop them from being better than ever. *See page 69.*

tertiary identity A sense of self that simultaneously addressed an illness and a person's alignment toward it (e.g. breast cancer survivor). *See page 68.*

Tuskegee Syphilis Study An infamous study conducted in which African American men were enrolled without their knowledge in a medical experiment, and many were allowed to experience the devastating effects of syphilis even after a cure had been discovered for it. *See page 74.*

Voice of Lifeworld A way of communicating (often by patients) that is primarily concerned with health and illness as they relate to everyday experiences. *See page 65.*

Discussion Questions

1. Write a paragraph about a health concern you or someone you know has experienced. Does your description mostly reflect the Voice of Lifeworld or the Voice of Medicine? How?

2. If you were a care provider and a patient felt the treatment advice you gave her was unlikely to work, would you want to know about her reservations? Why or why not? What is the best way the patient might express her disagreement?

3. Imagine a scenario in which someone you love has been having agonizing headaches and doctors cannot figure out what is wrong. Write down several communication options that incorporate Jerome Groopman's (2007) advice to patients.

4. Think of the most dissatisfying health experience you have ever experienced. Create two columns on a sheet of paper. On the left side, write down what happened. On the right side, rewrite the experience to be more satisfying. What would you change? Why?

5. Have you ever stopped taking prescription medicine before you were supposed to or missed a dosage? Have you engaged in unhealthy habits you would rather not admit to your doctor? If so, what factors affected your decision? Do any of the factors covered in this chapter apply to your situation? If so, which ones?

6. Imagine that someone close to you is diagnosed with diabetes and will have to radically alter his diet and take insulin injections every day. How might this affect his personal identity? His tertiary identity? If he perceives this to be a serious threat to his identity, what phases might he experience, as reflected in Charmaz's (1987) model of identity management?

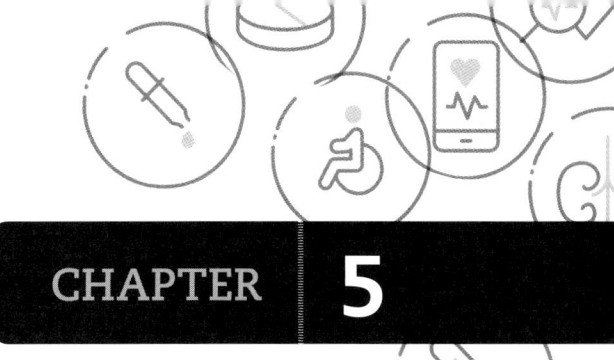

CHAPTER 5

Care Provider Perspectives

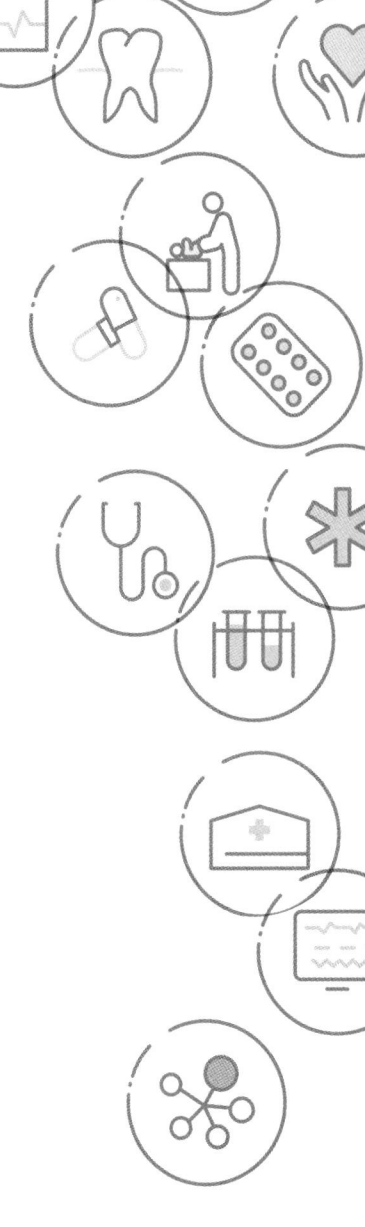

Health care executive Fred Lee remembers a moment when a nurse's comment made the difference between despair and hope. His mother had been badly injured in an automobile accident, and as Lee stood by her bed, he feared that the intensive care team might forbid him from remaining there. Instead, the nurse smiled and said, "My, my, my, you should see what your touch just did to your mother's vital signs. It's amazing. We need you here all of the time!" (Lee, 2004, pp. 61–62)

This story illustrates many facets of modern-day medicine. Health care is a mix of life-saving technology, institutional rules and guidelines, and, at its best, a deep appreciation for the role that compassion, love, and touch play. The example also points to the powerful role of communication. Lee reflects: "Could she [the nurse] have come up with a more perfectly timed thing to say? It was as if she had read my mind and in one gracious comment had made me feel needed and welcome, an essential part of the healing team" (p. 62).

Lee's experience brings to mind the privileges and challenges of working every day with human life. Health care providers—whether they are technicians, physical therapists, dentists, pharmacists, physicians, or another of the many professionals we will discuss in this chapter—experience many of the same challenges and rewards while communicating with people who need their help. (See Box 5.1 for career options in patient care.)

In this chapter we look at health care from the diverse perspectives of professional care providers. We begin at the beginning, following the path of care providers-in-training through educational experiences and into the professional domain. Along the way we focus on the ways that communication is influenced by time, maturity, mindfulness, confidence, and satisfaction. Then we conclude with discussion of three key issues: stress and burnout, medical mistakes, and interprofessional teamwork.

BOX 5.1 Career Opportunities

Care Providers

Dentists, Hygienists, and Assistants
The number of jobs for *dental hygienists* and *dental assistants* is expected to increase 11% (much higher than average) by the year 2028. A 7% increase in demand (higher than average) is expected for *dentists*.

Doctors of Medicine and Osteopathy
Job growth for *medical doctors, osteopaths,* and *surgeons* is expected to increase by 7%. Need is particularly high in low-income communities.

Emergency Personnel
The job outlook for *emergency medical technicians* and *paramedics* is good, with the need expected to rise 7% by 2028.

Midlevel Providers
Demand for *physician assistants* and *nurse practitioners* is especially high, with a 26% increase expected.

Mental Health Professionals
An 14% increase is expected for *psychologists*, an 11% increase for *social workers*, and a 29% increase for *substance abuse, behavioral disorder, and mental health counselors*.

Nurses
Employment growth of 12% is expected for *registered nurses* (RNs), reflecting the demand for prevention, care for chronic conditions, and aging patients. RNs have associate's or bachelor's degrees in nursing and are state licensed. Demand will increase 11% for *licensed practical nurses* (LPN) and *licensed vocational nurses* (LVN), who usually complete a year or so of specialized training after high school.

Physical Rehabilitation Professionals
Physical, recreational, occupational, respiratory, and *speech-language therapy* positions are expected to increase by 18% to 27%. Positions for *assistants* and *aides* in these fields should increase as much as 26%.

Physical Fitness and Diet Specialists
The number of jobs for *dieticians, nutritionists,* and *exercise physiologists* is expected to grow at least 10%, along with 19% growth for *athletic trainers*, and 22% growth for *massage therapists*.

Pharmacists and Pharmacy Technicians
Jobs for *pharmacists* are expected to hold steady at current levels, and jobs for *pharmacy technicians* to increase by about 7%.

Technicians and Technologists
Job growth between 9% and 12% is predicted for *medical records* and *health information technicians, psychiatric technicians, surgical technologists, radiation technologists,* and *clinical laboratory technicians*.

Source: U.S. Bureau of Labor Statistics. (2019). *Healthcare occupations*. Washington, DC: Author. Retrieved from https://www.bls.gov/ooh/healthcare/home.htm

Care Provider Preparation

"It was one of the most anxiety-inducing moments I'd experienced in my medical training—my first real patient interview. I had interviewed mock patients and had rehearsed questions and physical exams many times. I had trained for it, but this was different. This was real. A 65-year-old Vietnam veteran looked back at me when I entered the exam room. Could he trust me, a 23-year old medical student, to diagnose and treat him? Would I do a good job?"

These musings by physician Fisayo Ositelu (2015) evoke the hopes and uncertainties of learning to be a professional care provider. In this section, we consider how educational experiences influence the way health professionals communicate.

Historical Perspective

To understand the care provider education system, let's rewind history a bit. In the United States prior to 1900, most medical schools were run as private businesses, oriented more toward profit than to providing high-quality education (Cassedy, 1991).

Things changed in the early 1990s, when reformers called for a more rigorous focus on biology and other sciences, as well as more hands-on experience with patients. About two-thirds of medical schools closed, unable to meet the reform standards (Twaddle

& Hessler, 1987). Most that remained open were incorporated within universities. Curricula began to focus intensely on organic aspects of disease as well as clinical and laboratory experience.

University-based nursing schools started becoming widely available in the early 1900s as well. Previously, nurses (mostly women) had been expected to care for loved ones at home or to learn on the job without much formal training (Judd & Sitzman, 2014). Specialized knowledge paved the way for them to become more active partners in patient care.

Scientific aptitude became a key consideration in medical and nursing schools, and to varying degrees, in other care provider education programs. Few people question the value of that, but many critics feel that medical programs have not always devoted enough attention to communication skills such as listening, sharing bad news (Zakrzewski, Ho, & Braga-Mele, 2008), shared decision making (D'Agostino et al., 2017; Rodriguez et al., 2008), and cultural sensitivity (Joo, Jimenez, Xu, & Park, 2019).

The Role of Communication

"Effective communication skills are at the heart of quality patient care" and are essential to relationship building, leadership, and teamwork, say spokespersons for the Accreditation Council on Graduate Medical Education (ACGME, 2015, p. 20). As you learned in Chapter 4, communication skills are essential to building trust, sharing information, diagnosing what is wrong, and partnering with patients in prevention and treatment efforts. As you will see in this chapter, communication is important for other reasons as well. Health professionals who do not feel confident about their communication skills are more likely than others to experience frustration and burnout, to be sued, and to leave the profession (Boodman, 1997; Brett, Branstetter, & Wagner, 2014; Tourangeau & Cranley, 2005).

Communication can't work miracles, but it can make a substantial difference. Patient satisfaction scores tend to rise when care providers take part in communication training, because those who take part tend to provide clearer information, show more empathy, and address a greater variety of patients' lifestyle behaviors than others (Allenbaugh, Corbelli, Rack, Rubio, & Spagnoletti, 2019; Haskard et al., 2008; H. Wang et al., 2018). Likewise, after training, care providers are typically more confident about their ability to interact effectively with patients, even in difficult conversations (Jin et al., 2019). As a result of such factors, effective communication can help reduce costs, improve patient satisfaction, and minimize mistakes and misunderstandings (Epstein, Fiscella, Lesser, & Stange, 2010).

At the end of this section, we consider curriculum reforms and teaching techniques that place a greater emphasis on communication than in years past. But first, let's consider the socialization process involved in becoming a professional care provider.

Socialization

> "Dental school feels like flying a fighter jet, while undergrad was like riding a bicycle. Each week we have new materials and more exams coming at us. It is important not to fall behind, because it would just create the snowball effect."
> —Kai Ta Huang (2017, para. 4)

Becoming a health care provider is partly a matter of studying hard. It's also a process of **socialization**—learning to behave appropriately within a specific community. School is often the first place people begin to learn what it means to act and talk like

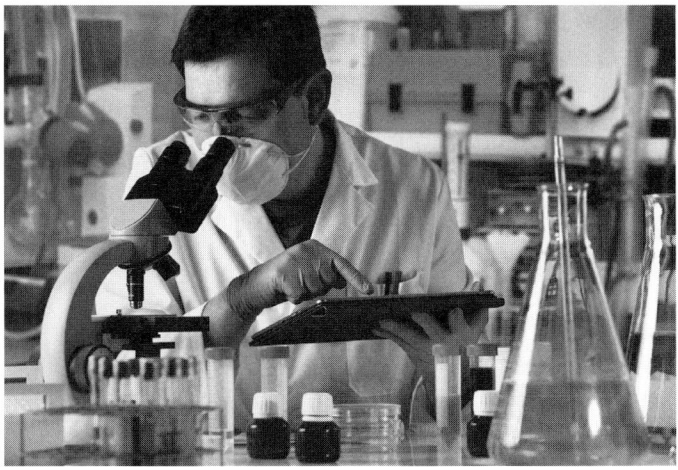

In the early 1990s, medicine came to be viewed mostly in terms of science.

Taking nothing away from science, what other skills would you like care providers to be good at?

a professional caregiver. Few other experiences are so extensive and life altering. The intensity, uniqueness, and isolation make high-intensity caregiver education programs especially hospitable arenas for socialization.

VOICE OF MEDICINE

One impact of socialization into a specialized community such as health care is that members, once socialized, may have expectations and practices that differ substantially from other people's. In Chapter 3 we talked about the Voice of Lifeworld that is typically spoken by patients. In contrast, care providers in the United States are expected to be proficient in what Elliot Mishler (1984) calls the **Voice of Medicine**. As the vocabulary of traditional biomedicine, this voice is characterized by carefully controlled compassion and a concern for accuracy and expediency.

The Voice of Medicine is designed to help people. One limitation, however, is that it is not designed to facilitate emotional expression. Instead, it focuses mostly on medical terminology and physical details. For the most part, patients' individuality is treated as less important than their bodily conditions. However impersonal it may sound, the Voice of Medicine answers to the extraordinary demands of time and emotion exacted from health professionals and suits society's image of them as stoically objective and in control.

The Voice of Lifeworld and the Voice of Medicine sometimes complement each other. A patient's account of an illness may be consistent with a biomedical focus on symptoms and functioning. At other times, the two perspectives present what some scholars call *dualism*, a tension between conceptually incompatible ways of thinking or behaving. Care providers may find themselves in a quandary about whether to focus on patients' "stories" (e.g., narratives and lived experiences) or their "data" (e.g., test results and vital signs) (Olufowote & Wang, 2017, p. 679). Focusing on both may be ideal, but it's not always easy. As one medical school educator tells medical students, "We don't [just] want you to take a medical history we want you to be curious about what it's like for them to have cancer" (p. 680).

This medicine/lifeworld dualism is sometimes conceptualized as the difference between the science of medicine and the art of medicine. Some care providers feel that honoring both yields the most satisfying results for all involved. Physician Denis Cortese puts it this way:

> The artist knows when the patient needs a warm smile, reassuring words, or a gentle hug. It's the artists who make every patient feel welcome, comfortable, secure, hopeful. The artist sees the anxiety and reassures the new mother that her baby's fever is nothing to worry about. . . . The artist knows when there's nothing more the engineer can do and helps the patient and family cope at the end of life. What the artist does is why I became a physician. (quoted by Berry & Seltman, 2008)

Let's trace some of the factors that influence the socialization process as we move out of the classroom and into clinical environments. As you will see, this going-public phase is an important step in donning the identity of professional care provider.

HIDDEN CURRICULUM

Socialization occurs partly as a result of the **hidden curriculum**—that is, the attitudes and practices that others model, even though they do not explicitly teach them. As medical professor Michael Wilkes says:

> We can teach extensively about the appropriateness of respecting different cultures, different beliefs and different health practices, but when the student hears a resident dissing a patient's mistaken notions of disease, or hears them making fun of a patient's body, the lesson is clear—to be a part of the "club," this is the expected behavior. (quoted by Lauer, 2008, p. 50)

Wilkes and others warn that, very often, seeing is doing when it comes to shaping new professionals. Students are likely to adopt the behaviors and mindset of their mentors.

ISOLATION

Intense training programs typically involve both physical and experiential isolation. Long hours mean less time in the company of family and friends. At the same time, the uniqueness of students' experiences can make them feel different from others.

Emily Transue (2004) recalls the initial shock of clinical work. "I had woken up that morning having never seen a death, and by lunchtime I had been part of one," she says. "Nothing in medical school or in life had prepared me for that moment. . . . I felt wrenchingly and terribly alone" (p. 1). As she felt herself being transformed by the experience, Transue wondered if the people she loved could still relate to her. "Would they understand what I had just seen and done? Would I be inevitably separated from them by this experience and those that would follow it?" (p. 1).

Being different from others can be a special feeling. It can also interfere with relationships and with communication, particularly when people are still figuring out the roles they should play.

IDENTITY IN LIMBO

The process of framing a new identity typically involves a phase during which people experience a sense of limbo. Care providers-in-training are no longer laypersons, but they are not yet full-fledged professionals either.

As in the military, health care typically observes a strict hierarchy, and those at the bottom levels are reminded in many ways of their lowly status. Medical interns are sometimes referred to as "the dirt on which the ladder stands" (Hirschmann, 2008, p. 59) and as those who get "pimped first, blamed first, and thanked last" (Jauhar, 2008, p. 201). Dietician students in a Canadian study described a dynamic in which preceptors asserted that they had superior power by withholding information and demoralizing them (MacLellan & Lordly, 2008). Said one student in the study, "Sometimes it feels as though interns, we are put at the bottom of the priority list. . . . I sometimes feel as though my ideas and input are disregarded without any consideration" (p. E87).

By most accounts, 40% to 60% of medical school students in the United States say they have been mistreated—typically in the form of public humiliation or racist or sexist comments (American Association of Medical Colleges, 2018; Chung, Thang, Vermillion, Fried, & Uijtdehaage, 2018; Fried, Vermillion, Parker, & Uijtdehaage, 2012). Novice nurses face many of the same challenges. "The phrase 'nurses eat their young' describes bullying imposed by senior nurses on new nurses or student nurses as an initiation into the profession," write Sandra Henley and colleagues (2018, para. 8), who studied patterns of mistreatment.

Role theory explains such behavior by proposing that positions within a society are defined by unique sets of rights, responsibilities, and privileges (Mead, 1934). By asserting their power, preceptors may be sending the message that initiates have not yet earned the privileges and rights of bona fide practitioners. Students and interns are reminded of their place with public pop quizzes in which personnel of higher status can publicly challenge them to answer questions and make diagnoses. They may also be called on to do menial chores that no one else wants to do. It is commonly accepted that some of these chores are assigned mainly to punish or humiliate the newcomers.

Although students often have immense responsibility, they have less experience than the professionals around them. In the midst of this, there is usually little time for students to get their bearings. The expectation that they will move expeditiously from being observers to participants is reflected in the traditional clinical battle cry, "Watch one, do one, teach one" (Conrad, 1988, p. 326). Learning on the job can be a frightening experience when human lives (including one's own) are at stake. But, gradually, even as they are being cast as peons within the system, students may begin to see themselves as different, even superior, to those *outside* it.

PRIVILEGES

It can be exhilarating to be part of the action and learning at a rapid pace. Medical interns sometimes say that, as much as they long for a day off, when it comes they feel adrift and left out. When things got really tough, Transue (2004) reminded herself, "I will never learn as much in any year of my life as I will in this one. I may never have the same intensity of experience. I intend to make the most of it" (p. 34).

To be granted access to wonders seldom witnessed can also be a heady experience. Perri Klass (1987) recalls a sense of wonder dissecting cadavers, reflecting that she was doing something "normal people never do" (p. 37). Klass compared the sensation to initiation into a priesthood.

In these ways and others, students get an early dose of the responsibilities, but also the privileges, that go along with professional status. Sometimes, as they begin to feel more like professionals and less like students, the emotional distance between them and their patients can widen, as we discuss next.

LOSS OF EMPATHY

The rigors of clinical experience can lead to darker aspects of socialization. Confronted by overwhelming demands, it is not surprising that students sometimes begin to regard patients as adversaries. Phillip Reilly (1987) remembers the extreme exhaustion during his residency that led him to resent the neediness of a comatose patient: "He was an enemy, part of the plot to deprive me of sleep. If he died, I could sleep for another hour. If he lived, I would be up all night" (p. 226).

Medical professionals sometimes refer to patients in derogatory terms, such as *drain circlers* and *gomers*. The first is a reference to patients who are expected to die (go down the drain) soon. The second, an acronym for "get out of my emergency room," generally refers to older patients who have little chance of recovering and are seen as wasting valuable time and space.

If students are persuaded by the curriculum and mentors that disease is best understood in physical terms, depersonalizing patients begins to feel acceptable. Focusing on specific, organic concerns is more familiar and less emotionally exhausting than thinking in terms of unique individuals.

Nursing and midwifery students have typically not experienced the same level of empathy-loss as medical students. Analysts speculate that this is because their training typically involves closer, ongoing relationships with patients (Williams et al., 2014).

IMPLICATIONS

It's natural to feel a mixture of awe and outrage over what some people go through on the way to becoming professional care providers. One limitation of the Voice of Medicine is that it does not provide caregivers with much of a vehicle for sharing their emotions or focusing on patients' unique experiences.

Communication Training and Integrated Approaches

Some analysts point to a new wave of reform in provider education, with greater emphasis on person-centered care, teamwork, and cultural awareness (Smith, 2017). Here are a few examples of emerging programs and perspectives.

INTERPROFESSIONAL EDUCATION

One model gaining popularity is **interprofessional education (IPE)**, in which students develop expertise in two or more fields such as medicine, pharmacology,

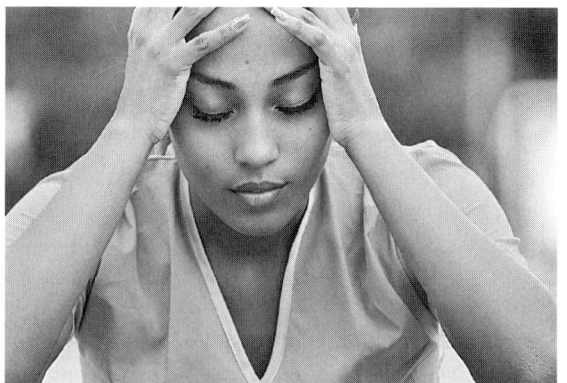

The emotional and physical demands on care providers and providers in training can be intense.

Have you ever seen care providers who seem to resent the demands of patients or who depersonalize them? If so, what have you observed? Why do you think it happened?

nursing, physical therapy, social work, midwifery, and so on. The idea is that well-rounded practitioners will be better prepared to fill multiple roles, address complex health needs, and collaborate with diverse colleagues (WHO, 2013).

In one program, students studying to be athletic trainers, nurses, and occupation therapists collaborated to provide care for a simulated patient who had suffered a spinal cord injury. The students engaged in shared decision making as they imagined themselves at the site of the injury (a football field), through the ambulance ride, during emergency treatment, and while the patient received inpatient hospital care (Morrell et al., 2018). The students say the experience helped them better appreciate the value of interprofessional communication and respect.

Research supports that IPE graduates often take a more active role than others in multidisciplinary teamwork and are usually more open and respectful toward colleagues with diverse backgrounds (D. Morris & Matthews, 2014). They also tend to be particularly adaptive and confident when communicating with patients (Defenbaugh & Chikotas, 2015; Hagemeier, Hess, Hagen, & Sorah, 2014). We'll talk more about the challenges and rewards of interprofessional teamwork at the end of the chapter.

PROBLEM-BASED LEARNING

Another evolving method is the use of **problem-based learning (PBL)**, a process in which students apply information to actual scenarios rather than simply memorizing it. For instance, they might be presented with a case study, then asked to analyze the patient's condition and identify factors relevant to the person's health. PBL is positively correlated with improved performance and knowledge among pharmacology students (Dube, Ghadlinge, Mungal, Saleem, & Kulkarni, 2014) and with health professionals' competence after graduation, particularly in terms of their ability to communicate about complex health matters (Li, Wang, Zhu, Zhu, & Sun, 2019).

Another PBL technique involves interactions with so-called standardized patients—people who are trained to play the part of patients, with realistic symptoms and emotional concerns. These interactions are usually video-recorded so that students can review them later, with feedback from their professors and the mock patients who were involved.

BIOPSYCHOSOCIAL FOCUS

Some schools have made awareness of personal and social factors part of the curriculum. For example, the Northeastern University School of Pharmacy in Boston implemented a program in which pharmacy students learn about nutrition and weight management and then, for a week, model the behaviors they would recommend to an obese or diabetic person (Trujillo & Hardy, 2009). The students are asked to calculate what portion of a limited family budget would be available for food purchases after subtracting medical costs, and then design a grocery list and shop for the recommended foods. Five months after the exercise, the students reported that the experience was still with them. They felt more confident counseling people about dietary matters and more sympathetic toward people with weight problems, especially those trying to buy healthy foods with limited financial means. Said one student, "This activity really made me realize how important it is to understand someone's culture and income level before recommending lifestyle changes" (p. 6).

A program at Harvard Medical School requires students to participate in a three-year course on patient relationships. The program is designed to create "humanistic physicians" who appreciate social and psychological aspects of illness and embody ethics, warmth, and sensitivity. The course makes use of small-group discussions to help students explore their own feelings and philosophies and work together to develop communication skills.

Pediatric residents at the University of California (UC), Davis, don't only train in hospitals and clinics. They also work as advocates in the community, actively partnering with various groups to improve the overall health of children. "Physicians have a greater responsibility to their patients beyond telling them what will keep them healthy," says Richard Pan, a UC physician who developed the program. "We need to be in our patients' communities and neighborhoods working with families" (UC Davis Health, "Getting Doctors Out," 2002, para. 3). The program has won numerous awards, and research shows that physicians tend to maintain their community-oriented focus after they transition into licensed medical practice (Paterniti, Pan, Smith, Horan, & West, 2006).

Next, let's move from the education phase to professional practice to examine other factors that affect the way care providers communicate.

Systems-Level Influences on Care Providers

Once they join the ranks of health professionals, care providers are influenced by a range of factors, including organizational protocols and time constraints. These factors can be both enabling and frustrating. On the good side, most care providers say the frustrations are tempered by unforgettable moments in which they connect with people and know they are making a difference. Real-life examples throughout this chapter highlight the impact that health professionals have on peoples' lives.

Let's start our discussion of system theory with an example.

Organizational Culture

The cancer center administrators were stunned. A Japanese sensei *(master or teacher) with Toyota had handed them a map of their medical center and asked them to illustrate, with blue yarn, the path patients usually took in the process of receiving care there. By the time they were done, representatives from the Virginia Mason Cancer Center in Seattle had created a maze-like web of yarn that went back and forth, up and down various floors, circled back over itself, and demonstrated clearly that the staff was putting patients under ridiculous emotional and physical stress to get treatment (Mars, 2011).*

Charles Kenny, who wrote a book about the Virginia Mason experience, observes that the team members were horrified to realize that "they were taking these patients, for whom time is absolutely the most precious thing in their lives, and they were wasting huge amounts of it" (quoted by Weinberg, 2011, para. 6).

Systems theory awakens us to the presence of **organizational processes**, which are habitual or prescribed ways of doing things, and **organizational culture**, which comprises members' basic beliefs and assumptions about an organization, its members, and the organization's place in the larger environment (Schein, 1986). To the extent that these behaviors and assumptions become part of everyday thinking, they contribute to the culture of an organization and the socially constructed identities of people within it.

Familiar routines and structures often have a taken-for-granted quality that blinds people to alternatives. Organizational members become, as systems theorist Peter Senge (2006) puts it, "prisoners of systems" that they themselves create. No one at Virginia Mason wanted patients to exhaust themselves traversing the large facility, but they had probably never questioned the necessity of it. Once awakened to the problem, they realized that individual action would not be enough to solve it. A more productive option would be to redesign the system itself.

The staff of Virginia Mason did just that. They converted the perimeter of the building into a sunny pathway with waterfront views that patients can follow in a logical progression when it is necessary for them to move from one area to another. They also created a central corridor that allows care providers to easily move from one treatment room to another so that patients don't have to. These and other changes have reduced the average time that patients spend in the medical center by 50% and made it possible to eliminate waiting rooms. Because of the changes, Virginia Mason skyrocketed to the top 1% in the nation in terms of safety and efficiency and earned a 37% reduction in insurance premiums (Kenney, 2010; Weinberg, 2011). The system continues to evolve, but it is both kinder and more efficient than it used to be. The staff now treats more patients in less time, which is good for patients and for the bottom line. Profits are up, but the greatest satisfaction, say team members, is doing what's right for the patients.

Although people often assume that health professionals call the shots, in reality, they are constrained in many ways by the systems in which they operate.

Many of the conditions that influence what happens in patient–provider communication are established at a systemic, not an individual, level. The Virginia Mason example demonstrates this and perhaps offers some encouragement that, if people are not happy with a system, they may be able to improve it. After all, as Senge (2006) reminds us, even small changes to a system can have potent implications.

Next, let's examine some of the systems-level factors that influence care providers' communication and satisfaction.

Time Constraints

Sharon Spalding, an avid runner and cyclist, felt like an unlikely candidate for breast cancer. "I was in the best shape of my life and had just run a marathon," she says (Augusta Health, n.d., para. 3). In the months following her diagnosis, chemotherapy made Spalding feel tired, yet she yearned for physical activity. Fortunately, her caregivers had time to get to know her.

Spalding's care team designed a treatment plan specific to her needs and lifestyle, including consultations with a certified cancer exercise trainer. The trainer helped her develop light workout routines that eased her lethargy when she was sickest, and then as she improved, more vigorous regimens so she could resume running and biking as she had before.

A critical element in this real-life scenario is time—time to listen and time to respond effectively. When time is short, health professionals may seem rushed and impatient. Although it is tempting to blame them for this less-than-hospitable demeanor, care providers usually dislike time constraints as much as patients do. Like patients, providers typically feel most satisfied when they have time to develop trust and share information unhurriedly (Bell, Bringman, Bush, & Phillips, 2006; Kisa, Kawabata, Itou, Nishimoto, & Maezawa, 2011; Tellis-Nayak, 2005).

Health professionals who are worried about time constraints may limit talk to specific physical indicators—perhaps reasoning that friends, family members, clergy, counselors, and others are available to offer emotional support, but they alone are uniquely qualified to diagnose physical conditions and prescribe treatments. They may also reason that a fast pace is the only alternative to turning away people in need. As a nurse in one study explained it, although it is rewarding to spend time with individual patients, doing so may mean less time for other patients and more work for one's colleagues (Chan, Jones, & Wong, 2013). However, rushing may be counterproductive in that it often results in follow-up visits that might have been avoided, poorly developed relationships, misunderstandings, and other time-intensive outcomes.

One option is to make the most of care providers at every level. For example, midlevel providers such as nurse practitioners (NPs) and physician assistants (PAs) now handle routine and minor concerns in some medical offices, which frees physicians to spend more time with seriously ill patients. Patients are typically satisfied with NPs and PAs because they are often less rushed than doctors and they tend to focus on social and personal concerns in addition to biomedical matters (Budzi, Lurie, Singh, & Hooker, 2010; Charlton, Dearing, Berry, & Johnson, 2008).

Researcher and psychologist Jeffrey Rudolph (2008) offers the following tips for bonding with patients when time is limited:

- *Start strong.* Say hello, look the patient in the eye, inspire trust from the beginning.
- *Do not interrupt, and do not multitask.* Give the patient your full attention.
- *Empower patients.* Provide information, web links, follow-up phone calls, and other means of encouraging the patient's active involvement during and after the encounter.
- *Don't end the visit before you ask if the patient has other questions or concerns.* You are not actually saving time if the patient leaves without knowing what to do next. And even if you make a note to address some of the concerns on the next visit, it is ultimately more efficient to encourage full disclosure than to remain in the dark about what a patient wants and needs.

Now that we have looked at some of the external factors that influence care providers, let's shift our focus to their emotional health.

Psychological Influences on Caregivers

The patient had once attempted to stab a nurse. But when mental health social worker Peb Johal met the woman, she was "incredibly gentle," no longer in a delusional state in which she thought people were trying to harm her. Johal earned the woman's trust, worked with her family, and collaborated with other members of the care team to identify helpful medication. Johal reflects that social work "can be a tough profession with its own challenges, but I believe it does come with the power to make a positive difference" (Johal, 2016, last paragraph).

Health care can be emotionally rewarding and challenging. Care providers are charged with helping others, but it may feel that few people are looking out for them. In this section, we discuss how they are affected by emotional preparedness, mindfulness, confidence, and satisfaction.

Emotional Preparedness

Patients look to health professionals not only for technical advice but also for wisdom and understanding. Such a high expectation is difficult to satisfy. As Weston and Lipkin put it, we "may know precise drug treatment but stand empty-handed and mute before the patient who desperately needs counsel and support" (1989, p. 45).

As a result, providers may avoid emotional matters or offer stiff platitudes such as "It will all be fine." Patients are likely to sense the insincerity and may feel that their concerns have been brushed aside as unimportant. Seldom do patients realize that care providers may not *know* how to respond. The sheer number and breadth of patients' concerns can be overwhelming,

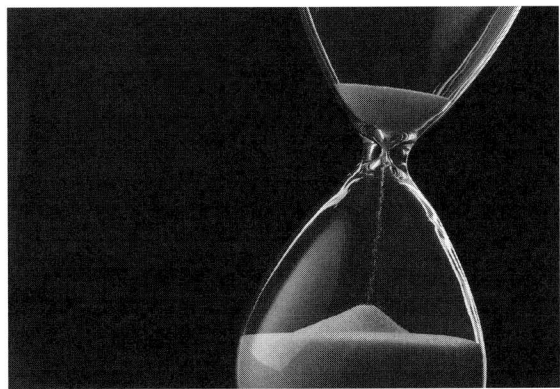

Patients have an obligation to communicate openly but not to monopolize care providers' time.

In your opinion, how can patients collaborate with care providers to manage time effectively?

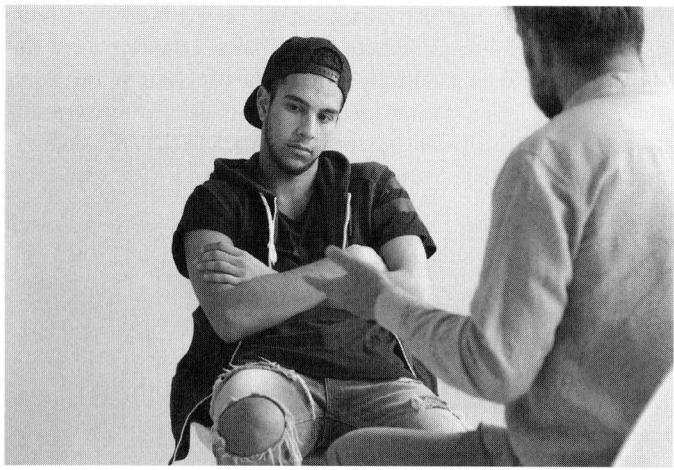

Health encounters often stir up intense emotions. Even if the concern seems to be relatively minor, it may hit emotional hot buttons for one or more people involved.

Even if you did not show it outwardly, have you ever been surprised by your emotional reaction in a health care experience? If so, what caused you to feel that way?

and providers may not feel well trained to meet their emotional needs.

A complicating factor is that we all have emotional hot buttons. When one of these sore spots is touched, the emotional response can surprise the care provider and the patient, although neither may understand it (Novack et al., 1997). For example, a health professional may feel resentment, disgust, or sexual attraction for a patient, may become overly protective, or may wish to have nothing to do with the person. Novack and coauthors (1997) point out that personal biases are unavoidable, but professionals will have a hard time putting their feelings in perspective if they don't take time to acknowledge and understand them. We consider ways to do that at the end of this section.

Mindfulness

> When negative feelings start to creep in, says a first-year nursing and midwifery student, "I acknowledge that and I go: Oh no, stop . . . try and be positive. I think that has helped me more than anything" (quoted by van der Riet, Rossiter, Kirby, Dluzewska, & Harmon, 2015, p. 46).

The student developed this response in a seven-week program to cultivate **mindfulness, which is defined** as awareness of one's self and others and a nonjudgmental respect for diversity (Epstein, 1999).

Research about the effects of mindful health communication is encouraging. Nurses in the program just described reported that the mindful techniques they learned have helped them focus, manage stress, sleep better, and be more fully present with people (van der Riet et al., 2015). In a similar way, physicians who took part in small-group interactions to increase mindfulness experienced an increased sense of empowerment and engagement (West et al., 2014). The positive effects go both ways. Patients report feeling satisfied with highly mindful health professionals and say that mindful care providers seem more patient centered and affiliative than others (Beach et al., 2013).

Marleah Dean and Richard Street, Jr. (2014) presented a three-part model to guide health professionals in being mindful with people in distress.

- The model involves, first, *recognizing* the person's feelings with a statement such as, "It sounds like you are overwhelmed with all the possible options for treatment" (Dean & Street, Table 1).
- The second stage is *exploring* those feelings together by actively listening and encouraging the distressed person to describe how they feel.
- The final stage involves *therapeutic action* in which the people involved collaborate to determine the most helpful course of action. This stage may involve statements such as, "We will figure this out together," "Would you like to . . . ?" and "We are here to help you" (Dean & Street, Table 1).

Dean and Street emphasize that this model is not simply about what professionals say to people who are distressed, but about developing genuine awareness and compassion for peoples' feelings.

Confidence

"What gives me the right to be here?" wondered a psychology doctorate student about his first encounters with patients (Weir, 2013, para. 3). It's natural to feel like an imposter when one adopts a new role. Health professionals say they sometimes doubt their capacity to cure and understand the people they treat, and they wonder what gives them the right to make decisions and know others' most intimate secrets.

Their confidence may also be shaken by mistakes, a topic we cover later in the chapter.

Socialized to be confident and in control, care providers may hide their self-doubt behind a protective gruffness or arrogance. The message is, "Don't get too close," not because they dislike people but because they are at a loss or are intimidated by peoples' appraisals of them. Patients may misinterpret this behavior as cold and distant.

Caregivers' self-doubt may be more of an issue as patients become more knowledgeable and assertive. While it was once assumed that patients could not understand the details of their conditions, today patients may know more than their care providers about particular experimental procedures or the latest research. Professionals cannot be expected to know offhand the latest details of every medical condition. Still, they may feel defensive or inadequate when they do not.

Satisfaction

Most people seem to take it for granted that health professionals' satisfaction is either guaranteed or irrelevant. However, dissatisfaction among professionals correlates with stress, burnout, and high employee turnover rates. For these reasons, scholars such as Ashley Duggan (2006) urge researchers to give more attention to caregivers' emotional well-being.

Care providers' satisfaction is bolstered when patients are friendly and up front about their needs (J. Halbesleben, 2006), when the providers are confident about their communication skills (McKinley & Perino, 2013), and when they feel appreciated and proud of the work they do (Brett, Branstetter, & Wagner, 2014). Health professionals are also sensitive to issues of autonomy and respect. For example, nurses are most likely to stay in the profession if they feel that people recognize and honor their efforts and involve them in decision making (Tourangeau & Cranley, 2005).

A common frustration involves the nonmedical aspects of health care. The term "administrative fatigue" describes care providers' frustration with paperwork, red tape, hassles over reimbursement, and other aspects of the job that can drain their energy and divert effort from patient care ("Frustrated by Bureaucracy," 2017; Olson 2017). One implication is that, if health professionals seem tired and rushed, it may be more because of bureaucratic demands than the challenges of patient care. In a survey of 5,000 physicians, nearly 9 in 10 said that their relationships with patients are positive and are a key source of their satisfaction (Saley, 2019).

We focus now on two issues that can be distressing to care providers—burnout and mistakes—and one that holds promise for improving the first two: interdisciplinary teamwork.

Stress and Burnout

"People think that burnout means you weren't working hard enough, but I'm here to tell you that the opposite is true," says physician Errin Weisman (n.d., para. 4). Despite being a leader among her peers and an energetic advocate for medical care, Weisman became burnt out. "I felt I that I was alone in a cave, had dropped my flashlight and couldn't find the way back out," she says (para. 6).

Weisman is not alone. "Helping people can be extremely hazardous to your physical and mental health," attests psychiatrist James Gill (quoted by Wicks, 2008, p. 21). Burnout is higher in health care than in other fields, and it may manifest in harmful ways, such as depression and substance abuse. (See Box 5.2 for a true story about one physician's substance abuse.)

Burnout is a combination of factors, including emotional exhaustion, depersonalization, and a reduced sense of personal accomplishment (Maslach, 1982). **Emotional exhaustion** is the feeling of being "drained and used up" (Maslach, p. 3). People experiencing emotional exhaustion feel that they can no longer summon motivation or compassion. **Depersonalization** is the tendency to treat people in an unfeeling, impersonal way. From this perspective, people may seem contemptible and weak, and the individual experiencing burnout may resent their requests. A **reduced sense of personal accomplishment** involves feeling like a failure. People who feel this way may become depressed, experience low self-esteem, and leave their jobs or avoid certain tasks.

People experiencing burnout are at elevated risk for heart disease, depression, and accidents. They are also more likely than others to be apathetic, to miss work, and to leave the profession (Paris & Hoge, 2010). What's more, burnout is linked to poor patient outcomes and medical errors (Hall, Johnson, Watt, Tsipa, & O'Connor, 2016).

BOX 5.2 PERSPECTIVES

Blowing the Whistle on an Impaired Physician

As manager of a small community clinic, having to identify an impaired physician was not on my agenda. Clinic operations were going smoothly and patients seemed to like the clinic and the physician, Dr. Havard (not his real name). I knew things about Dr. Havard, such as his turbulent relationship with his ex-wife and his constant financial difficulties. However, he seemed to be a caring and sensitive doctor. Several months into his employment at the clinic, I started noticing strange behavioral changes in Dr. Havard, such as being chronically late for work and his inability to account for missing narcotic samples.

I thought Dr. Havard's actions were suspicious, but I did not know they were signs of an impending problem until I received a phone call from a representative of an internet pharmaceutical company. The woman on the other end of the phone explained to me that large quantities of a prescription narcotic had been ordered for the clinic. I explained to her that the physician does not dispense narcotics on the premises because of the potential of robbery. After several similar phone calls from various companies, I approached Dr. Havard with the information. He said, "It's all a mistake. I'll take care of it."

I knew that he was not going to resolve the situation, and the phone calls became more frequent, demanding payment in excess of $20,000. I notified the clinic administrator, whose office is in a neighboring city. When I originally reported the problem, the administrator told me to "watch and listen." A week later, while working in my office, I received a phone call from a local pharmacist, who explained to me that a clinic patient presented a prescription for the same narcotic with authorization for three refills from Dr. Havard. She called because she knew it was rare for Dr. Havard to write prescriptions for such a large quantity of narcotics. When I asked for a description of the patient, she described Dr. Havard to a "T." After my initial shock, I called the administrator back and explained the situation. The next day, the administrator confronted Dr. Havard and asked if he had written the prescription. He denied it and said he didn't know who the patient was. I was given the "go-ahead" to treat the prescription as stolen and contact the Sheriff's Department.

Soon after the incident, Dr. Havard was drug tested and suspended from employment because he tested positive for narcotics and could not produce a legitimate prescription. When sheriff's deputies caught up with him, he confessed to writing the prescription for a "relative." He was offered assistance through the state's impaired-practitioners program. The program offers confidential counseling and assistance and the chance to resume practice.

I felt that I was ruining Dr. Havard's career by turning him in. However, I had an ethical and moral obligation to report him to protect his patients.

—DENISE

What Do You Think?

1. If you discovered that your doctor was abusing narcotics, would it change your opinion of them?
2. Would you want the doctor to undergo counseling and have a second chance to practice medicine? Why or why not?

Causes

Some of the most common causes of stress and burnout among health professionals involve conflict, emotional fatigue, and excessive workload. We discuss those factors here, and then review communication tips for maintaining one's sense of enthusiasm and purpose, even when the job is challenging.

CONFLICT

Care providers of all types can probably relate to the nurses who say they feel stressed when they are faced with conflicting demands, such as responding to multiple requests at the same time or interrupting patient care to answer phones or fill out paperwork (Happell et al., 2013; Rosenstein & O'Daniel, 2008).

The frustration is exacerbated, the nurses say, if supervisors and colleagues do not appreciate their efforts.

Another stressor arises when care providers are required to carry out treatment decisions they believe to be inappropriate or harmful to patients (Catlin et al., 2008). These situations place them in a **double bind**, meaning there are negative consequences no matter which option they choose. They may feel that it is unacceptable to challenge the orders they have been given. At the same time, it may seem insupportable to put patients in danger.

EMOTIONS

Intense emotions can cause stress and lead to emotional exhaustion. Although care providers work in emotionally charged situations, they are required to remain calm (Pincus, 1995). (See Box 5.3 for tips on dealing with difficult patients.) In the same vein, they are expected to be caring and compassionate yet keep their emotions in check. To cope with these challenges, they often develop what Harold Lief and Renée Fox (1963) call **detached concern**,

---

BOX 5.3 COMMUNICATION SKILL BUILDER

Dealing with Difficult Patients

Some patients bring out the best in their care providers. Others—a small percentage but powerful nonetheless—evoke defensiveness and anger. Experts offer the following tips for communicating effectively with people who are stressed, tired, and worried, without becoming too frustrated yourself.

- *Treat complaints as opportunities.* Frustrated patients and family members may want or need something they are afraid to ask for outright. Their emotion can be a signpost calling your attention to it. Physician Calvin Martin recalls an aggressive patient who threw things at the staff and yelled at everyone around him. "He knew he was dying, but everyone else was denying it," he says. Once the doctor learned the problem and was honest with the patient, his entire demeanor changed. "He was wonderful after that," Martin recalls (quoted by Magee & D'Antonio, 2003, p. 163). He says, "In medical school they tell you that 75% of the people you are going to see have nothing really wrong with them. That's not true. I think they all have something real, but we are just not finding it" (p. 164).
- *Empower team members to handle problems before they grow.* Most nonclinical problems start as minor annoyances—a phone call not returned, an appointment mix-up. A quick and thoughtful response (even if the patient has not complained) may save a great deal of time and stress down the line.
- *Invest in patient relationships.* In *The Field Guide to the Difficult Patient Interview,* Platt and Gordon (2004) propose that "engaging our patients in a partnership with us" and "enlisting them in following our recommendations" are the hallmarks of effective communication (p. 3). They encourage caregivers to take the time to know patients and establish mutual trust and rapport. "Spending more time early in our patient encounters saves time in the long run," they maintain (p. 3).
- *Show empathy.* Demonstrate through words and nonverbal cues that you understand what the patient is experiencing. Listen attentively, paraphrase to check your understanding, and ask for clarification until the patient confirms that you understand what they are trying to express (Platt & Gordon, 2004).
- *Display curiosity.* If a patient hints at a grievance or a concern that they are reluctant to share, show interest in hearing more. Platt and Gordon (2004) use the example of a patient who refuses to say how much she smokes. They propose saying, "That is really interesting! Of course you don't have to tell me. But I am enormously curious to understand why you don't want to tell me. Can you help me understand that?" (p. 118).
- *Try a little humor.* If the patient shows an inclination toward it, you can sometimes use gentle humor to clear the air. Transue (2004) recalls a hospital patient who did nothing but complain about the food, the service, and the interruptions. She recalls thinking to herself, "I'm pretty sure there's humor under his crabbiness, but I can never quite pin it down" (p. 100). One day the man declared that he wouldn't leave the hospital until the food there improved. Several days later, after checking his lab results and vital signs, Transue was prepared to discharge him, but she asked first, "Has the food gotten any better?" She recalls: "He stares at me for a long moment. Finally he bursts out laughing. 'How do you think I'll answer that . . . Has the food gotten any better. You get out of here—' . . . I wave and walk away, listening to him laugh" (p. 101).

a sense of caring about other people without becoming emotionally involved in the process. Some degree of detachment is useful to keep from feeling overwhelmed. However, the expectation that health professionals will squelch or avoid their own emotions may lead them to become apathetic, cynical, and confused.

WORKLOAD

An excessive workload or a highly monotonous one can cause stress. Because of funding structures and limited resources, hospital patients are said to be "quicker and sicker" than in the past, meaning that overnight stays are now limited to people who are very sick or badly hurt. As a consequence, hospital personnel are likely to be involved in difficult, intense situations most of the time.

At the other end of the spectrum, some caregivers must cope with monotonous, repetitive tasks. Laura Ellingson (2007) studied staff members at a dialysis care center, where they are required to perform the same routines over and over. Many of the caregivers said they break the monotony by focusing on the unique qualities of each patient. As one put it: "Our job is repetitious, but the patients are not. Yeah, they all have the same illness, they have kidney failure, but each person is different, so that's what makes it different every day" (p. 109).

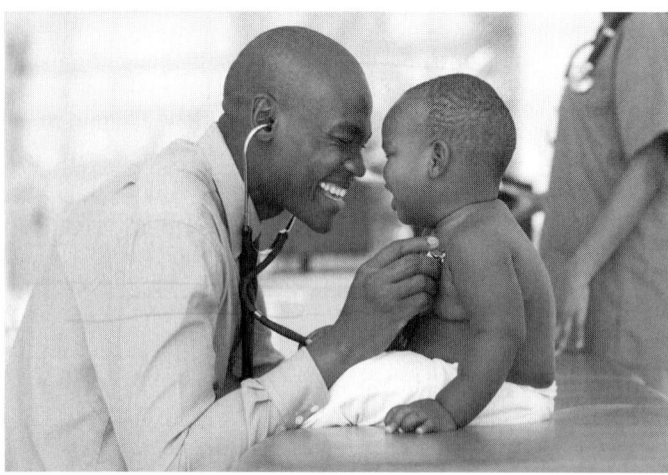

Like patients, health professionals are most satisfied when they have time to make personal connections with patients.

Who is your favorite care provider and why?

Healthy Strategies

Ironically, the very qualities that draw people to careers in health care make them especially prone to burnout. The **empathic communication model of burnout** suggests that health care is appealing to people who are concerned about others and are able to imagine others' joy and pain (Miller, Birkholt, Scott, & Stage, 1995; Miller, Stiff, & Ellis, 1988). These people are typically responsive communicators (able to communicate well with people in distress), but they may easily feel overwhelmed by constant exposure to emotional situations.

Regrettably, care providers usually receive little instruction on how to care for themselves, and the symptoms of burnout may creep up on them before they know it. "The causes of burnout are often so quiet and insidious that we fail to notice them until they have caused a great deal of harm," observes Robert Wicks (2008, p. 18). Here are some suggestions for avoiding burnout, mostly drawn from Wicks's (2008) book *The Resilient Clinician*:

- *Hold daily debriefings with yourself.* Honestly assess your own emotions and hot buttons. Reflect on such questions as: *What made me sad? Overwhelmed me? Sexually aroused me? Made me extremely happy or even confused me?* (Wicks, 2008, p. 31).
  - *Resist the urge to put off the "good stuff."* Wicks (2008) recommends making time for quiet walks, meditation, laughter, listening to enjoyable music, having friends over for dinner, daydreaming, being in nature, making love, and journaling.
  - *Be mindful about what makes you happy.* Frequently consider your answers to the following questions: *What is my heart's desire? What is truly important to me? How do I most want to live?* (Wicks, 2008).
  - *Invest in gratifying relationships.* The **Relational Health Communication Competence Model** observes that communication, social support, and emotional resilience are positively associated with each other (Kreps, 1988; Query & Kreps, 1996). Research bears out that providers' stress is eased when patients and colleagues

are supportive of one another (Fiabane, Giorgi, Sguazzin, & Argentero, 2013; Gelsema et al., 2006).

- *Design your own time pie.* What amount of your time do you (or would you like) to devote to each of the following—being with loved ones, working, learning new things, spending time alone, being creative?
- *Seek the company of people whose presence replenishes you.* A good friend who listens without judgment or who helps you find the humor in a tense situation can ward off burnout. Transue (2004) remembers a playful conversation with a fellow intern who asked her, "Do you really want to be a doctor for the rest of your life?" Transue joked, "I don't even want to be a doctor for the rest of the week, especially" (p. 75).

Errin Weisman, the discouraged physician whose story began this section, says she learned to find a healthy balance again with help from a mentor and coach. "I go to the clinic or hospital now in a good mood, wanting to do this work," she says, adding, "I work my shift, I engage with my patients, and I feel that my work is meaningful. And when I come home, I can shift gears and be present with my family" (Weisman, n.d., para. 7). She is now a coach for other health care providers and is creator of the Doctor Me First podcast and the Truth Prescriptions website.

Let's turn to a topic of particular stress for caregivers—one that often boils down to an issue of communication.

Medical Mistakes

"Doctor Amputates Wrong Leg"

The headlines told a shocking story. Tampa surgeon Rolando Sanchez had mistakenly removed Willie King's left leg rather than his right one. It is easy to imagine the anguish of a patient with one good leg and one bad leg, awakening to realize the good leg is gone. "Now he'll be without any legs at all," mourned the patient's brother ("Florida Hospital," 1995, para. 4).

The Willie King case is horrifying. But the public did not hear the whole story.

Why Mistakes Happen

In his book *Medical Errors and Medical Narcissism*, clinical ethicist John Banja (2005) relates the behind-the-scenes facts of the Willie King case. First, King did not have one good leg and one bad leg. He suffered from diabetes and related vascular diseases to such an extent that open sores on both legs had developed gangrene, his skin was cold to the touch, and it was nearly impossible to detect a pulse in either leg. The left leg (which was mistakenly amputated) was actually worse than the right, and King was aware that he would lose both legs before long. He chose to have the right leg amputated first because it was the more painful of the two. So it was not an easy choice between good leg and bad leg. But a cascade of communication errors contributed to the mistake as well.

Someone dropped the ball. Who? There's no easy answer, says Banja (2005). The public might imagine a distracted, careless, or bumbling surgeon. However, Dr. Sanchez was anything but. He was "at the height of a sterling medical career" (Banja, 2005, p. 9), having served as chief resident among his colleagues at New York University School of Medicine and professor at Albert Einstein College of Medicine before returning to practice in his native Tampa. The mistake ended with him, but it began much earlier.

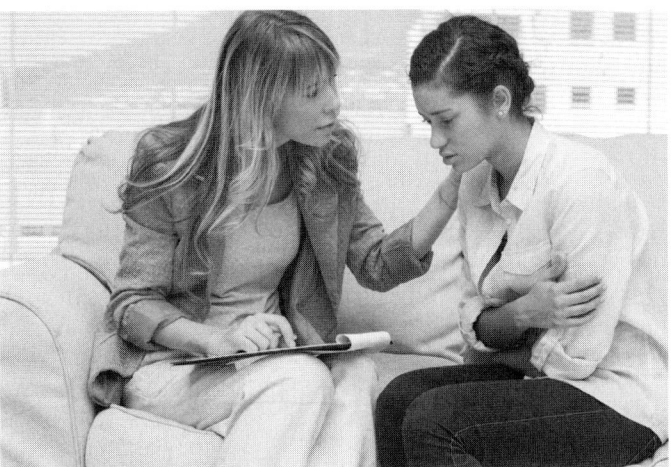

Caregivers often experience grief and withdrawal after serious mistakes, many of which stem from miscommunication in the context of time pressures.

Have you ever made a mistake because you were rushed or misunderstood someone else? If so, what happened? What might you do to minimize the chance of a similar mistake happening again?

Because of a miscommunication between Dr. Sanchez's office staff and the surgery department at the hospital, the surgical staff incorrectly listed the procedure as a left-leg amputation. A hospital nurse detected the error and told another nurse about it. That nurse put a surgery-schedule correction notice on a clipboard, which she gave to another nurse. Each nurse began a sequence of remedial events. But the sequence was somehow interrupted. The correction never made it to the official surgical log or to the blackboard in the surgery unit.

Yet another correction opportunity arose just prior to surgery, when King told a nurse that his right leg was to be amputated. She noted this on his record but prepared his left leg. When the surgeon entered the room, King's body was draped, except for the left leg, which was braced and ready for the operation. Sanchez confirmed, by looking at the blackboard, that this was the intended leg, and he was nearly done with the surgery before the medical team realized the error.

It is easy to see, in retrospect, that the mistake might not have happened if people had communicated more clearly with each other or if the surgical team had consulted King's consent form (which correctly indicated his right leg) rather than relying on the blackboard or surgery schedule. But at the time, people were following standard procedure, and the error occurred because of system and communication breakdowns that were beyond any one person's control (Banja, 2005).

Banja (2005) points out the systemic nature of this mistake and others like it. "Well-trained, well-motivated people make errors all the time," he says (p. 11). Medical mistakes are often the result of ineffective communication—sloppy handwriting, forgotten or delayed instructions, busy shift changes in which there is not time to talk about everything in a patient's chart, and so on (Pham et al., 2011; Ross et al., 2013). Small omissions and misunderstandings can quickly lead to critical breakdowns.

What Happens After a Mistake?

People who are hurt by medical mistakes often say they just want an apology, to feel that they are getting the full story, and reassurance that the organization is taking steps to avoid similar errors in the future. It can be agonizing not to know exactly what caused a loved one's death or suffering. Dale Ann Micalizzi (2008) recalls her own bewildered grief when her 11-year-old son died following a relatively minor surgery to treat an infected cut on his ankle.

Micalizzi says her family did not want to sue. She works for an HMO herself and understands the intricacies of medical settings. But otherwise, no one would tell them what happened. "We were owed the truth," she says. "Money wasn't an issue for us" (2008, para. 12). Micalizzi describes sitting in a courtroom three years later, seeing the defense team consult a 6-inch-thick binder containing her son's medical records and reports from the hospital investigation. "This was information that I had begged to see for such a long time and have still never seen," she says. "In the intervening time I had searched for the truth, only to hit my head against walls of silence" (para. 8).

Errors can happen in any organization, in or out of health care. But medical mistakes are particularly hard to handle because the stakes are so high and because caregivers are not expected to commit errors. When health professionals' mistakes are brought to light, they may suffer more than people in other occupations from feelings of guilt and inadequacy, recriminations from others, and legal action. Even if others are involved in medical mistakes, it is typically physicians who are sued. And they may feel personally responsible, even when events were out of their control.

On the one hand, it is hard to deal with guilt and self-blame in isolation. Ethical guidelines and a sense of fair play encourage health professionals to make full disclosure to patients and their loved ones, to apologize, and to take corrective action. Likewise, hospitals' contracts with insurers typically stipulate that the hospital will promptly report medical errors when they occur. However, care providers may be discouraged from admitting mistakes by their own sense of distress, by fears about their reputation, by ego needs that make them reluctant to admit fallibility, and by reluctance either to blame others or to accept blame for what is often a systemic chain of events involving numerous people (Banja, 2005).

Banja (2005) proposes that health professionals may rationalize not saying anything because they believe no permanent harm was done, the error probably did not change the outcome (e.g., "the patient would have died anyway"), knowing about the mistake would only make the family feel worse, or the mistake was not anyone's fault, just something that happened.

Added to people's natural reluctance to admit mistakes are more tangible considerations, such as *Who will be held responsible?* and *Who will pay?* Malpractice insurance policies sometimes include a clause that revokes coverage if the physician admits culpability. Thus, although patients yearn for apologies and explanations, and health professionals may want to provide them, they may feel that, if they own up to mistakes, they are on their own if lawsuits ensue.

The issue is not only who will pay for a malpractice judgment, it is also who will pay for remedial care. For example, if a hospital stay is extended or a patient is transferred to an intensive care unit because of a medical error, who pays for the extra care? In recent years, many insurance companies have declared that they will not pay costs associated with what they call *never events*. **Never events** are loosely defined as clear, preventable errors with serious consequences. "Think wrong-side surgery," says Dennis Murray (2007, p. 18). The idea is that hospitals with a strong financial incentive to avoid never events will be more diligent about preventing them, identifying their root causes if they do occur, and avoiding future tragedies.

But the issue is not clear cut. A gray zone surrounds less obvious avoidable outcomes, such as infections. If a patient contracts an infection in the hospital, was the staff negligent? In many cases it is hard to say what constitutes negligence versus a reasonable (but imperfect) standard of care. David Burda (2008) worries that insurers may become so stringent that medical professionals will be afraid to try new procedures. Even if the standard options are not working, professionals may feel they cannot step out of bounds for fear of being either sued or refused payment. And Burda warns that care providers who are terrified of making mistakes will not learn very much, and will probably order so many precautionary tests that precious medical resources will be squandered.

Medical mistakes (and perceived mistakes) are not only expensive, they can be demoralizing and humiliating. Family physician Steven Erickson (2008) remembers being sued over a difficult birth that resulted in the baby's having brain damage. In the courtroom, he weathered aggressive questioning by the plaintiff's attorney, all the while worrying that his colleagues, family, and friends would think less of him and doubt his judgment. Erickson won the case, but embarrassment and fear of future lawsuits shadowed him for a year, until he met a new patient, Roger. Roger had just moved to town, and he and his wife had chosen Erickson to be their doctor based on their son's recommendation. A year earlier, their son had served on the jury that heard the malpractice case against Erickson. Roger said that, as a farmer, his son had explained to fellow jurors that births do not always go perfectly, even when the doctor is honest, competent, and doing their best. Writes Erickson:

> I thanked him for his candor and finished up the visit, all the while fighting to maintain my composure. But as I walked back to my office, my eyes welled up and I was crying. After all the embarrassment and self-doubt my malpractice case had engendered in me, there was a juror who not only believed my defense, but trusted me enough to refer his elderly father and mother to me. (p. 33)

Erickson's words remind us that while we should guard citizens' right to reasonable legal recourse if they have been badly treated, lawsuits have many costs, emotional and financial. Very often, patients wish to avoid lawsuits just as much as medical professionals do, but a variety of human and systemic restraints may stand between them. When it comes down to it, the factors that lead to mistakes—and the factors that determine what will happen afterward if mistakes are made—involve mostly one thing: communication. Effective communication has the potential to save lives and prevent some of the anguish that bereaved families and guilt-ridden professionals feel as a result of errors.

Communication Skill Builder: Managing Medical Mistakes

> "I felt like the right thing to do was to go talk to them and tell them and if they felt like they needed to sue me then you know we would just have to deal with that," says a physician describing a medical error (Plews-Ogan, Owens, & May, 2013, p. 238).

It's natural to feel a range of emotions in such a situation. Plews-Ogan and colleagues (2013) identified five stages common among health professionals coping with serious medical mistakes.

- The first stage is *acceptance*, which involves recognizing a mistake and its effects.
- The second stage, *stepping in*, involves taking responsibility for the mistake, often by telling colleagues, patients, and their loved ones about the error and apologizing. Although difficult, this stage was turning point for many care providers

studied, who said they coped more effectively afterward (Plews-Ogan et al., 2013).

- In the third stage, *integration*, health care providers assimilate what they have learned from the mistake and admit to themselves that they are capable of making errors that have tragic consequences. Faced with this, some physicians interviewed by Plews-Ogan and colleagues (2013) left medicine temporarily in the wake of mistakes.
- The fourth stages involves the emergence of a *new narrative*, in which professionals typically emerge as more humble and cautious than before.
- The final stage, *wisdom*, involves knowledge mixed with compassion and understanding. As one doctor put it, "I certainly am absolutely more understanding and forgiving of the frailties of others, whether my coworkers or the nurses" (Plews-Ogan et al., p. 240).

Following are some tips from the experts on how to avoid misunderstandings, disappointments, and lawsuits, and how to respond when mistakes occur.

FROM THE BEGINNING

- *Establish trust*. Invest in open and trusting relationships with patients from the very beginning. Be sincere, polite, friendly, and engaging. Patients are less likely to sue providers they like and trust (Boodman, 1997), and it is easier to share decisions and to admit mistakes with people one knows and trusts.
- *Invite feedback*. Patients who play an active role in deciding on treatment options are more likely to consider them worthwhile, even if things do not work out perfectly.
- *Respond to complaints and requests as quickly as possible*. Patients who perceive that you do not care or are not paying attention are more likely to assume you have neglected other aspects of their care. When you are unavoidably delayed, apologize, explain why, and express your sincere concern.
- *Show that you care*. Do not assume that patients know you care. Be explicit, as in "I don't know if we can eliminate 100% of your pain. But I think, if we work together, we can do a lot. It would make me happy to see you smiling and walking again."
- *Create realistic expectations*. Brushing aside patients' concerns, as in saying, "There's nothing to worry about," may set them up to be disappointed and even to file lawsuits down the line. Attorney S. Allan Adelman (2008) suggests, "You can't always prevent undesirable outcomes, but you can help create realistic expectations" (p. 14).
- *Put it in writing*. "Document, ad nauseam," recommends Ralph Caldroney (2008), a family physician who has never been sued in 30 years of practice.
- *Do not be shy about giving referrals*. If another doctor can help, or the patient wants a second opinion, be supportive. Do not cast yourself as the roadblock that kept the patient from exploring all avenues (Caldroney, 2008).
- *Do not forget the family*. Keep in mind that the patient's loved ones often have opinions and fears of their own. Invite their input, and nurture those relationships.
- *Own up to small mistakes*. Showing that you have nothing to hide can engender trust.

IF AN ERROR DOES OCCUR

John Banja and Geri Amori (2005, p. 178) recommend the following five-step guide to telling patients and their loved ones about a medical mistake:

- Rehearse how you will disclose the information.
- Deliver it as simply, truthfully, and clearly as possible.
- Stop talking and listen.
- Assess how the news is being received.
- Respond empathically.

Banja and Amori recommend using the word *error* or *mistake* rather than blurring the issue with terms such as *unintended outcome* or *unexpected occurrence*. They also coach health professionals to tell the people affected: (1) when and where the error occurred, (2) what harm resulted, (3) what actions have been taken to offset the harm, (4) actions being taken to prevent future errors, (5) who will be caring for the patient and how, (6) a description of systemic factors that contributed to the error, (7) the costs of responding to the error and how they will be handled, and (8) information about counseling and support resources. They also recommend that the speaker "apologize profusely" and mean it (p. 185).

Finally, do not let doubt and remorse erode your confidence. It is easy to obsess about what might have happened—if only you had stopped by one more time, ordered one more test, put a request in writing rather than called it in, and so on. These are not necessarily errors, just limitations in the amount a person can do.

The chapter concludes with a communication strategy that has the potential to ease some of the pressure on health care professionals.

Interprofessional Teamwork

Mr. S,[1] age 65, is retired from the automotive industry. Although he lives alone, he joins close friends for breakfast twice a week, a tradition they have maintained for 15 years. In the last two weeks, however, his health has deteriorated to the point where he can barely walk and it is difficult for him to talk. He is a smoker and has been treated in the past for heart disease and emphysema, but he has never felt this sick, tired, or discouraged. He worries that he will no longer be able to spend time with his friends.

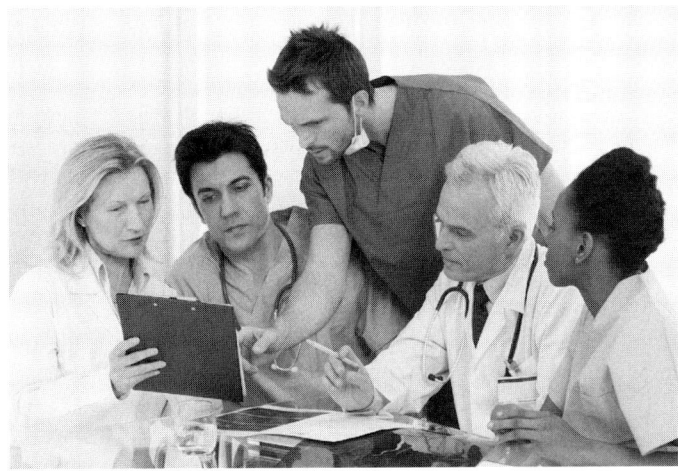

The advantages of multidisciplinary teamwork in health care are powerful, but so are the communication challenges.

Describe the most successful team of which you have ever been part. Describe the least successful one. What made the difference?

What is the best approach for optimizing Mr. S's health? A team of students at the University of Utah addressed this question in a program designed to prepare them for multidisciplinary teamwork as health professionals (Barnett, Hollister, & Hall, 2011). Mr. S is a hypothetical patient created by medical school professor Caroline Milne, complete with vital signs, health history, socioeconomic profile, and more. The students—preparing for careers in pharmacology, nursing, medicine, audiology, nutrition, physical therapy, and occupational therapy—formed interprofessional teams to meet with a trained actor who portrayed Mr. S and devise a plan for his care.

Students who participated in the program gave it high marks. Most said that it impressed upon them the benefits of involving diverse perspectives in patient care. They also said that the experience made them more comfortable interacting with people in other medical disciplines. This is important, since a common barrier to teamwork is lack of trust and communication between people in different fields (Bindler, Richardson, Daratha, & Wordell, 2012).

As we mentioned at the beginning of the chapter, there is a move toward more interprofessional teamwork in health care, both to meet patients' diverse needs and to make the most of health resources. Teams may include social workers, recreational therapy, psychologists, dieticians, pain specialists, and people in many other fields.

Simply defined, a **team** is "a set of individuals who work together to achieve common objectives" (Unsworth, 1996, p. 483). Teamwork is nothing new to health care, but the rules and reasons for teamwork are changing. To apply the terminology of management guru Peter Drucker, health care teams used to function like baseball teams, but now they must act like doubles tennis partners. Drucker (1993) writes that (managerially speaking) a doubles tennis game is different from a baseball game. In baseball, each player is assigned a position, with a specific set of tasks to perform. The pitcher pitches, the catcher catches, the batter bats, and so on. The game is specialized and precise. Doubles tennis is different—faster, less precise. Players have basic positions but must always be poised to help each other, and there is scarcely time to stand still.

Health professionals used to play their positions with little overlap (like baseball players). A patient might see a physical therapist, a nurse, a doctor, and a laboratory technician—but one at a time, never all together. Technically, the caregivers were working toward the same goal, but they contributed in specialized ways, independently. The problem is that team members who do not communicate with each other are likely to drop the ball. Lack of communication can lead to duplicated efforts, costly (and sometimes life-threatening) delays, frustration, and wasted time. Teamwork can minimize the waste and frustration. However, teamwork is not always easy to accomplish.

---

[1] I assigned the patient this name simply to make him easier to discuss. The research report itself does not name him.

An organization famous for teamwork is Mayo Clinic. There's a saying at Mayo that "teamwork is not an option," it's the rule (Berry & Seltman, 2008, p. 51). The medical center is unusual in that, although it is one of the largest in the world, it is a truly integrated system. To appreciate how, let's consider a patient-care scenario somewhere else. Typically, a patient with a serious health concern schedules an appointment with a primary care physician, who refers her to a separate facility for diagnostic tests, where the staff sends her back to the doctor for results, who refers her to a specialist in a different location, who might recommend surgery at still a different place, and so on. The patient probably has to make appointments with each provider separately, supply her health history and insurance information at each office, and perhaps wait weeks or months between appointments. The physicians involved with the patient's care probably do not work directly for the hospital, nor are they likely to have an easy or quick way to communicate with each other or to review an overall medical chart for the patient. (In many cases, there is no overall patient chart. Instead, each doctor maintains a separate chart detailing their work with the patient.)

In contrast, Mayo Clinic is a fully integrated system of doctors, specialists, therapists, hospitals, laboratories, and everyone and everything else needed to provide comprehensive medical care. Everyone involved—including the physicians—works for the clinic. They are linked with sophisticated communication technology and, very often, close enough proximity to allow face-to-face conversations about patients. The Mayo team practices what they call "destination medicine." When patients go there for serious health concerns, they should be prepared to stay in town for a few days. In that time, they will probably be seen by several specialists, have diagnostic tests done, and undergo treatment—all on the same campus. Even surgeries are typically scheduled on a next-day basis. The whole process—from the initial consultation, through visits with specialists, diagnostic tests, and even surgery and recovery—might take three to five days, compared to weeks or months elsewhere.

Mayo's streamlined efficiency is supported by an organizational culture that values and rewards teamwork as well as a carefully designed infrastructure. All appointments are made through one centralized system. This saves time and energy and allows the staff to coordinate the timing and sequence of tests and treatments. Pathologists and radiologists immediately evaluate diagnostic test data, usually before the patient leaves the office, in case more data is required. The results are immediately posted in the patient's electronic medical record. Every care provider has instant, online access to the patient's comprehensive medical record, including all test results and other physicians' notes. This makes it feasible for everyone to get the full picture, to avoid delays or duplications, and to work effectively as a team. All the while, physicians are free to collaborate and to refer patients to each other without loss of income because they are all on salaries and are all part of the same team. "It's like you are working in an organism; you are not a single cell out there practicing," says Mayo physician Nina Schwenk. "I have access to the best minds on any topic, any disease or problem I come up with and they're one phone call away" (quoted by Berry & Seltman, 2008, p. 53).

Advantages

One advantage of teamwork is that members are able to apply multiple perspectives to a problem, enhancing innovation and creativity. This applies to overarching issues, such as new cost-cutting measures and service lines, and to everyday dilemmas. A second advantage is that interprofessional teamwork blurs the lines between departments and presents new opportunities for diverse employees to take part in decision making, which is linked to job satisfaction and retention.

Third, teamwork reduces costly errors and duplications that may occur when people are devoted to highly specialized tasks. Health care organizations can no longer afford, if ever they could, the oversights that result when team members do not communicate well with each other. Ask any hospital employee about patients who have gotten "lost in the system." Usually the story is that the patient is scheduled for a series of treatments or tests, but somewhere along the way everyone assumes that the patient is with someone else—until they realize the poor soul has spent hours lying on a gurney in the hallway.

Bureaucracies are especially vulnerable to these kinds of oversights because many tasks do not fall squarely within the boundaries of any job description. Teamwork encourages people to look at the larger picture and pitch in, even with tasks that are not specifically assigned to them. For example, nurses who notice that lab results have not arrived on time may take the initiative to find out if tests were run and why results are delayed. This extra effort can save time and money in the long run.

Fourth, teamwork is well suited to biopsychosocial care. Members of some organizations have concluded that the best way to keep patients healthy is to pay attention to their broad range of concerns. As physician Alan R. Zwerner advises:

> The dog ate a 100-year-old patient's glasses, and she's not eligible for a covered pair for another year? Give her a pair. Free. It could prevent a fall that would break her hip. There is a reward for quality care, patient satisfaction, and doing the right thing at the right time. (quoted by Azevedo, 1996, para. 22)

Teams can help provide care that simultaneously addresses a variety of issues such as patients' personal resources, nutrition, exercise, psychological well-being, and more.

Finally, team members may benefit from their involvement with coworkers. Teamwork allows professionals to share the immense responsibilities of health care, provide mutual support, and learn from each other.

Difficulties and Drawbacks

None of this means teamwork is easy. Although it presents many advantages, there are potential disadvantages as well.

For one thing, teamwork takes time. If a quick decision is needed, an individual may be better qualified to make it. Some nurses in Julie Apker's (2001) study appreciated opportunities to be part of shared-governance teams. Others felt overwhelmed. Said one nurse, "I don't feel it's fair to give someone a project if they don't have time" (quoted by Apker, 2001, p. 125).

Second, especially if they are rushed or intimidated, team members may resort to **groupthink**—going along with ideas they would not normally support (Janis, 1972). Third, busy schedules make it hard to schedule meetings, especially if the organization is not supportive in allowing time for teamwork.

Finally, teamwork can also be particularly difficult because health professionals from different disciplines often have very different ideas about health, which creates the potential for competition and conflict. Status differences can also cause rifts and intolerance. Health care is often characterized by what Kreps (1990) calls **professional prejudice**. Some professions are considered more prestigious than others, which means that people without impressive titles (including patients) may be excluded from discussions even though they have valuable information and ideas to share.

Communication Skill Builder: Working in Teams

Following are some of experts' tips for working through the tricky communication dilemmas just described.

- *Honor the contributions of every individual.* Few organizations honor this ideal more than Mayo Clinic. Denis Cortese remembers his early experiences as a physician at the clinic (related by Berry & Seltman, 2008, p. 44). "I was unaccustomed to have a desk attendant tell me, a physician, that I needed to adjust my schedule to see a patient right away," Cortese says. But then another physician pulled him aside. "He explained that at Mayo Clinic, the focus is always on the patient. And whichever member of the staff is interacting with the patient deserves our full support," Cortese recalls. "I've never forgotten that lesson."
- *Take time to build trust and camaraderie.* When quick or important decisions are needed, the investment may pay off.
- *Conduct team meetings with the goal of involving everyone.* Minimize distractions, and whenever possible sit together (in person or via video conference) in real time so that all members can see each other. Encourage all group members to contribute ideas, and strive to find creative options that meet numerous goals simultaneously. Summarize group discussions and decisions out loud to clarify the group's viewpoints and perspectives.
- *Establish ground rules.* These might involve expectations for attendance, discussions, and decision making.
- *Develop an understanding of what each team member has to offer.* People bring unique talents and perspectives as well as diverse professional backgrounds.
- *Be aware that conflict is a natural part of group work.* Group members who remain committed to the task often work through the conflict to achieve a mutual sense of accomplishment.
- *Monitor the health of the team.* "Diagnose communication errors as you would any illness," recommend Eduardo Salas and colleagues (2008, p. 333), adding, "Examine the team and look for symptoms, then treat the symptoms through team learning and self-correction."

Summary

Care Provider Preparation

- In the early 1990s, medical schools began to focus on science and clinical experience, as did many other training programs.
- Communication skills are essential in that they help care providers build trust, share information, diagnose what is wrong, and partner with patients in prevention and treatment efforts.
- Many care providers learn to speak the Voice of Medicine, which emphasizes a biomedical, scientific approach.
- The extraordinary demands of being a student can lead to social isolation, a sense of privilege, and a loss of empathy, at least temporarily.
- Emerging trends involve coursework and experience in interprofessional teamwork and problem-based learning with a biopsychosocial focus.

Systems-Level Influences

- Habitual and prescribed ways of doing things influence how care providers are expected to behave.
- Well-designed systems can save time and improve the health care experience for everyone involved.
- Although patients may be quick to assume that care providers don't want to spend time with them, time constraints are often as frustrating to professionals as they are to patients.

Psychological Influences

- Care providers may avoid discussion of highly emotional topics because they do not know how to respond or they feel overwhelmed themselves.
- Mindfulness is one way to help patients feel valued and appreciated, and at the same time, help health professionals manage stress.
- Health professionals say they sometimes doubt their capacity to cure and understand the people they treat, and they wonder what gives them the right to make decisions and know others' most intimate secrets.

Stress and Burnout

- Care providers are expected to be quick but thorough, strong but emotionally accessible, always available but never tired, and honest but infallible. It's no wonder that stress and burnout are often a problem.
- Stress often results when providers are expected to manage an excessive workload, do many things at one time, or carry out orders they believe to be detrimental to patients.
- When dealing with difficult patients, providers may benefit from looking for root causes of the patient's dissatisfaction, empowering team members to deal with problems before they grow, building strong relationships, displaying empathy and curiosity, and when appropriate, using humor.
- Following are a few of the strategies that may be useful in managing stress: stay in touch with your emotions, do things that make you happy and allow you to relax, and build strong relationships with people whose presence revives you.

Medical Mistakes

- Mistakes typically result from miscommunication.
- When mistakes do occur, disclosing them compassionately and fully can prevent lawsuits, provide comfort to those affected, and relieve some of the guilt that care providers feel.

Interprofessional Teamwork

- Interprofessional teamwork is not always easy, but it offers extraordinary rewards in terms of quality decision making, shared responsibility, and biopsychosocial perspectives of people's health.
- It is recommended that team members take time to get to know one another, honor each person's contributions, establish clear ground rules, and monitor the health of the team.

Glossary

burnout A combination of factors, including emotional exhaustion, depersonalization, and a reduced sense of personal accomplishment. *See page 92.*

depersonalization The tendency to treat people in an unfeeling, impersonal way, often as a result of feeling depleted oneself. *See page 89.*

detached concern A sense of caring about other people without becoming emotionally involved in the process. *See page 91.*

double bind A situation in which there are negative consequences no matter which option a person chooses. *See page 91.*

emotional exhaustion A feeling of being drained with little left to give. *See page 89.*

empathic communication model of burnout The proposition that health care is appealing to people who are concerned about others and are able to imagine others' joy and pain, but this same sensitivity may lead them to feel overwhelmed by being constantly exposed to intense emotions. *See page 92.*

groupthink A tendency for members to go along with ideas they would not normally support as individuals. *See page 99.*

hidden curriculum The attitudes and practices that others model, even though they do not explicitly teach them. *See page 82.*

interprofessional education (IPE) A model in which students develop expertise in two or more fields such as medicine, pharmacology, nursing, physical therapy, social work, midwifery, and so on. *See page 84.*

mindfulness Awareness of one's self and others and a nonjudgmental respect for diversity. *See page 88.*

never events A term insurance companies use to describe preventable errors with serious consequences (which are usually not covered by insurance). *See page 95.*

organizational culture Members' basic beliefs and assumptions about an organization, its members, and the organization's place in the larger environment. *See page 86.*

organizational processes Habitual or prescribed ways of doing things (e.g., what people typically talk about, when, and with whom). *See page 86.*

problem-based learning (PBL) A process in which students apply information to actual scenarios rather than simply memorizing it. *See page 84.*

professional prejudice A pattern in which some professions are considered more prestigious or important than others. *See page 99.*

reduced sense of personal accomplishment Feeling that one is failing others. A common component of burnout. *See page 89.*

Relational Health Communication Competence Model The theory that communication, social support, and emotional resilience are positively associated with one another. *See page 92.*

role theory The perspective that positions within a society (e.g., healer, patient) are defined by unique sets of rights, responsibilities, and privileges. *See page 83.*

socialization A process of learning to behave appropriately within a specific community. *See page 81.*

team A set of individuals who work together to achieve common objectives. *See page 97.*

Voice of Medicine A style of communicating about health that is characterized by carefully controlled compassion and a concern for accuracy and expediency. *See page 82.*

Discussion Questions

1. If you were designing a communication course all care providers would take, what five communication skills would you emphasize most and why?

2. Considering the transformation at Virginia Mason Cancer Center, what would you do to improve the environment and reduce wait times at your doctor's or dentist's office? Be creative.

3. How do you respond to some care providers' argument that they must limit patient's input so they can keep exams within a particular time limit? How might organizational leaders help with this? How might patients help?

4. Name some strategies for avoiding burnout as a care provider. Which of these do you, or might you, incorporate into your own life whether you are a care provider or not?

5. In the case of Willie King, whom do you believe should be held responsible for amputating the wrong leg? Why? Whom, if anyone, should be sued? Who should pay the extra medical bills?

6. What do you say to health professionals who are devastated by a mistake and want to apologize, yet are afraid that doing so will invalidate their malpractice coverage and possibly destroy their careers?

7. Imagine that your grandfather is the hypothetical patient described in the chapter as Mr. S. What types of professionals would you choose to be on his care team? What factors would you like them to focus on mostly? Why?

Sociocultural Issues

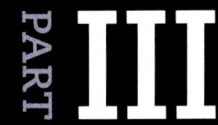

We can become so caught up in our own view of health and healing that we forget that these are largely cultural constructs. In some cultures, *healing* evokes images of science and technology; in others, the power of Mother Nature and meditation. Bernie Siegel has taught us that love and laughter should be part of the mix as well. Sadly, diversity sometimes becomes the basis for discrimination and exclusion, such that the color of our skin is a factor in how long we are likely to live—not because we are born with different genetic blueprints, but because inequitable resources and discrimination affect our health. In this section, we sample a rich variety of cultural perspectives about health and healing. We also look at the link between health and race, socioeconomic status, literacy, and other factors. As you will see, effective communication is our most promising means of learning about, celebrating, and integrating diverse ideas.

If you watch how nature deals with adversity, continually renewing itself, you can't help but learn.

—BERNIE SEIGEL, MD

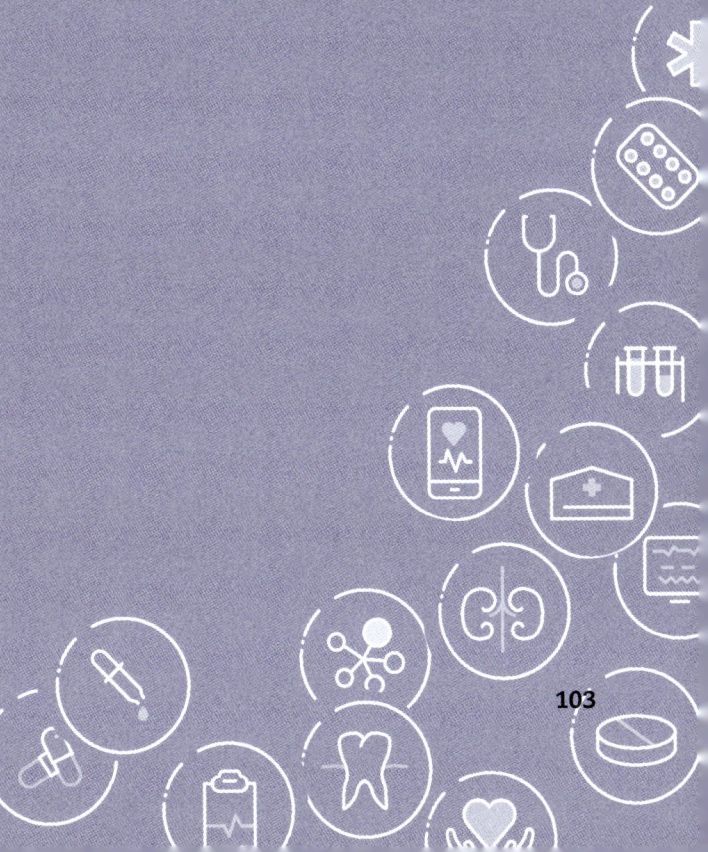

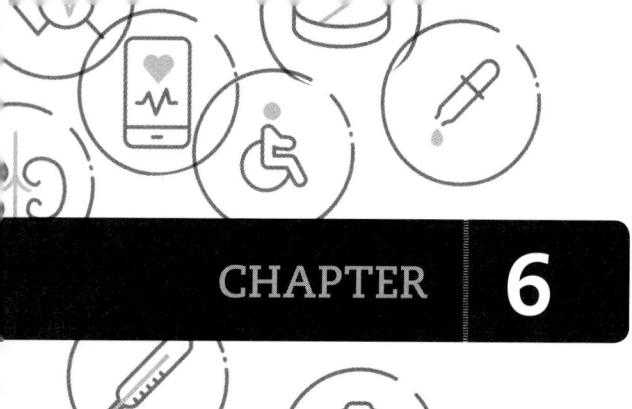
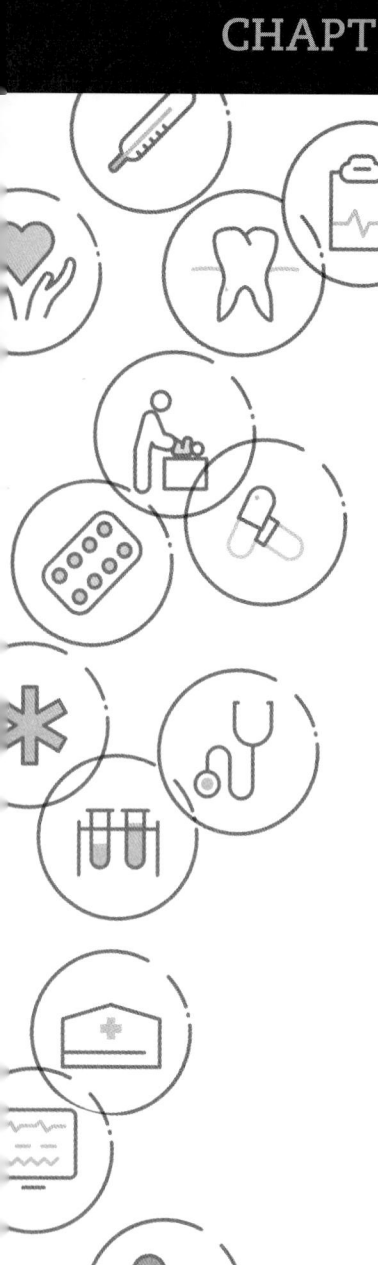

CHAPTER 6

Diversity in Health Care

She was in a motorized wheelchair that she controlled with her only usable finger. I could not understand her guttural speech or her facial contortions. She could not consistently hold her head up or control her drooling. After a few desperate moments, I asked her if she knew how to use a typewriter. She managed to make me understand a "yes" answer, and I ran out of the room to locate a typewriter on a movable stand. Pleased with my ingenuity, I stood next to her expecting some limited request. My smugness gave way to sheer awe as she painstakingly, letter by letter, tapped out with her left fourth finger the question: "What are the risks for me taking the birth control pill?"

In this account, Lucy Candib (1994, p. 139) recalls a young woman who taught her anew to respect each patient as an individual. It may be tempting to group people within impersonal categories. However, there is extraordinary diversity among the people who seek health care.

Since diversity among health professionals still does not reflect the diversity in the population overall, people are likely to see caregivers whose experiences are different from their own. This can be an opportunity for growth and connection. It can also be an occasion for misunderstandings. The difference often lies in the quality of communication they share.

In this chapter we explore diversity among both patients and caregivers in terms of socioeconomic status and literacy, sexual orientation, race and ethnicity, language, disabilities, and age. As you will see, factors such as these interconnect in unique ways to influence health and the way we communicate about it.

Intersectionality Theory

"Human lives cannot be reduced to single characteristics," writes theorist Olena Hankivsky (2012, p. 1713). No one is simply a man or a woman, heterosexual or gay, rich or poor, or so on. Instead, individuals are influenced by how these identities (and many others) intersect within the context of larger environments. These points are central to **intersectionality theory**, which proposes that a person's social position emerges within the interface of micro-level personal identities and macro-level sociocultural patterns (Bauer, 2014). Each of these levels is dynamic and complex. Personal identity may reflect age, race, sexual orientation, physical ability, and education, to name just a few. Sociocultural variables may include sexism, racism, power, resources, public policies, and so on (Crenshaw, 1989, 1991).

One implication of intersectionality theory is that social position is not simply the sum total of different identities. Lisa Bowleg (2008) offers the example that "Black + Lesbian + Woman ≠ Black Lesbian Woman" (p. 312). Indeed, the theory emerged in the late 1980s, when Kimberlé Crenshaw (1989) made a similar observation—that issues facing Black women were not well represented in either the civil rights movement, which focused mostly on Black men, or the women's movement, which focused mostly on White women.

Another implication is that it is infeasible to rank-order the variables that influence social position. This becomes obvious if you try to answer the question, "Which influences your life more—your sex or your race?" You would probably say, "I can't compare them" or "It depends." As Bowleg (2012) points out, "no social category or form of social inequality is more salient than another from an intersectionality perspective" (p. 1271). In the end, the *intersection* of complex micro- and macro-level factors is different and more impactful than any factor on its own.

When applied to health communication, intersectionality theory reminds us that categorizations such as *older adults, persons with disabilities*, and *the poor* mean very little by themselves. The theory also draws attention to people who are exceptionally disadvantaged by the multiplicity of factors that influence them. For example, Hispanic immigrants in a New Mexico community say they are aware that diabetes may kill them one day, but many of them struggle daily just to feed their families, do not have health insurance, and feel that health professionals resent it when they use the community clinic. In the context of all these factors, many of the immigrants believe, or at least hope, that they can manage diabetes on their own with folk remedies (Page-Reeves et al., 2013). A health campaign that addresses only one of these issues is unlikely to change their circumstances very much.

Intersectionality theory also emphasizes that guesses and generalizations often have harmful consequences. There is no substitute for getting to know people (be they coworkers, patients, members of at-risk communities, or anyone else) in terms of the overlapping identities and social structures that define life as they experience it. Achieving this level of localized knowledge may seem like a daunting challenge, but evidence suggests that it can be both rewarding and effective in terms of carrying out research, creating high-impact health campaigns, and developing effective health policies (Hankivsky, 2012; Hankivksy et al., 2014; Turpin, 2013).

The remainder of this chapter explores aspects of personal identity most often referenced in intersectionality theory. (Chapter 8 broadens the scope to explore more macro-level considerations.) As you read, keep in mind that, although it is most manageable to talk about these dimensions of identity one at a time, they are not experienced that way and their effects are not the same for everyone.

Socioeconomic Status

Chaquita Turner lives two blocks from a neighborhood park, but she seldom brings her children there because of gang violence, prostitution, open drug use, broken glass, and the threat of being mugged. In addition to the daily stress of living in that environment, she and her family have few opportunities to exercise or enjoy the outdoors.

Turner says that change is needed, but because her neighborhood is "at the bottom of the totem pole" public officials mostly consider it a lost cause (quoted by Seervai, 2018a, para. 10). Her story reflects elements of **socioeconomic status** (SES), an overarching term that factors in education, income, employment level, and similar variables.

The link between health and SES is a strong one. In the United States, a 40-year-old woman in the top income bracket is likely to live 10 years longer than a woman in the bottom income bracket, and the life-span differential among men is even larger, at 14.6 years (Chetty, Stepner, & Abraham, 2016).

Many factors play into the link between health and SES. Theorists use the term **health inequities** to describe structural and systematic factors that put some groups at a disadvantage compared to others

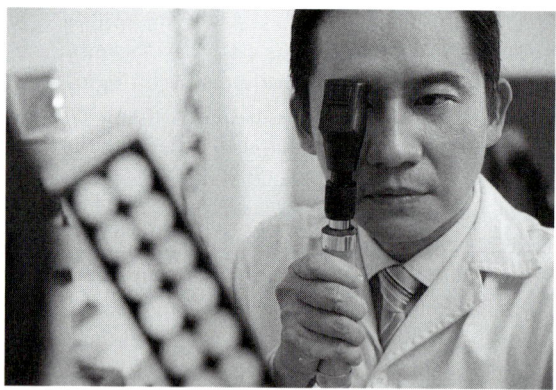

By virtue of their specialized knowledge, tools, and institutional settings, care providers sometimes seem intimidating even when they don't mean to be.

Have you ever perceived a status difference between yourself and a health care provider? If so, how did that affect the way you communicated with them?

(Braveman, 2006). Low-SES individuals often live in neighborhoods affected by pollution, crime, violence, financial strain, discrimination, inadequate public transportation, and a shortage of educational opportunities and health services (WHO, 2017). These environments are often *food deserts* in which fresh, healthy food is unavailable or unaffordable ("USDA Defines," 2011). Largely as a consequence, people of low SES are more likely than others to suffer from depression, to have attention-deficit/hyperactivity disorder, be obese, smoke, have poor oral health or various forms of cancer, and more (Cruz, 2014; National Center for Health Statistics, 2012; Peretti-Watel et al., 2014).

As of this writing, about 1 in 10 Americans under age 65 has neither private nor state-sponsored insurance (Garfield & Orgera, 2019). As one person of limited means reflects, that forces difficult decisions such as "do you want your teeth, or do you want your heart to continue beating? You've got to figure out which one" (quoted by Lewis, Abrams, & Seervia, 2017, para. 1). Since survival relies on balancing very tight budgets, people may forsake immunizations and health screenings, particularly if they don't know the costs involved. Researchers suggests that, whenever possible, health promoters state upfront what patients will be expected to pay for public health services (Chen, Moran, Frank, Ball-Rokeach, & Murphy, 2018; Maertens, Jimenez-Zambrano, Albright, & Dempsey, 2017).

Even when health care is accessible, it can be tricky to negotiate treatment decisions. Physicians surveyed by Susannah Bernheim and associates (2008) said that, ideally, SES should not be a factor when making treatment decisions, but practically speaking it often *is*. That's because patients of low SES may lack reliable transportation, have rigid or unpredictable work schedules, be incapable of paying for medications, or have a hard time finding specialists or therapists who will take them on as clients. Said one doctor in the study:

> *He [a patient] was a trucker ... we really had to tailor the medication. He did not have any proper time to eat, and you know, he did not have time to come to his appointments. We have to tailor his appointments according to his travel schedule. It is not optimal, but we do the best we can. (p. 56)*

In this and other ways, physicians surveyed said they try hard, but they are often constrained by factors outside their control (Bernheim, Ross, Krumholz, & Bradley, 2008).

Other barriers are conveyed largely through communication. People of low SES are more likely than others to perceive that care providers are disrespectful, unconcerned, and don't understand their circumstances (Arpey, Gaglioti, & Rosenbaum, 2017; Horowitz et al., 2012; Singh, Evans, Williams, Sezginis, & Baryeh, 2018). Part of the problem involves different expectations and vocabularies. For example, Hispanic patients with diabetes may follow doctors' advice not to eat "white bread" to the letter, but they may be unaware that flour tortillas are also bad for them (Vardeman-Winter, 2017).

Preconceived notions can also be a stumbling block. A meta-analysis of 10 years of research suggests that, like members of the larger population, health professionals often display an *implicit bias* (behavior based on unconscious stereotypes) toward some individuals on the basis of their race, ethnicity, gender, and socioeconomic status. For example, providers may assume that hardship is the result of weakness or laziness. Many of the general practitioners Sara Willems and colleagues (2005) interviewed consider that people are impoverished mostly because they do not try hard enough to overcome their circumstances. Said one doctor, "[Low income individuals] are not interested in their health. They don't see the advantage of, for example, healthy food" (p. 180). It's easy to understand how patients may pick up on such attitudes and feel judged and misunderstood.

Communication gaps also arise when participants have different expectations about a health care visit. Physicians in the United States typically consider patients to be proactive if they are assertive, ask questions, and engage actively in conversations (Verlinde, De Laender, De Maesschalck, Deveugele, & Willems, 2012). However, people of low SES are typically less assertive than other patients. They tend to ask fewer questions and reveal less about their health concerns (Fleming et al., 2017; Fowler, 2006). This may be because they are not highly knowledgeable about health issues, they are intimidated by health professionals, and/or they consider it disrespectful to question or challenge them (Bao, Fox, & Escarce, 2007). Whatever the reasons, a downward spiral often results from these mismatched expectations. Health professionals may perceive that low-SES patients are uninterested or apathetic. As a result, they themselves may come off as less attentive and less immediate than they normally would, which can further heighten patients' anxiety and reticence, and so on.

Barriers to effective care are especially regrettable considering that low-SES patients are less likely than others to feel confident reading health information and understanding health statistics (Smith, Wolf, & Wagner, 2010). They are also less likely to seek out health information online (Hovick, Liang, & Kahlor, 2014; Lee, Ramírez, Lewis, Gray, & Hornik, 2012). As a result, they tend to rely mostly on television and people they know for health information, which contributes to a knowledge gap since those sources do not offer as much information as the web (Seo & Matsaganis, 2013). On the bright side, some health promoters are using mobile devices to convey information to people who might not otherwise get it. As you will see in Chapter 9, mobile technology is now prevalent, even among people who don't have computers.

Although we have been talking in generalities, keep in mind that there is enormous diversity among people who fall into the category of low SES. For example, some people have low-income jobs but are highly educated. Evidence suggests that these individuals are even more dissatisfied than others when they feel rushed or belittled during health care encounters (Jensen, King, Guntzviller, & Davis, 2010).

There is also diversity among care providers. Some are vigorous advocates for impoverished patients and actively try to help them improve their health, neighborhoods, and living conditions (Willems, Swinnen, & De Maeseneer, 2005). Care providers who devote themselves to helping low-SES individuals often say they are gratified to be part of communities that appreciate their efforts, even when resources and salaries are limited. "When you live in a small town like this and somebody runs up to you at a baseball game or in the grocery store and gives you a hug because of something you did for them, I think that is all the pay that you need sometimes," says one physician (quoted by Seervai, 2018b, para. 19).

Issues of socioeconomic status point to the dangers of stereotyping and categorizing. As you will see next, people who suffer from health literacy challenges also work hard to avoid feeling judged and alienated.

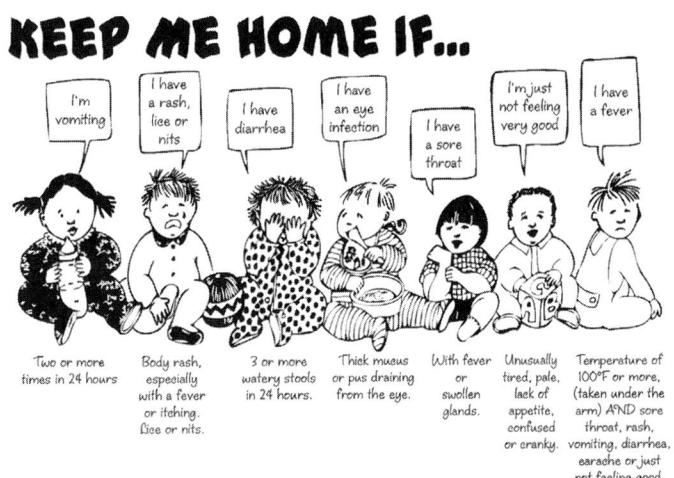

This page from the booklet *What to Do When Your Child Is Sick* provides easy-to-understand advice for parents about children's minor health concerns.

Have you ever wondered whether to stay home from school or work, or whether to seek professional attention for a health concern? If so, how did you resolve your uncertainty?

Health Literacy

The hospital staff uses an orange to teach a patient how to give himself daily insulin shots for diabetes. Later, when his blood sugar is worse than ever, the staff realizes the communication breakdown: The man has been injecting insulin into oranges at home and then eating them (Boodman, 2011).

. . .

A tired mother misunderstands the instructions "3 tsps" on a cough syrup bottle. She uses tablespoons rather than teaspoons, thereby giving her child the equivalent of 9 teaspoons of medicine.

. . .

When a man sees that the results of his biopsy for prostate cancer are "positive," he is relieved. He doesn't realize that "positive" means he has cancer.

. . .

Health literacy refers to individuals' ability to access health information, to understand it, and to apply it in ways that promote good health (WHO, 1998). The conventional idea of literacy as the ability to read is part of the equation. But health literacy involves a great deal more than that. To be health literate, people must also:

- understand the language in which information is conveyed (be it English, Spanish, statistical jargon, legal talk, or some other language variant),
- have access to reliable and relevant information,
- be interested in health-related information,
- have the social skills to discuss health matters with others,
- have adequate hearing and/or vision to get the information,
- understand how to apply the information, and
- be willing and able to put health information to effective use.

Regarded in this way, it's clear that being health literate is no simple matter. Medical information is often baffling, even to well-educated individuals. The man who thought "positive" meant he was cancer free was an attorney and former mayor of New York (Boodman, 2011). Such a misunderstanding could happen to anyone.

To the 32 million adults in the United States with serious health literacy challenges, misunderstandings can have tragic consequences (U.S. Department of Education, 2015). They are less likely than other people to get flu shots and to undergo cancer screenings, and they are more likely to miss appointments, to misuse medication, to prepare improperly for procedures, to be hospitalized, and to die prematurely (Berkman et al., 2011).

Part of the problem is that health tends to have a language of its own, and health professionals may forget how foreign it is to most people. For example, "Why do hospitals have signs for the 'nephrology department' when patients with kidney disease who need that department's services are unlikely to know what the word nephrology means?" asks a representative of Harvard University's school of public health ("Improving Americans', health literacy" 2011, para. 1). (See Table 6.1 for a list of other words that can easily baffle people, and suggestions for expressing the same ideas more clearly.)

Of course, people who are not strong readers are at a distinct disadvantage. About 1 in 5 adults in the United States reads below a fifth-grade level ("National Assessment of Adult Literacy," 2014). However, most health information is written at a much higher level (Ryan et al., 2014). That includes instructions on prescription bottles and medical consent forms.

In the United States, literacy is a special challenge for people who do not speak English well. Researchers in California found that residents with limited English were more than three times more likely than others to have health literacy challenges and poor health status as a result (Sentell & Braun, 2012). (We talk more about language barriers later in the chapter.)

Emotions play a role as well. People who are otherwise highly literate may feel so overwhelmed by medical information that they cannot pay close attention to it. For example, imagine that a health professional is teaching you to provide care at home for a loved one with a ventricular assist device, which involves a wire extending from inside your loved one's chest to a bank of complicated electronics, says patient advocate Diana Dilger (2013):

> *You're in charge of making sure the wire stays clean. It if doesn't, it could mean infection and possible death. . . . You might pay an obscene amount of attention every time she shows you how to do it. But maybe the enormity of this responsibility blocks you from really remembering every step. (para. 2 and 4)*

Dilger recommends that health professionals acknowledge the emotional intensity of encounters such as these, provide written or online instructions, and schedule follow-up conversations to make sure people

TABLE 6.1 Words That Can Baffle

Following are some of the "words to watch" in the American Medical Association's free Ask Me 3 health literacy toolkit, along with suggestions for being more easily understood.

COULD BE CONFUSING	A CLEARER ALTERNATIVE
Adverse (reaction)	Bad
Ailment	Sickness, illness, problem with your health
Benign	Will not cause harm; is not cancer
Cognitive	Learning; thinking
Excessive	Too much
Intake	What you eat or drink; what goes into your body
Lesion	Wound; sore; infected patch of skin
Noncancerous	Not cancer
Oral	By mouth
Progressive	Gets worse
Referral	Ask you to see another doctor; get a second opinion

have a chance to ask questions when they are thinking more clearly.

Literacy challenges may be masked by embarrassment. People are often too ashamed to admit they cannot read or understand medical information (Mackert, Donovan, Mabry, Guadagno, & Stout, 2014). Even friends and family members may not realize it. At a briefing to launch the American Medical Association's (AMA) new health literacy initiative, physician David W. Baker said:

> We find that a lot of people have gone through their lives and listen to the radio, watch television and don't read their newspapers too often but can get by pretty well with minimal reading skills.... They come into the health care setting and they are all of a sudden faced with medications and instructions and all of this information written at too high a level for easy comprehension. (AMA, 2003, para. 7)

People in this situation may be mortified to admit that they do not understand. As a result, they are more likely than others to avoid medical care, to take medicine incorrectly, to overlook health risk factors, and to miss out on important information. Avoidable health care costs attributed to health literacy are estimated at $106 billion to $238 billion a year in the United States—enough money to insure more than 40 million people (Vernon, Trujillo, Rosenbaum, & DeBuono, 2007).

The unfortunate result of status- and literacy-related communication barriers is that the neediest people often receive the least amount of information and attention. In an effort to overcome that, experts offer the following tips for public health professionals, caregivers, and patients.

Skill Builders for Public Health Care Professionals

- *Watch your language.* Words such as *pandemic, influenza,* and *prevalence* can frighten and confuse rather than inform. Use everyday language instead (USDHHS, n.d.-a).
- *Use multiple formats.* A combination of words, diagrams, and videos helps to appeal to people with diverse learning styles and literacy resources.
- *Evaluate messages for effectiveness and cultural appropriateness.* Audience reaction is the ultimate gauge of how effective messages are. Pilot health messages with target audience members before disseminating them, and then assess their impact afterward.
- *Focus on action.* Specific suggestions for health behavior can be more valuable than lengthy explanations.

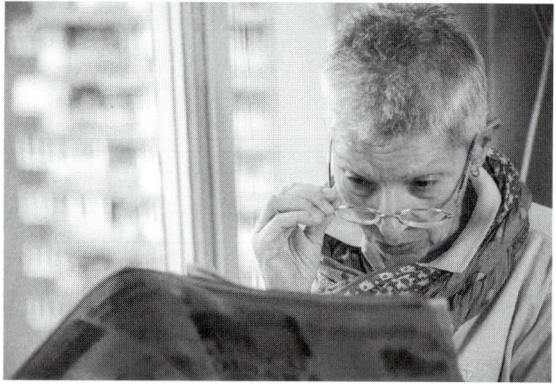

For people with significant health literacy challenges, it can be challenging to read the label on a prescription bottle, understand instructions, and keep appointments straight.

What would you say to patients who are ashamed to admit they cannot understand information? What might we do to make them feel less anxious?

Skill Builders for Health Care Providers

- *Create shame-free environments.* Make it easy for patients who do not understand information to get assistance without embarrassment. For example, routinely offer to help patients fill out intake paperwork rather than simply handing it to them. A statement such as, "These forms can be confusing. The nurse will help you, if you like," signals that it is okay and normal to need assistance.
- *Gauge literacy levels.* Although it's difficult for most people to admit literacy challenges aloud, about 90% of patients say it would be helpful if their doctors understood their limitations (Wolf et al., 2007). Most are in favor of simple questionnaires that allow them to disclose reading and math challenges in a face-saving way (Ferguson, Lowman, & DeWalt, 2011; Vangeest, Welch, & Weiner, 2010).
- *Be attentive and respectful.* Try to identify patients' needs and respect their contributions. Do not assume they are uninterested if they are quiet.
- *Let patients know what is expected.* Patients may be tongue tied by intimidation or simply be unaware of what is expected of them. Explain routines and encourage them to participate in discussions.
- *Use metaphors and pictures to help explain complex ideas.* Remember that words and concepts you consider familiar may be baffling to nonprofessionals. Comparing pneumonia to a saturated sponge or arthritis to creaky hinges can help bridge the gap between health information and concepts that people already understand.
- *Use the teach-back method to make sure patients understand.* Physician Howard J. Zeitz describes his approach: "The way I do it is to ask, 'When you get home tonight, your husband or wife will probably want to know what happened. What are you going to tell him or her about what you and I agreed to in the office today?'" (quoted by O'Reilly, 2012, section 3). Asking "Do you understand?" or "Do you have any questions?" is notoriously ineffective. Most people will simply say "yes" and "no" to avoid sounding foolish. Unless patients can explain aloud what you have told them, you cannot be sure they understand.

Skill Builders for Patients

- *Be explicit about your feelings.* Don't assume that health professionals understand your concerns. Statements such as, "I'm embarrassed to say this but . . ." or "I feel scared about . . ." will help them know how you feel.
- *Ask three key questions.* The American Medical Association and cosponsors of the Ask Me 3 program encourage patients to ask the following questions: *What is my main problem? What do I need to do?* and *Why is it important for me to do this?* (Ask Me 3, n.d.).
- *Admit it if you don't understand.* "You are not alone if you find things confusing at times," says a spokesperson for Ask Me 3. You might say, "This is new to me. Will you please explain that one more time?" (Ask Me 3, n.d.).

Gender Identity and Sexual Orientation

"You always reach that moment in the conversation with the doctor where they ask you the birth control question. 'Are you sexually active?' 'Yes.' 'Are you using birth control?' 'No.' And then they stare at you."

This is a common predicament among people in same-sex relationships. The woman quoted summarizes the options this way: simply say "no" and give the impression that you are irresponsible; or divulge your sexual orientation, even if you are not yet comfortable doing so (Venetis et al., 2017, p. 582).

A related dilemma often confronts people with queer identity while completing intake forms at health care visits. **Queer theory** challenges the notion of static identities and rigid social categories (Butler, 1999). It represents the idea that binary labels such as *man* and *woman* underrepresent the multitude and complexity of gender identities that people actually experience. Nevertheless, medical forms often give only two options—male or female (Redfern & Sinclair, 2014). The implication is that anything else is invalid or abnormal, and people may have a literal sense of being "marginalized" if they write something different on the edge of the paper.

It's more than semantics. Although it can feel risky to divulge one's gender identity or sexual orientation, people may receive substandard care if providers are not aware of them (Potter, 2002). For example, a transgender woman with male genitalia may be at risk for prostate issues and other concerns that are not immediately apparent. Or care providers may overlook a lesbian woman's need for information about sexually transmitted infections if she says she doesn't have "sexual intercourse" (Goins & Pye, 2013).

Moreover, staying quiet may rob people of valuable health information and guidance. When researchers surveyed African American men who have sex with men, they found that those who communicated openly with their care providers were more likely than others to be aware of their hepatitis risk and to be vaccinated for it. However, their numbers were small: only 34% of the men in the study had been vaccinated (Rhodes, Yee, & Hergenrather, 2003).

Although the internet may be one way for LGBTQ+ individuals to find information they are not comfortable asking about in person, accurate online sources are still fairly scarce (Rose & Friedman, 2013). A study of websites about lesbian sexual health revealed that they were often difficult for the average person to understand, and that they focused mostly on HIV and AIDS and very little on preventive measures such as mammograms and gynecological care (Lindley, Friedman, & Struble, 2012).

Another risk of staying quiet is that it deprives people of opportunities to feel valued for who they are. Jennifer Potter, a physician who is gay, says she has sometimes passed as heterosexual. "On the face of it, maintaining silence makes almost everyone happy," she reflects—everyone, that is, except herself and her closest friends (2002, p. 342). In periods in which she allowed people to believe she was heterosexual, Potter says she felt she was lying by omission. Pretending to be straight eroded her self-respect and put her in cahoots with people who wished to ignore and invalidate multiple gender orientations. It also isolated her socially. She could not introduce her long-term partner to friends or invite her to professional and social gatherings. Now, although Potter is open with her close friends and associates, some people still presume she is heterosexual. "Coming out is a process that never ends," she says. "Every time I meet someone new I must decide if, how, and when I will reveal my sexual orientation" (p. 342).

A third danger is that, if partners are not acknowledged or if they are not married, they may be denied visiting privileges and information when one of them is sick or injured. This point hit home with internist Suzanne Koven when she had shoulder surgery. "My husband of 30 years did all the things a loving spouse would be expected to do: He fluffed my pillows and put toothpaste on my toothbrush (try doing that with one arm!) and overlooked my crankiness," she remembers. It saddens her, she says, to think of "lesbian and gay couples who are as deeply committed as my husband and I are" but who are not allowed the same opportunity to support their loved ones during health crises (Koven, 2012, para. 1–3).

In summary, a person is adversely affected when they feel they cannot be open with health care providers. For their part, health professionals who avoid talking about gender and sexuality are not necessarily prejudiced. They may be embarrassed or uncomfortable with the subject or feel that it lies outside their expertise, especially because their training may not have

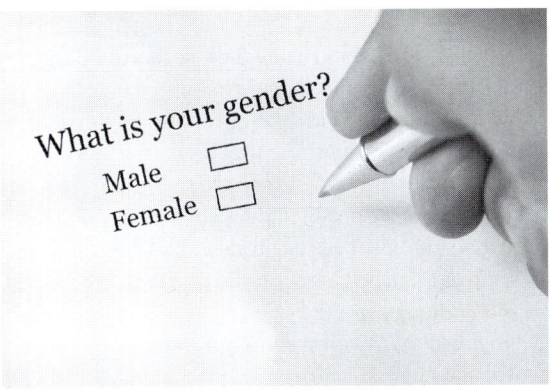

Many health questionnaires don't provide options for people to accurately describe their gender identity or sexual orientation.

What are the implications for health communication and health outcomes if people feel they cannot be honest about their identity and sexual practices?

addressed issues of diverse gender identity (Levine, 2013).

Experts offer the following suggestions for health professionals.

- *Practice aloud*. People who rehearse conversations about sex and gender with friends and colleagues may feel more comfortable conversing about these topics with patients. Care providers who are comfortable with the topic are more likely to help patients feel at ease as well (Gamlin, 1999).
- *Consider the questions you ask*. On written forms, include an option for patients to write in (if they wish) their gender; sexual orientation; name and pronouns; and if they have sex with men, women, or both (Goins & Pye, 2013). (It's most useful to let people describe themselves rather than providing a fixed number of options.) Consider the same issues when you ask questions in person.
- *Use the person's name and pronouns*. Addressing a person as *Mr.*, *Ms.*, *he*, or *she* when they identify another way can cause them to feel disconfirmed and uncomfortable (Ross & Bell, 2017). Likewise, summoning a patient from the waiting room with a name or honorific they do not use may have the embarrassing effect of "outing" them in front of others.
- *Don't ignore the issue*. Research suggests that most individuals would like health providers to know about their sexual identity, but they tend to wait for providers to ask.
- *Don't be "nosy."* People with diverse gender identities say that it's fine for health providers to ask questions such as "What do you identify with?" and "What are your pronouns?" Beyond that, however, they urge providers to focus on sex and gender only when they are relevant to their health. Overly personal questions meant only to satisfy the speaker's curiosity can feel nosy and embarrassing (Ross & Bell, 2017).
- *Avoid judgment*. Transgender individuals report that health providers sometimes make judgmental statements such as "It's my job as a Christian to save you" and "What the hell is this?" (Ross & Bell, 2017, p. 736). Even more subtle signs of disapproval can discourage patients from sharing information and concerns that are integral to their care (Redfern & Sinclair, 2014).

As you will see in the next sections, a fear of discrimination also influences people of different races and ethnicities.

Race and Ethnicity

During clinical rotation as a medical student, Jennifer Adaeze Okwerekwu often felt that she was treated differently because she is Black. Once "a patient called me a 'colored girl' three times in front of the attending physician," she recalls, adding that, "the doctor did not correct the patient, nor did she address the incident with me privately. . . . Her silence in this circumstance diminished my presence. I wondered if she thought of me as a 'colored girl' too" (Okwerekwu, 2016, para. 14).

Okwerekwu is now a physician and a columnist for the online publication *STAT*. Interested in the intersection of social ideas and health care, she has worked with CNN, *The Dr. Oz Show*, Radio Disney, and the Kaiser Family Foundation Health Reporting Program. She has degrees from Harvard, Columbia University, and the University of Virginia ("Columnist, Off the Charts," n.d.). She is no stranger to the idea that racism can make you sick.

Racism is discrimination based on a person's race. Race is an imprecise term, loosely defined in terms of social identity and hereditary background. Practically speaking, people often judge race by visible characteristics, such as skin color, although appearance is not a reliable indication of race. *Ethnicity* reflects cultural identity such as shared language, religion, and customs. The terms *race* and *ethnicity* are often used together, but they are not synonymous. For example, if you are the children of immigrants, you may be of the same race as your parents but identify with a different set of beliefs and customs. Or perhaps you identify with more than one ethnic group, as many people do.

For the most part, there is no biological reason that people of different races and ethnicities should fare differently in life (Kaufman, Dolman, Rushani, & Cooper, 2015). Nevertheless, members of many minority groups in the United States are in poorer-than-average health. Black Americans are twice as likely to die from preventable heart disease and strokes as White Americans are (CDC, 2014), Hispanic Americans are 50% more likely to die of diabetes (CDC, 2015), and the list goes on. Compared to others of the same sex, Black men typically die four years sooner than the national average, and Black women three years sooner (CDC, 2014). In this section we consider why these differences exist and the implications for health communication.

There are several reasons why people of different races and ethnicities may receive different medical care and respond to it differently. Overall, the differences are mostly rooted in distrust, high risk, lack of knowledge, limited access, and ineffective patient–provider communication.

Distrust

Some people steer clear of health care because they distrust the medical establishment based on historic patterns of discrimination such as the Tuskegee Syphilis Study described in Chapter 4 (Meredith, Eisenman, Rhodes, Ryan, & Long, 2007). In the United States, members of racial and ethnic minorities are more likely than others to feel that their doctors fail to listen, to show respect, or to explain things clearly (Commonwealth Fund, 2008; Hwang et al., 2017; Singh, Evans, Williams, Sezginis, & Baryeh, 2018).

Distrust may cause people to underutilize health services and to doubt the validity of medical advice (Armstrong et al., 2013). This could contribute to the comparatively low number of medical interventions among African Americans and Hispanics. They may be approved for prescriptions they never fill and may decline to undergo medical procedures if they distrust health professionals. Or they may avoid seeking care at all.

High Risk, Low Knowledge

Members of some nondominant racial and ethnic groups often are not well informed about health issues even though they are at high risk for them. One health-eroding factor is the daily stress of social discrimination. Medical research shows higher than average incidence of hypertension and heart disease among people who are subjected to everyday discrimination, such as poor service, insults, and being treated as inferior or stupid (Szanton et al., 2012).

People of color may also be at high risk because a disproportionate number of them are of low socioeconomic status. With limited resources, they may suffer from poor living conditions, stress, unhealthy diets, and insufficient access to health information and health services (Dinwiddie, Zambrana, & Garza, 2014).

Despite their high-risk status, people of color may be relatively unaware of health issues because, on average, they do not use or trust mainstream media as much as White audiences and because many health messages are not designed to appeal to them. For example, illnesses related to smoking are the leading cause of death among Hispanic/Latinx individuals (CDC, 2018), but few stop-smoking programs are designed for them (Piñeiro et al., 2018).

Individuals who are not well informed about health services and disease warning signs are more likely than others to become seriously ill before they seek medical attention (Ginossar, 2014). If people are sicker than others when they seek medical care, that might explain, in part, why they do not respond to treatment as well and why they do not undergo the same procedures as other patients.

Limited Access

A third explanation is that members of some minority groups have comparatively low access to advanced medical facilities. Below the age of 65 (when Medicare coverage begins), about 1 in 3 Hispanic Americans and Native Americans and 1 in 5 Black Americans are uninsured, compared to about 1 in 10 non-Hispanic White Americans (Artiga & Orgera, 2019). In the United States, people without health insurance are about half as likely as others to be screened for cancer (Collins, Rasmussen, Doty, & Beutel, 2015). They are also less likely to qualify for care in medical centers that offer high-tech and advanced-care treatment (Venkatesh et al., 2019), and they are more likely to go without needed care and to be financially devastated by medical bills (Henry J. Kaiser Family Foundation, 2018).

"Your health care depends on who you are," conclude researchers for the Robert Wood Johnson Foundation who studied the different care received by members of racial and ethnic minorities in the United States ("Reducing Disparities," 2014, para. 1). Data over the last 14 years consistently show that members of ethnic minorities, especially if they are of low-income, receive less care and lower quality care than others (USDHHS, 2016). Physicians agree. Some 55% of those surveyed say they believe White patients receive better care than minority patients, and nearly 2 out of 3 have personally witnessed such episodes (American Medical Association, 2005). When Clara Manfredi and colleagues (2010) studied nearly 500 American cancer patients, they found that, all else being equal, the Black patients were less often referred to cancer specialists than the White patients were (Manfredi, Kaiser, Matthews, & Johnson, 2010).

It's a familiar theme. A decade earlier, Schulman and colleagues (1999) videotaped actor/patients describing chest pains using the same words and gestures, wearing identical clothing (hospital gowns), in the same setting. The patients differed only in terms of age, sex, and race. Doctors who viewed the patients' videotaped presentations of symptoms were significantly more likely to recommend heart catheterization for White male patients than for female or Black patients. (See Box 6.1 for a discussion of ethical principles when allocating health resources.)

BOX 6.1 Ethical Considerations

Who Gets What Care?

Doctor, do everything you can!

Is it ever justified for a care provider to do less than everything possible? Conventional American wisdom says no. Americans have come to expect that physicians will provide the best possible care, cost notwithstanding. However, it has become too expensive to do everything possible for every person.

At the same time, many people feel that if the U.S. health system is to survive, it is necessary to make judgments about who gets what care. Health care leaders are being called on to eliminate excessive and unnecessary procedures. The question is: *Where is the line between necessary and unnecessary?*

One option is to provide care to those people who can afford it. This option places underprivileged persons at a disadvantage and may create a deeper schism between people of high and low socioeconomic status. All in all, few people are willing to allow low-income citizens to suffer in ill health.

Another option is to give priority to procedures that are known to have high success rates. For instance, a procedure that gives patients a 30% chance of survival may be granted priority over one with a 20% survival rate. This seems logical, but as Norman Levinsky (1995) points out, statistics are merely generalizations, and every patient is unique. There is no guarantee that a risky procedure will fail or that a tried-and-true one will succeed. Moreover, statistics vary, and sticking with well-established procedures diminishes the chances of developing new, better ones.

Still another option is to provide care for people who are likely to enjoy the highest quality of life as a result. From that perspective, it might be more important to fund expensive treatment to help a young child walk than to help an 85-year-old use his legs again following a stroke. Levinsky (1995) warns that such judgment calls are likely to lead to unfair discrimination. He wonders how it is possible to judge people's quality of life, and warns that such judgments are likely to be biased against people who hold values different from those of the medical decision maker.

As you can see, deciding how health resources will be allocated is no simple matter. To get an idea of how difficult it is, try answering the following questions.

What Do You Think?

1. If one person can afford expensive treatment but another cannot, is it okay to refuse care to the less affluent person?
2. If there is a slight chance that an expensive experimental drug will prolong a dying person's life, should the insurance company or health organization pay for use of the drug? Why or why not?
3. If two people have the same condition, should they be treated differently? What if one is a child and one is very old? What if one is famous and the other is unknown? What if one is homeless and the other is a community leader?
4. If you could fund only two of the following procedures, which would you choose? On what criteria would you base your choices?
   a. Surgery to help an infertile couple conceive a child
   b. Plastic surgery to improve the appearance of a person born with a facial deformity
   c. Chemotherapy for a person with cancer
   d. Drug therapy that might prevent a person from getting AIDS

continued

5. Who should decide which care will be funded? Doctors? Funding agencies? Community members? Patients? Legislators? Explain your answer.
6. If researchers are able to develop improved treatment options but the cost of the research significantly raises health care costs, should the system continue to fund research? What if higher costs mean some people will lose their insurance?
7. Doctors say one reason they overtreat patients is because they may be sued for malpractice if they don't do everything possible. How would you resolve this dilemma?

Stereotypes

As we mentioned in Chapter 2, care providers do not yet reflect diversity in the overall population. Although Black and Latinx individuals make up about 31% of the U.S. population, only about 16% of the country's dentists, 14% of pharmacists, 15% of physicians, and 20% of registered nurses are from these groups (U.S. Bureau of Labor Statistics, 2014, 2019; U.S. Census Bureau, 2014; U.S. Census Bureau News, 2018). These differences can lead to stereotypes and communication gaps.

There is a history in the United States of treating patients differently because of prejudice. An African American participant in Meredith Grady and Tim Edgar's (2003) study remembers being diagnosed with diabetes and the diagnosing physician's reaction:

> *He said, "I need to write this prescription for these pills, but you'll never take them and you'll come back and tell me you're still eating pig's feet and everything.... Then why do I still need to write this prescription?" And I'm like, "I don't eat pig's feet." (p. 393)*

The patient was left to wonder how the doctor's prejudicial assumptions affected other decisions.

Of course, the effects go both ways. Jennifer Adaeze Okwerekwu, the physician described at the beginning of this section, says she and colleagues experience the sting of "everyday racism" (Okwerekwu, 2017). Other care providers describe patients who take one look at their Muslim headscarf and make insulting comments or insist on being cared for by someone else (Saadi, 2016). Care providers are sensitive to discrimination, just as patients are. Physician Jerome Groopman (2007) urges people to consider that patients and their loved ones are responsible for showing health professionals the same respect they wish to be shown themselves.

Intercultural Health Communication

Ethnic concordance is the perception of cultural similarities between oneself and another. When patients and care providers are of similar ethnicities, the patients tend to say more, be more trusting, and remember more about the encounter (Alegría et al., 2013; Arendt & Karadas, 2019). The effects are especially strong among patients who have trouble understanding health information in general (Arendt & Karadas, 2019).

When patients and providers have different communication styles, it's easy to misunderstand one another and overlook important cues. For example, researchers point to a so-called happy migrant effect that occurs when patients (particularly those who are new to a culture) act as if they are happy and satisfied with their health care to appear polite and respectful, even when they have serious concerns (Garret, Dickson, Young, & Klinken Whelan, 2008). A person familiar with their culture might pick up on signs of pain or distress, but someone from a different culture might underestimate the severity of a patient's symptoms, anxiety, or reservations about care options.

Similar patterns are present in health messages communicated to larger audiences. For example, health campaigns that encourage Hispanic parents to have their teens vaccinated for the sexually transmitted human papillomavirus (HPV) may be ineffective if they don't take into account a general cultural preference for warm (as opposed to clinical) language and if they don't address a widespread fear in that culture that vaccinated teens will feel encouraged to have sex (Maertens, Jimenez-Zambrano, Albright, & Dempsey, 2017).

Professionals from underserved groups are more willing than their peers to provide care for underprivileged patients. About 49% of non-White minority medical students say they plan to provide care for the underserved, compared to 19% of White students, and

16% of Asian Americans and Americans with ancestry from India, Pakistan, and the Pacific Islands (Saha, Guiton, Wimmers, & Wilkerson, 2008). Personal heritage is not the only factor, however. Medical students whose classmates are of highly diverse backgrounds are more likely than others to feel confident in their ability to care for minority patients and to advocate for equitable care for everyone (Saha et al., 2008). Based on evidence such as this, some people feel that recruiting more minority health professionals should be a priority.

We have spoken a good deal in this section about racial and ethnic identities. But, of course, people differ on an even deeper level as well. A new type of discrimination—based on health conditions that have not even surfaced yet—may loom ahead. See Box 6.2 for information about the pros and cons of genetic profiling.

BOX 6.2

Genetic Profiling: A View Into Your Health Future

"The crystal ball says you will live a long and healthy life."

It's hard to put much stock in such a prediction. But scientists have come up with something better. They did it by unlocking the codes that make up individuals' genetic blueprints (Human Genome Project Information Archive, 2008).

These days you might have genetic testing done to find out if you are predisposed to various forms of cancer, liver disease, Alzheimer's disease, or other conditions known to have a genetic link. Being predisposed to these diseases doesn't mean you'll necessarily get them. In fact, one promise of genetic testing is that you might find out in time to lower your odds. For example, you might engage in more preventive behaviors if you know you are at high risk of certain disorders, and be screened for them more regularly than usual.

One reservation concerning genetic testing is people's fear that the results will be used against them or their family members. The Genetic Information Nondiscrimination Act of 2008 (better known as GINA) stipulates that health insurance companies cannot refuse health coverage on the basis of genetic test results, nor can they require people to undergo genetic testing. By extension, GINA rules out informal genetic profiling, such as basing a person's insurance rates on a family history of heart disease. In the past, health insurance companies could figure family history into the price of your coverage. GINA now forbids that practice.

GINA also stipulates that employers cannot judge job applicants or current employees on the basis of genetic profiles. That is, they cannot hire, fire, promote, or refuse to promote anyone because of genetic propensities. Nor can employers require, request, or purchase genetic test results on any employee. (This does not apply to tests designed to monitor the effects of workplace exposure to dangerous materials. Those are still allowed.)

It is important to note what GINA does not cover, however. The stipulations don't apply to life insurance, long-term care insurance, or disability insurance. And GINA doesn't apply to the U.S. military, the Veterans Administration, or the Indian Health Service, because they are governed by a different set of laws.

What Do You Think?

1. If it were affordable, would you undergo genetic testing? Why or why not?
2. Are you worried that genetic test results may be used to discriminate unfairly against individuals or groups of people? Why or why not?
3. Suppose your test results show a genetic propensity for a disease that, so far, we don't know how to prevent. Would you want to know? Why or why not?
4. Do you think genetic test results would strengthen your resolve to engage in healthy behaviors? Why or why not?

Language Differences

Physician Harold Jenkins set a goal for himself to learn at least un poquito *(a little bit) of Spanish. He began writing several new Spanish words on index cards every day and studying them. While driving to work, he challenged himself to read traffic signs and license plate numbers aloud in Spanish. "I even rolled my Rs," he says (Jenkins, 2008, p. 42).*

Spanish-speaking nurses who work with Jenkins have encouraged him. They aren't put off that he can only speak Spanish in present tense or that his pronunciation is sometimes a bit off. (One nurse was amused when he asked a patient to "vacuum deeply" instead of inhaling.) They give Jenkins a thumbs-up for trying. His patients appreciate the effort as well. Jenkins says he feels like a better doctor when he can understand and speak at least a bit of the patients' language. He's right. It's hard to offer quality care across a language gap. And that gap is notable.

About 1 in 5 residents of the United States speaks a language other than English at home (Batalova & Alperin, 2018). Even when their English is adequate for most activities, medical settings can present linguistic challenges. Although health care agencies that receive federal aid are required by Title VI of the Civil Rights Act to "take reasonable steps" to make health care information understandable to people who are not proficient in English, it's often unclear who should pay for health care interpreters (USDHHS, n.d.-b, para. 1). In many cases, family members and multilingual employees fill in as untrained interpreters, even if they speak English poorly themselves and have little knowledge of medical terminology (Juckett & Unger, 2014).

Medical interpreting is difficult. Even people who are fluent in both languages may have a hard time fully conveying the speakers' tone and intent. Sometimes a direct translation is not easy or possible. For example, members of the Hmong culture do not have a word for cancer. In Chinese, the word for "voices" also means "noises," so a patient being evaluated for mental illness may indicate that they hear "voices," when they actually just mean that they can hear sounds (Fisher, n.d.).

Even colloquial terms such as "okey dokey," "under the weather," and "going under the knife" can cause confusion (Vickers & Goble, 2011). As one person struggling to master a new language says: "You think you understand what all the individual words in the phrase mean—but put together, they lose all meaning" (Moffatt, n.d., para. 2). For example, if you're not a native Japanese speaker, imagine how you might struggle to interpret idioms such as "eight-tenths full keeps the doctor away" and "if you speak of tomorrow, the rats in the ceiling will laugh." (The first suggests that moderation is healthy, the second that it's foolish to try to predict the future [Moffatt, n.d.]).

Language barriers can compromise the quality of care people receive. It's difficult to make an accurate diagnosis if a care provider cannot fully understand what a patient is experiencing. And even if the diagnosis is correct, it's hard to ensure that patients are fully informed concerning their medical options. (Box 6.3 describes the experiences of a Spanish-speaking woman in a U.S. hospital.)

A physician at Maimonides Medical Center in New York asserts that language differences increase a patient's risk factor by about 25%. "When you walk up to a person

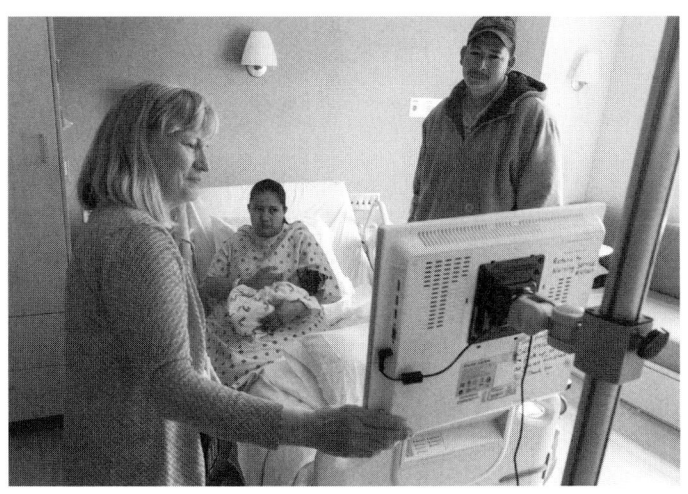

A social worker communicates with a Spanish-speaking family with the help of a remote interpreter available in the hospital via video technology.

Have you ever had trouble understanding health-related information because the terms used were unfamiliar to you? If so, what did you do?

BOX 6.3 PERSPECTIVES

Language Barriers in a Health Care Emergency

Picture yourself in Mexico at a hospital trying to get someone, anyone, to help make a terrible pain in your stomach go away. You hear: "Tú no hablas español, y nadie te puede entender." In other words, "You don't speak Spanish, and no one can understand you." Finally, you find a first-year English student, a schoolboy, who attempts to translate. Next, you find yourself in a room, half-clothed, wearing a hospital robe, wondering: *Did the boy understand me? Did the doctors understand him? What is wrong with me? What is happening?*

Perhaps this will give you some idea what it's like for Spanish speakers in the United States health care system. This is a true story about my mother, Maria, and her mother, Consuelo, Cuban Americans trying to deal with the frustrations, anxieties, and fears of communicating with medical professionals who speak a different language.

The Story

Consuelo had been showing symptoms for some time before finally agreeing to see a doctor. Now that she had moved to a new city with little to no Hispanic culture, she wondered fearfully if she would be able to communicate with doctors. But this time the pain was intense, and at least she had her daughter, Maria, to help her communicate. Consuelo wanted very much to be understood, and maybe this time she would be. That thought finally gave her the courage to see a doctor.

At the doctor's office Consuelo could tell something was wrong. She was now in her early sixties and knew her diabetes was not getting any better. She understood enough of the conversations between the doctors and her daughter to gather that she needed a heart catheterization. Maria was not giving her all the details, but Consuelo could sense from her body language that the procedure was serious. She was right. A few moments later she found herself being wheeled off to the operating room for an emergency cardiac catheterization—without Maria. Now she felt more scared and afraid, knowing she had no means of communicating with the people around her and unsure what they were doing or why.

Before the procedure, the surgeon needed Consuelo to understand the process and answer some questions. This was no easy task. Once again, as Consuelo had feared, she was unable to communicate. By this time, she began feeling extremely anxious and frustrated that neither the surgeon nor any of his assistants could understand what she was saying. Finally, after what seemed decades, the surgeon summoned Maria to the operating room after finding no one else who could translate.

For Maria, the experience involved mixed emotions. She had accompanied her mother many times before to the hospital but had never been allowed inside the operating room. Now that she was there, she felt more anxious than ever. First, she wanted to do a good job because she felt that her mother's life depended on it. Second, she felt uneasy being in the room because she was unfamiliar with the environment. Consequently, Maria did not know how she should act, what she should say, or what was expected of her. She also had to fight her emotional reactions at seeing her mother on the operating table. However, Maria was relieved to be able to be with her mother and decided to concentrate on positive feelings to get them both through the experience.

When Consuelo was back in a hospital room after the procedure, the doctor broke the news that Consuelo needed open-heart surgery and would soon be transferred to a larger hospital. Once again, Consuelo could tell something negative was being conveyed, but knew she would have to wait until the conversation was over to get the full story from Maria. Waiting only added to her anxiety. A few times, Consuelo tried to interrupt, but was only chastised by Maria for interfering with her efforts to understand the implications of what the doctor was trying to tell her.

Unfortunately, although the larger hospital was located within a predominantly Hispanic community, few doctors and nurses there could speak Spanish. That meant that Maria and her husband, Jesús, would have to take turns staying at the hospital to translate for Consuelo. But the difference in Consuelo's outlook was remarkable. After only a few hours in the new hospital, she started to feel better about herself and less depressed. This was because the new physicians, regardless of whether they spoke Spanish well

continued

or not, attempted to speak to her in Spanish and to understand what she was saying. Consuelo recalled one young physician who would walk into her room saying, "Buenos días," bringing a smile to her face, and then leave saying, "Buenas noches," despite the time of day, making her laugh. These small gestures made all the difference to Consuelo.

Maria noticed that her mother began to light up whenever a doctor entered the room. She also noted that the doctors were no longer looking at her but talking directly to her mother instead. Maria was still translating, but she was no longer the focus of their conversation. In return, she noticed that her mother seemed more attentive and willing to follow the doctors' advice. A few times, Consuelo even answered the physicians in English with responses such as "Yes" when she understood what they were saying. This in turn would make them laugh and rub her hand as a sign of acceptance and reward. And if this were not enough, Consuelo was introduced to a Spanish-speaking nurse at the hospital who would occasionally visit, making her feel even more at home.

The surgery went well, but following it, Consuelo was paired with a therapist who could not speak Spanish and made no effort to communicate with her. She began to feel depressed and frustrated again. But she learned to get over this new obstacle quickly after talking about her feelings with her family. They found a way to make her realize that her good experiences at the new hospital far outweighed the bad ones, and soon Consuelo was able to ignore the therapist's behavior and move on with her treatment.

Consuelo was in the hospital for about a month. In that time she learned a lot about what she liked and did not like. As a result, she asked Maria to help her look for doctors who would be as attentive with her as the hospital doctors had been. Now Consuelo has at least one doctor she likes very much who speaks Spanish.

—MARIE

What Do You Think?

1. How might you have acted if you were Consuelo? If you were Maria?
2. Do you think hospitals should do more to accommodate non–English speakers? Why or why not?
3. How could Consuelo have eliminated some of her anxiety?
4. What could the first surgeon have done to help both Maria and Consuelo feel more at ease?
5. Researchers have found that people are more fearful about medical visits if they feel socially alienated and disconnected from their environments. What might we do to ease these feelings?
6. Have you ever been in a situation in which you have had to communicate with someone who did not speak the same language as you? How did you handle the situation?

---

from another country who speaks another language, that is a risk—period. It's as much of a risk factor as diabetes or anything else," says the doctor (quoted by Salamon, 2008, para. 5).

Cognizant of the risk, Maimonides Medical Center employs more than 30 patient representatives who help families and interpret when needed. The medical center's president and CEO Pamela Brier has implemented a "Code of Mutual Respect," complete with staff training sessions on communication and diversity appreciation. The extra effort is worth it, says Brier:

> Communication problems are what cause mishaps that can harm patients. I mean communications between doctor and nurse, nurse and clerk, housekeeper to nurse or doctor, everybody. The idea of the "Code of Mutual Respect" for me was to make the place safer and medical care better. (quoted by Salamon, para. 9)

It is her conviction that good communication is good medicine and good business.

Other efforts are underway as well. Wake Forest University School of Medicine has had success helping physician assistants work effectively with interpreters and Spanish-speaking patients. After a four-hour training session, 97% of students were able to demonstrate proficiency in role-play scenarios that involved interpreters and non-English-speaking patients (Marion, Hildebrandt, Davis, Marin, & Crandall,

2008). Members of other organizations report success using trained interpreters who are either present in the exam room or linked via telephone or videoconference technology (Jones, Gill, Harrison, Meakin, & Wallace, 2003). (For more about careers related to language diversity in health care, see Box 6.4.)

Following are experts' strategies for communicating about health matters when language differences are an issue (Fisher, n.d.; "6 Tips," 2017; Squires, 2018).

- Learn at least a few key words in the other language.
- Try to avoid using idioms and slang, or at least explain their meaning.
- When using an interpreter, speak in full sentences. Stopping midstream to let the person "catch up" may alter their understanding of the message.
- Don't hesitate to talk more with the interpreter to clarify what you mean if they seem confused or uncertain about what you have said.

Disabilities

When Anna, who has Down's syndrome, was in the hospital with pneumonia, her care team worked with her to fill out a "health passport," which helped them learn more about Anna's physical condition and realize that she is afraid of the dark and loves Elvis Presley. Thereafter, they always left a lamp on in her room, and they frequently initiated conversations about Elvis to engage and soothe her. When Anna left the hospital, she was allowed to keep the health passport to share with health care providers in the future (Blair, Glaysher, & Cooper, 2010).

Health professionals have typically not received much training on how to communicate with people who have physical and cognitive challenges. Here we consider the interface between different abilities and health communication.

What It Means to Have a Disability

The World Health Organization (WHO, 2002) challenges us to abandon the notion that there are two types of people—those with disabilities and those without them—and to recognize, instead, that we all have disabilities in various forms and degrees. This perspective shifts the focus away from labels and more toward the goal of helping every person function optimally in life.

As you may remember from Chapter 1, the WHO's International Classification for Functioning (ICF) represents a biopsychosocial approach. To illustrate, imagine that you are unable to climb stairs. A *medical* approach, such as surgery or physical therapy, might be effective if it helps you regain the physical capacity to use stairs. That may or may not be possible. A *social* approach, on the other hand, focuses more on the environment and on people's attitudes. For example, decision makers at your school, workplace, or favorite grocery store might provide rails, ramps, elevators, or other features that allow you to use the space much like anyone else. A host of other personal and social factors are involved as well, such as resources, coping ability, public policies, and social support.

BOX 6.4 Career Opportunities

Diversity Awareness

Diversity officer
Equal Employment Opportunity (EEO) officer
Health care interpreter

Career Resources and Job Listings

- American Hospital Association's Institute for Diversity in Health Management: www.diversityconnection.org
- National Council on Interpreting in Health Care: www.ncihc.org
- Registry of Interpreters for the Deaf: www.rid.org
- U.S. Equal Employment Opportunity Commission: www.eeoc.gov
- U.S. Bureau of Labor Statistics Occupational Outlook Handbook: www.bls.gov/ooh

In the example that opens this section, the care team and Anna take an approach that allows them to minimize communication barriers. A **health passport** is a collection of information that allows people to express biopsychosocial needs and preferences in an easy-to-share format (Blair et al., 2010). A range of customizable templates are available. Anyone can download a health passport template online, respond to any prompts they wish, and print copies to share with others. Information might include biomedical details (such as medications, allergies, and immunizations) as well as psychosocial preferences (such as how the person prefers to communicate, their religious beliefs and cultural background, what helps them feel better, and what makes them feel anxious or afraid). Health passports are especially helpful for people with physical or intellectual challenges. But anyone can benefit from them, especially in emergencies and difficult situations. In a study by Marina Heifetz and Yona Lunsky (2018), one emergency room care provider said they are helpful for "anyone who goes to an appointment of any sort that might be nervous and forget things" (p. 27).

Communication Dilemmas

Individuals with significant disabilities are often confronted with frustrating dichotomies. For one, people tend either to treat their disabilities as the most important thing about them or self-consciously to avoid the issue entirely. For example, care providers often focus on the disability and ignore other concerns that are not directly related to it (Braithwaite & Thompson, 2000). In other situations, however, people may consider it taboo to talk about the disability. A woman described by Dawn Braithwaite and Lynn Harter (2000) said she initially appreciated it when her future husband did not make a big deal about her disability when they met. But after several months of getting to know each other, she was exasperated that he never even mentioned the subject. Eventually she brought it up to end the awkward silence about it.

Another dichotomy concerns the way persons with disabilities are regarded by society. Sally Nemeth, a health communication scholar who is blind, reflects that people with disabilities are often cast "either as heroic super crips or as tragic, usually embittered and angry, unfortunates worthy only of pity and charity" (Nemeth, 2000, p. 40). The reality is that people with disabilities are much like anyone else.

It's frustrating to be treated as helpless or unsophisticated. Health professionals (and others) sometimes treat individuals with disabilities as if they are childlike—speaking slowly and loudly to them even when that isn't necessary and giving instructions rather than asking for their opinions. People may also avoid talking to people with disabilities about sensitive subjects such as sex.

People whose disabilities are invisible to others may encounter unique difficulties. Some are loath to admit disabilities they think will make them seem dependent or pitiful (Moore & Miller, 2003). A study of people with heart disease revealed that they often consider themselves older than their same-age peers, largely because of physical limitations and attention to end-of-life issues typically associated with older people (Kundrat & Nussbaum, 2003). (For more about the frustration of invisible disabilities, see Box 6.5.)

On the bright side, even brief training sessions can help caregivers interact more confidently and sensitively. In a training program piloted by Ashley Duggan and colleagues (2009), medical students interacted with trained standardized-patient educators with disabilities, then took part in interactive feedback sessions about the experience. The medical students acknowledged that the patients' disabilities and appliances sometimes made them feel awkward and uncomfortable, they were unsure

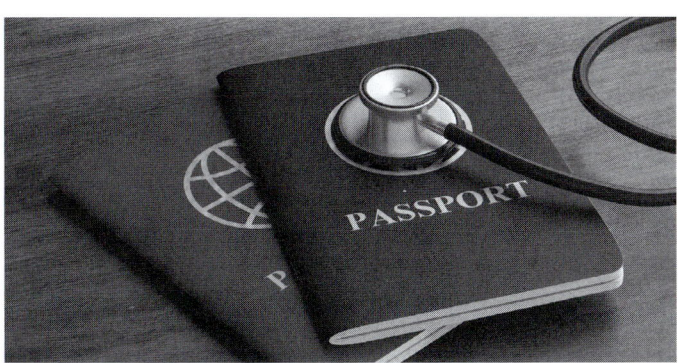

Health passports, easily downloaded online, help patients share information about their physical and emotional needs with health care providers.

Have you ever thought it would be helpful to provide information to a health professional in writing, perhaps because you might forget it or feel too rushed or nervous to say it aloud? Is the idea of a personal health passport appealing to you?

BOX 6.5 PERSPECTIVES

My Disability Doesn't Show

Dear Editor,

Since receiving my handicapped hangtag two years ago, I have been rudely approached by so many people that I've lost count.

I am a 44-year-old female, tall, thin, and do not walk with a cane, nor am I in need of a wheelchair. My handicap is internal, from two major back surgeries, and although I do have pain while walking, I walk with confidence. By simply looking at me, one would not know that I have a handicap.

Since using my handicapped hangtag, I have been rudely approached by, not only people off campus, but from just as many students on campus. I have heard it all, from "You sure look handicapped" or "You must really be handicapped from driving a car like that (a 1992 Firebird)," to "How can I get one of those (a handicapped hangtag)?" These comments not only hurt my feelings but are truly insulting, especially since I received my back injuries from serving my country while in the military, and the scar on my back extends from my neck to my buttocks.

I would like to educate everyone on campus, as well as people off campus, that not all handicaps are visible. Not everyone with a handicap is over 60, nor do they have to walk with a cane, nor do they have to be in a wheelchair.

In order to receive a handicapped hangtag, the Department of Motor Vehicles requires that one must have limitations of walking because of arthritic, neurological or orthopedic (which I have) conditions, and one must have a disability rating of 50% or greater. My disability rating is 80% and is permanent.

The last comment came January 28th by a student getting into his blue truck, which was parked next to me in front of the campus police station. The young man made the normal comment that I did not look handicapped. Normally I usually just tell people if they have a problem with me to take my license plate number and report me, but this time, I lost it and told this guy to mind his own business, and added a few explicit words to boot.

I would like to see people stop stereotyping others based on their looks and think before they inadvertently insult someone, because it really does make me feel bad, and I have every right to use my handicapped tag.

—BEVERLY DAVIS

Source: Copyright © 2003 by The Voyager, the student newspaper at the University of West Florida. Reprinted by permission from The Voyager *and Ms. Davis.*

---

whether to talk about the disability or ignore it, and their advice was sometimes off the mark, as when one medical student advised a wheelchair user to ease the symptoms of her tendonitis by not using her shoulder. The student later told the mock patient, with chagrin: "Your arms are your mobility and independence, and I'm telling you to stop you using them" (Duggan, Bradshaw, Carroll, Rattigan, & Altman, 2009, p. 804).

Following are some tips from the experts.

Communication Skill Builder: Interacting with People Who Have Disabilities

- Talk to people with disabilities directly, not to their interpreters or companions.
- Remember to identify yourself to sight-impaired persons.
- Treat adults with disabilities as adults.
- When a person with a disability is difficult to understand, listen attentively, and then paraphrase to make sure you heard correctly.
- Whenever possible, sit down when conversing with people in wheelchairs so that you can communicate at eye level.
- Relax! For example, don't be embarrassed if you accidentally say "See you later" to a blind person.
- Don't insist on helping people with disabilities. If they don't ask for help or if they decline your offer of assistance, respect their wishes (Soule & Roloff, 2000). (It's okay to extend the same courtesies you would offer an able-bodied friend, such as holding a door open.)
- Heed the wisdom of Thuy-Phuong Do and Patricia Geist (2000), who remind us: "Everyone is othered to some extent; we all possess disabilities, whether visible or invisible" (p. 60).

As you have probably gathered by now, the concept of being "othered," or treated as if you do not belong, is demoralizing in everyday life and particularly in health care interactions. As the following section shows, age can be a source of "othering" as well.

Age

Aging alone is rarely viewed in a positive light and thus has led many to depict aging as a time of great loss and decline. —Jon Nussbaum (2007, p. 1)

In his presidential address to members of the International Communication Association, Nussbaum (2007) challenged scholars to reconsider social assumptions about aging. "Aging alone has also been a favorite of the great poets, playwrights, and novelists, who love to make us feel the 'horribleness' of our lonely human existence," he said (p. 1). But that idea, he argued, is more cultural myth than objective reality: "My mission is to spread the news that we are not purely or even remotely organisms that exist only within our own skins" (p. 1). Nussbaum proposed that it is possible to age happily and that the nexus of sustained quality of life is effective communication, as evidenced by people's ability to manage interpersonal conflict, develop relationships, manage uncertainty, share thoughts and ideas, and more.

In this section we examine the communication practices that affect people throughout their lives. We focus first on children and then more extensively on older adults. As you will see, both groups use health care services a great deal, and their communication is profoundly affected by the assumptions of people around them.

Children

"She gots bad monsters inside her tummy that try to eat her up,"—said 4-year-old Sophit explaining her mother's breast cancer.

This quote, from Jenifer Kopfman and Eileen Berlin Ray's (2005) case study "Talking to Children About Illness" (p. 113), helps to illustrate the way children make sense of illness. Although their conceptualizations may seem naive, children are often remarkably attuned to the ramifications of illness experiences. When Sophia's young friend Ethan asked her what color the monsters were, she said, "I think they're orange 'cause orange's a gross color" (p. 113). She went on to explain what happened when her mother received chemotherapy:

She always gives me lots of hugs and kisses before she gets her medicine from the doctor 'cause she says it makes her throw up and be tired after she takes it, and I hafta be quiet and let her sleep and not ask for too many hugs and kisses until she feels better again. (p. 113)

After that, Ethan showed Sophia his "scary monster face" and they dashed off to play.

Communicating with children can be challenging because their perceptions are often different from those of adults. For example, children may perceive that painful medical treatments are a means of punishment (Ryan-Wenger & Gardner, 2012). Moreover, children may be unsure how to express their feelings or may be afraid to speak freely in front of people they don't know.

Bryan Whaley and Tim Edgar (2008) outline the phases of development in which children conceptualize illness with increasing degrees of sophistication.

- In the **prelogical conceptualization** phase (roughly ages 2–6), children define illness as something caused by a tangible, external agent, such as a monster or the sun.
- In the **concrete-logical conceptualization** phase (roughly ages 7–10), children begin to differentiate between external causes, such as wind and cold, and internal manifestations, such as sneezing and talking funny.
- In the **formal-logical conceptualization** phase (roughly age 11 and older), children are remarkably adept at envisioning the complex influence of agents they cannot readily see.

In contrast to the "monsters inside her tummy" explanation, older children may be capable of understanding and articulating sophisticated explanation of illness. Consider this example from Bibace and Walsh's (1981) study, in which they asked children older than 11 to explain various illnesses:

Have you ever been sick? "Yes." What was wrong? "My platelet count was down." What's that? "In the bloodstream they are like white blood cells. They help kill germs." Why did you get sick? "There were more germs than platelets. They killed the platelets off." (Bibace & Walsh, p. 37)

This is a good reminder that children's ideas typically evolve over time.

PARENTS' ROLE IN CHILDREN'S CARE

Parents can be both a help and a hindrance in caring for young patients. Many times, parents have valuable information about their children's conditions and are able to comfort them as no one else could. Parents may become especially frustrated if their concerns are not taken seriously or if they do not feel well informed about their children's health needs (Haskell, Mannix, James, & Mayer, 2012). And rightly so. Parents are the children's principal caregivers, and their responsibility does not end at the doctor's office or hospital. However, it can be difficult for caregivers to attend to young children *and* manage the complex emotions of their parents. Parents tend to be especially anxious, guilty, and uncertain where their children's health is concerned.

When children are hospitalized, parents and professional caregivers may have conflicting ideas about what care each of them should provide. It may be unclear who is to feed the child, change bandages, and perform other tasks. With nurses' input, Rebecca Adams and Roxanne Parrott (1994) drafted a list of tasks parents should perform for their hospitalized children. By sharing the list with parents (orally and in writing), the nurses were able to reduce parents' uncertainty and their own. As a result, the nurses were more satisfied with their jobs, and the parents were more confident in the care their children received.

COMMUNICATION SKILL BUILDER: TALKING WITH CHILDREN ABOUT ILLNESS

Bryan Whaley, who has conducted extensive research about children in health situations, and colleagues offer the following advice for explaining illnesses to children.

- *Let children set the tone*. Determine what the child wants and needs to know before launching into explanations they may find incomprehensible, distressing, or irrelevant (Nussbaum, Ragan, & Whaley, 2003; Whaley, 1999; Whaley & Edgar, 2008).
- *Pay attention*. Notice how the child conceives of illness and medical care. Ask questions and invite the child to describe (and perhaps to draw) what is wrong (Whaley, 2000).
- *Go easy on medical terminology*. Usually, children are more interested in how an illness will influence their lives and activities than in the precise germs, tests, and scientific names involved. As Whaley (1999) puts it, "Disease and etiology appear inconsequential or of negligible concern to children," at least when they are young (p. 190).
- *Talk about illness as something normal*. Children are typically reassured to know that their illnesses are normal and manageable. Speaking of an illness as a crisis or mystery may interfere with the child's coping ability (Whaley, 1999).

Buchholz (1992) adds that children benefit from honesty. Like adults, children usually cope better if they have a realistic idea of what to expect from health care experiences. Adults should also keep in mind that prior experience with medical procedures may not diminish children's fear and anxiety (Buchholz, 1992). Experienced youngsters may be all too aware of how frightening and painful procedures can be.

Older Adults

> When a physician told James McCague's 85-year-old aunt that she was not a candidate for bypass surgery because she was "quite functional" for her age, she objected. "I am the sole caretaker of my 90-year-old sister," she said. "I can't be just 'functional.' I want to be as healthy as I can be" (McCague, 2001, p. 104). Her doctor saw her point and performed the procedure.

A physician himself, McCague reflects on changes among elderly patients:

> The elderly patient does not report symptoms with resignation; the questions ask for a solution. The elderly patient does not want [their] questions taken within the context of [their] age and, more important, is angry when the physician does so. (p. 104)

McCague advises fellow health professionals to consider that, while it may sometimes be necessary to shape and moderate expectations, people's desire to be healthy whatever their age is real and laudable. "We must never ignore or ridicule it," he says. "And my aunt? She had her revascularization several years ago. I called her last week to say hello, but she wasn't home; she was in town getting her passport photo" (p. 104).

Experts predict that about 1 in 5 Americans will be 65 or older by the year 2050 (Ortman, Velkoff, & Hogan, 2014). Population shifts will likely change health care needs and transform our understanding of the aging process. As with all stereotypes, the belief that all members of a group are alike in some way (e.g., sad, fun, weak, jovial) never holds up. **Ageism is discrimination based on a person's age.** It occurs when people judge others by preconceived notions about their age group, as when managers refuse to hire people over 65 because they believe employees of that age are not productive.

Ageism results largely from negative stereotypes of older adults. Health personnel sometimes reinforce these stereotypes by referring to older patients in such derogatory terms as "coffin dodgers" and "digging for worms" (Fowler & Nussbaum, 2008). Older adults are often portrayed in the media as unhealthy, lonely, unhappy, and irritable (Robinson, Callister, Magoffin, & Moore, 2006). Of 84 Facebook groups that talked about older adults, only one presented them in a positive light. Most described older adults as annoying, grouchy, and incompetent (Levy, Chung, Bedford, & Navrazhina, 2014).

People with ageist beliefs are unlikely to regard older adults as unique individuals who can change, learn, react, and grow physically stronger. Instead, they tend to patronize older adults by speaking slowly to them, using baby talk, and restricting conversations to happy subjects (Cavallaro, Seilhamer, Chee, & Ng, 2016; Hummert & Shaner, 1994). They may even avoid communicating with older adults (Giles, Ballard, & McCann, 2002).

Social beliefs about growing older often have profound implications for people's identity. When Laura Hurd Clarke and Meredith Griffin (2008) interviewed women ages 50 to 70, many of them said they actively engage in beauty work to maintain a youthful appearance because they believe that, if they do not, they will become "invisible" in society's eyes. As one woman in the study put it: "Be young or you're not counted" (p. 660). Another expounded:

> We won't love women if they're not lovely. . . . And as you get older, you get less and less okay, and people look at you less and less. . . . It gets down to "Well, you're old. You can't look good anyway." So, I think it's about trying to look young, youthful, perky, and put on this "See I'm lovely, you can love me" kind of thing. (pp. 660–661)

Women in the study said they feel immense pressure, both from the idea that women's worth is inherent in their appearance, and from the notion that feminine beauty is inherently youthful.

Based on the idea that getting older is a process of decline, people often assume that natural signs of aging (hearing loss, vocal changes) indicate cognitive deficits. Young adults tend to underestimate the cognitive abilities of older adults with known hearing loss, although they score them highly on wisdom and visual memory (Ryan, Anas, & Vuckovich, 2007).

Despite Western society's cynical views about aging, many older adults enjoy good health, rewarding relationships, and a positive outlook on life (Nussbaum, Ragan, & Whaley, 2003). When Laurie Schur and Lisa Thompson interviewed women 80 and older for the video documentaries *Greedy for Life* (2008) and *The Beauty of Aging* (2012), they found that some of the women were frustrated with the effects of aging, but most said they were having the time of their lives. A 97-year-old woman in the video said, "A few years ago someone asked me what time of my life did I like best and I said 'now.'" Another one said, "I see women 50 and 60 decide to give up on life and go sit down somewhere, don't look forward to a future. Even at 82 years old I've still got things that I want to do."

The baby boomers may change popular notions about aging. Actress Helen Mirren, for one, is defying the adage that women above a certain age cannot be sexy or adventurous. Now in her seventies, Mirren continues to play action roles and allow herself to be depicted in the nude or partially clothed. What's more, she insists that the images be portrayed realistically, not computer enhanced to make her appear younger than she is (Overton, du Pré, & Pecchioni, 2015).

COMMUNICATION ACCOMMODATION THEORY

To **accommodate** is to adapt to another person's style or (perceived) needs. When people believe, rightly or wrongly, that older adults have diminished capacities, they tend to change their behavior toward them. For instance, people may speak more loudly or move closer. Despite changing trends, reconciling Western society's negative view of aging with new ideas about getting older is still a challenging enterprise with numerous implications for health communication.

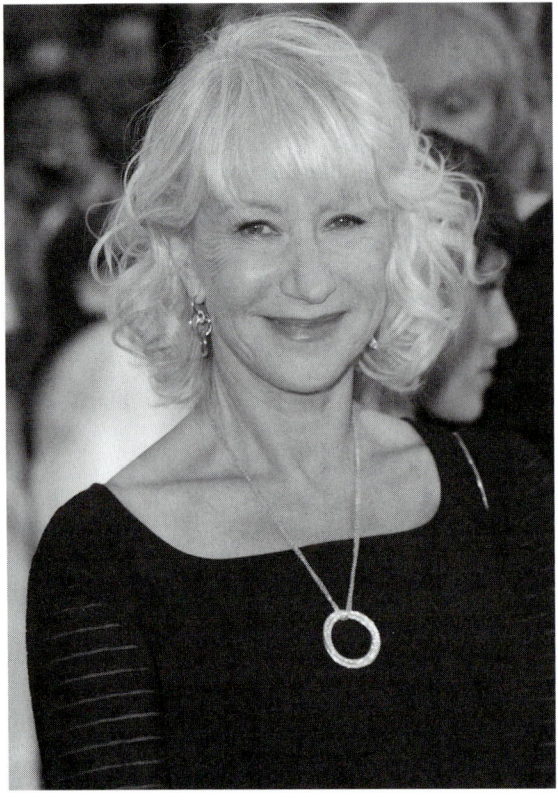

Helen Mirren is challenging the notion that women can only be sexy if they are young. She continues to play femme fatales in her 70s. Some people predict that she and other baby boomers will transform society's view of aging.

As you get older, how do you expect your identity to change, if at all? What role do you think communication will play in establishing the identity you envision for yourself?

In some cases, accommodation is useful and appreciated. According to **communication accommodation theory**, people tend to mirror each other's communication styles to display liking and respect (Coupland, Coupland, & Giles, 1991). **Convergence** occurs when partners use similar gestures, tone of voice, vocabulary, and so on. On the other hand, **divergence** involves acting differently from the other person, as in whispering when the other shouts. Divergence implies that the partners are socially distant. They may be asserting uniqueness, pursuing different goals, or displaying that they don't understand or don't like each other.

To illustrate, patients who are baffled by their doctors' rapid explanations may converge by speaking rapidly themselves or by being silent to accommodate the physicians' speech. However, patients may diverge by paraphrasing the explanations more slowly to make sure they understand them. Socially speaking, divergence is risky, in that it shows the participants to be somewhat out of sync. Extreme divergence may seem disrespectful or rude.

People often mirror the behaviors of their conversational partners without really thinking about it, especially if they like each other. Accommodation can spiral, however, so that feedback encourages people to escalate their behaviors toward each other. For instance, when a dear friend speaks loudly and slowly to an older adult, the older person may respond in a similar way, which may reinforce the friend's belief that the older person is a bit slow and hard of hearing. In turn, the friend may accommodate even more, and so on. Thus, what was intended to be accommodation has become **overaccommodation**, an exaggerated response to a perceived need.

Especially if the overaccommodation is pervasive (everybody seems to do it), older individuals may begin to believe that they are indeed of diminished capacity, and they may behave in line with that expectation (Ryan & Butler, 1996). In short, they start to "do" being old, as society has defined it.

Older adults usually have no control over the cues that suggest to others that they are aging. An older-sounding voice is one example. People whose voices sound old are often perceived by others to be older than their contemporaries and may even perceive *themselves* to be older (Moyse, 2014; Mulac & Giles, 1996). An "old" voice is quivery and breathy, with prolonged vowel sounds and extended pauses between words. These characteristics are certainly not signs that the speaker is less intelligent or is physically impaired in any significant way, but they may be enough to spur accommodation and overaccommodation.

Ironically, a great number of accommodating behaviors are unnecessary. Older adults tend to compensate for communication deficiencies in some areas by becoming stronger in others. For example, many become especially good at reading nonverbal cues if their hearing diminishes (Fowler & Nussbaum, 2008). "What's important to remember about people over age 65 is that while many begin to experience some physical limitations, they learn to live with them and lead happy and productive lives," says a spokesperson for the American Psychological Association ("Older Adults," n.d., p. 1). Today's older adults are more diverse, better educated, healthier, and more affluent than any generation before them (Howe, 2018; U.S. Census Bureau, 2011). Only 3% of people ages 75 to 84 live in nursing homes (USDHHS, 2017). The reality is that communication accommodating behaviors are often unnecessary.

Ageism and overaccommodation present several implications for health communication. For one, older adults are usually treated by care providers who are significantly younger than they are. If they are unfamiliar with the diversity of the older generation, young people tend to rely on stereotypes. They may lump older adults into simplistic categories, such as frail, mild-mannered grandparents, or worse, cantankerous grumps.

Second, people may not try very hard to maintain or restore older people's health. Research indicates that people expect older adults to be ill and confused. As a result, they tend to shrug off illnesses and emotional distress as unavoidable and untreatable. In short, if they do not believe older people can change, people don't try very hard to help them.

Third, studies support that treating people as if they are helpless encourages them to believe it. Margaret Baltes and Hans-Werner Wahl (1996) found that, in one nursing home, caregivers encouraged older adults to be dependent by being attentive and supportive when the residents needed help but discouraging or ignoring them when they seemed independent. By contrast, researchers in another nursing home coached residents to take an active role in their health and encouraged the staff to support those efforts. The older adults in that setting experienced significantly higher levels of self-efficacy and perceived health benefits (Yeon-Hwan & HeeKyung, 2014).

Fourth, care providers tend to underestimate older adults' desire for information. Providers may assume they are not interested in medical details, are incapable of understanding them, or will be unduly frightened by risk factors. However, research suggests that most older adults are interested in and capable of understanding and assessing risks. In fact, because of long-standing experience, older adults often have more extensive medical vocabularies than younger people. Reflecting this, older adults' satisfaction with medical care is most closely linked to how well health professionals listen, how concerned and attentive they are, and how actively they include patients in decision making (Atherly, Kane, & Smith, 2004; Finkelstein, Carmel, & Bachner, 2015).

COMMUNICATION PATTERNS

Although older and younger adults are not as different from one another as people may think, it's worth noting several communication patterns that distinguish older adults' behavior in medical contexts. For example, because they may have been taught to respect authority figures by not interrupting, older adults may be reluctant to ask questions and assert themselves with health professionals, despite their desire to participate and be well informed (Nussbaum, Ragan, & Whaley, 2003).

Conversely, some older adults become what Fowler and Nussbaum (2008) call *extreme talkers,* chatting incessantly about topics that may seem irrelevant to their health concerns. Given time constraints in medical organizations, "it is quite easy to imagine communication with patients who have a tendency to stray from the matter at hand being quite frustrating" to doctors and others (Fowler & Nussbaum, p. 165).

Third, caregivers may be put off by the presence of loved ones who often accompany older adults to medical visits. According to Nussbaum, Ragan, and Whaley (2003), very often "the companion will ask more questions, will cause the medical encounter to last significantly longer, and will expect more information regarding the health of the older patient than the older patient normally seeks" (p. 192).

Finally, the fast pace of medical contexts may be incompatible with older adults' health needs, which (although they are not necessarily debilitating) are likely to be more numerous and chronic than those of younger patients, making it infeasible to cover them during quick visits (Nussbaum, Pecchioni, Grant, & Folwell, 2000).

The good news is that even brief training sessions have been effective in dispelling ageist assumptions among medical students and health professionals (Christmas, Park, Schmaltz, Gozu, & Durso, 2008). Such educational programs may help change the way older adults are treated in medical situations.

Technology provides another resource. The next section discusses communication technology as it affects older adults.

COMMUNICATION TECHNOLOGY AND OLDER ADULTS

Advanced technology can be a benefit or a liability for older adults. From one perspective, access to online health information and interaction expands opportunities for adults with limited mobility. On the other hand, older adults who do not keep up with technology may have difficulty finding and keeping jobs and staying in the mainstream of a technology-savvy society. There is some evidence that older adults are rising to the challenge.

"It's clear that older adults, like their younger counterparts, don't want to be left behind on the information highway," writes Donald Lindberg (2002, p. 13). About two-thirds of people age 65 and older use the internet (Anderson & Perrin, 2017).

Evidence suggests that many older adults who are proficient at using online resources benefit from a sense of control over their environment and personal fate. They also feel less isolated and more informed about choices and options than they might otherwise. Based on these ideals, Douglas McConatha (2002) proposed what he called the **e-quality theory of aging**, which posits that older adults benefit as both teachers and learners when they "use, contribute to, influence, and express themselves" in electronic environments (p. 38).

Based on experience working with older adults in an assisted living facility, David Lansdale (2002) notes that residents often experience a new sense of freedom when they learn new modalities online. Lansdale applies the metaphors of "driving" and "going back to school" when he writes:

> Driving *is the antidote to helplessness. One of the most exciting events in adolescence comes with access to the keys to the car, and the freedom it promises. At the other end of life's continuum, an elder is often forced to relinquish the keys, often one of the more trying transitions of a lifetime.* (p. 135)

Lansdale says that older adults who are proficient using computers are free to "go" where they please and choose their own paths and experiences. At the same time, they can relieve boredom and feel that they are participating in life beyond the facility's borders. Similarly, by "going back to school" via the internet, many older adults find pleasure in expanding their knowledge and skills. This provides a striking contrast to the view of aging as a steady decline in intellect and abilities.

The web may even serve as a modern equivalent to a house call. In their study of internet use among people ages 63 to 83, Wendy Macias and Sally McMillan (2008) report that many older adults are "bringing the physician and health information into their homes through the Internet" (p. 38). The web allows them to take their time, learning as much or as little as they like about a health concern without being constrained by someone else's timetable. One woman in the study said:

> *When my husband had his shoulder replacement, he could not get in to therapy right away, and that's when I went in to the websites and was able to print actual diagrams and information about what . . . to do, so then when we finally got in to the therapy and back to the doctor, he said this was very good.* (p. 38)

Although participants in the study sometimes felt overwhelmed by the volume of online information and unsure what information to trust, they generally appreciated the opportunity to research their own concerns and issues affecting their friends and family members.

Summary

Intersectionality Theory

- A person's social position reflects a dynamic, multidimensional interface between many factors.
- It is more effective for policy-makers and health professionals to become acquainted with people than to make assumptions based on nebulous or isolated categories.

Socioeconomic Status

- Patients of low socioeconomic status are typically more fearful and less informed than others.
- In addition, practical considerations such as financial constraints, inflexible work schedules, and lack of transportation may limit the care they are able to receive.

Health Literacy

- The adverse effects of health literacy include unnecessary suffering, misunderstandings, reduced productivity, shame, premature death, and billions spent on avoidable health needs.
- People can most effectively bridge literacy gaps if they develop trust, acknowledge and reconsider stereotypes, make the most of face-to-face communication, and encourage questions and open dialogue.

Gender Identity and Sexual Orientation

- Health professionals may feel out of their depth discussing sexual issues, although ignoring them may compromise care because some health risks are related to sex and because close relationships are crucial to coping.
- Patients may be reluctant to bring up gender identity and sexual orientation for fear of being negatively judged negatively.

Race and Ethnicity

- The health of racial and ethnic minorities may suffer because they don't trust doctors and because they have limited access to health care and health information.
- The United States has yet to fully transcend decades of racist and segregationist thinking, and the impact is realized in worse health and shorter lives for members of racial and ethnic minorities.

Language Differences

- Patients baffled by language differences may agree to procedures they don't understand or may be so frustrated that they don't return for further care. Care providers may be held liable if adverse outcomes result.
- Interpreters can be helpful, but it's not always clear who will pay for them.

Disabilities

- Many people treat individuals with disabilities as if they are childlike or incapable of contributing to conversations and decisions. These assumptions may seriously limit communication with care providers.
- Even when people mean well, their actions may stigmatize and isolate individuals with disabilities.

Age

- Children may be frightened by the foreign atmosphere, strangers, and threat of pain that health care poses. Parents can help, but their role is somewhat ambiguous. Health professionals may feel that parents are either too demanding or not helpful enough.
- Ageist assumptions that older people are less healthy and less intelligent than others may cause people to write off legitimate health concerns as unavoidable signs of old age. Communication accommodation behaviors are often unnecessary and can be stigmatizing, especially if carried to extremes.

Glossary

accommodate To adapt to another person's style or (perceived) needs. *See page 125.*

ageism Discrimination based on a person's age. *See page 125.*

communication accommodation theory The proposition that people tend to mirror each other's communication styles to display liking and respect. *See page 126.*

concrete-logical conceptualization A stage of development among children (roughly ages 7–10) in which they begin to differentiate between external causes, such as wind and cold, and internal manifestations, such as sneezing and talking funny. *See page 123.*

convergence Using gestures, tone of voice, and vocabulary, and so on similar to one's communication partner. *See page 126.*

divergence Acting differently from another person, as in whispering when they shout. *See page 126.*

e-quality theory of aging The idea that older adults benefit as both teachers and learners when they use communication technology. *See page 128.*

ethnic concordance The perception of cultural similarities between oneself and another person. *See page 115.*

formal-logical conceptualization A stage of development among children (roughly age 11 and older) when they are adept at envisioning the complex influence of agents they cannot readily see. *See page 123.*

health inequities Structural and systematic factors that put some groups at a disadvantage compared to others. *See page 105.*

health literacy The ability to access health information, understand it, and apply it. *See page 108.*

health passport A collection of information that allows people to express biopsychosocial needs and preferences in an easy-to-share format. *See page 121.*

intersectionality theory The idea that a person's social position emerges within the interface of micro-level personal identities (e.g., age, race, sexual orientation, physical ability, education level) and macro-level sociocultural patterns (e.g., sexism, racism, power, resources, public policies). *See page 105.*

overaccommodation An exaggerated response to a perceived need, as when someone speaks loudly and slowly to an older person when they can hear fine without those behaviors. *See page 126.*

prelogical conceptualization A stage of development among children (roughly ages 2–6) in which they define illness as something caused by a tangible, external agent, such as a monster or the sun. *See page 123.*

queer theory A perspective that challenges the notion of static identities and rigid social categories. *See page 111.*

racism Discrimination based on a person's race. *See page 112.*

Discussion Questions

1. Consider the brief scenario described by Lucy Candib at the beginning of the chapter. What elements of intersectionality theory can you apply to the patient she describes? What micro- and macro-level factors intersect to define your own social position?

2. How might you apply the factors relevant to socioeconomic status to yourself? In what ways are you privileged? In what ways are you disadvantaged? How do these affect your health and the way you communicate about it?

3. We are all more literate in some ways than others. What types of information do you find easy to understand? What types are difficult for you? How might someone best help you understand information you find challenging?

4. List at least 10 words that describe your gender identity. Does your gender identity influence your health and the way you communicate about it? If so, how?

5. What are some explanations of why people of different races seem to achieve different health outcomes? Have you ever witnessed or experienced any of these factors? If so, which ones?

6. Are you interested in knowing your genetic profile? Why or why not? Are you concerned that, if you have a genetic profile, the information might be used against you? Why or why not?

7. What did you learn from the case study "Language Barriers in a Health Care Emergency" (Box 6.3)? Have you ever been in a situation in which it was difficult to understand or convey important information? If so, what happened?

8. Researchers make the point that we all have abilities and disabilities of different sorts. What do you consider your greatest abilities? Your greatest challenges? Do these influence your identity and the way people treat you? If so, how?

9. Imagine that you must explain to a child what it means to have cancer. What language and metaphors might you use? How would you change the way you communicate based on the child's age and ability to conceptualize illness?

10. Think carefully about the way you communicate with older adults. Does your communication exhibit accommodation in any way? If so, how? Do you think the accommodation is necessary or might you be overaccommodating?

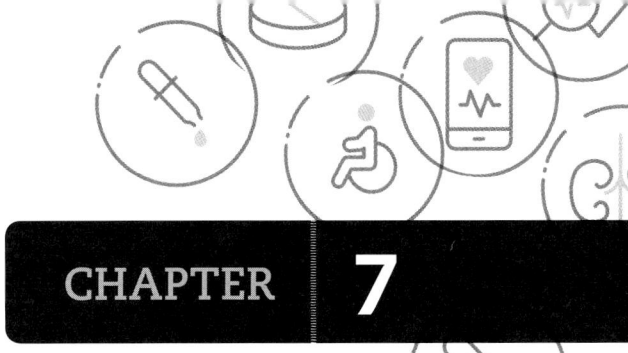

CHAPTER 7

Cultural Conceptions of Health and Illness

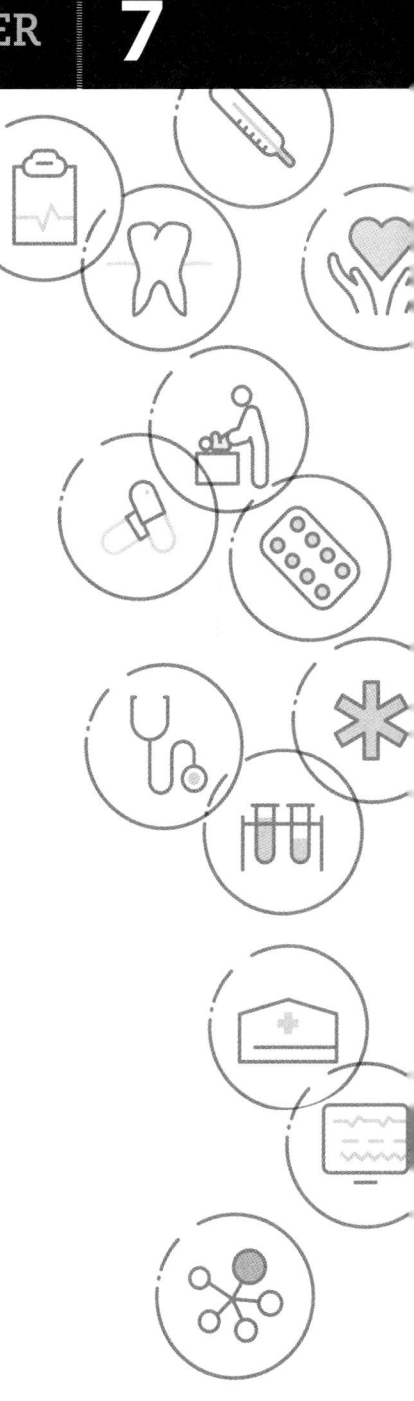

Ella, a labor and delivery nurse, is puzzled when a woman who has just given birth refuses an ice pack to ease her swelling and leaves a glass of cold water untouched, even though she is very thirsty.

Logan, a hospice volunteer, arrives at a client's home to find it crowded with friends and family members. They are welcoming and polite, but they are firm in insisting that Logan not speak with the ill person.

Devorah keeps her breast cancer diagnosis a secret, even from her close friends. However, she suspects that some people have found out because they avoid talking to her or making eye contact when they pass on the street.

Each of these episodes illustrates a cultural view of health and healing. In the first, the new mother is a Caribbean immigrant. Based on traditional beliefs, she considers it unhealthy to touch anything cold just after a birth. However, if the nurse offers hot tea, she would gratefully accept it to soothe her thirst (Winkelman, 2009).

Logan has arrived at the home of a Hispanic family whose members pride themselves on caring for loved ones personally. They fear that the presence of a hospice volunteer will make their loved one think they feel burdened by his care (Evans & Ume, 2012).

Devorah is a member of a charedi Jewish community in which it is considered immodest to speak about breasts, even to close friends. Members of this community may also consider her unappealing as a wife or mother because they believe her children will be genetically predisposed to cancer (Coleman, 2009).

In this chapter we examine the impact of culture on health and healing. We explore cultures associated with Asian, Hispanic, Arab, Native American, African American, Cambodian, and Canadian communities, among others. The list seems long, but it barely scratches the surface. Entire books are dedicated to the topic of health and diverse cultural perspectives. As you read, bear in mind that this review can offer only a broad look at cultural customs. People vary widely from each other, even within the same culture.

131

The chapter begins with a discussion of culture and adaptability. It then describes the influence of sex roles and family involvement on health, followed by cultural perspectives on what it means to be healthy, to be sick, and to help others. The chapter concludes with a focus on holistic medicine.

Culture and Health Communication

Culture refers to a set of beliefs, rules, and practices that are shared by a group of people. Cultural assumptions suggest how members should behave, what roles they are expected to play, and how various events and actions should be interpreted (Samovar & Porter, 2007). As the opening examples illustrate, cultural assumptions can affect what people consider acceptable, admirable, and shameful regarding health. In a deeper sense, culture may even define what it means to be healthy, as you will see later in the chapter. Culture is not limited to particular nationalities or regions, but may reflect shared expectations in terms of age, education level, family background, gender identity, occupation, and many other factors.

Cultural beliefs often have a taken-for-granted quality that makes it difficult to imagine or accept alternatives. **Ethnocentrism** is the attitude that one's own culture is better than others. Even when people mean well, it's easy to feel slighted by the implication that others hold a different view. After an administrator at a Canadian hospital suggested that staff members not wish patients "Merry Christmas," one nurse fumed, "Why should we worry that it offends someone of a non-Christian culture? That really is too bad. I think the administrator was hoping to be politically correct, but it happened to offend a lot of people" (Kirkham, 2003, p. 768). The nurse felt that Canada was a "Christian country" and people should honor that perspective.

Contrast that with the anguish of a Cambodian family in an American hospital where the staff insists on cutting off silk threads that encircle the patient's wrist. The threads were tied on by a holy person in a traditional *Baci* ceremony as a way to "tie in the soul." To the family, cutting these threads renders a person vulnerable and invites bad luck (Galanti, 2014). Although that view is not the dominant perspective in the United States, it is immensely important to the family.

Appreciation for cultural diversity can occur on many levels. Health communication theorist Mohan Dutta (2009) calls attention to the distinction between being culturally sensitive and culture-centered. As he uses the terms, those who take a **culturally sensitive approach** craft messages based on an awareness of cultural characteristics. For example, health promoters who are aware that a target audience values collective identity might craft messages that emphasize the social ramifications of a health-related behavior. By contrast, a **culture-centered approach** is a more collaborative endeavor situated within a specific community. Community members are treated as active agents in defining, understanding, and addressing health-related issues within the context of culture, socioeconomic structures, and other factors that affect them (Dutta, 2009). From this perspective, the role of scholars, health professionals, and others is mainly to help create spaces for collaboration and capacity building and to assist as needed with message design (Dutta et al., 2016). For example, when researchers led by Haijuan Gao conducted in-depth interviews with Chinese immigrants working in restaurants in the midwestern United States, they learned that many of them were dissuaded from seeking medical attention because of uncertainty about the health care system, the costs involved, and their eligibility to receive care (Gao, Dutta, & Okoror, 2016). One implication is that communication may be a means of increasing their capacity to navigate the health system.

The Challenge of Multiculturalism

It's difficult to discuss diversity and health responsibly. For one thing, culture is not a fixed construct, but an evolving and complex one. Even within the same culture, what's considered appropriate for one person, in one situation, may be unacceptable for another. No amount of cultural knowledge allows us to predict accurately how an individual will think or behave. Furthermore, speaking in terms of people's differences can overshadow the ways in which they are alike, and it can inadvertently distance the people being described. As David Napier and colleagues (2014) observe, talking about diversity can feel divisive rather than inclusive. At the same time, it is negligent and insensitive to ignore the influence of culture. The tenets of cultural adaptability can help us navigate this tricky landscape.

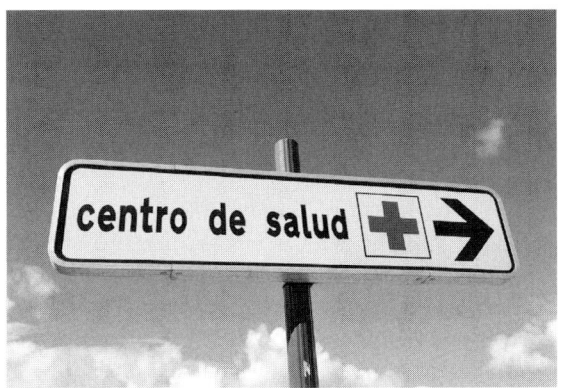

Have you ever experienced health care in a culture different from your own? If so, how was it similar to the health care you experience at home? How was it different?

CULTURAL ADAPTABILITY IN HEALTH CARE

As manager of a community health center in Australia, Jeffery Fuller puzzled over how to interact respectfully with a diverse array of clients. He worried that staff members would be insensitive to patients' wishes. But he also worried that they would clam up around diverse patients or abandon important medical goals so as not to offend. After studying research about the issue and trying different approaches, Fuller and his team decided to avoid assumptions as much as possible, and instead, to communicate openly with patients about their cultural and personal viewpoints. He subsequently published a model of cultural adaptability in health care that reflects that perspective.

Fuller's **reflective negotiation model** involves two enacted commitments and an end goal (Fuller, 2003). The commitments involve sensitivity to cultural differences and to self-awareness. The goal is that, together, these will foster a collaborative "space for negotiation," in which patients and professionals can respectfully exchange ideas without feeling constrained by status or cultural differences.

Sensitivity to cultural differences involves knowledge, which emerges to varying extents when people seek out information and when they interact with people from different cultures. Knowledge is helpful, but it is an insufficient measure of cultural adaptability for three main reasons (Fuller, 2003). One, health professionals cannot know the ins and outs of every culture with which they come in contact. For another, people operate within complex webs of cultural significance, and it's impossible to know which of them are most salient in a particular situation: *Is it more germane that a patient identifies as female or that she is Himalayan? Does it matter more that she is a CEO now or that she grew up in a low-income housing project?* Of course, it is impossible to say. Third, as we have already established, people differ from one another, even within the same culture.

This presents a rather daunting prospect: If knowledge isn't enough, what else is there? Fuller (2003) proposes that cultural adaptability involves inquisitiveness. In other words, it *embraces* ambiguity. Rather than making presumptions, health professionals might attentively observe and inquire. Toward that end, Geri-Ann Galanti (2014) recommends that care providers ask patients three critical questions: *What do you think is wrong? What do you think caused your problem?* and *How do you cope with your condition?* The answers, she says, reveal a great deal about how patients define their conditions and the impact of those conditions on their lives.

At the same time, culturally adaptive individuals look inward to become aware of their own emotional hot buttons and ego threats. For example, a nurse in Fuller's (2003) study said:

> I'm a white male in a society that's increasingly worried about diversity, feminism, and respecting homeless people. I'm none of those things, and I think it's an area where it would be easy for me to be fearful if I wanted to be. (p. 788)

The nurse said he listens to his inner voice so he can recognize when he feels threatened or bothered. He finds that this awareness allows him to make conscious choices rather than isolating himself or being judgmental. Thus, in the same way that being sensitive to others involves asking questions, self-awareness involves honest introspection: *What am I feeling? What am I afraid of? Are my feelings rational? What are my options?*

It is important to note that effective cultural adaptation does not privilege one perspective over another. Consider the experience of a health professional prepping a Sikh child for surgery. Religious edicts prohibit cutting or shaving one's hair, which is considered a gift from God. On the other hand, medical experts recommend that surgical sites be shaved to reduce the risk of infection. Sensitive to the parents' distress, the care provider tells the parents that she understands the rule about not cutting hair. If she has their permission, she will shave only a small area at the surgical site to protect the child's health. The parents consent, and both sides are comfortable moving forward (Galanti, 2014).

From Fuller's (2003) perspective, cultural adaptability involves respect for one another's viewpoints. However, especially when the stakes are high, it also embraces reflective negotiation. For example, physicians find themselves in a difficult position when patients seem chronically depressed but feel that it would be shameful to admit those feelings. One option is to campaign for a mutually acceptable interpretation, as when one doctor said to a patient: "If you had diabetes, you would say to me, 'Please help me fix this.' And this is no different. It's just chemicals in your brain instead of chemicals in your liver or your kidney" (Patel, Schnall, Little, Lewis-Fernández, & Pincus, 2014, p. 1265).

All in all, Fuller's (2003) reflective negotiation model recognizes that health care occurs within an intricate constellation of beliefs. The model presents cultural adaptability as an ongoing process in which we must be both introspective and interested in other people. Fuller recognizes that diversity can stir up powerful emotions but proposes that the mutual benefits of negotiation are worth the effort.

With these commitments in mind, we next examine two sociocultural factors that help to shape our identities and influence the nature of health communication: gender and family.

Cultural Conceptions of Health

A patient describes a perplexing set of symptoms, including a sense of heaviness and insomnia. Physical tests can detect nothing wrong. The patient attributes his illness to "too much wind" and "not enough blood" as a result of his past immoral behavior. A folk healer has been treating him with meditation and herbal therapies (Kleinman, Eisenberg, & Good, 1978).

A health professional might conclude that the man is delusional or uneducated. However, if she is familiar with traditional Chinese medicine, she may discern that "too much wind" and "not enough blood" refer to a sense of being tired, dull, and out of sorts (Dharmananda, 2010). Considering the man's reference to "heaviness" and "insomnia," his account may be a face-saving way of implying that he is depressed.

Examples such as this one highlight that well-meaning people can trip over cultural gaps, sometimes with harmful consequences. This section describes two cultural perspectives on health—one that conceives of health in mostly organic terms, and one that interprets health as harmony between many factors.

Health as Organic

In the mid-1800s, a chemistry professor in France developed a new procedure to stop wine from souring before consumers could enjoy it. A few years later, the same professor helped to keep the silk industry alive by discovering what was killing off silkworms (Swazey & Reeds, 1978). He couldn't know it at the time, but these efforts would lead the professor, Louis Pasteur, to revolutionize medicine.

Pasteur realized that the wine was souring and the silkworms were dying because of tiny organisms called germs. He didn't discover germs. A Dutch biologist had done that nearly 200 years earlier. But Pasteur was the first to recognize that germs could be killed and, with effort, be kept out of sterile environments. (His discovery would lead him to *pasteurize* milk, among other things.) Prior to Pasteur's discovery, scientists believed that germs spontaneously generated and could not be contained or avoided (Zimmerman & Zimmerman, 2002).

Simply put, **germ theory** states that disease is caused by microscopic organisms, such as bacteria and viruses (Twaddle & Hessler, 1987). Pasteur's breakthrough helped hospitals and medical centers become safer than in the past. Staff members began to sterilize medical instruments and environments and to separate people with contagious diseases from others (Marwick, 1997).

Pasteur's ideas seeped into popular culture, as well. An **organic model** of health took root, based on the assumption that health can be understood in terms of the presence (or absence) of physical indicators. Care providers and researchers began to rely heavily on scientific tests to diagnose patients and to conduct medical research (Raffel & Raffel, 1989). At the core of the organic approach is the conviction that, if health professionals are vigilant enough, they can minimize or eradicate most illnesses. Indeed, an awareness of microscopic agents has allowed communities to remove the threat of many contagious diseases, reduce the incidence of infection, and develop inoculations against smallpox, measles, polio, and many other harmful conditions.

If you grew up in an environment that reveres biomedicine, it may seem strange to consider the organic perspective a matter of culture. One quality of cultural assumptions is that, over time, they tend to assume the authority of universal truth. That's not to say that biomedicine is wrong or false. But it is certainly not the only perspective on health, and like all perspectives, it has limitations.

One limitation is the biomedical model's inability to account for conditions that cannot be physically verified. People with undetectable conditions, such as chronic fatigue syndrome, sometimes say the worst part is that so many people regard their condition as "not real" (Komaroff & Fagioli, 1996). A similar phenomenon affects people with mental illness. In the United States, mental illness has long been regarded as less authentic than physical illness—an assumption that changed (at least somewhat) only when researchers identified a chemical basis for some mental disorders (Byck, 1986). Objectively speaking, mental illness did not become any more *real*, at that point. It simply became more culturally acceptable.

Another limitation is that the organic approach largely excludes social, spiritual, and psychological factors that may be relevant to the lived experience of health and illness. Since the Industrial Revolution, many doctors in the United States have been reluctant to bring up spiritual concerns during medical visits, perhaps because they are uncomfortable with them or they seem irrelevant. This is understandable to some people, but it can seem cold and impersonal to those who are accustomed to a different style of care. Members of some African American and Latinx communities, for example, are often dissatisfied with health care because they perceive that providers are distant and uninterested compared to the close sense of community they value (Mead et al., 2013).

A third limitation is that, although classifying people as either healthy or sick feels logical in a binary way, it is an oversimplification. As Charles Rossiter (1975) points out, *sick* and *healthy* are inadequate to describe all aspects of the human condition. There are varying levels of sickness and varying levels of health. Moreover, some people are unhealthy although they do not have specific diseases.

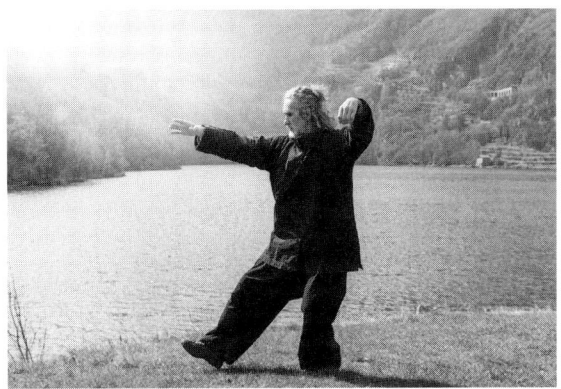

Describe ways in which your health is affected by organic factors and ways in which it is influenced by your emotions and mental state.

Health as Harmonic Balance

As you may remember from Chapter 1, the World Health Organization defines health as "a state of complete physical, mental, and social well-being and not merely the absence of disease or infirmity" (WHO, 1948, p. 1). From this perspective, health exists at the nexus of many factors, including personal beliefs, contact with other people, aspects of the environment, physical strength, and many more. From the **harmonic balance perspective**, health is not simply the absence of physical signs of disease. Rather, it is a sense of overall well-being and equilibrium. This perspective is in keeping with biopsychosocial and sociocultural perspectives (Chapter 1). Following are a few examples that illustrate cultural perspectives on health as a harmonic balance.

PHYSICAL, EMOTIONAL, AND SPIRITUAL

Members of many cultures do not perceive the mind/body dualism popular in Western thought. Instead, they regard the mind and body as an interwoven whole and perceive that one affects the other.

The Hispanic concepts of *susto* and *coraje* are examples. Both refer to emotionally intense and unpleasant episodes. The idea is that a traumatizing experience can diminish one's spiritual vitality and upset the link between body and soul (Durà-Vilà & Hodes, 2012). In most Mexican cultures, *susto* (SOO-sto) means *fright* and *coraje* (core-AH-hey) means *anger*. In one study of Mexican American immigrants, the majority felt their diabetes was at least partly caused by experiencing either extreme *susto* or *coraje* (Mendenhall, Fernandez, Adler, & Jacobs, 2012).

Members of some traditional Navajo cultures also honor a connection between mind, body, and soul. They believe that the best way to remain healthy is to balance physical strength, social interactions, and spiritual beliefs ("Native American Religions," 2010). Concentrating on only one factor can upset the delicate balance between them. For example, striving for physical strength without also seeking spiritual growth is not healthy, and a person may become ill because of the imbalance. This is not to say that Navajo deny the existence of germs. They accept that germs cause some diseases. But they also observe that some people are less vulnerable than others to them. If several people are exposed to a contagious disease, some of them are likely to get sick, but others may not. Based on Navajo beliefs, people who live balanced lives are more likely to remain well, even when they are exposed to physical threats.

HARMONY WITH NATURE

> *[Mother Earth] is something that heals you if you let it. You don't always feel it. You have to be thinking about it. You can't just go out for a walk and feel it. You have to be spiritually connected to feel her. (Wilson, 2003, third section, para. 8)*

This statement, by a member of the Odawa aboriginal community in Canada, emphasizes the therapeutic value of living in harmony with nature. Similar beliefs are common in Caribbean communities and many others.

Illustrative of this idea, the renowned biologist Edward O. Wilson proposed the **biophilia hypothesis** that people have an inherent affinity for nature and often derive a sense of well-being from contact with it. A good deal of research suggests that people typically experience decreased stress, elevated moods, and other positive benefits from activities such as gardening, dog walking, and hiking (Chen, Tu, & Ho, 2013; McCune, Beck, & Johnson, 2011). Based on this evidence, urban planning coalitions such as Eco advocate for at least a 20% increase in parks, public gardens, and other green spaces to bolster community health (Hall, 2014).

HOT AND COLD

In one of the examples that opens this chapter, a new mother refuses an ice pack and cold water because she has just given birth. In many traditional Caribbean, Chinese, and Latin American cultures, health is considered in terms of "hot" and "cold" (Sobo & Loustaunau, 2010; Winkelman, 2009). Bodily conditions are associated with different temperatures, as are foods, drinks, and other elements of the environment. For example, childbirth is considered hot. To counteract it with something cold might interfere with the body's natural healing process. In other circumstances—such as when a person feels lethargic (a cold condition)—hot substances such as coffee and chocolate can counter that and help restore a healthy balance.

"Hot" and "cold" are not always literal temperatures (coffee is hot, but so are chocolate, cinnamon, and tobacco). The real determinant is a substance's effect on the body, which can also be metaphoric. Hot foods are energizing. By contrast, low-calorie foods, such as fruits and vegetables, are cold. Health professionals sensitive to this perspective can recommend remedies that are both helpful and culturally suitable. For instance, cold juice might be regarded as inappropriate to counteract the flu (which is considered cold), but hot tea may be a useful and appealing alternative (Winkelman, 2009).

Heat and cold are interwoven with the Chinese conception of **Qi**, which we will discuss next. But before moving on, it's worth noting that even people not raised in the cultures mentioned here may rely on thermal metaphors. For example, people in the United States may describe a personable care provider as *warm* and friendly, bemoan the misery of catching a *cold*, and long for the healing value of *hot* chicken soup.

ENERGY

Around the world, members of many cultures conceive of health primarily in terms of energy. For example, a traditional Hindu individual from Asian India may believe that accidents are caused by **karma**—energy that results from either good or bad deeds in the past. From this viewpoint, a disabling injury may be regarded as the inevitable consequence of bad karma. Recovery may involve not only physical healing, but a resolve to be more altruistic in the future (Gupta, 2010).

According to the Chinese Tao, **yin** and **yang** are polar energies whose cyclical forces define all living things (Uba, 1992). *Yin* is associated with coolness and reflection, and *yang* with brightness and warmth. Cycles and combinations of yin and yang define human life and unite all forms of existence.

Within this belief, one's central life energy is called **Qi** (pronounced *chee*, sometimes spelled "chi"). Illness and even death may result if *Qi* is wasted or if yin and yang are not balanced. Life energy is sustained and balanced by awareness, rhythmic breathing, physical regimens, and meditation.

Qi is often difficult to grasp and study from an empirical perspective because it is invisible. *Qi* is sensed rather than measured or directly observed (Ho, 2006). Unlike in organic medicine, in which the practitioner and the patient are treated as distinctly separate entities, *Qi* is a force that flows through them both. As one practitioner described it, an acupuncturist is "the conduit between the heavenly and the earthly *Qi* and it comes through you and through your hands and into the needle and the point" (Ho, 2006, p. 426). Some highly experienced people are said to know what is wrong with a person by sensing the person's *Qi* visually or through touch.

There is sometimes a perceived tension between traditional methods and biomedicine. One tension is between technology and tradition. A traditional Chinese medicine practitioner reflects that people accustomed to biomedicine often value "the newest, latest things," therefore "to them, old things are considered outdated" (Chang & Lim, 2019, p. 241). At the same time, organic and harmonic balance approaches overlap and coexist. Physical health is a significant component of both perspectives. Moreover, each model may be appropriate in different situations, and sometimes they are useful together. Amos Deinard, a pediatrician at the University of Minnesota Hospital, says, "Our attitude is, you bring your shaman and we'll bring our surgeon and let's see if we can work on this problem together" (quoted by Goode, 1993, para. 7).

Making Sense of Health Experiences

Two friends, one Jamaican and one American, watch a woman cross the street. The American thinks, "Look how slender she is. She must have a healthy diet." The Jamaican thinks, "I wonder what sort of stress has caused her to be so thin. She is unwell" (adapted from Sobo & Loustaunau, 2010, p. 86).

As mentioned, one function of culture is to make sense of the world. In this example, a slender physique is interpreted as healthy to one friend and unhealthy to another. In a similar way, depending on one's culture and circumstances, death might be interpreted as a glorious ascension to the afterlife or as a tragic and regrettable occurrence. An illness may be regarded as an unfair and random affliction or as a valuable opportunity for renewed awareness. (See Box 7.1 for more about that idea.)

This section explores how members of various cultures make sense of health conditions.

BOX 7.1 THEORETICAL FOUNDATIONS

Theory of Health as Expanded Consciousness

The majority of us spend our lives trying to stay healthy, and when we get sick we want nothing more than to be well again. We may be missing the point. According to Margaret Newman's **theory of health as expanded consciousness**, a health crisis is not necessarily negative or undesirable (Newman, 2000). Instead, health events are integral parts of life that provide opportunities for growth and change.

Newman was inspired by David Bohm's (1980) concept that our everyday life is influenced by underlying patterns that characterize who we are and what we experience. Bohm conceived of two types of order—the *explicate order*, made up of the tangible elements of our existence, and the *implicate order*, composed of patterns beneath the surface. Although the tangible elements of our lives may seem like the "real thing" because we can see, hear, taste, and feel them, the meaning of what we do often lies within the underlying, implicate order. Bohm compares the dual nature of life to waves on the ocean. We can see the waves, but we won't really understand what causes them unless we explore the underwater currents that give rise to them.

continued

continued

Within this metaphor, a health event makes waves. It disrupts what might otherwise seem to be a peaceful, unremarkable existence. As nurse and nurse educator, Newman (2000) observes:

> *The thing that brings people to the attention of a nurse is a situation that they do not know how to handle. They are at a choice point. Each of us at some time in our lives is brought to a point when the "old rules" do not work anymore, when what we have considered progress does not work anymore. We have done everything "right" but things still do not work. (p. 99)*

You might ask: And this is a *good* thing? According to Newman, yes. In her view, life is a process of attaining greater levels of understanding and awareness. When things stop working well, we experience a sense of chaos. But, she says, if we "hang in there," the uncertainty and ambiguity of a health crisis may become a means of seeing underlying patterns and transcending previous limitations. This can be a richly rewarding and liberating experience (Newman, 2000).

Imagine a person who has worked throughout her life to support others. She has devoted her energy and time to doing well at work, caring for her family, running errands, serving on committees, cleaning the house and yard, and so on. She is lauded with thanks and awards. Meanwhile, she appears less physically fit than she used to be. Her hair and clothing are not as carefully groomed and tended. But this is nothing compared to what is happening within her. In fulfilling so many outward "obligations," she neglects her own spiritual and emotional growth. Although she interacts frequently with people, she doesn't share much of herself or appreciate the uniqueness of the people around her.

Suddenly (or what appears to be suddenly), the woman comes down with the flu and must cancel her commitments for several days. Faced with this prospect, she might put all her energy into fighting the illness, frustrated that it has interrupted her life. Or she might look for a deeper level of meaning. What does the illness (an outward manifestation) suggest about what is happening within her? And at an even deeper level, what does this disruption signal about the underlying pattern of her life? Perhaps this is an opportunity to reevaluate a pattern that appears virtuous on the surface but is harmful to her and others in the larger scheme of things. Perhaps understanding the pattern will allow her to restructure her life in a way that is more functional and adaptive, allowing her to develop her inner self as well as perform helpful tasks in the tangible world. Or perhaps she will ignore the underlying currents until they give rise to a much bigger, harder-to-ignore "wave," such as a stroke or a heart attack.

Seen this way, health events are opportunities for developing higher levels of understanding and more effective interactions with our environments. Greater harmony between inner and outer levels of existence provides the means for seeing beyond one's self and transcending old habits and assumptions. As Newman learned from her mentor, Martha Rogers, "health and illness should be viewed equally as expressions of the life process in its totality" (Newman, 2000, p. 7).

Newman (2000) coaches nurses to help people find the meanings and patterns revealed by their health experiences, whether or not their diseases are eradicated. She writes:

> *Transcendence of the limitations of the disease does not necessarily mean more freedom from the disease; it does mean more meaningful relationships and greater freedom in a spiritual sense. These factors are considered an expansion of consciousness. (p. 65)*

Furthermore, a health crisis is not merely a senseless or regrettable circumstance. Newman (1986) writes that, since she began to regard health as the expansion of consciousness,

> *illness and disease have lost their demoralizing power. . . . The expansion of consciousness never ends. In this way aging has lost its power. Death has lost its power. There is peace and meaning in suffering. We are free from the things we have feared—loss, death, dependency. We can let go of fear. (p. 3)*

What Do You Think?

1. Have you ever learned something valuable about yourself as the result of a health crisis?
2. What can care providers and loved ones do to help people evaluate their life circumstances when an illness occurs?
3. In what ways are your health and outward, everyday life (explicate order) influenced by underlying factors (implicate order)?

Health Condition as Social Asset

By now it should be clear that interpretations of illness and health are not absolute. What members of one culture consider tragic others may revere. For example, Native American folklore is rich with examples of spirit leaders who fall into sleep-like trances that last for several days (Neihardt, 1932). A biomedical practitioner might classify these episodes as comas, but in some Native American cultures they are regarded as sacred opportunities for the person to leave the body and experience the spiritual realm. The person's dreams in this state are often carefully noted and used as the basis for ceremonial dances and rituals.

Another famous example is described in the book *The Spirit Catches You and You Fall Down*, which describes the life of Lia, a young Hmong girl in California who had frequent seizures (Fadiman, 1997). Her family considered Lia special because the episodes allowed her to have contact with the divine. However, biomedical practitioners diagnosed her with epilepsy and charged the parents with negligence for not keeping Lia on antiseizure medication. The book chronicles the intercultural struggle to define what was healthy, what was holy, and what was best for Lia.

Less extreme examples of the illness-or-asset dilemma involve people whose "deformities" and "diseases" make them especially good at what they do. For example, doctors believe that the legendary violinist Niccolò Paganini probably had a genetic disorder that affected collagen in his body (S. Kean, 2012). As a result, his health was always fragile, but Paganini was able to hyperextend his thumbs in ways that other violinists couldn't. Likewise, some professional basketball players probably have gigantism, a condition that results in the overproduction of growth hormone (Caba, 2016). Evidence also suggests that many fashion models have eating disorders that may benefit them professionally but damage their health (Murgatroyd, 2015; National Eating Disorders Association, 2015).

On the flip side are health conditions that society regards with fear or revulsion. We discuss those next.

Health Condition as Social Liability

At different times in history, epilepsy, cancer, tuberculosis, mental illness, AIDS, and other ailments have been viewed so negatively that people with these conditions were shunned or even imprisoned (H. Friedman & DiMatteo, 1979). Sick people may be regarded as a threat to the moral order because behaviors associated with their conditions are considered immoral or because their conditions seem contagious or frightening.

Many times, public reaction is not based on facts but on fears or cultural assumptions. Prior to 1950, people were so fearful of cancer that they typically avoided telling anyone outside the family if a loved one was diagnosed with it (Holland & Zittoun, 1990). They often chose not to tell the patient either. As more accurate information about the disease surfaced, namely that it is not contagious, public opinion and communication about it changed as well.

As you will see here, ill health often has negative social connotations in that the affected person may be treated as cursed, unappealing, negligent, or victimized.

DISEASE AS CURSE

When other explanatory models fail, people may reason that illness is caused by God or witches. During the Middle Ages in England, mentally ill individuals were incarcerated as criminals and thereafter denied the right to marry or own property (MacDonald, 1981). Still today, in many areas of the world, mental illness is considered God's punishment, and people make great efforts to deny and conceal it (Purnell, 2008). As White (1896/1925) puts it, "In those periods when man sees everywhere miracle and nowhere law . . . he naturally ascribes his diseases either to the wrath of a good being or to the malice of an evil being" (p. 1).

During the bubonic plague of the fourteenth century, more than one-third of the European population died (Slack, 1991). Struggling to make sense of this devastating epidemic, people killed tens of thousands of women, accusing them of using witchcraft to make their neighbors ill (Nelkin & Gilman, 1991). Others attributed the plague to God's wrath over women's fashions, blasphemy, drunkenness, improper religious observances, and other behaviors (Slack, 1991).

If people believe illness is a curse, they may try to keep their health conditions secret and write off efforts at prevention and treatment. In Europe in the late 1700s, some people refused the smallpox vaccination because it was regarded as interference with God's way (Nelkin & Gilman, 1991). For similar reasons, some Kashmiri men in India, although at high risk for diabetes, frequently decline treatment or lifestyle changes because they feel that the disease is Allah's will and they should enjoy life (including eating what they want) until it is their fate to die (Naeem, 2003).

STIGMA

Nisha, a native of India, caught HIV at age 19 from the man her parents had arranged for her to marry (de Souza, 2009). When her husband became seriously ill, Nisha was beaten and disowned by her husband's family, who blamed her for his misfortune. Nisha returned to live with her parents and younger sisters, but when they found out she was HIV positive, they shunned her as well. Nisha now works for a nonprofit organization that provides care for people with HIV and AIDS and educates the public about these conditions.

For those whose conditions stir society's fears and prejudices, disease is clearly more than a physical phenomenon. People may be considered frightening, corrupt, or immoral on the basis of health-related factors. As Erving Goffman (1963) used the term, **stigma** refers to social rejection in which a person is treated as dishonorable or is ignored altogether. A striking example of this involves mental illness. A meta-analysis of research on the topic revealed that people with mental illness are stigmatized in regions as far-reaching and diverse as Finland, Africa, Japan, the United States, and Estonia (Boyd, Adler, Otilingam, & Peters, 2014). So great is the stigma that many people with mental illness internalize the harsh judgments and suffer reduced self-esteem and a sense of helplessness as a result (Boyd et al.).

One effect of social stigma is that people's individuality, even their humanity, is overshadowed by a particular characteristic. Activist and educator Stacy Bias (2015) wrote about a shaming episode (one of many) on a public train during which a passenger goaded her by loudly lambasting what he called "fat slobs" as being "lazy" and "irresponsible" and "like drunks." Bias considered saying to him, "Hi! I'm a real live fat person. . . . I'm up here in front of you being an actual human being" (para. 7). In the end, Bias's efforts to inspire the man's understanding and compassion only resulted in him bullying her more aggressively. She reflects that "stigma kills people. It make us sick, silent, and afraid to advocate for ourselves. It isolates us, turns us against ourselves, and breaks down our mental health" (para. 26). Because the issue of weight is so socially sensitive, people who are considered obese may find that health professionals either focus mostly on their weight, avoid the issue, or address it awkwardly (Knight-Agarwal, Kaur, Williams, Davey, & Davis, 2014). That is especially regrettable since people who have been subjected to ridicule may feel that there are few trustworthy confidants to whom they can talk openly (Puhl & Heuer, 2010). Stacy Bias is challenging the stigma, however, with blog posts, speaking engagements, and events designed to shed the shame and challenge the notion that beauty and health equate to being "thin, beautiful, white, and heterosexual" (Bias, 2014). (Read more about her work at stacybias.net/blog.)

Stigma can be heightened or minimized by the stories people tell. One man remembers that, when his uncles would become belligerent at family get-togethers, his mother would say, "Your uncles were at war, and they've seen some stuff and can't forget it. And now, the only way they cope is with drugs and

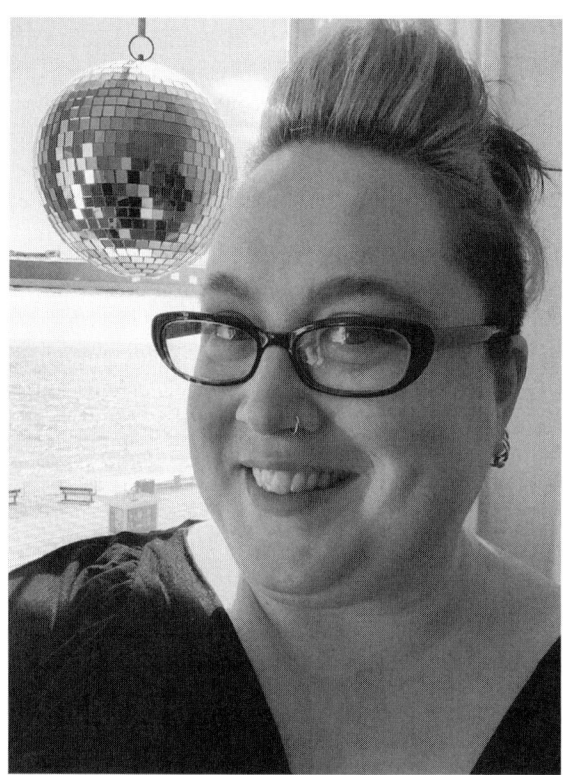

Stacy Bias, self-proclaimed fat activist and educator, has taken a stand against stigmatizing behaviors and bullying. She founded FatGirls Speak, a conference featuring performances and fashion shows that celebrate women of all sizes, as well as the BelliesAreBeautiful.com website at which she invites people to post photos in celebration of size diversity.

In what way, if any, does your appearance privilege you in the communities to which you belong? In what ways, if any, does it put you at a disadvantage?

alcohol" (Flood-Grady & Koenig Kellas, 2019, p. 611). Researchers reflect that, on the one hand, the mother's narrative shielded the uncles from being directly "to blame," but on the other, it supported a stigmatized view of mentally ill individuals as out of control and unwilling to seek treatment.

People with socially sensitive conditions such as inflammatory bowel disease face a dilemma as well. Members of their social circles often respond less judgmentally when they know about the diagnosis than when they don't (Rohde et al., 2018), but risk and vulnerability are involved in disclosing a condition that others may consider stigmatizing.

THE MORALITY OF PREVENTION

It seemed for a time that reframing disease in scientific terms would shield sufferers from moral judgment. Ironically, Western society has attributed a moral quality to science, with the effect that people who get sick are often considered to be lazy or ignorant.

The news is filled with health warnings and risk factors. Such information enables people to make healthy choices, enhancing their own well-being and assuring themselves of long, healthy lives. At least that's one implication: Take care of yourself and there is no reason you should become ill. But taken too far, the same idea can lead to prejudice against ill persons.

One backlash of the prevention movement is the presumption that, if illness can be avoided, ill people have not tried very hard to stay healthy. "Why isn't it possible to just get sick without it also being your fault?" asked physician/essayist Paul Marantz (1990, p. 1186). Marantz described the smug comments surrounding a young friend's unexpected death from heart failure. A medical resident minimized the man's death by dubbing him "a real couch potato" (Marantz, 1990, p. 1186). Marantz was angry that onlookers would judge his friend, even to the extent of making his premature death seem okay or deserved.

The fallacy that only the lazy or indifferent get sick compounds the hardship of being ill. People fall ill for reasons that are hard to explain, even though they have worked hard to stay healthy. Marantz (1990) and others propose that suffering is often made worse by the assumption that ill persons engineer their own misfortunes.

One alternative to blaming ill persons is to see them as victims of circumstances beyond their control. As you will see, however, there are also social implications to playing the victim role.

VICTIM ROLE

As the average life span has increased, so has the duration of chronic diseases. These days, many people with serious diseases survive and lead relatively normal lives. This has created a semantic dilemma. These people are not accurately described as "patients."

So what do you call a person with AIDS or cancer or emphysema? A common practice is to call them victims, as in "AIDS victims" or "cancer victims." However, many people so described resent the implications of that characterization. When Laura Barnes, a life coach in Arizona, posted her original poem "I Am Not a Victim of Breast Cancer" online, it went viral, apparently striking a chord with many people. Here are a few lines from the poem:

> I am not a victim of breast cancer.
> I am experiencing breast cancer.
> I am not dying.
> I am living. . . .
> I am not weak or diminished.
> I am strong and whole and complete. . . .
> I am not powerless.
> I am powerful beyond measure.

You can read the entire poem by searching for "Laura Barnes" and "I Am Not a Victim" online (Barnes, n.d.).

In closing, this section offers a powerful reminder that serious health concerns have social and cultural implications. In some cases, a person enjoys social benefits as a result of the condition. More often, however, serious health issues—particularly if they are frightening or baffling—are interpreted as a punishment, a sign of depravity, or as bad luck. As the next section illustrates, culture not only helps to conceptualize what health and illness mean, but also how we should behave in the context of social structures.

Social Roles and Health

"He was very uncooperative and refused to do anything for himself. He would ring for the nurses and demand, 'You get here right now and do this.' He would not, however, accept anything he had not specifically requested, including lunch trays and medication. He posted a sign on his door that read, 'Do not enter without knocking, including the nurses.'"

This is a nurse's description of a 25-year-old male patient in their care (Sobo & Loustaunau, 2010, p. 32). Eventually, a relative of one of the nurses provided an explanation. The patient was a wealthy man from Iran, accustomed to having servants and not accustomed to having women (such as female nurses) tell him what to do. Most of the staff came from a different background. They took it as a given that women should be treated as equals and that patients should accept the rituals and products of medical care as they knew it. Some of the nurses may also have felt slighted about being "bossed around" by someone younger than them. The staff felt badly treated, but so did the patient, who interpreted the staff's behavior toward him as disrespectful and belittling.

As this episode illustrates, health communication is influenced by the social roles that people play in a larger sense. Some of the most powerful influences on social identity, and therefore on health communication, involve gender and family.

Sex, Gender, and Health

It is oversimplified to consider *male* and *female* an either-or dichotomy. As we discussed in Chapter 6, intersex individuals embody physical characteristics of both, and most of us identify both with traits culturally defined as feminine and those considered masculine. As you read the following section, keep in mind that the real issue is not one's biological sex, but rather cultural constructs about what it means to be masculine, feminine, or some mixture of both.

FEMALE IDENTITY AND HEALTH

In many cultures, women are economically dependent on men and considered subordinate to them. Partly because of this, women worldwide are less likely than men to have regular access to health care, and the gap is even greater if the women are economically impoverished (Gustavo et al., 2013). The perception that women are less powerful than men sometimes fosters a patriarchal pattern in which women are treated as less active agents than men in making health-related decisions. For example, a Canadian study showed that physicians discussed a patient's preferences for knee surgery 57% of the time when the patient was male but only 15% of the time when the patient was female (Borkhoff et al., 2013).

There is also a tendency in some cultures to consider women's primary role to be childbearing and childrearing. In the United States, breast cancer gets more attention than other women's health topics, although heart disease is actually the number-one cause of death among women, just as it is among men (CDC, 2015).

A cultural focus on motherhood puts women at a disadvantage in some ways, but privileges them in others. Among some members of the Muslim faith, female fertility is revered to such an extent that a woman's inability to bear children, and even the onset of menopause, can be seen as shameful (Douki, Zineb, Nacef, & Halbreich, 2007). On the other hand, a Jordanian man interviewed about his wife's health said, "She is the one who nurtures the young generation while the man is busy outside the home. . . . her health is a higher priority than my health" (Taha, Al-Qutob, Nyström, Wahlström, & Berggren, 2013, p. 9).

Ironically, although women are often valued in terms of their reproductive capacity, expectations about female modesty and chastity may shield them from gynecological health information. Women may avoid or dread "shameful" and "embarrassing" medical examinations. In some African American and Appalachian cultures, talk about reproductive health and sexually transmitted diseases is considered so taboo that girls do not learn much about these issues from their parents (Studts, Tarasenko, & Schoenberg, 2013; Warren-Jeanpiere, Miller, & Warren, 2010).

Women also suffer disproportionately from domestic violence. About 12 million women a year in the United States, and 1 in 3 women worldwide, are physically assaulted by intimate partners, stalked, or raped (CDC, 2014; WHO, 2014). As a consequence, women in the United States are two to three times more likely than men to experience the recurring nightmares, fear, and emotional agitation of posttraumatic stress disorder (PTSD) (Vogt, 2013).

Because intimate-partner violence is a difficult issue to talk about, health professionals may not ask about it and may not even realize that women wish they would. A study of Lebanese women revealed that they would rather talk about abuse with health professionals than with friends or neighbors, if the professionals are nonjudgmental and keep the information confidential. The women suggested that doctors and social workers ask them directly if they are experiencing violence at home. Said one woman in the study, "I trust my doctor more than I trust my neighbor, I talk to him and he usually guides me what is best for me to do" (Usta, Antoun, Ambuel, & Khawaja, 2012, p. 216).

MALE IDENTITY AND HEALTH

In many cultures, men are expected to be strong, stoic, and virile. This can be empowering, as when they are considered active agents in making decisions about their health. However, it can also shame men who feel that their health concerns are signs of weakness. The expectation that they be "strong" and "protective" can also put them in harm's way.

In some traditional Latin American and Arab communities, among many others, men's worth is defined largely in terms of their career success and how well they provide for their families (Kumar, Warnke, & Karabenick, 2014; Rubenstein & Macías-González, 2012). A downward emotional spiral can result when men perceive that they do not measure up to these expectations. However, few people may know it. Admitting to others that they feel ashamed or depressed can make men feel even weaker and more vulnerable. Rico, a middle-aged man of Mexican descent, admitted in counseling that he felt constantly criticized and belittled, imagining his father saying he should be "working harder," his boss saying he was "not working fast enough," and his own self-critical voice saying, "I am stupid and everyone might find out if I don't hide it" (Shepard & Rabinowitz, 2013, p. 456). Rico reflected on how difficult it was to voice those feelings aloud, even in a group therapy session with other men.

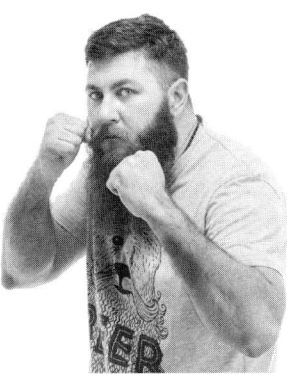

In the United States, men are four times more likely than women to be murdered and four times more likely to commit suicide, partly because of cultural expectations that they fight for honor and that they keep quiet about depression.

How do people in your culture regard depression? Is the topic openly discussed or not? What effect do you think that has on people's health?

The social implications of ill health can be especially hard on men who consider their conditions to be emasculating. For example, men experiencing erectile dysfunction, incontinence, sexually transmitted infections, and eating disorders may have a hard time admitting their concerns to loved ones or seeking treatment (respectively, Peate, 2012; Hrisanfow & Hägglund, 2013; Morris et al., 2014; Dalgliesh & Nutt, 2013).

Whereas women are more likely than men to experience violence in the home, men more often encounter it in social settings and in battle. In the United States, men are nearly four times more likely than women to be murdered, most often by firearms (CDC, 2013). This is partly because men in some cultures are expected to fight. For example, in parts of the southern and western United States, men feel duty bound to respond aggressively and even violently if they perceive that someone has insulted their honor or that of their family or religion (Crowder & Kemmelmeier, 2014). Homicide rates tend to be higher than normal in these communities, but so do suicides, especially among men who feel they have been publicly shamed (Crowder & Kemmelmeier). In the United States, men are four times more likely to commit suicide than women are (CDC, 2012).

In summary, the importance of health communication is underscored by patterns that cast women and men in narrowly defined roles and discourage them from talking about some health concerns. The issue is not so much that some cultural expectations are wrong, as that they can be very restrictive. Gender roles are becoming less rigid in some regions of the world, as evidenced by the increasing visibility of women as educated professionals and the relatively small but growing number of men who are stay-at-home fathers (Krajewski & Beach Slatten, 2013; Rampell, 2014).

Next we discuss another type of social identity that affects nearly everyone: the roles we play as family members.

Family Roles and Health Communication

Family members are often involved in caring for one another on a daily basis. But it is sometimes unclear how, and to what extent, loved ones should be involved in health care rituals and decisions when health professionals are involved.

Since family is particularly important in many Hispanic and Latinx communities, misunderstandings can occur when loved ones' presence clashes with health professionals' notions of efficiency and privacy.

A hospital nurse in one study expressed frustration that some families insist on being always present, saying, "The patient is perfectly fine, they don't need to have anybody stay in overnight, but they will insist and make a big fuss" (Kirkham, 2003, p. 771).

The very notion of family is open to interpretation. It is common for a traditional Arab household to include several generations as well as uncles, cousins, and others. Men are largely expected to provide for the family and women to raise the children and perform domestic tasks. In this collectivistic culture, a dishonorable action by one member may bring shame on the entire family. This means that some health conditions, such as mental illness and out-of-marriage pregnancies, may have powerful implications for the entire family. Health care professionals are encouraged to approach these matters delicately. Even when the issue is not a shameful one, many traditional Arabs prefer that doctors not tell the patient directly about a serious and terminal illness, but instead give the news to the nearest relative or the male head of the family, who, in turn, will share it with the others (Ahmad, 2004).

For individuals, such as immigrants, who may not have extensive family nearby, even the presence of caring strangers can be comforting in a health crisis. Part of the Muslim creed involves caring for people in need (Padela, Killawi, Forman, DeMonner, & Heisler, 2012). Therefore they may wish to be at the bedside of Muslim community members, even if they did not previously know them.

All in all, experts encourage health professionals to honor patients' wishes about family involvement as much as possible, since loved ones may be crucial to healing, coping, and decision making (Zoucha & Broome, 2008). We talk more about family caregivers in Chapter 8. (See Box 7.2 for more about a Thai family providing caring for a loved one.)

BOX 7.2 PERSPECTIVES

Thai Customs and a Son's Duty

Absolutely nothing in Thai culture is as important as a son's duty to take care of his elderly parents. My paternal grandmother came to live with my family when I was 15 years old. She left Chonburi, a small city in the eastern part of Thailand, and moved to Bangkok after my grandfather died of a heart attack. Grandmother Kim had been paralyzed for 20 years because of a bad fall, so my father insisted she must come to live with us so we could take proper care of her and so she wouldn't be lonely.

Grandmother Kim was 91 years old then, but she still had a great memory, especially about finances. Even though she had no expenses of her own, she insisted that my father give her a monthly allowance. She kept perfect mental notes on the status of her money so that she could distribute it as she pleased. For example, every day before I left for school, Grandmother gave me some money to give to the monk she watched on television each day. She was looking after her future by buying merit enough to go to heaven when she died. Grandmother also gave me money for myself each morning, and she gave other people money as well.

Although she required a lot of care and assistance, Grandmother was not depressed. Instead, she seemed happy and content with her financial projects and with providing advice to our family. Still, my mother and I watched over her constantly and we hired a private nurse to help take care of her. My mother was a very skillful and competent caregiver since she had taken classes at the hospital to prepare her to take care of Grandmother Kim.

After I graduated from high school, I pursued a bachelor's degree at a university far from home. I would go back every weekend, however. When she was 95, Grandmother began to get weak. The doctor said she might have lung cancer. I didn't think she had any diseases; instead, I believed it was her time to go to heaven. My father didn't think she had lung cancer, either. He was convinced her lungs were perfect because she had no symptoms of any lung problem. No matter how strongly my father opposed the doctor's opinion, the doctor insisted on a lung biopsy as soon as possible. We agreed not to tell my grandmother about any suspicion of cancer, since we thought it might be too hard for her to know. We agreed only to tell her she had suffered a stroke. As we waited during the surgery, my father confided in

continued

me that he was unsure he had made the right decision to let the doctor do a biopsy.

When the results came back, my grandmother didn't have cancer. After she came home, everyone expected her to feel better. Unfortunately, Grandmother got worse. We took her to another doctor, who said that, since a biopsy could make an elderly patient weaker, it had been inappropriate to do the procedure. My father asked the doctor how much time his mother had left in this world. He told us that Grandmother could not be expected to live longer than one year. She died within several weeks.

Although I was away at the university when Grandmother died, I quickly returned. It is Thai custom that kin and family have to see the dead person before the body is placed in the coffin. Therefore I had a chance to see her for the last time in the mortuary. As my mother and I got her dressed and cut her hair, I noticed that Grandmother's body was small and cold. I told my mother that Grandmother had kissed me and told me to be a good girl the last time I saw her. Up to this day, I still remember every single word she told me. I think she knew her time to go was close. However, she didn't show any signs that she was afraid of death.

My father blamed the first doctor for his mother's death, but he blamed himself most of all. He thought that if he had insisted the doctor not perform the biopsy, she would have stayed with us longer. My mother and I both tried to comfort Father. I thought the best way to relieve him of some of his sorrow was to tell him that it was time for Grandmother to go. She had stayed longer than most other people could; also she had suffered from a stroke and had been paralyzed for a long time. However, I do understand my father's feeling because he is a son, and his responsibility is to do everything to keep his mother alive and healthy.

—PEM

Illness and Coping Metaphors

When Robin Williams died by suicide in 2014, CNN explained that the star "was battling depression" and *People* magazine proposed that he "fought, and lost, his battles with addiction and depression" (respectively, Duke, 2014; Tauber, 2014, headline). In many cultures, military metaphors such as these are common. They imply that "fighting" is the most effective and admirable way to respond to illness. In other cultures, however, responding to illness more closely resembles a peace initiative. We explore both perspectives here.

"Fight for Your Life"

The battle metaphor of ill health is bolstered by an organic, scientific perspective. The body, especially when ill, is regarded as a complex and unpredictable space vulnerable to invasion by enemy forces (bacteria, viruses, allergens) beyond most people's

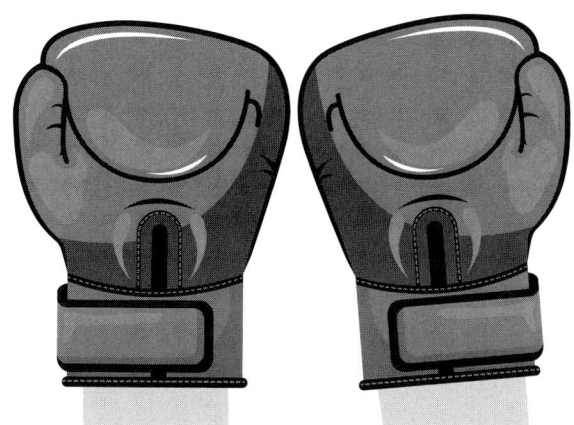

When someone becomes seriously ill, they are often admired for "fighting the disease," and if they die, people often say they "lost the battle."

Are there ways in which the military metaphor is appealing to you? Are there ways in which the peace and flexibility perspective is appealing to you? On balance, which feels more appealing to you and why?

understanding. An analysis of media coverage conducted by Juanne Nancarrow Clarke and Jeannine Binns (2006) helps to illustrate this idea.

A sense that the human body is on the verge of war or disaster is evident in terms such as *heart attack, asthma attack,* and *risk factors* (Clarke & Binns, 2006). From that perspective, it is recommended that people be vigilant (*watch for warning signs*) and ready to engage in combat (*fight* disease). When illness does occur, it is often portrayed as an invader that has attacked the body-as-fortress (Clarke & Binns, 2006). Ill individuals are encouraged to *be strong* and to *fight for their lives.* Within this metaphoric landscape, medical care is described as *life-saving, state of the art,* and *tried, tested, and true.* Some medications (such as Viagra) are even heralded as "miracle drugs" (Baglia, 2005, p. 28).

If people recover, they are said to *triumph* over disease. Otherwise, they *lose their battle* with heart disease, cancer, or any number of other conditions. The implication is clear: Death represents defeat.

"Strive for Peace and Flexibility"

In contrast to the military metaphor, members of some cultures in Korea and China, for example, believe in making peace with the body, especially when a serious health concern emerges.

They may engage in meditation and yoga to bring the mind and body into harmony and to evoke a sense of calm (Woodyard, 2011). These activities are consistent with other cultural customs, such as taking part in tai chi, qigong, karate, and tae kwon do—all designed to enhance spiritual and bodily awareness, flexibility, and fluid strength.

This perspective portrays the body not as a battlefield, but as a place of natural harmony. It follows that the best way to maintain good health is to honor the body and follow its rhythms.

In traditional Chinese medicine, for example, interventions are typically mild and designed to enhance the body's natural functioning. Aggressive interventions, such as surgery and strong drugs, may be viewed suspiciously as interfering with the body's natural rhythms. Some people depict traditional Eastern medicine as *health from within* and Western medicine as a *cure from without.*

Of course, the dichotomy between military and peace metaphors is not absolute. There is evidence to support both. People may embrace harmony-enhancing activities *and* the stance of a warrior. Still, it is helpful to highlight the essential differences between these perspectives so we can better understand the shades between them.

Sick Roles and Healer Roles

Culturally speaking, there are right and wrong ways to "do" being ill and providing assistance. For example, members of some Arab cultures expect women to cry out in pain during labor and delivery (Ahmad, 2004), whereas members of some Hispanic cultures believe that pain should be endured stoically because it is God's wish (Duggleby, 2003). Likewise, people might be expected to remain "respectfully" quiet in medical encounters or to take a "responsible" role by sharing their thoughts. The rules for being a good patient and a good care provider may be contradictory and confusing. Nevertheless, with people's health hanging in the balance, participants may fervently wish to behave correctly.

A **role** is a set of expectations that applies to people performing various functions in the culture. For example, people may play the roles of patient, doctor, sister, friend, employee, and parent. Each role is guided by a set of culturally approved rules. Typically, one role exists in relation to another: patient–caregiver, student–teacher, parent–child, and so on. A role may lose meaning without its counterpart (e.g., a teacher is not a teacher without students). Therefore, role-playing is a collaborative endeavor, and people usually adjust their performances to form meaningful combinations. This can be so compelling that people sometimes feel forced into roles they would rather not assume. For example, if your conversational partner adopts a parental role, you may feel like a child, and you may act that way even if you would rather not. To do otherwise might seem uncooperative and rude.

As you will see in this section, patients and care providers often play complementary roles—as mechanics and machines, providers and consumers, parents and children, and so on. Keep in mind that these roles are collaborative achievements, supported by participants' mutual efforts. This does not mean the participants always like the roles they assume. They may be motivated by a sense of cultural appropriateness or the perceived need to "play the scene" as the other person is playing it.

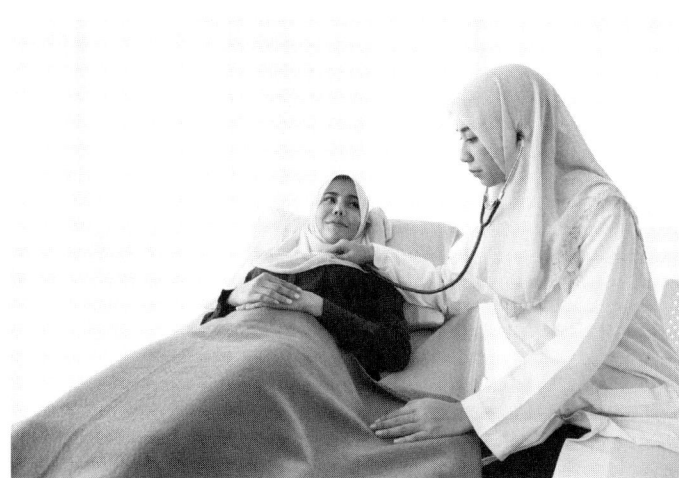

The traditional Muslim diet forbids the consumption of pork or alcohol. This can make hospital food, including foods fried in animal lard, unacceptable and can be an issue with some medications.

If you are ever hospitalized, what personal and cultural preferences would you like your care providers to know about?

Mechanics and Machines

From one perspective, care providers are similar to mechanics and patients to machines. The implication is that patients are relatively passive and care providers are expected to be analytical and capable of fixing the problems that are presented.

This perspective does not encourage emotional communication between patients and health professionals. The focus is more on identifying physical abnormalities and fixing them. When providers take on a mechanic role, they are typically more concerned with what they can observe and change than what a patient might be feeling.

Some people feel that scientific medicine is relatively mechanistic. That is, when health professionals take on the role of scientists, they are much like mechanics—concerned with the orderly physical functioning of the human body. As mechanics or scientists, care providers are expected to be objective, value neutral, and capable of collecting information, diagnosing a problem, and fixing it. It may seem inappropriate for them to display emotions or to call into play such intangible notions as faith and spirituality. Eric Cassell (1991) puts it this way: "Adjectives like warm, tall, swollen, or painful exist only for persons but, ideally, science deals only with measurable quantities like temperature, vertical dimensions, diameters" (p. 18).

One advantage of the mechanic-scientist role is that it reduces the emotional drain on health professionals. If patients are like machines who simply need fixing, emotions need not become part of the process (Bonsteel, 1997). At the same time, the confidence that people *can* be fixed may seem comforting and neat.

Of course, patients may not appreciate being treated like machines. Some people argue that ignoring patients' descriptions and considering them passive in their own care casts them as little more than a set of parts. In Richard Swiderski's (1976) analysis of medicine through the ages, he concludes that doctors have often considered patients less relevant than their pulse rates, blood, and urine. This is an image the public has embraced as well, as evidenced by patients' disappointment when their physicians do not run tests or prescribe medications. One reason for overuse of antibiotics is patients' insistence that treatment be embodied in some physical form, even when pharmacology suggests it will have no effect (Fisher, 1994). Moreover, the unrealistic belief that doctors can fix anything may lead to disappointment and even lawsuits.

Parents and Children

The popular expression "doctor's orders" suggests a relationship in which physicians issue directions that patients are expected to obey. This approach is consistent with **paternalism**, the idea that patients are like children and care providers are like parents.

The dynamic that "health providers know best" may be enacted in cultures common in Japan, India, and Venezuela that honor a high **power distance**—that is, the degree to which they defer to people of greater power or status (Hofstede, 2001). Members of these cultures may consider it rude to disagree with or question an authority figure such as a health professional. In these cultures, patients have traditionally declined to take part in treatment decisions, preferring that professionals make decisions on their behalf ("Reducing Health Disparities," 2005). It is risky to assume that this is always the case, though. When Dana Lathan Alden et al. (2010) interviewed urban Vietnamese women, most of them indicated that they would like a say in choices regarding their contraception use, even though it is common in their culture to honor the judgment of physicians without question (Alden, Merz, & Thi, 2010).

One challenge of the paternalistic model is that professionals may misunderstand how much patients understand and agree with them. For example, Japanese individuals may use the word "yes" to signal politely that they understand the speaker, not as a sign that they agree. If they have questions, they may not ask them, for this might be seen as criticism.

Another challenge is that health professionals may be expected to know what is best for their patients. Some theorists believe this is a dubious assumption because patients may have many feelings and desires unknown to their care providers (Bealieu-Volk, 2014). Expecting providers to anticipate and act on patients' wishes may place an unrealistic burden on them and unfairly rob patients of opportunities to make their own decisions. (See Box 7.3 for more on this issue.)

Spiritualists and Believers

Care providers may be cast as spiritualists who use their powers on behalf of faithful patients. The image of providers as spiritual figures (and even as gods) was established thousands of years ago. Jesus has been called "the great physician" and is revered for legendary acts of curing the sick (Moore, Van Arsdale, Glittenberg, & Aldrich, 1987). Throughout history, physicians have been described as "little gods," a celestial metaphor that extends to nurses, often portrayed as "angels of mercy" (Moore et al., 1987, p. 232).

Anthropologists have compared the physician's role to that of a priest, a powerful and somewhat mysterious authority figure. This awe-inspiring image may be strengthened by patients' reverence and physicians' displays of power. Pendleton and colleagues (1984) point to doctors' laboratory coats, specialized vocabulary, and honorific titles as supporting props in this image. They also suggest that the image is bolstered by an information imbalance that makes physicians' knowledge seem all the more marvelous: "Powerful

---

BOX 7.3 **Ethical Considerations**

Physician as Parent or Partner?

Medical ethicist Robert Veatch (1983) reflects that physicians are often criticized as being "aloof and unconcerned" rather than concerned and attentive, as people would like them to be. In short, physicians often act like strangers when patients wish they would act like friends or family members.

Paternalism (the idea that doctors are like parents) is a long-standing tradition. The Hippocratic oath, written approximately 2,500 years ago, beseeches physicians to use their best "ability and judgment" on each patient's behalf. This presumes that physicians are well acquainted with medicine *and* with the particular needs and preferences of each patient. Paternalism is also based on the belief that physicians are more capable of making medical decisions than patients are.

Some people feel that paternalism is outdated. Veatch (1983) points out that it is difficult to know patients well in the current age of large patient loads, specialization, and emergency and outpatient care. These factors make it unlikely that doctors will understand the unique needs and preferences of each patient. The paternalistic model is also criticized as inconsistent with patient empowerment, which presumes that patients are knowledgeable and active agents in their own health care (Emanuel & Emanuel, 1995).

What Do You Think?

1. Do you feel it is realistic or preferable for health care providers to know their patients' feelings and values? If so, how might they accomplish this? If not, what alternatives would you suggest?
2. Can you think of circumstances in which you would want your physician to know your feelings and life circumstances?
3. Can you think of circumstances in which you would rather your physician did not know you well?
4. Do you feel patients are capable of making decisions about their own care?

rituals, such as examining and prescribing, are the more charismatic in the absence of adequate explanations" (p. 9).

By contrast, folk healing is typically oriented toward lifeworld concerns (Chapter 4). Usually, a folk healer's role is to integrate social support with spiritual faith and physical treatment. Among the most well-known healers and spiritualists are the shamans and hand-tremblers of Native American cultures and the *curanderos* (coo-ran-DARE-ohs) of Mexican American cultures. These folk healers are usually well-known members of their communities. As such, they are familiar and accessible, without institutional boundaries or technical jargon.

A shaman is believed to coax a patient's disease into their own body and then expel it through strength of will (Hutch, 2013). The assumption is that illness is an invasion of magical or supernatural forces. The faithful believe shamans can communicate with beings beyond the physical world, which gives them magical abilities and healing powers.

Folk medicine's focus on sense-making and social support addresses the distinction between healing and curing. McWhinney (1989, p. 29) calls *healing* a "restoration of wholeness," which includes spiritual and moral consideration, as opposed to purely physical *curing*, which he says may still leave a patient in "anguish of spirit" about the causes, effects, and fears associated with the illness.

Another spiritualist group is the Christian Science Church. Some members of this religion believe that conventional medicine is anti-Christian and that illness is an illusion and can be cured only through prayer (Christian Science Board of Directors, n.d.). Thus, they may refuse biomedical therapies, including surgery. This has raised controversy across the nation, especially when children's lives are involved. Currently, the church's website presents examples of people who were cured by prayer and mind control but says health-related decisions are up to individual members.

A focus on the supernatural also characterizes the health beliefs of some southern Appalachians. In that culture, spiritual ceremonies involving faith healing and glossolalia (speaking in tongues) are believed to restore health. **Faith healers** are expected to channel the curative power of the Holy Spirit, which they pass to believers through ceremonies such as the laying on of hands. **Glossolalia** involves a trancelike state during which a worshipper seems to speak in a foreign language. It is believed that the language is known only to God, or that it is a foreign tongue known to some but unknown to the worshipper, except through divine inspiration.

The success of a spiritual ceremony is often said to rely on the patient's faith in the healer and the greater spiritual force that has accepted the healer as a medium. One result of this assumption is that failure to recover may be construed as an indication of the patient's insufficient faith (Kearney, 1978). For this reason, patients may be particularly trusting and may benefit from the power of positive thinking. However, if their conditions do not improve, they may be reluctant to admit it.

Even scientists acknowledge the power of faith, although they are not likely to regard it as the central focus of their work. Evidence supports that people who expect to be cured sometimes are, even when the "treatment" is an inactive **placebo** such as flavored water or sugar. Placebo effects are so common that medical researchers routinely give some research participants an actual treatment and give other people a placebo. If the treatment group does not experience greater effects than the placebo group, the researchers cannot be sure they are measuring anything more than the power of suggestion. The reverse is sometimes true as well. People who have no confidence in a treatment may be unaffected by it. These examples do not prove that all disease can be reduced to the effects of faith and emotions. However, they demonstrate that there is more to disease than meets the (microscopic) eye.

A religious-like faith in care providers serves multiple goals. It inspires confidence on the part of patient and provider, which may be an important part of healing. It also honors the extraordinary role health professionals play in managing life and health. There is a downside, though, in dashed hopes and exorbitant malpractice claims. With the expectation that medicine can work miracles if done correctly, people may feel particularly angry when things do not go well, and they may rightly or wrongly charge that their care providers are incompetent (Kreps, 1990).

Providers and Consumers

It has become popular to describe health care in terms of consumerism. Patients are regarded as shoppers or clients who pay care providers primarily to provide information and carry out the patients' wishes. Consumerism is partly fueled by internet resources.

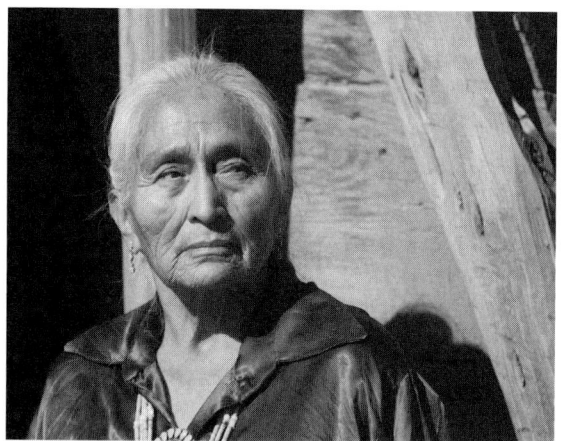

Some members of Navajo communities believe it is bad luck to discuss potentially negative outcomes of a medical procedure.

As a patient, does it make you uneasy to talk about what might go wrong, or do you feel better knowing the worst case scenario?

People can now look up extensive health information for themselves. Websites such as ConsumerReportsHealth.org, DoctorScorecard.com, and AngiesList.com offer reviews of hospitals, treatments, products, and professionals—including consumer reviews of doctors' bedside manner, perceived quality of care, price, the cleanliness of their offices, the courteousness of their staff members, and more.

Competitiveness has made many care providers especially mindful of patient satisfaction. However, some who see themselves as serving a higher purpose than profit margins find the marketplace metaphors disturbing. Analysts warn that consumer websites can have a backlash. For one, anyone can file comments online but most people don't. As a result, the comments that appear may not represent most patients' opinions.

Years ago, Howard Friedman and M. Robin DiMatteo (1979) cautioned that consumerism may be a risky conceptualization for all involved. If the customer is always right, they wondered, will medical centers that respect patients' treatment decisions later be held liable if adverse outcomes result? Friedman and DiMatteo also worried that pleasing patients may sometimes be at odds with helping them. Considering that the most effective medical options are sometimes the most unpleasant, how far will care providers go to avoid upsetting their patients?

Similarly, consumerism seems to place cost as a top priority. Richard Glass (1996) is concerned that physicians may choose less aggressive treatment options if they are forced to be more mindful of cost than care. A physician himself, Glass maintains that patients "rightly expect something different from their doctors than from consumer goods salespersons" (p. 148). He argues that a marketplace mentality may have "perverse effects" on medical care, and he beseeches health care managers not to interfere unduly in medical decision making.

There is some evidence that people who are well informed about health information do not view their doctors in quite the same way as before. Unlike generations past, people are unlikely to believe that doctors have all the answers (Lowrey & Anderson, 2006). This may diminish physicians' professional status. Or it may simply fuel a different kind of relationship, such as the one we will discuss next.

Partners

Only as partners do patients and care providers assume roles of roughly equal power. Of course, they each bring something different to the encounter in terms of experiences and expertise. But as partners, they orient themselves to identifying mutually satisfying solutions, acting as peers in the process. The partner role is consistent with collaborative medical talk (Chapter 5).

The success of health care managed in this way hinges largely on the quality of patient–caregiver relationships. In 1996, the *Journal of the American Medical Association* introduced a column called "The Patient–Physician Relationship." In an article launching the new feature, Richard Glass (1996) proclaimed the doctor–patient link to be the "center of medicine," a covenant not to be compromised by impersonal reliance on technology or profit-oriented decisions. This emphasis underscores the importance of trusting communication between patients and care providers.

Some people find the partnership model appealing because it allows both patients and health professionals to have influence over medical decisions, as opposed to being strictly patient centered or provider centered. Hufford (1997) attests that patients have important and relevant statements to make about their own health: "Sick people, it turns out, often do know exactly what has been happening to them, what it feels like, and when it happens, and there is nothing fictional about it" (p. 118). (See Box 7.4 for an example.)

One way to encourage patients' active participation is to follow the lead of Myra Skluth (2007) and

BOX 7.4 PERSPECTIVES

Partners in Care

Tina, a middle-aged mother of two, has been referred to a hemodialysis center for treatment. When she arrives for her first visit, an advanced nurse practitioner notices that she is upset and takes the time to speak with her. Tina says she has long had diabetes, but she does not understand why her doctor wants her to undergo dialysis. She feels fine and her family relies on her to work full time.

Recognizing that Tina needs to be an active agent in making decisions about her own care, the nurse practitioner listens attentively to her concerns and helps her better understand her medical condition, which involves kidney disease that might kill her without treatment. Together, they devise a regimen in which Tina is able to undergo dialysis for about a year until she receives a donor kidney.

Debra Hain and Dainne Sandy (2013) write about Tina in an article on the value of being a partner, rather than a parent, when it comes to patients. They reflect that a paternalistic model probably would not have helped Tina understand the need for dialysis or coordinate her care in light of her other responsibilities.

"Tina is forever grateful for the support she received at a time she desperately needed it," the authors write, reflecting that, when the nurse practitioner asked Tina what had made her start dialysis, she replied warmly, "It's the way you spoke to me" (Hain & Sandy, 2013. p. 156).

What Do You Think?

1. In what circumstances, if any, might you follow a doctor's advice without question?
2. In what circumstances, if any, would you rather be treated as a partner in making decisions about your care?

---

create patient to-do lists. She and patients negotiate the terms of the to-do lists, and then each keeps a copy. "This approach works very well," she says (p. 16). Because the to-do lists are in patients' charts, "if they call with questions, the nurses know exactly what I told them. I can also review the items with them at the beginning of the next visit—what they accomplished, and what they didn't and why. I find my patients really appreciate this" (p. 16).

Few people criticize the idea of patients and health professionals as partners. However, this may be a difficult transition to make. Both sides have traditionally upheld the expectation that professionals will guide medical discussions and patients will be relatively quiet and passive in their presence. A shift is possible, and indeed we see some evidence of it, but it will require continued change and cooperation on both sides.

In closing this section, note that these interaction models characterize various aspects of medical discourse, yet they are not as simple as they appear. Transactions often, perhaps always, involve elements of several models, even if one is dominant. The following discussion of holistic medicine involves a treatment model that draws upon many of the ideas we have discussed about health as harmonic balance and can employ, at times, any of the relationship types described here (Ho & Bylund, 2008).

Holistic Care

> Lisa immediately notices the differences between this setting and her doctor's office. Soft music is playing, and the lights and colors are soothing. She lies on a massage table and Jing, an acupuncturist, encourages her to relax. Despite her fear of needles, Lisa finds the experience mostly painless. "I could barely feel the needles go in," she says. "There was the slightest of sensations, followed by a feeling of energy flowing."

This story, adapted from Lisa Rosenthal's blog ("Fertility Acupuncture," 2012), describes an initial experience with holistic care. In the United States, options such as acupuncture, meditation, and chiropractic—once derided as quackery—are gaining acceptance. There are a number of reasons for this,

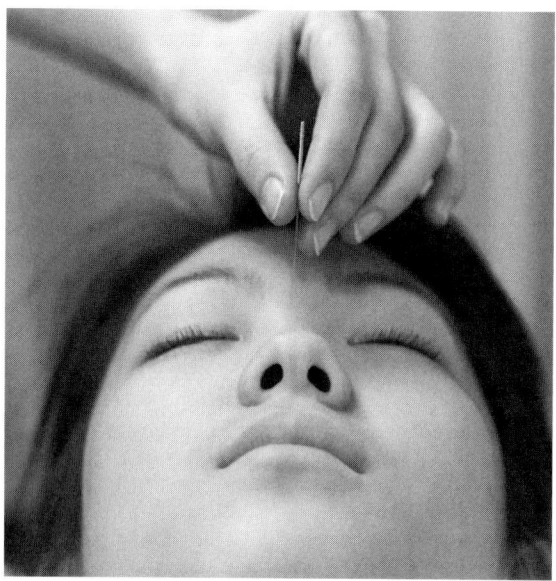

Holistic therapies such as acupuncture have gained acceptance in recent years, partly because they are typically less expensive and invasive than many biomedical procedures. *Have you taken part in holistic approaches such as acupuncture, homeopathy, or meditation? If so, how would you compare the experience to other health care encounters?*

including their emphasis on open communication. The following section describes holistic forms of medicine, factors fueling recent interest in them, and their advantages and drawbacks.

Terminology

The term *alternative medicine* has traditionally been applied to therapies that have not been scientifically researched and consequently approved by professional associations such as the American Medical Association. However, "alternative" is not a particularly accurate description of these therapies. As Lisa Schreiber (2005) points out, it is not an either/or proposition. Many people use "alternative" therapies in conjunction with other treatments. For example, meditation, prayer, and yoga are not biomedical means of treating cancer, but most oncologists agree that, if they are useful in promoting emotional well-being, they are valuable components of a treatment regimen.

Some people have adopted the term *complementary medicine* or *complementary and alternative medicine (CAM)*. These are somewhat problematic as well, in that they define these therapies not by what they *are* but simply in terms of their (implicitly peripheral) relation to biomedicine. Another semantic alternative is the term *traditional medicine,* used in parts of the world such as Africa, Asia, and Latin America. However, this term seems to exclude recent innovations. For lack of a better term, this section follows Schreiber's suggestion and uses the term *holistic medicine.* Some make a good point that not all methods that fall within this rubric are holistic. However, for the most part, their approach is more holistic than biomedical therapies, which are largely grounded in identifying specific causes and cures of illness. The glossary in Box 7.5 explains the wide variety of holistic therapies.

Popularity

There are several reasons for the recent popularity of holistic medicine. For one, an increasing number of people are receptive to the idea. About 38% of U.S adults and 12% of children use holistic therapies such as acupuncture, chiropractic, Ayurveda, meditation, massage, yoga, and hypnosis (National Center for Complementary, 2012). Acceptance is even greater in some areas of the world. In some parts of Asia and Africa, 80% of citizens rely primarily on holistic care (WHO, 2008).

Second, well-trained providers are becoming more plentiful. In the United States, chiropractic is one of the fastest-growing occupations. There are currently about 47,400 chiropractors in the United States, and the number is expected to rise 7% between 2018 and 2028 (U.S. Bureau of Labor Statistics, 2019).

Third, research dollars are more available than in the past. In 1997, the U.S. Congress voted to fund a new Office of Alternative Medicine as part of the National Institutes of Health (NIH). It offers funding for researchers interested in testing the efficacy of diverse therapies. For example, acupuncture has been shown in clinical trials to help some people lose weight, relieve chronic depression, diminish some forms of pain, and meet a range of other treatment goals, particularly when combined with other forms of care (Cho, Lee, Thabane, & Lee, 2009; Tough & White, 2011; Zhang, Chen, Yip, Ng, & Wong, 2010).

Finally, many insurance companies and physicians are now giving the go-ahead to nonbiomedical treatments, and Medicare and workers' compensation plans in all 50 states reimburse chiropractic care. (For more about careers in holistic medicine, see Box 7.6.)

Advantages

There are several reasons for the growing popularity of holistic care. For one, such care typically involves low-cost and low-tech methods. If these are useful, they stand to reduce health care costs. That is good news for insurance

BOX 7.5

Holistic Medicine at a Glance

Acupuncture is believed to stimulate and balance the body's energy flow (Qi) through tiny needles inserted in the skin.

Ayurveda is based on ancient Indian practices, including yoga, diet, and meditation.

Biofeedback involves learning to recognize the body's physiological states (such as tension) and to control them.

Chiropractic medicine focuses on the physical alignment of the spine, muscles, and nerves.

Herbal therapies use plant extracts such as chamomile, licorice, and St. John's wort to treat ailments ranging from skin conditions to asthma and depression.

Holistic care emphasizes overall well-being (physical and emotional), with an emphasis on maintaining health, not just curing ailments.

Homeopathic medicine uses very small doses to escalate symptoms in an effort to stimulate the body's immune system. (In contrast, most mainstream medical care is *allopathic*, relying on remedies that counteract symptoms.) *Homeo* is derived from the Greek word meaning "same," and *allo* comes from the Greek word for "other."

Integrative medicine combines biomedical and naturopathic therapies.

Naturopathic medicine focuses on diet and the use of herbal therapies to help people maintain good health.

Osteopathic medicine is taught in traditional medical schools. This branch of medicine focuses on the muscular and skeletal system, treating the body as an integrated unit.

Reiki (pronounced RAY-kee) is based on the Japanese tradition of channeling energy through the healer's hands to increase the patient's spiritual strength.

Traditional Asian medicine includes therapies such as herbal remedies, acupuncture, and massage. It is based on establishing a healthy flow of energy through the body and achieving harmony between mind, body, spirit, and surroundings.

---

companies and managed care, if people simultaneously maintain their involvement in conventional care, which they seem inclined to do. The World Health Organization is supporting research to see if low-cost herbal remedies can effectively treat malaria, AIDS, diabetes, and other conditions in impoverished areas of the world.

Second, holistic methods are usually based on simple principles that may be more understandable and less frightening to patients than conventional medicine. People who use holistic therapies often do so with the goal of maintaining health in everyday ways (National Institute of Medicine, 2005). For the most part, these people also see biomedical practitioners, although they tend not to tell doctors about holistic methods they are also using.

Third, holistic practitioners often spend more time with their patients and develop closer relationships with them than do biomedical practitioners. This may suit people who feel that most medical settings are too impersonal. As a holistic practitioner in Geist-Martin and Bell's (2009) study expressed it, "The most important thing is to listen. If I listen to the patient I am able to know what worries him, what he needs, what bothers him, and from there I can better maneuver the process" (p. 636).

Fourth, holistic therapies are usually more directed to health maintenance than biomedicine, which has traditionally focused on curing and treating. The new imperative to conserve health care resources and money makes prevention appealing.

Finally, people may turn to holistic therapies if other methods offer little or no help. For example, symptoms of anxiety that are not alleviated by medication may sometimes be managed with relaxation and biofeedback.

Drawbacks

Many holistic therapies are nonthreatening. Energy work, relaxation, and minute traces of natural substances (as in homeopathy) are unlikely to hurt anyone. However, some therapies involve the use of herbs and other natural products. Because they are considered dietary supplements rather than drugs, the U.S. Food and Drug Administration (FDA) does not require manufacturers to register them or prove their safety before they go on the market. Consequently, many supplements are not thoroughly researched. This is worrisome, first, because significant health risks are associated with some natural therapies. Taken by the wrong person or in the wrong amount, they can be deadly. Some natural remedies have caused lead poisoning, hepatitis, and renal failure. The herb germander, often included in herbal teas and tablets, has been linked to acute nonviral hepatitis. Before it was banned, the herb ephedra, sold as an enhancement for bodybuilding, was linked to at least 17 deaths (Capriotti, 1999; WHO, 2003, Update 83).

Another concern is that people may be swindled into buying useless products. Cancer patients, for instance, are vulnerable to advertisers who claim to provide the latest life-saving serums. The FDA cautions consumers to beware of wording such as "treats all forms of cancer," "skin cancers disappear," and "shrinks malignant tumors" (U.S. FDA, 2008). Such claims signal a scam, not a bona fide product. Consumers should also realize that "actual patients" and spokespersons who appear to be physicians actually may be actors hired to sell the product.

Third, endangered plant species may be wiped out in the zeal to provide health benefits (and reap the financial awards) associated with high-demand herbal remedies. Already, harvesters have endangered rain forests in Malaysia, Africa, and the Amazon. Environmentalists urge world citizens to consider regulations, herbal farming, and ocean-based cultivation to protect the planet's wildlife.

A final drawback involves a lack of communication. Only about one-third of Americans who use holistic therapies tell their physicians about them (Kennedy, Chi-Chuan, & Wu, 2007). One woman in the United Kingdom described her doctors' reaction to acupuncture: "They didn't actually ridicule it, but they said, 'hmmm' [frowns]. I felt like they didn't really want to talk about it" (Tovey & Broom, 2007, p. 2556). All the same, when doctors do not know about other treatments, they may prescribe medications that interact with them in dangerous ways.

In summary, considering both the potential advantages and drawbacks of holistic therapies, it's important that people become comfortable talking about them. Lisa's experience, which began this section, was a positive one. Once the needles were in place, Jing wrapped her in a warm blanket and said she should close her eyes and relax. "The best way that I can describe the experience is to relate it to twinkling lights," Lisa recalls. "It was a lovely, subtle feeling. . . . The rest of the day I felt relaxed, calm, and as serene as I feel after a restorative yoga class" ("Fertility Acupuncture," 2012).

BOX 7.6 Career Opportunities

Holistic Medicine

Acupuncturist
Chiropractor
Holistic nurse
Massage therapist
Midwife
Naturopathic physician
Nutritionist/dietician
Reiki practitioner
Yoga instructor

Career Resources and Job Listings

- Academy of Nutrition and Dietetics: http://www.eatright.org
- Accrediting Bureau of Health Education Schools: http://www.abhes.org
- American Association of Naturopathic Physicians: https://naturopathic.org/page/AboutUs
- American Chiropractic Association: http://www.acatoday.org
- American College of Nurse-Midwives: http://www.midwife.org
- American Council on Exercise: http://www.acefitness.org
- American Massage Therapy Association: http://www.amtamassage.org/index.html
- Associated Bodywork and Massage Professionals: http://www.abmp.com/home
- Association of Chiropractic Colleges: http://www.chirocolleges.org
- Commission on Dietetic Registration: http://www.cdrnet.org
- International Association of Reiki Professionals: http://www.iarp.org
- U.S. Bureau of Labor Statistics Occupational Outlook Handbook: http://www.bls.gov/ooh

Summary

Culture and Health Communication

- Ethnocentrism undermines cultural adaptability.
- As Dutta uses the terms, a *culturally sensitive* approach involves being aware of cultural beliefs and practices, whereas a *culture-centered* approach is a collaborative endeavor in which health advocates work actively with members of a culture.
- Fuller's reflective negotiation model of cultural adaptability proposes that cultural adaptability involves a continual process of asking and listening—both to others and to oneself.

Cultural Conceptions of Health

- From one perspective, disease is an organic phenomenon, and what shows up under a microscope may be more to the point than a patient's subjective experiences.
- From another perspective, health is affected by harmonic balance among factors such as relationships, spiritual forces, the environment, behavior, and energy fields within the body.

Making Sense of Health Experiences

- The theory of health as expanded consciousness proposes that a health disruption can be a valuable opportunity for reflection and change.
- Especially when a condition is threatening or difficult to understand, it is common to blame ill persons for their conditions or to see them as cursed or lazy.

Social Roles and Health

- In many cultures, women are encouraged to be dependent and to focus mostly on motherhood.
- Whereas women are more likely than men to experience violent assaults from intimate partners, men are more likely to die in fights or battles.
- Partly because men are often expected to be aggressive and to avoid showing emotional distress, they are more likely than women to feel shamed by emotional concerns and to avoid communicating about them.

Illness and Coping Metaphors

- In some cultures, a military metaphor of health characterizes "fighting" as the most effective and admirable way to respond to illness.
- In other cultures, people are encouraged to pursue peace and flexibility as a means to health.

Sick Roles and Healer Roles

- If disease is regarded as a physical phenomenon, patients may be like passive machines and care providers like mechanics or scientists.
- Patients may be considered incapable if they are cast as children seeking the guidance of parent-like providers who know what is best.
- Care providers have been deified to varying extents through the ages for their ability to understand and treat illness.
- In some cultures, healers are spiritual leaders, expected to channel supernatural powers for the benefit of patients.
- Some worry that medical care may suffer if it is forced to uphold the rules of the marketplace.
- As partners, patients and care providers work to build mutually satisfying relationships and care plans.

Holistic Care

- Holistic care specialists focus primarily on lifestyle changes and natural remedies.
- Some people seek holistic care when they are not satisfied with the results or nature of biomedicine. In the majority of cases, however, people continue to see physicians and other practitioners as well.
- It's a good idea to become knowledgeable about herbs and supplements before trying them.

Glossary

biophilia hypothesis The idea that people have an inherent affinity for nature and often derive a sense of well-being from contact with it. *See page 136.*

culturally sensitive approach Involves an awareness of cultural characteristics (by comparison, see *culture-centered approach*). *See page 132.*

culture A set of beliefs, rules, and practices that are shared by a group of people. *See page 132.*

culture-centered approach Involves a collaborative endeavor situated within a specific community's characteristics (by comparison, see *culturally sensitive approach*). *See page 132.*

ethnocentrism The attitude that one's own culture is better than others. *See page 132.*

faith healers People believed to channel the curative power of the Holy Spirit, which they pass to believers through ceremonies such as the laying on of hands. *See page 149.*

germ theory The scientific principle that disease is caused by microscopic organisms, such as bacteria and viruses. *See page 134.*

glossolalia A trancelike state during which a worshipper seems to speak in a foreign language; believed by some to have curative power. *See page 149.*

harmonic balance perspective The perspective that health is not simply the absence of physical signs of disease, but rather is a sense of overall well-being and equilibrium. *See page 135.*

karma Energy believed to result from either good or bad deeds in the past. *See page 136.*

organic model The perspective that health can be understood in terms of the presence (or absence) of physical indicators. *See page 134.*

paternalism The idea (as it pertains to health care) that patients are like children and care providers are like parents. *See page 147.*

placebo A harmless but ineffective "treatment" such as flavored water or sugar; often used in medical trials for comparison purposes. *See page 149.*

power distance The degree to which people defer to people of greater power or status. *See page 147.*

Qi One's central life energy; a component of traditional Chinese medicine. *See page 137.*

reflective negotiation model A perspective that involves two commitments (sensitivity to cultural differences and self-awareness) and with the goal of fostering respectful, collaborative interactions. *See page 133.*

role A set of expectations that applies to various people performing various functions in the culture. *See page 146.*

stigma Social rejection in which a person is treated as dishonorable and/or is shunned. *See page 140.*

theory of health as expanded consciousness The idea that health events are integral parts of life that provide opportunities for growth and change. *See page 137.*

yin and **yang** Polar energies whose cyclical forces are believed to define all living things; a component of traditional Chinese medicine. *See page 136.*

Discussion Questions

1. Consider the quote on page 132 by the nurse who was offended by the suggestion that staff members avoid telling patients "Merry Christmas." If she were to follow the principles of Fuller's reflective negotiation model, what questions might she ask other people? What questions might she ask herself? What might be a good outcome in that situation?

2. What aspects of your health are well explained by an organic approach? By a harmonic approach? If you made a list of healthy behaviors you would like to adopt, what, if anything, would you list in terms of organic factors? What, if anything, would reflect the desire for balance? Why?

3. If you were to schedule a day's worth of activities in which you would experience a balance of yin and yang energy, what might that day include? Do you think living that way on a consistent basis would influence your health? Why or why not?

4. Think of a health episode you or someone you know has experienced. In what way did explicate-level factors play a role? In what way did implicate-level factors influence what happened? Do you think these factors have a significant impact on health overall?

5. Reread the "I Am Not a Victim of Breast Cancer" poem on page 141 or go online and read the entire poem. In what ways does the author seem to be addressing the stigma of disease? What do her words suggest about the notion that people with cancer are "victims?"

6. In what ways is your life affected by your gender identity? By your role as a family member? Do any of these factors influence your health or the way you communicate about health? If so, how?

7. Are you more inclined to respond to illness as a "fighter" or as a "peacekeeper" or as a bit of both? What behaviors reflect your approach? Do you believe they are effective? Why or why not?

8. Which of the patient–care provider role sets best describes your health care experiences? Which do you prefer? Why?

9. Have you participated in holistic care, either as a patient or a practitioner? If so, describe the role of communication in your experience. What were the potential advantages and disadvantages, in your opinion?

PART IV
Coping and Health Resources

Two of the most powerful means we have for staying healthy and happy have little in common with each other on the surface.

One is the love and support of people around us. Research overwhelmingly confirms that people who have close and supportive relationships with others consider themselves healthier, cope with adversity better, and tend to live longer than others. Communication is the means through which we foster and maintain those ties. In Chapter 8, we will talk about the role of social support, including how we can be effective listeners and good friends, and what it means to cope, together, with health crises and end-of-life experiences. We will also look at a few social support disasters, when efforts that are meant to be helpful turn out to be hurtful instead. The lessons from those experiences can help us avoid the same outcomes.

The second resource is communication technology. At first glance, technology feels far removed from the warmth of companionship and social support. But we find that it can help us to establish and maintain supportive relationships, become well informed, and feel that we have the resources to cope with health issues. The possibilities are expanding faster than we ever imagined, as you will see in Chapter 9.

This unlikely combination of health resources reminds us that—in its many forms—communication is a powerful part of what allows us to be happy in good times and in the midst of life's great challenges.

> *We all need each other.*
> —LEO BUSCAGLIA

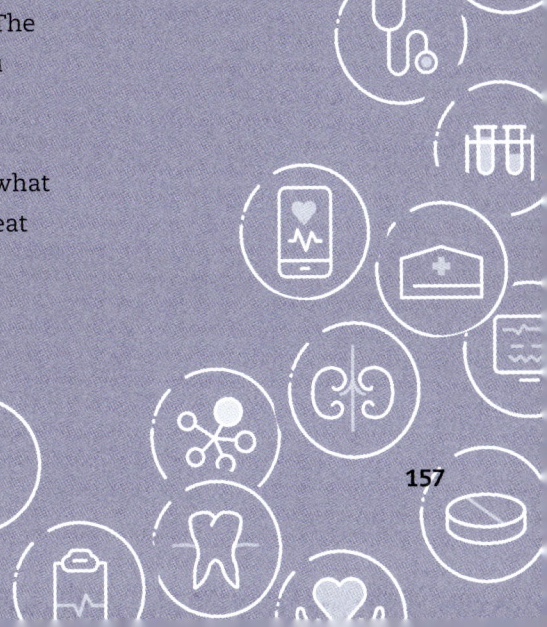

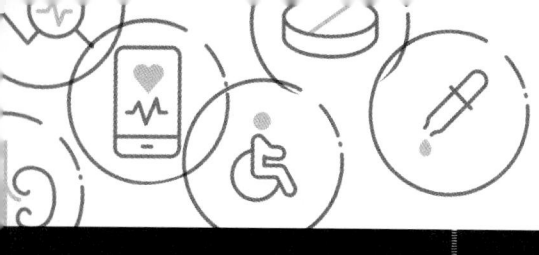

CHAPTER 8

Social Support, Family Caregiving, and End of Life

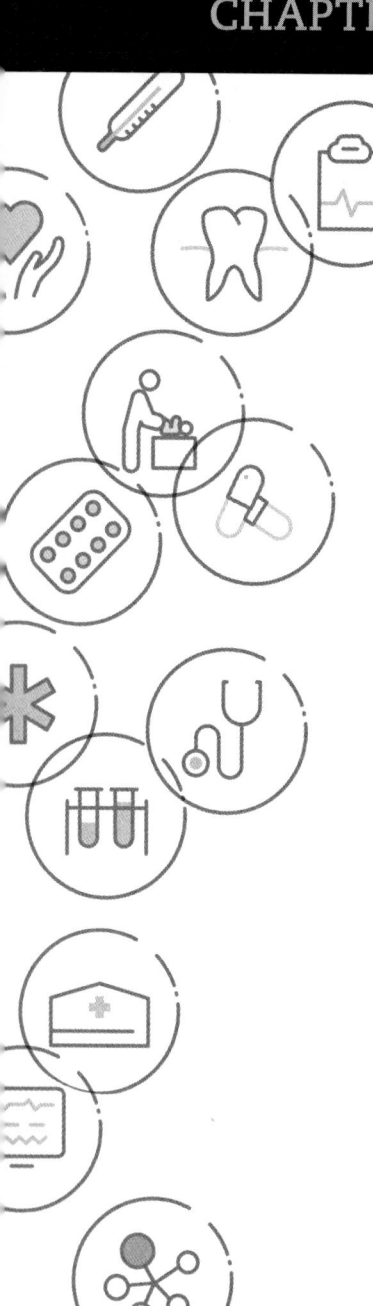

Struggling to be strong after the death of his young daughter, Alonzo is hurt and mystified when friends' first question is, "How is your wife?"

Margie misses the normal times, when people talked to her about the weather, boys, and school. Now they just hold doors for her and try not to stare at her wheelchair.

Everyone knows Drew's illness is very serious, but no one speaks of it to him. Drew wonders how he is supposed to cope with such an emotional topic in silence.

Lucy spends two hours each morning and three hours each evening caring for her three children and her elderly mother. In between, she maintains a full-time job outside the home. Lucy is glad she can help, but she wonders how many years it will be before she can take a vacation or spend a quiet day alone. Such thoughts make her feel sad and guilty.

Mario is pleased with life and himself. Things have not been easy, but he appreciates the pleasures of life like never before. Friends and loved ones are closer, and he is at peace with himself. He marvels that dying has brought about some of the best days of his life.

As these scenarios suggest, the majority of communication about health does not occur in a doctor's office or hospital. It occurs at home, at the grocery store, on the telephone, and in other settings of everyday life. Spouses, children, friends, and coworkers often have as much influence as doctors and nurses.

Social support includes a broad range of activities, from comforting a friend after a romantic disappointment, to listening while a grieving father tells and retells his story, to performing an internet data search, to acknowledging that an individual with physical or intellectual challenges is a normal person.

Most people perform more supportive behaviors than they realize and, as a consequence, have positive effects on people's health and moods. Research shows that supportive communication can help speed healing, reduce loneliness, reduce symptoms and stress, lessen pain, and build self-esteem (see, e.g., Chia, 2009; Segrin & Domschke, 2011; Thomtén, Soares, & Sundin, 2011). And the benefits go both ways. People who provide social support often feel an enhanced sense of well-being themselves (Robinson & Tian, 2009).

This chapter begins with a conceptual overview of coping and social support, including the role that communication plays as we demonstrate caring for others, strive for a sense of control, and negotiate uncertainties. We will talk about the benefits of social support, but also what happens when well-intentioned efforts hurt more than they help. Then we briefly explore the role of animal companions and the idea of health crises as transformative experiences before we examine social support in two contexts—family caregiving and end-of-life experiences.

Conceptual Overview

In the simplest sense, support involves people helping people. Melanie Barnes and Steve Duck (1994) define **social support** as "behaviors that, whether directly or indirectly, communicate to an individual that they are valued and cared for by others" (p. 176). Some theorists (e.g., Albrecht & Adelman, 1987) consider that the central function of social support is increasing a person's sense of control. Their viewpoint is substantiated by research (covered in this chapter) that people cope best when they feel well informed and actively involved. This section describes different coping mechanisms and the role social support plays in helping people through crisis situations.

Theoretical Perspectives

The **buffering hypothesis** holds that social support is most important when we encounter potentially stressful experiences, in which case knowing that other people are there for us can cushion (buffer) us from feeling overwhelmed or helpless (Cohen & Wills, 1985). For example, your ability to cope with bad news may be strengthened by the conviction that loved ones will stick by you no matter what, will be understanding listeners, will help with information and assistance, and so on. The buffering process is likely to be especially meaningful if the support offered matches the support you feel you need. One college student said that, when he tore the anterior cruciate ligament (ACL) in his knee on vacation, he was relatively calm about it because his girlfriend, a physical therapy assistant, was by his side, telling him what to expect in terms of pain, treatment, and recovery. He says her presence and knowledge made the experience feel "doable."

In another sense, social support is like money in the bank. It is nice to know it is there, even if we don't spend it. The **direct-effect** or **main-effect model** proposes that social support is beneficial even when we are not encountering notable stressors. A strong social network helps us feel valued every day and is a reassuring reminder that loved ones' support is always available (Barnes & Duck, 1994). Joann Reinhardt and colleagues (2006) found that adults age 65 and older who were experiencing vision loss were least likely to be depressed and most likely to adapt well to lifestyle changes if they perceived that they had strong emotional support. For them, actually receiving support was less important than knowing it was there if they needed it (Reinhardt, Boerner, & Horowitz, 2006).

Indeed, the main-effect model suggests that we may encounter fewer stressful episodes and enjoy greater overall health if we have strong social networks (Cohen & Wills, 1985). Older adults who are unsatisfied with the amount of emotional support they receive from friends and family members are twice as likely to rate their health only "fair" or "poor" as their peers who feel emotionally supported (White, Philogene, Fine, & Sinha, 2009). They may even live longer. In an Australian study of people 70 and older, those with the most active social networks (in the top third as compared to their peers) were 22% more likely to live another 10 years than those with the least active networks (Giles, Glonek, Luszcz, & Andrews, 2005). This is no surprise to older adults who have experienced the death of a spouse. They typically say that the best coping strategy is to keep busy and interact with others, and the worst coping strategy is to isolate oneself at home (Bergstrom & Holmes, 2000).

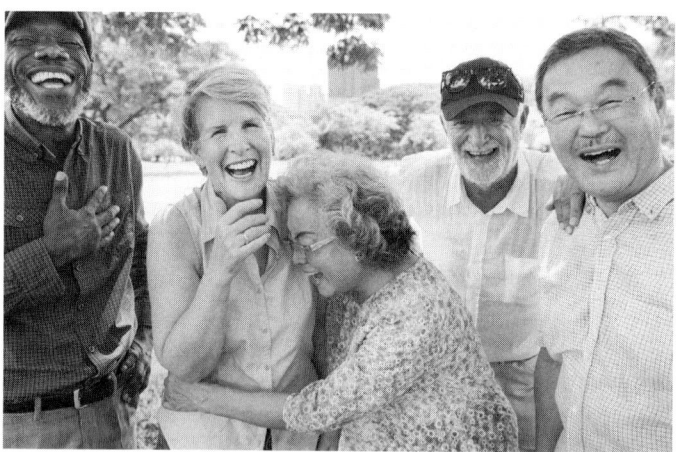

Evidence suggests that older adults with active social networks may outlive their less socially active peers by as many as 10 years.

Social support is important at every age. How would you rate the quality of your social support network on a scale of 1 to 10? How supportive are you of others?

There are several reasons for the link between social ties and good health. One is that we learn from others and develop confidence through interactions. Teens are most likely to negotiate safer-sex options with their partners (Troth & Peterson, 2000) and avoid eating disorders (Botta & Dumlao, 2002; Miller-Day & Marks, 2006) if they come from families that display a collaborative problem-solving orientation rather than a distant or conflict-avoidant orientation. Others' actions are informative guides to behavior, especially in intense and uncertain times. For example, when news that Patrick Swayze had pancreatic cancer broke at about the same time that health communication scholar Barbara Sharf learned that her childhood friend Rita had been diagnosed with the disease, Sharf says that Swayze's narrative became part of their experience as well. Sharf (2010) writes that she scanned newsstands for tidbits, enthralled by Swayze's resolve to keep working and his frank descriptions about both the tolerable and the "hellish" aspects of the disease. When she heard news of Swayze's death four months after Rita's, she says that the news brought fresh waves of grief.

Second, strong social ties are associated with physical benefits. Resting blood pressure and blood glucose levels are lower (healthier) among people who express a great deal of affection compared to those who do not (Floyd, Hesse, & Haynes, 2007), and shared humor tends to reduce tension, enhance mood, and boost immunity (Alston, 2007; Lockwood & Yoshimura, 2014; Wanzer, Sparks, & Frymier, 2009). In contrast, lonely individuals are more likely than others to sleep poorly, to feel stressed, and to have poor health (Hawkley, Masi, Berry, & Cacioppo, 2006; Segrin & Passalacqua, 2010).

Third, loved ones may support us in making healthy decisions. Teenagers are most likely to be effective when confronting their peers about alcohol abuse if both parties perceive that they are good friends and that the concern is legitimate (Malis & Roloff, 2007). Likewise, romantic partners with whom we share a high sense of intimacy are more likely than others to convince us to improve our diets and engage in other healthy behaviors (Dennis, 2006).

It's important to note that the quality of our relationships is more important than the quantity. Having a few close friends and loved ones is typically healthier than an active social life without much intimacy (Segrin & Passalacqua, 2010). And it matters why people support us. Friends' attention is flattering partly because it is freely given, whereas family members are more obliged. When individuals studied by Metts and Manns (1996) told loved ones they had HIV or AIDS, friends were typically more supportive than family, perhaps because the family members were more overwhelmed by their own emotions.

Friendship quality is especially important in later life. After age 70 or so, we are likely to put stock in a small number of very close friends and family members (Nussbaum, Baringer, Fisher, & Kundrat, 2008). These smaller, more intimate networks are well suited to situations in which we may have limited mobility, when close friends are likely to rely extensively on each other, and when changes in hearing and vision may impact our communication abilities (Nussbaum et al., 2008). (See Box 8.1 for more about the effects of communication impairments.)

In short, the buffering hypothesis and main-effects model suggest that social support is helpful both during major life events and the challenges of everyday life. For many reasons, in ways that change throughout our lives, having strong social ties is good for our health. Later in the chapter, we will discuss other theoretical perspectives, including dialectics and problematic integration theory. But to establish a basis for those, let us first shift to the more specific topic of coping.

BOX 8.1

When Communication Ability Is Compromised

Unfortunately, health concerns can interfere with social interaction and friendships, particularly when an individual's ability to communicate is affected. When researchers led by Jennifer Bute (2007) interviewed friends and loved ones of people with compromised communication abilities, they found that some of them continued to feel an easy and even improved camaraderie despite communication limits. But many experienced it as a profound loss, particularly if dementia was involved (Bute, Donovan-Kicken, & Martins, 2007). Said one woman in the study, "It is a different relationship. . . . I have lost the friend I used to have before" (p. 239).

What Do You Think?

1. Have you ever experienced difficulty communicating with someone because of a disability? If so, how did you handle the situation?
2. Has your ability to communicate ever been compromised, even temporarily? Did people respond to you differently? If so, how?
3. What would you do if a loved one could no longer communicate easily with you? Do you think it would change your relationship? If so, how?

Coping

To understand social support, it is useful to consider what it means to cope. As Sandra Metts and Heather Manns (1996) define it, **coping** is "the process of managing stressful situations" (p. 356) that range from everyday hassles to life-threatening occurrences.

Coping usually involves two efforts: changing what can be changed (**problem solving**) and adapting to what cannot be changed (**emotional adjustment**) (Tardy, 1994). Of course, it is not always easy to know when to solve a problem and when to adjust to it. The options vary according to the people and the circumstances involved. Often, coping strategies depend on how much control people believe they have over their situations.

Sometimes attaining a sense of control requires reevaluating ideas about one's body. Canadian researchers Jennifer English and colleagues (2008) interviewed women about the strategies they used to heal emotionally and physically from the effects of breast cancer. From the respondents' stories, the researchers conceptualized the body as a "therapeutic landscape." Often, they say, that term is used to describe places and physical environments such as spas, gardens, and nature that foster a sense of peace and well-being. In this case, English and colleagues applied the same idea to the body, regarding it as a place of illness but also of healing and recovery.

Breast cancer is particularly relevant to the landscape image, of course, because mastectomies represent a physical redefinition of the body-physical. Although the women interviewed were unaware of the landscape concept, their stories naturally illustrated it. For example, one woman described her body as a damaged object:

> It was feeling like I had been broken. . . . My body was cut up and I took all these chemical drugs and I was radiated, and you know what I mean. I just sort of in my mind felt like I was coming from a not very good physical place. (p. 71)

Another described the realization that radiation was permeating the very cells of her body. She felt the experience was simultaneously taking her into the depths of her unconscious. The women also spoke of the physical changes in their bodies—hair loss, weight gain, and their new awareness of the food, air, and other elements around them. In a therapeutic sense, they spoke about the healing properties of time spent with friends, exercising, and enjoying nature. Many of the women said that such pleasures were more intense because life had lost some of the taken-for-granted quality it used to have. The authors conclude:

> The body, being the smallest and most personal landscape, represents the embodiment of illness for women living with breast cancer. In other words, the body is both an everyday site of illness but also an everyday landscape of healing. (English, Wilson, & Keller-Olaman, 2008, p. 76)

In this way and many others, illness, coping, and healing occupy the same spaces in human experience.

Sense of Control

When people believe they can manage their health successfully, they are said to have **health self-efficacy** (Bandura, 1986). Efficacy is derived from the Latin term for "change-producing." People with high self-efficacy are more likely than others to maintain healthy lifestyles because they are confident in their ability to make changes that have positive consequences. A sense of self-efficacy may be fostered by positive experiences in the past, encouragement from others, and an **internal locus of control**, which is the belief that people control their own destinies. Locus of control is more general than health self-efficacy, although the two are often related. Many North Americans have an internal locus of control. As a result, they tend to be change oriented and hard-working, but they may be frustrated by failure and may feel baffled and betrayed when things do not work out as they had planned. People who believe they control their own fate may be reluctant to ask for help and may believe they are responsible for what happens—both good and bad. Faced with ill health, they might ask, "What did I do to cause this?" Even assured that no one is to blame, these people may feel guilty and ineffectual.

Sometimes making sense of a health event involves comparing it to something familiar. In a study of American and Puerto Rican male veterans recovering from strokes, many of the men compared having a stroke to a crash or a hurricane because it was unexpected and destructive (Boylstein, Rittman, & Hinojosa, 2007). However, the men typically chose a different metaphor—war—to describe their recovery. Like war, they said, recovery requires immense courage, determination, and active engagement. "I've always been a fighter," said one man (p. 284). Another said, "You quit, they're gonna win. Now where's the fight in you?" (p. 284). The researchers note that, in the men's stories, the "enemy" was typically a body part (an arm, a leg, or a hand) that no longer worked like it did before and that required diligent therapy and exercise. The men's explanations revealed that, although their strokes seemed to have come from out of the blue, they considered themselves active agents in getting well again.

In contrast, people who do not believe they can change their health for the better have low health self-efficacy. That's common in cultures in which people have an **external locus of control**: the belief that events are controlled mostly by outside forces. Because of their belief in fate, these people are sometimes characterized as **fatalistic**. They are likely to regard events as God's will or the natural order of things.

People with low health self-efficacy may not be motivated to take personal action regarding health matters. For example, even if they are aware of healthy dietary recommendations, they may not change their diets because they do not feel they have control over their health (Rimal, 2000). In fatalistic cultures, people may reason, "It makes no sense to change my lifestyle. I will die when it's my time, no sooner or later," or "I am sick because God willed it. Therefore, it's not right to seek a medical cure."

People with a fatalistic worldview are significantly more likely than others to feel that cancer is unpreventable and to avoid seeking information about the subject (Ramanadhan & Viswanath, 2006). And, as you might expect, adolescents with an external locus of control are more apt to "follow the crowd" and smoke if their friends do (Booth-Butterfield, Anderson, & Booth-Butterfield, 2000).

Our locus of control may also influence how we interpret other people's actions and health. For example, do people become overweight because of behavioral choices or because of factors beyond their control? As information surfaces about a genetic tendency toward obesity in some people, the public is likely to feel more sympathetic toward overweight people (Jeong, 2007). But at the same time, people may become more lax about health behaviors, concluding that obesity either is or is not their genetic destiny and there's not much they can do about it (Jeong, 2007).

As with most things, the extremes are typically dysfunctional. People at either end of the internal/external locus-of-control scale are likely to have trouble coping. One moderating effect, at least for fatalists, is a healthy dose of confidence. Some researchers have found that people are less likely to avoid threatening health messages if they are well informed and confident about prevention methods (Fry & Prentice-Dunn, 2005).

People with high self-efficacy are typically problem solvers, highly motivated to protect their own health. However, they may be at a loss when illness reduces their sense of control. In some situations, people are powerless to change their health status or to repay their caregivers' kindness. One man adapting to physical limitations after a stroke described his frustration this way: "It's hard to depend on other people to take you places. Because, you know, they have things they have to do, and they need to get done, and you don't want to interfere with their schedule" (Egbert, Koch, Coeling, & Ayers, 2006, p. 49). Forced dependence may be especially demoralizing for people who have always believed they can control their health. In these situations, a belief in fate may help people accept what they cannot change. All in all, effective coping seems to combine elements of both problem solving and acceptance.

Dialectics

Of course, no one perceives an entirely internal or external locus of control. We occupy a perspective somewhere between the two, and we may shift perspectives over time. This is an observation well explained by **dialectics**, which describes the ongoing tension of meaning between coexisting but contradictory constructs such as "hopeless" and "hopeful" (Baxter, 1988; Rawlins, 1989).

We continually navigate meaning within dialectic continua based on our circumstances, beliefs, and interactions with others. For example, family caregivers often describe ongoing efforts to balance the dialectic between attending to their own needs and sacrificing themselves to care for loved ones (Brann, Himes, Dillow, & Weber, 2010). In a similar way, hospice nurses say they strive for a balance between being honest with families and at least temporarily shielding them from information that would overwhelm them (Gilstrap & White, 2015).

People also manage the dialectic between being hopeful and realistic. Many people consider it adaptive to be optimistic, and it sometimes is. But the dialectic perspective challenges the notion that there is one right or static way to think. Instead, meaning is adaptive and changing. For example, a man caring for his wife following a stroke said that, after several years of determined optimism, they began to accept that she would never use her arm and leg again. As he put it, "We backed off . . . We're not expecting miracles anymore" (Brann et al., 2010, p. 327). That sense of acceptance can sometimes bring peace and can lead to more effective, realistic coping strategies.

Communication scholar Brittany Peterson (2019) describes the multiple levels of dialectical "push and pull" she experienced while her 2-year-old daughter received care in a pediatric intensive care unit (PICU) following major surgery. Peterson says she felt compelled to be with her daughter night and day. At the same time, the exhaustion and emotional distress of always being there diminished her effectiveness as a parent/caregiver. This situation reflects a common dilemma: Dialectical tensions can feel both diametrically opposed and mutually dependent (Baxter & Montgomery, 1996). "Either-or" decision making is typically inadequate to manage the dynamic complexities involved. At one point, a concerned doctor strongly urged Peterson to leave the hospital for a while to get some sleep, which she reluctantly did. She found that the brief absence enhanced her ability to cope and to care for her daughter. "After this event, my management of the dialectic changed," reflects Peterson. "I was more open to embracing the necessity of absence to be more authentically and completely present when I was in the PICU" (p. 3).

We cope with some degree of stress every day. But crises test our limits. Next we take a closer look at what's involved when that happens.

Crisis

At every crisis in one's life, it is absolute salvation to have some sympathetic friend to whom you can think aloud without restraint or misgiving. —Woodrow Wilson

A **crisis** is an occurrence that exceeds a person's normal coping ability. The first sign of crisis is usually a sense that events are out of control. This may

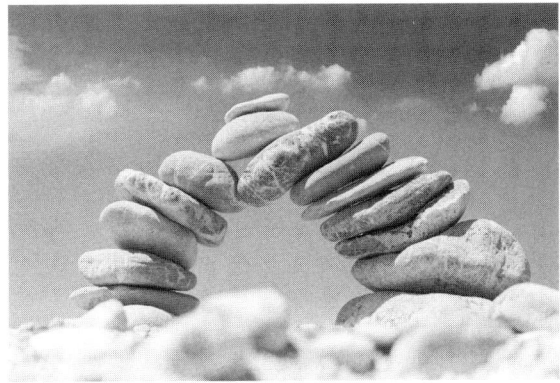

Based on the principles of dialectics, people continually navigate a place between interdependent opposites.

Can you identify examples in your own experience in which you have managed the dialectics between being hopeful and realistic, attending to self and sacrificing self, or expressing emotions and suppressing emotional displays?

give rise to panic or denial. For example, the parent of a seriously ill child remembers, "I didn't want to talk about it because it was something I wanted to shut in the back of my mind and have go away" (Chesler & Barbarin, 1984, p. 123).

People in crisis are likely to feel that things have changed, perhaps forever. During difficult times, people often yearn for the simple routines that characterized everyday life. It may seem that things will never be the same again. Following a death, for example, grieving loved ones may wonder how they will ever resume daily activities when they feel so sad and disconnected to the things that used to seem normal. It's common for people in intense grief to forget momentarily how to perform simple routines or drive familiar routes.

One of the most distressing aspects of a crisis can be the sense that one is helpless and not in control. Health professionals can help by actively involving patients in making decisions and expressing their preferences. Patients who feel that they can ask questions and be assertive tend to experience less anxiety and more optimism than those who feel that their input is not valued (Venetis, Robinson, & Kearney, 2015).

A major crisis may serve as a turning point or dividing line. People affected by serious illnesses often feel their life has two parts, before the diagnosis and after it (Tiedtke, de Rijk, Donceel, Christiaens, & Dierckx de Casterl, 2012). Circumstances are so radically altered that nothing seems the same. The change is not always negative. People who learn to cope with terminal illnesses or near-death experiences sometimes say they are happier than before, appreciating pleasures they used to disregard. A cancer survivor interviewed by Jennifer Anderson and Patricia Geist Martin (2003) reflects on the strength and courage she has discovered while undergoing surgery and radiation treatments:

> *I wear my scar as a badge of courage but I've never thought of myself as a courageous person. But I am, I am a courageous person. People notice the scar. But you know, I don't mind the scar. Years ago, I decided that I wanted to change my name, to pick out who I wanted to be. Ivy came to mind because I liked the plant. It's a vine, it is strong, you can cut it down and it comes back. There's a lot of strength in Ivy. (p. 138)*

We'll talk more about transformative health experiences later in the chapter.

Normalcy

A sense of crisis does not usually abate until it seems that life is normal again. **Normalcy** is essentially the sense that things are comfortable, predictable, and familiar. Being normal is not always as easy as it sounds. It requires the cooperation of other people, even strangers (Barnes & Duck, 1994). Consider the dilemma of individuals with physical disabilities. Often, their toughest challenge is not learning to use wheelchairs or other appliances. It is resuming a sense of life as usual. Without that, they are trapped in a crisis-like state, excluded from the comfortable give and take of everyday transactions with people (Braithwaite, 1996). Persons with disabilities may be inundated with people willing to help them but with very few who engage them in casual conversation or friendly debates over politics or sports. When people behave as if individuals with disabilities are unlike other people (even by being unusually kind or helpful toward them), they perpetuate a sense of crisis and alienation (Braithwaite, 1996).

A return to normal is not guaranteed, even when an illness is considered to be "in the past." "One of the hardest things about treatment is not knowing what happens next," says a spokesperson for the National Cancer Institute (NCI, 2019, para. 3). Even after good health is restored, a person's body, perspective on life, diet, routines, fears, and hopes may be different from before. "It's not so much 'getting back to normal' as it is finding out what's normal for you now," says the NCI representative, who suggests the following strategies for managing a "new normal":

- *It's okay to feel afraid.* Don't be dismayed if you feel alarmed about aches and pains you might have shrugged off prior to your illness.
- *Share your concerns with health providers.* They may provide information, monitoring, and reassurance.
- *Take care of yourself.* Commit to regular relaxation, exercise, a good diet, and healthy social interaction.
- *Focus on mental as well as physical health.* Counselors, therapists, loved ones, and people who have had similar health concerns may be able to help you process what you are feeling.

Establishing a "new normal" can be stressful, but it sometimes has benefits as well. Toni Bernhard, who copes with long-term chronic fatigue syndrome, says

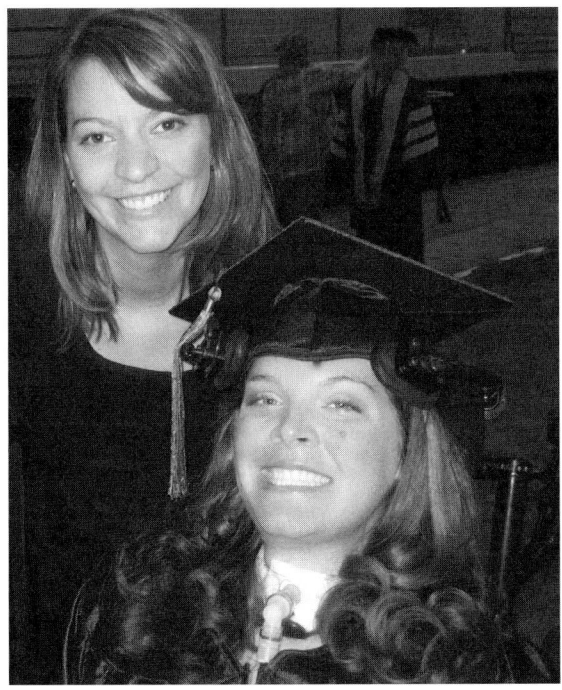

Following an automobile accident that left her paralyzed from the neck down, Samantha Rodzwicz was eager to return to college and her philanthropic efforts as soon as possible. During college, she helped to raise more than $40,000 to help others. Rodzwicz is shown here at her college graduation with her sister Veronica. She went on to earn a master's degree in communication.

Even less profound hardships can present obstacles. What have you had to overcome to be where you are today?

her illness is difficult to manage, but it has deepened her appreciation for the human body, friends, her dog, and the ability to take a walk (albeit a slow one) on good days (Bernhard, 2019).

We have talked about the value of social support and personal coping strategies. But how do the two intersect? Here are some of the communication strategies involved.

Coping and Communication

Coping strategies and social support often look very much alike in that they tend to fall into two main categories: **action-facilitating**, performing tasks and collecting information; and **nurturing**, building self-esteem, acknowledging and expressing emotions, and providing companionship (Cutrona & Suhr, 1994). Here is an overview of communication strategies based on these categories.

Action-Facilitating Support

Two types of action-facilitating support are performing tasks and favors and providing information. For instance, people might support someone trying to lose weight by sharing fitness information, buying healthy foods, and serving as exercise companions.

Tasks and favors are called **instrumental support** (Cutrona & Suhr, 1994). Instrumental support is usually most appreciated when care receivers feel they are active participants in the process and are involved in decision making (Forsythe et al., 2014). **Informational support** might involve performing an internet data search, sharing personal experiences, passing along news clips, and so on. In some cases, information can help people increase their understanding and make wise decisions. A cancer survivor in one study said she worries about every change in her body, so she appreciates her physicians' willingness to run tests to be sure nothing is wrong. "Otherwise, I'm going to sit here freaking out all the time," reflects the woman (Miller, 2014, p. 236).

Even when people cannot change their circumstances, those who are knowledgeable about what is happening usually feel more in control, experience less pain, and recover more quickly than others. Margo Charchuk describes the sense of hopelessness and impotence she felt as the mother of a seriously ill child (Connor) in a neonatal intensive care unit (NICU). "I felt that I was an outsider looking in with no voice in the care of my child," she writes (Charchuk & Simpson, 2005, p. 198). When she felt uninformed, she says she felt helpless and hopeless. Charchuk urges health providers to foster hope, even when the outcome is uncertain:

> *In my experience, health care providers can help parents to enjoy their child and find hope in the moment even if the child will not ultimately survive. . . . I hoped that he would live, but I also had hope that I was being a good mother and that I was doing all that I could to ensure his health and safety. When I was involved in his care, my hopes increased, as this enabled me to feel I was being a good parent. I did not lose hope when the information was bad; I only lost hope when I was given no information at all. (pp. 194–195)*

Charchuk describes a dilemma that many people feel in health care situations. She sensed that, if she showed emotion, health professionals would consider that she was incapable of hearing the hard truths and making important decisions, but if she did not show emotion, they might overlook her fervent concern and desire to know more. One of the most hope-enhancing events of Charchuk's account occurred when a NICU nurse invited her to rub the baby's back to soothe him. "The importance of this small amount of control that I was able to take helped restore my hope," she remembers (p. 199).

Although most people, like Charchuk, say it feels better to be well informed, sometimes too much information can feel overwhelming and compromise a person's coping ability (L. Miller, 2014). The theory of problematic integration (Box 8.2) describes how and why people manage ambiguous, contradictory, and complex information.

Nurturing Support

Nurturing typically involves three types of support: esteem support, emotional support, and social network support. These are not directly oriented to task goals but, rather, to helping people feel better about themselves and their situations.

Esteem support involves efforts to make another person feel valued and competent. Here's an example from a study by Maria Carpiac-Claver and Lené Levy-Storms (2007) in a long-term care facility:

> A nurse aide stands next to the resident after delivering her tray of food and says in a soft and moderately pitched voice, Hi [resident's name]. Okay. Want a spoon? *The resident, with laughter in her voice, says,* Thank you *and smiles broadly at the nurse aide. The nurse aide gives the resident a spoon and says,* Here you go. *The resident thanks the nurse aide while shaking her head and pulling the nurse aide down to give her a kiss on the cheek.* (p. 61)

The researchers observed other nurse aides laughing and singing with residents and helping those with cognitive impairments keep their memories active. Carpiac-Claver and Levy-Storms identified four themes of the nurse aides' affective communication: *personal conversation,* pleasantries and talk not directed to any particular task; *addressing the resident,* using the person's name or a term of endearment; *checking in,* asking and looking to see if the resident is feeling okay or needs anything; and *emotional support/praise,* as in saying, "You look beautiful today!" or "Congratulations!"

Encouraging words may ease feelings of helplessness and despair. People often report that unconditional approval is the most helpful form of support. Statements such as "We're behind you no matter what you decide" are comforting reminders that loved ones will not leave if the situation is difficult to handle. Listening is also important. Studies show that most distressed individuals are not looking for advice; they just want to talk and be heard (Lehman, Ellard, & Wortman, 1986). Following are some tips from the experts on listening well.

COMMUNICATION SKILL BUILDER: SUPPORTIVE LISTENING

Brant Burleson, a leading authority on social support, offered the following tips for being a supportive listener (based on Burleson, 1990, 1994).

- *Focus on the other person.* Give the person a chance to talk freely. Focus on what they are saying rather than on your own feelings and experiences.
- *Remain neutral.* Resist the urge to label people and experiences as good or bad. Likewise, encourage the speaker to describe experiences rather than label them.
- *Concentrate on feelings.* It's usually more supportive to explore why someone feels a certain way than to focus on events themselves.
- *Legitimize the other person's emotions.* Statements such as "I understand how you might feel that way" are typically more helpful than telling the other person how to feel or how not to feel.
- *Summarize what you hear.* Calmly summarizing the speaker's statements can help clarify the situation and help the distressed individual understand what they are feeling. As Burleson (1994) explained, "Due to the intensity and immediacy of their feelings, distressed persons may lack understanding of these feelings" (p. 13).

Emotional support includes efforts to acknowledge and understand what another person is feeling. This support is particularly valuable when people must adapt to what they cannot change. In a health

BOX 8.2

Theory of Problematic Integration

Imagine that you will go through life knowing with relative certainty what to expect and how to feel. Perhaps you will graduate, establish a rewarding career, stay healthy and fit until retirement, and enjoy your later years with the money you have wisely saved along the way. At least this is what you expect and what you hope will happen.

The **theory of problematic integration** is based on the idea that we orient to life in terms of *expectations* (what we think will probably happen) and *evaluations* (whether occurrences are good or bad) (Babrow, 2001). However, our expectations and values are challenged almost constantly in large and small ways. (Although this sounds regrettable, the challenges are actually opportunities for greater development, a point to be discussed presently.)

As defined by Austin Babrow and colleagues, the theory of problematic integration describes a process in which communication serves to establish a relatively stable orientation to the world but also to challenge and transform that orientation (Babrow, 1992; Brashers & Babrow, 1996; Ford, Babrow, & Stohl, 1996; Russell & Babrow, 2011). *Problematic integration* (PI) occurs when expectations and evaluations are at odds, uncertain, changing, or impossible to fulfill. The disruption may be relatively minor (perhaps a setback that delays graduation) or major (someone close to you is diagnosed with a life-changing illness). Whatever the case, communication will play a pivotal role at every stage of your experience. As Babrow (2001) puts it:

> Communication shapes conceptions of our world—both its composition and meaning, particularly its values. [Problematic integration theory] also suggests that communication shapes and reflects problematic formulations of these conceptions and orientations to experience. (p. 556)

In recognizing that communication helps to define, challenge, and transform our experiences, Babrow (2001) makes the point that uncertainty is not inherently bad or good, and we are not always able to extinguish uncertainty by dousing it with information. Sometimes uncertainty exists because we have too little or too much information or because we are not sure what to make of the information presented to us.

We make sense of the world partly through the stories we tell and partly through our efforts to achieve coherence between our narratives and other accounts, or what Russell and Babrow (2011) call "preexisting narrative frames," such as media depictions of environmental hazards and terrorism. As we both construct and confront narrative themes, we assess risk by selectively evaluating, bracketing, integrating, and comparing information from many sources within what philosophers call the blooming, buzzing confusion of experience (Russell & Babrow, 2011).

Uncertainty and ambivalence may also be inherent in the information we receive about our health and threats to it. Scientific findings change, and every promise of relief is accompanied by some degree of risk and side effects (Gill & Babrow, 2007; Russell & Babrow, 2011). Furthermore, resolving one uncertainty may produce others. Babrow writes that "PI permeates human experience" (p. 564), although it is difficult to predict when and how uncertainties will arise. Going back to Babrow's first point, the notion of uncertainty is not necessarily undesirable. Indeed, he suggests that uncertainty presents an "opportunity for self-exploration" (p. 563).

Consider the example of advance-care planning provided by Stephen Hines (2001). Medical professionals have typically been disappointed by patients' disinclination to specify what care they wish to have (or forgo) should they become too ill to express their wishes. Hines observes that people may shy away from the issue because health care professionals, in their desire to reduce their own uncertainty in end-of-life situations, have not been very sensitive to the uncertainties experienced by prospective patients and their loved ones. In short, people may neglect to file advance-care directives, not because they are indifferent or stubborn, but because the uncertainty surrounding them feels unmanageable.

This brief review does not encompass all the facets of problematic integration theory, but hopefully it illustrates something about the ways people constitute, challenge, and transform their understandings, particularly in health-related crises.

crisis it's common to feel angry, baffled, afraid, depressed, or even unexpectedly relieved or giddy.

Emotions are a natural part of coping with health crises, yet many people are uncomfortable with emotional displays—theirs or others people's. They may be afraid to appear weak or may be reluctant to upset others. The result is that people tend to present the appearance that things are going well, even when they are not. In interviews with grieving parents, fathers were more likely than mothers to use work as a distractive coping mechanism, whereas the women were more likely than the men to talk about their feelings and stay close to family members. Partly as a result, the women reported feeling more in control of their grieving process than the men did six months after the loss of a child (Alam, Barrera, D'Agostino, Nicholas, & Schneiderman, 2012). Although it was probably not obvious to others, the men no doubt needed support as much as their wives did.

Problems may arise when people find themselves feigning a cheerfulness they do not feel or avoiding subjects they actually wish to discuss. Suppressing emotions commonly leads to depression, especially among men (Flynn, Hollenstein, & Mackey, 2010). When asked, people (patients, care providers, and others) often say they avoid sensitive topics because they don't want to distress the people around them (Bevan, Rogers, Andrews, & Sparks, 2012). However, when interviewed individually, people usually express the private wish that subjects such as death be brought into the open. In the long run, it's usually easier to cope when emotions can be expressed and discussed without trepidation. Following are some tips for accomplishing this.

COMMUNICATION SKILL BUILDER: ALLOWING EMOTIONAL EXPRESSION

- *Look for "affective moments."* Physician Frederic Platt (1995) encourages care providers to stay tuned for signs of strong feelings such as anger, sadness, fear, and helplessness. These are opportunities to understand something important about the other person and their coping status, he says.

- *When necessary, give yourself a moment.* Emotions often flood out other thoughts, making it difficult to respond effectively. A helpful strategy is to say, "Let me stop and think about what you've been telling me for a moment" (Platt, 1995, p. 25).

- *Keep in mind that people usually benefit from opportunities to talk openly and honestly.* For example, people with advanced cancer who feel they can talk about subjects like death and pain with their loved ones typically cope better than people who consider those topics taboo (Thomsen, Rydahl-Hansen, & Wagner, 2010).

- *People in grief often find it insensitive and unhelpful when others try to minimize their losses or get them to cheer up.* One cancer survivor put it this way: "The emotions went up and down, up and down. I talked to Jack and he listened. There was a point where Jack's optimism got to me. It was like stop, you're not listening to me. I could die, stop" (Anderson & Geist-Martin, 2003, p. 137).

- *Acknowledge and respect emotions.* Branch, Levinson, and Platt (1996, para. 15) suggest the following communication tools for responding

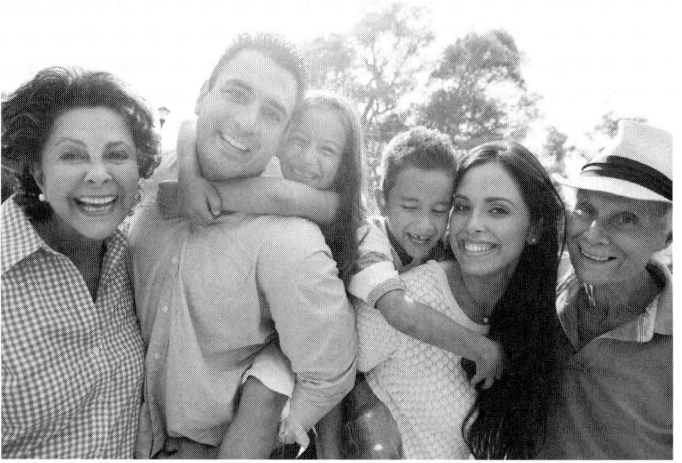

A paradox puzzles researchers: Hispanic Americans are more likely than average to suffer from unfair discrimination, low incomes, poor living conditions, and limited education—factors that typically contribute to poor health. However, they tend to live several years longer than Black and non-Hispanic White Americans. Some researchers feel that a cultural emphasis on family relationships and close-knit communities partly accounts for Hispanic Americans' comparatively good health and longer lives.

In what ways might having a strong family network improve a person's coping ability and overall health?

to emotions: (1) Acknowledge the emotion ("I can understand how upsetting it must be"); (2) show respect ("You've been doing your best to cope"); (3) reflect ("It sounds as though you are really feeling overwhelmed"); and (4) support and partner ("Maybe we can work together on these things.")

All in all, it's important to remember that emotions are a natural part of the coping process and that the person who displays strong and even conflicting emotions may be coping more effectively than the one who keeps a stiff upper lip.

SOCIAL NETWORKS

Common sources of social-network support include family members, friends, professionals, support groups, virtual communities, and self-help literature. Each source is likely to provide a somewhat different form of assistance. Since we have said a good deal already about the value of social networks, we will focus here on support groups.

Support groups are made up of people with similar concerns who meet regularly to discuss their feelings and experiences. They range from informal self-help groups to treatment groups facilitated by trained professionals and from groups that meet in person to virtual groups conducted entirely online.

In their various forms, support groups are popular around the world. More than 24,000 Al-Anon/Alateen group meetings are conducted in 30 languages in 130 countries (Al-Anon.org). There are also support groups for people dealing with grief, codependence, an enormous variety of illnesses and addictions, and other concerns. The effort may be justified. Support group members tend to experience fewer symptoms and less stress, and they may even live longer than similar people who are not members ("Living With Cancer," 1997; Wright, 2002).

Support groups have several advantages. Communicating with similar others may help people feel that they are not alone or abnormal. People going through similar experiences can also give firsthand information on what to expect and how to behave. At the same time, support group members may feel better about themselves because they are able to both express empathy with others and receive empathic messages themselves (Han et al., 2011). Another advantage of support groups is their convenience and low cost. Because they are made up mostly of laypersons, there are few or no fees, and for the most part, members can schedule meetings where and when they wish, even online. One plus of online support groups is the option to interact with people on a weak-tie basis—that is, to engage in relationships that do not require a great of time or emotional investment (Han, Hou, Kim, & Gustafson, 2014). Members of computer-mediated support communities often perceive that they feel less afraid of being judged online, and the information gleaned from others often seems more objective than what loved ones might provide (Wright & Rains, 2014).

The greatest dangers are that support groups will become counterproductive gripe sessions or that members will develop an us-versus-them viewpoint. They may begin to feel that no one outside the group understands them as well as they understand each other, a form of oversupport we will discuss next.

When Social Support Goes Wrong

Lucinda has seemed depressed for weeks. Some of her friends are attentive and sympathetic, but others are frustrated because they think Lucinda is not trying very hard to improve her outlook and is exaggerating her distress to get attention.

Interpretations such as these are personal and cultural. When people in one study were asked to consider a hypothetical case in which a person close to them was depressed, Hispanic respondents were likely to be sympathetic if they felt the person was helpless and trying to get attention, whereas other respondents more often reacted negatively to the idea that a person might play up her symptoms to gain the spotlight (Siegel et al., 2012).

Although it's often difficult to know when social support will be helpful and when it might make a problem worse, following are some scenarios in which ineffective social support seems to hurt more than it helps.

Friends Disappear

When Suleika Jaouad was diagnosed with leukemia at age 22, everything in her life changed. She was forced to give up her new job in Paris and return to the United States to

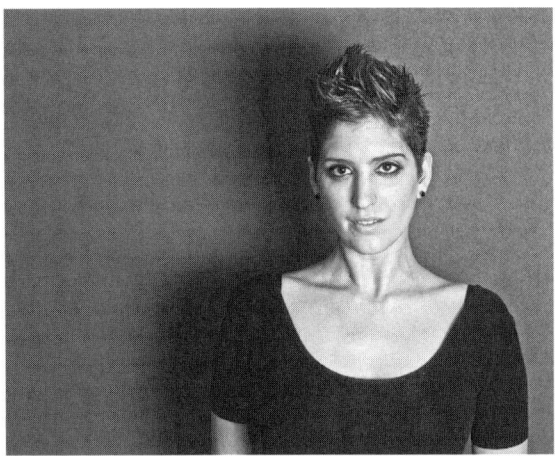

When Suleika Jaouad was diagnosed with leukemia at age 22, she says that many of her friends were at a loss for what to say or do around her. (Photo by Ashley Woo)

Have you ever felt at a loss when trying to comfort someone? If so, what did you do? What happened? Have you ever felt that people abandoned you when you needed social support?

> move back in with her parents, spend months in the hospital, and cope with treatments that were painful and frightening and that will make it difficult for her to conceive children in the future.

Amidst all of this, Jaouad says, she was shocked that many of her friends suddenly disappeared from her life. She explains:

> I think another aspect of being a young adult with cancer is that most of your friends, hopefully, you know, have never had to experience life-threatening illnesses themselves. . . . So a lot of my friends had no idea how to respond and found it really difficult not just to find the right words, but sometimes to find any words at all. ("Life Interrupted," 2012, para. 1)

Hurtful Jests

Here's another example, shared by Sherianne Shuler, who learned a great deal about effective and ineffective social support efforts when her 15-month-old daughter Lily was hospitalized with a rare, life-threatening infection. For example, an acquaintance who visited her in the hospital joked insensitively: "Nice hair, Shuler! . . . That's what you've got to love about Sheri Shuler, you don't care about things like that! If it were me, I'd be worried about my hair. But you just don't care!" Hurt, Shuler replied, "I think if you had a daughter in a coma and on a ventilator you wouldn't care." Inwardly, she says, she was silently screaming, "SHE'S SERIOUSLY STILL TALKING ABOUT HOW SHITTY I LOOK?" (Shuler, 2011, p. 200). The comments made her self-conscious at a time when she already felt vulnerable and overwhelmed.

Shuler also remembers feeling overwhelmed by the number of phone calls and emails she received and grateful that she could post information on a blog, since the process was therapeutic and took less energy than talking to everyone separately. Phone messages with offers such as "Call if you need . . ." were also

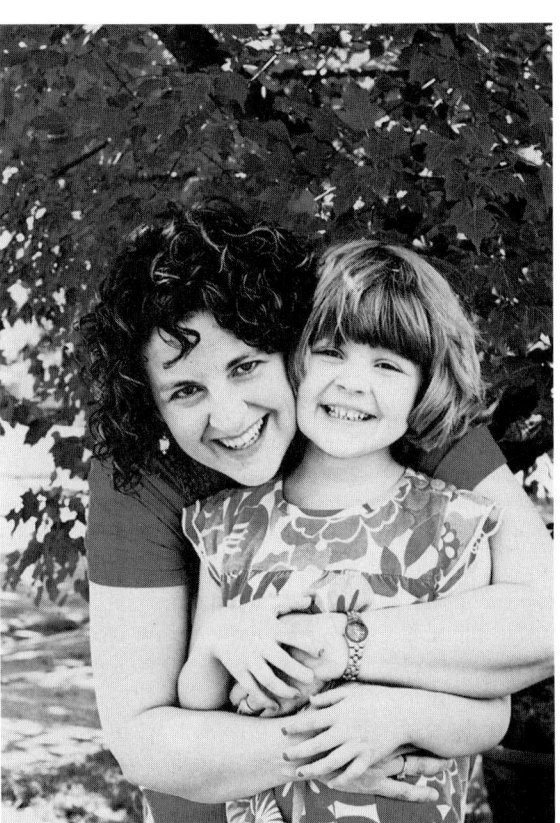

Sheri Shuler enjoys time with daughter Lily, shown here at age 6. A health scare when Lily was a toddler taught her a great deal about social support efforts that are helpful and those that are not.

Based on the experiences described in this section, what are some things a person might do to support a friend going through a difficult time? What things should they avoid doing?

unhelpful. Although people meant well, the energy and temerity it took to make such requests during a difficult time were prohibitive. Shuler observes, "As we learned, there are plenty of ways to offer well-meaning but ineffective support" (p. 199).

On the other hand, Shuler says it was immensely comforting when friends sent cards, letters, snacks, and healthy meals without being asked and without expecting anything in return. And she was grateful for people who took turns being present with her in the hospital waiting room without expecting her to talk or play hostess. Says Shuler, "I was floored by this thoughtful support my friends were providing. It was the gift of space and company simultaneously" (p. 199). Fortunately, Lily made a full recovery.

Too Much Support

Especially if "supportive" efforts are offered inappropriately or profusely, they can impair people's coping abilities. **Oversupport** is defined as excessive and unnecessary help (Edwards & Noller, 1998). Following is a discussion of three types of oversupport: overhelping, overinforming, and overempathizing.

Overhelping is providing too much instrumental assistance. This can make people feel like children or shield them from life experiences. People who are overhelped may perceive a loss of control, especially if others take on tasks for them without their consent (Morgan & Brazda, 2013).

Forcing information on people when they are too distraught to understand it or accept it (**overinforming**) may only heighten their stress. Philip Muskin (1998) calls this "truth dumping" and warns people against it. Health-related information can be confusing and frightening. Facts change and outlooks vary. People may shy away from the truth, preferring to preserve hope or minimize their confusion.

Overempathizing is actually something of a misnomer, because it applies only to a particular type of empathy, called *emotional contagion*. In a general sense, **empathy** is the ability to show that you understand how someone else is feeling. Katherine Miller et al. (1995) identified two components of empathy: **empathic concern**, which is an intellectual appreciation of someone's feelings; and **emotional contagion**, which involves actually feeling emotions similar to the other person's. Research shows that the second kind, emotional contagion, can be overdone.

Taken to extremes, emotional contagion can be detrimental to both support providers and recipients. For example, support group members sometimes empathize so much with each other that they distance themselves from others (Vilhauer, 2011). Another danger is that people may hesitate to express themselves to listeners who are likely to become upset. In Eric Zook's (1993) case study, a man who cared for his dying partner at home remembers, "As long as I was kind of detached and logical about it, he would take it [his declining health] very well" (p. 117).

Finally, some people find emotional empathy overwhelming or belittling. They may avoid scenes in which others seem to pity them. Wayne Beach (2002) describes the "stoic orientation" adopted by a father and son discussing the news that the mother was diagnosed with cancer. The son received the news calmly. Rather than reacting emotionally, he initially responded with a series of "OKs" and technical questions such as, "That's the one above her kidney?" (p. 279). Beach speculates that this factual, stoic orientation saved the father and son from immediately "flooding out." In this way, they were able both to maintain composure and to display that they were knowledgeable and capable of coping with the news.

A Note of Encouragement

Before you become too self-conscious about offering social support, consider that, although some of these examples were hurtful, the lessons behind them are fairly simple.

- *Don't overwhelm a distressed individual with requests for information*. If it's important for people to stay informed, appoint one person to convey news to them.
- *Be careful with humor, and avoid making jokes at others' expense*. People may not feel like laughing during a tense situation, and joking put-downs can be devastating when people are already feeling vulnerable.
- *"Call me if you need me" is usually not helpful*. It puts the onus for action on the distressed individual at a time when they are probably not up to the effort.
- *It's okay if you do not know what to say*. Just say something gentle or be available to listen.
- *Take a no-strings-attached approach*. When uncertain what to do, provide a quiet favor such as mowing the lawn, leaving a casserole, or simply being present without requiring anything from the distressed individual.

Here's a follow-up to the story about Suleika Jaouad, who was initially hurt by her friends' silence. Jaouad says their dilemma began to dawn on her when she remembered how she felt, just a few years before, when a friend phoned her to say that he had testicular cancer. She says:

> I remembered feeling so afraid when he called me and shared his diagnosis with me. And following that phone call, I, you know, I sat down and tried to compose an email, and I just didn't feel like I had the right words. I couldn't find the perfect words, so I said nothing. And I wasn't there for him at all during his cancer treatment. And I tried to remember that, and it's helped me forgive and understand the reactions of certain friends in my life and to realize that generally it's not that people don't care. It's that they're afraid or that they don't know what to say. (para. 3)

Jaouad's advice to people who want to offer comfort but aren't sure what to say is to forget about finding "the perfect words" and just say something. For her part, she says a highlight of her year was apologizing to the friend she had been unable to comfort several years before. "He understood, and he said, 'I know that you understand now,'" she says (para. 4).

On that note, we turn to a form of love and comfort that communicates a great deal but requires no words at all.

Animal Companions

> At Sunrise Hospital in Las Vegas, Nevada, care sometimes comes with four legs and floppy ears. About 12 dogs visit the hospital every few days through Pet Partners, a nonprofit organization that provides training and coordination for more than 10,000 carefully trained animal–volunteer teams throughout the world. The animals serve as therapeutic companions to people with health concerns.

Pet Partners leaders say the animals (mostly dogs and cats, but also a few horses) provide stress relief, a break from boredom, inspiration, and health benefits. The furry friends have been known to inspire people to keep up difficult physical therapy routines and to distract and calm children undergoing medical procedures. The staff at Sunrise Hospital reports that the animals are some patients' only visitors and they are a fun pick-me-up for people who choose to take part. "Often time, you'll see a patient who is really down in the dumps, and the dogs will show up in the room and their eyes light up," says Tracy Netherton, the hospital's volunteer coordinator (quoted by DeLucia, 2011, para. 4).

Animal companions often have positive effects on people's anxiety levels (Barker & Dawson, 1998), blood pressure (Allen, Blascovich, & Mendes, 2002), recovery time (Allen et al., 2002), and survival rates after heart attacks (Friedmann & Thomas, 1995); and trained dogs can even help with the diagnosis and treatment of conditions such as diabetes, cancer, and epilepsy (Wells, 2009).

Oncologist Edward Creagan of Mayo Clinic is a believer. He includes the names of people's pets in their medical history notes. In his experience, pets can be people's reason for living, and talking about pets is often calming for staff members as well as patients. Creagan attests, "None of us can speak about their pets without smiling" (Pet Partners video, n.d.).

We turn now to a type of experience that may occur when you least expect it and may have profound consequences for coping.

Transformative Experiences

Carol Bishop Mills remembers the day her daughter Maren was born:

> Dr. Jacobs, the NICU doctor, approached my bed about 15 minutes later and handed me a gorgeous baby girl. He was very pleasant and smiled when he told us all about her. "Mr. and Mrs. Mills, your daughter is quite healthy. She seems to have a strong heart, and her kidneys will be fine. There was some fluid pooled, but it will eliminate itself naturally. Her APGAR scores [used to measure a newborn's health] were 8 and 9 [out of a possible 10]. She's a beautiful little girl. There are some preliminary indicators in her features that she might have trisomy 21, Down syndrome, but we need to run some blood work to confirm that." (Mills, 2005, p. 198)

The Mills were not surprised. They suspected that their baby might have special needs. But they *were* deeply grateful—grateful that the doctor had not said "I'm sorry" or labeled their daughter "abnormal." Instead he saw, as they did, a unique, perfect little girl in radiant good health with a condition not all children have.

Good health is often defined in terms of what is "normal" or "expected." A deviation from that can feel like a tragedy—meaningless and unfair. In reality, however, what looks on the surface like a "bad outcome" can turn out to be one of life's most valuable and important gifts. Mills (2005) attests that, although no one hopes to have a child with Down syndrome, "it is simply a gift we were given that we would have never known to ask for and probably would never have understood before our Little Miss Magic captivated our hearts" (p. 196).

In this section we explore instances in which, in the midst of what might seem to be great hardship, people discover unexpected rewards. From the perspective of social constructivism (e.g., Berger & Luckmann, 1966), life is defined largely by a quest for meaning that is shaped both by our experiences and our interactions with others. To illustrate the powerful effect of social interaction, let's return to Mills's (2005) case study, but this time look through the eyes of Kate, another mother, who has just given birth to Joshua:

We heard a cry, we saw our boy, and then heard the following from Dr. Lee, "I am so sorry to tell you this. This baby looks like a Down's. I'm so sorry. . . . In 20 years, I've never delivered a Down's. Didn't you have tests? . . . I'm sure it's a Down's. I am so, so sorry." (quoted by Mills, p. 199)

As you might imagine, Kate's experience was much different from the Mills's. "In my heart, I knew the Down syndrome was my fault, and it was clear the doctor was angry," Kate remembers thinking. "I didn't have a boy, in my mind, I had an 'it,' a Down's, one of those short, funny, retarded kids that work at grocery stores. My mind flooded with thoughts of drooling, retardation, the little yellow buses, the teasing, and the problems" (quoted by Mills, p. 199).

Mills (2005) reports that Kate and her husband Chris have come to realize that Down syndrome is only one feature—a relatively insignificant one—in the myriad qualities that make their son Joshua wonderful. But they have often had to overcome health professionals' hurtful comments in the process. Considering what people may learn from her experiences, Mills says, "I really hope that students realize that, often, it is not the diagnosis that is so scary, but the language we use to talk about it . . . is so embedded in cultural disdain that [it] taints our view."

We may all sometimes fall into the hurtful trap of believing, as Kate and Chris's doctor did, that there is a norm—a normal way to look, a normal life span, a normal reaction, and so on—and that what is "normal" is the "good" or "right" way to be. Most people who experience a crisis initially feel the same way, wondering: *Is this my fault? What did I do to deserve this? Why did this happen? Can I make it okay again?* In short, if the norm is "right," a deviation means something has gone wrong. This is a common assumption because the unknown is often frightening and because, as humans, we are continually involved in sense-making, and an unexpected occurrence can rob us of our sense of safety and meaning. For this reason, it's especially important to learn about diverse ways of being (in other words, shrink our distrust of the unknown) and to remind ourselves continually that, although it takes courage to embrace them, some of life's most enriching gifts lie beyond the status quo.

You might be surprised how frequently people who have been part of health crises (even to the extent of learning that they do not have long to live) ultimately consider themselves grateful for the experience. du Pré and Berlin Ray (2008) examined such episodes in a study of **transcendent experiences**, which they define as episodes in which people come to perceive an overarching meaning, or supra-meaning, within experiences that might otherwise seem senseless or unthinkable (p. 103). The term *supra-meaning* comes from psychologist Victor Frankl's (1959) reflections about life in a Nazi concentration camp during World War II. In the midst of suffering more horrific than most of us can imagine, Frankl observed that some of his fellow prisoners still found a reason to value life and to be optimistic about the future, largely because they perceived a meaning in life that was not bounded by the barbed-wire fences that kept them physically captive. Frankl came to believe that a quest for meaning is the primary motivation of human nature. From his perspective, write du Pré and Ray, "transcendence is not denial of one's circumstances, but an awareness that those circumstances exist within the framework of something more meaningful than one might previously have imagined" (p. 103).

In a similar way, people who don't have long to live sometimes say life takes on a new, larger meaning that makes everyday concerns seem trivial. As one cancer survivor put it:

> I am no longer concerned that someone might see me in the same outfit and I no longer have to have the same sweater in every color. I can now not finish a book if I don't like it. Every day is a guessing game. But that's okay. I'm still here to talk about it. (Brett, 2003, p. B1).

Others say they have been able to lay old grievances to rest and have developed a heightened appreciation for nature and loved ones. Many people facing life-altering circumstances say they have found larger meaning in a spiritual quest that involves helping others, dedicating themselves to causes larger than themselves, allowing themselves to be creative and have fun, and seeking to live up to their full awareness and potential (Egbert, Sparks, Kreps, & du Pré, 2008). Some people say the loss of a loved one was partly relieved by the knowledge that their organs helped save lives. (See Box 8.3 for more on this topic.)

This is not an easy or guaranteed process. Transcendence often happens when people least expect it. Being aware that what appears tragic on the surface may eventually yield something beautiful is a good start toward coping when things seem their darkest.

We turn next to two contexts with powerful implications for social support and coping: family caregiving and end of life.

Friends and Family as Caregivers

Carol Green rushes into the caregiver support group with her hair partly in curlers, her sweater buttoned crookedly, a smudge on her face, two different shoes, and a panicked look on her face. "I can't find my keys! We have an appointment, we're late, and I CAN'T FIND MY KEYS!" she exclaims, wildly tossing items from her overflowing handbag.

BOX 8.3

Organ Donations: The Nicholas Effect

Recently I strolled through a park in Rome with Andrea Mongiardo, a 23-year-old Italian whose heart once belonged to my own son.

With this comment, Reg Green (2003) introduces the Nicholas Green Foundation website, named in honor of 7-year-old Nicholas, who was killed near Naples by robbers who mistook the Greens' car for their own and fired into the vehicle. Even in their shock and grief over the sudden attack, Reg Green recalls, he and his wife agreed that Nicholas's organs should be donated to others. The family has since befriended the seven people whose lives were changed as a result. Reg Green remembers when he and his wife met these organ recipients for the first time:

> *Our grief was still agonizingly raw. But that meeting, which both of us had to steel ourselves to attend, was explosive. A door opened and in came this mass of humanity, some smiling, some tearful, some ebullient, some bashful, a stunning demonstration of the momentous consequences every donation can have. We now think of them as an extended family. We've watched the children grow and leave school and get their driver's licenses and the adults go back to work. One of them, 19-year-old Maria Pia Pedala, in a coma with liver failure on the day Nicholas died, bounced back to good health, married and has since had a baby boy. And, yes, they have called him Nicholas. (para. 11)*

Reg Green's (1999) book *The Nicholas Effect: A Boy's Gift to the World* and a video of the same title tell the family's story.

In the United States, an average of 20 people a day die waiting for organ transplants (American Transplant Foundation, 2019). The waiting list is more than 100,000 people long, and the greatest need is for kidneys (accounting for 76% of all transplants).

continued

The issue of organ donation is an emotional one. Based on sensationalized accounts on TV and in the movies, people may fear that medical professionals will allow them to die so they can have their organs, or that their organs will be sold on the underground market (Frates, Bohrer, & Thomas, 2006; Morgan, Harrison, Afifi, Long, & Stephenson, 2008).

In reality, the physicians who care for a patient are not involved in decisions about their organ donation. Those are handled by an entirely different staff and medical team. Moreover, strict U.S. laws prohibit the sale or purchase of organs as well as bribery for desired organs ("Organ Donation," 2008, para. 3). Another common myth is that organ donation will mar a deceased person's appearance such that the family cannot have an open casket at the funeral. That's not true. Doctors are able to maintain the person's appearance so that people cannot tell the difference ("Organ Donation," 2008).

What Do You Think?

1. What factors make you more (or less) inclined to register as an organ donor?
2. What is most frightening about the prospect? What is most appealing?
3. Unlike the Greens, who live in Italy, people in the United States are not usually given the opportunity to meet the people who receive a loved one's organs. Would you want to meet them? Why or why not?
4. Have you seen TV programs or movies in which people's organs are misused? Were the depictions realistic, in your opinion? Do you think such depictions affect people's attitudes about organ donation?

"The audience roars," Green says. "They recognize the situation. They are family caregivers." The scenario is a skit, but it is only partly satirical. The sense of being in disarray, trying to manage constantly changing situations involving medications, appointments, finances, companionship, insurance claims, bathing, dressing, food preparation, transportation, emotional support, organizing and apprising others, and so on, is real, she says.

Green facilitates a family caregiver support group through her local Council on Aging. At similar group meetings around the country, anyone interested may learn skills, share concerns, socialize, and take a breather from the everyday demands of family caregiving.

"At meetings, after we cover the essential information, I always say to people, 'If this is your only chance to get out this week, go now! Catch a movie, read a book, take some time for yourself,'" Green says. "Sometimes we need that permission to get away for a little while. My dream is I want to give something back to these people who give so much."

Green draws upon her years as a nurse and her personal experience caring for a parent who has dementia. The need for integrated support is rising along with the need for family caregivers. Reasons for the increase are manifold. For one, the number of people age 65 and older is expected to triple worldwide between 2009 and 2050, at which point about 1 in 5 Americans will be 65 or older (respectively, U.S. Census Bureau, 2009; Ortman, Velkoff, & Hogan,

The average family caregiver in the United States is a 49-year-old woman. To be a better caregiver, she has probably cut back on hours at work and has seen her income and savings decrease as a result. The challenges are immense, but most family caregivers say the process is rewarding as well.

If you have ever cared for a loved one in need, even temporarily, what were the rewards? The challenges? What role did communication play in the experience?

2014). Another factor is that hospital stays are shorter than they used to be. As Donna Laframboise (1998) put it, "Good news! You can go home from the hospital tomorrow. Bad news! You'll have to do everything yourself, even though you're still on crutches or full of stitches" (p. 26).

About 40 million people in the United States provide at-home care for a loved one (Stepler, 2015). The average age of family caregivers is 49, and about three-fourths of them are women (Family Caregiver Alliance, 2019).

As we review the rewards and challenges of family caregiving, keep in mind that loved ones are an important source of social support, but they also need support themselves. While the rewards of caregiving can be immensely gratifying, family caregivers experience grief, uncertainty, and exhaustion as well, and their needs are frequently overlooked in concern over the ill individuals. This section focuses on people who provide ongoing care for loved ones at home. Before we begin, note that although we often speak in terms of *family caregivers*—and the vast majority (86%) are indeed family members—the rest are actually honorary family members, friends and neighbors who pitch in as well ("Caregiving in the U.S.," 2009).

Stress and Burnout

Caregiving is no simple task. By some estimates, adults today will spend more time caring for their parents than they will raising their own children. In addition to providing medical care and assistance, family caregivers are frequently responsible for maintaining households and budgets, working at careers outside the home, and providing information and support to others.

Legislation passed in the 1990s helps career people provide care for needy family members. The **Family and Medical Leave Act of 1993** guarantees that employees can take up to 12 weeks off work to care for ailing family members, seek medical care themselves, or bring new children into their families (through birth, adoption, or foster parenting). However, the act does not require that employers pay workers while they are on leave, and it doesn't apply to all companies or all employees. To be eligible, employees must have worked at the company at least one year for an average of 25 hours or more per week. Only companies with at least 50 employees are obligated to provide medical and family leave.

Although most people juggling careers and caregiving say they feel good about what they do overall, it is easy to feel stressed, exhausted, and resentful at times. Said a woman caring for her 94-year-old grandmother, "It is hard to get out and just get my hair done or go to a doctor's appointment for myself, so I go without. But I feel so guilty if I ask for help" (Potter, n.d., para. 2).

Part of the strain is emotional. Caregivers may grieve over future plans that no longer seem possible. A 76-year-old woman caring for her ailing husband lamented, "This isn't how we planned to spend our retirement years. . . . Why did this happen to us?" (quoted by Ruppert, 1996, p. 40).

It is also painful to see a loved one suffer or change. The progression of Alzheimer's disease is particularly heart wrenching. Caregivers may grieve as the individual's personality and awareness gradually change. Sometimes Alzheimer's patients become belligerent or unable to recognize the people around them (see Box 8.4). To make matters worse, caregivers may feel guilty about their own frustration and resentment. It may seem wrong to be angry with a person who is ill and needy.

Family caregivers may also feel unprepared to perform the tasks delegated to them. Although they now perform many services once carried out by health professionals, they often receive only minimal instruction on what to do and what to expect. As a result, they may feel overwhelmed and may worry that they will do something wrong or will miss important warning signs. When a loved one's life is at stake, the pressure can be as exhausting as the physical demands of caregiving.

Family caregivers may jeopardize their own health if they overextend themselves. People are like elastic, says Geila Bar-David of the Caregiver Support Project in Toronto (Laframboise, 1998). If they are stretched too thin for too long, they will lose strength and may even snap. Caregivers who are reluctant to leave their posts may need reminding that they will be of no use unless they remain healthy (emotionally and physically) themselves.

Caring for Caregivers

We began this unit with information about a caregivers' support group. Family caregivers need time for themselves as well as assistance and education. They also need a break from the social isolation that can come with at-home caregiving. Friends and other family members are a promising source of support. In a meta-analysis of 50 studies about family caregiving, a prominent theme was that caregivers missed opportunities to socialize with others (Al-Janabi, Coast, & Flynn, 2008).

BOX 8.4 PERSPECTIVES

A Long Goodbye to Grandmother

A few years ago, I lost my grandmother to Alzheimer's disease. Until she died, I saw my grandmother every week of my life. We had a very close relationship.

Alzheimer's is not a disease that just appears one day and kills you. It causes gradual deterioration of a person's memory and sense of being. Minutes and days and years all seem the same or don't exist at all. My grandmother's condition started about one year before her death.

Before Grandma got Alzheimer's, our extended family was fairly close. No one wanted to put Grandma in a nursing home, but caring for her was not going to be easy. Her three daughters (including my mother) decided Grandma would stay with each of them for one week at a time.

Grandma and I had always enjoyed playing Scrabble and working crossword puzzles together. She always tried to get me to use my thinking skills. My favorite times were when she would tell me stories about when she was a young girl or a teenager. She was a very flirty girl, although she had a prissy attitude as an elderly person.

As Grandma's forgetfulness worsened, she often forgot what year it was. She would also forget to eat. Soon she could no longer remember conversations we had had. I could answer a question and five minutes later, she'd ask it again. I would tell her every week why and where I was going to school. We would talk about the world now compared to the world in her day. Sometimes she would talk out loud to her parents, who had been dead 50 or 60 years.

Her worst times were at night. She stayed up most of the night talking to people she thought were there. As much as I loved Grandma, I would get aggravated with her during those nights of constant talking. Several times a night, we'd go into her room to comfort her. She'd whine and cry like a child. It was difficult for me to deal with this. I started distancing myself from her during the day because she made me angry with the things she did at night. Even though I knew she had no idea what she was doing, it still aggravated me.

The stress started wearing on other family relationships as well. The daughters started finding fault with each other. No one said anything out loud, but the frustration was there under the surface. I was sad to see relationships start to disintegrate. I asked my grandmother to forgive me even if she didn't quite understand why.

Over the months, Grandma's condition deteriorated. She lost touch with reality and she lost trust in her family. One day she and I were home by ourselves and I got her a glass of water. When I gave it to her, she smelled it. Then she looked at me and said, "I never thought you would do this." I asked what she meant, and she said, "Of all people, I didn't think you would poison me. I expected the others, but not you." This hurt me very much. I took the glass of water and poured it down the sink and let her watch me pour a new glass. But she continued to believe I was trying to kill her.

By the time she died, Grandma weighed less than 95 pounds. The times that I could talk with her were over. She stayed with us for the last month of her life. She was in such bad condition we didn't want to move her. The night of her death my mom and dad left for church and I stayed behind. I read her the Bible and sang her some songs while I played my guitar. As I did this she began to cry a little. I didn't expect her to respond, but that was a special moment. About five hours later, she died in her bed, with her family in the room with her.

—NICHOLAS

Caregivers often say that a word of encouragement or thanks is their greatest reward. Said one man who cares for his wife at home:

Sometimes she'll look up to me and give me such a priceless lovely smile, which says it all, and then the other morning she laid down for a bit and looked up to me and said, "You're lovely. I love you." It came out clear as a bell. Well, you can't put a price on that, can you? (Al-Janabi et al., 2008, pp. 116–117)

All in all, supportive communication can sweeten the rewards of caregiving and lessen the demands.

End-of-Life Experiences

It was not my first time at the Cleveland Clinic—I had visited my sister-in-law, Annie, there before. But as I walked in this time, I knew that things were going to be different. I knew that Annie was dying of ovarian cancer that she had been fighting for the past 2½ years and that we were going to be facing a whole host of new issues this time. (Teresa Thompson, 2011, p. 177)

With this statement, Thompson begins an examination of what she calls "a delicate balance" between hope and information at the end of life. She describes Annie's experiences managing the need for both hope and frank information. When the two seemed contradictory, Thompson says, the warmth of the caregiver's demeanor often made the difference in Annie's ability to cope effectively with the information. Thompson concludes that "hope is best engendered by a combination of honesty and empathy" that encompasses faith, dignity, peace, humor, and meaning, as well as treatment goals (p. 185). In this section we explore the role of communication and social support at the end of life.

Death is an unpleasant topic to people in many Western cultures. "Death is un-American. It doesn't square with our philosophy of optimism, of progress," wrote Herbert Kramer, a terminally ill cancer patient (Kramer & Kramer, 1993, para. 21). Nevertheless, dying is inevitable, and it marks a stage of life during which social support is crucial. End-of-life experiences also can be more meaningful and beautiful than many people realize.

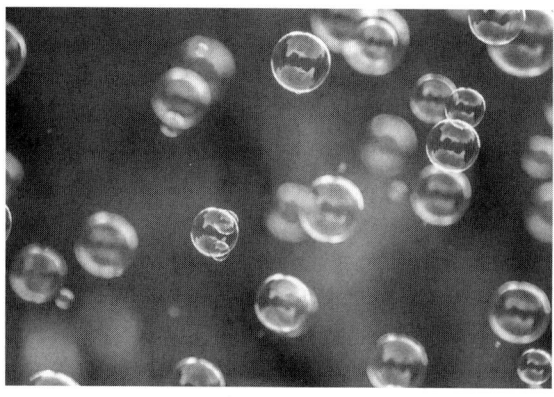

The Japanese concept of *pokkuri shinu* depicts death as popping gently like a soap bubble. By contrast, the ancient Greeks depicted death as the work of a grim reaper.

In your opinion, is there such thing as a good death? If so, how would you describe it?

To some people, the phrase "a good death" seems like an oxymoron. They do not believe there is such a thing. However, many people argue that dying can be a special (albeit emotional) experience with many positive aspects. This section analyzes these two perspectives, which are characterized as "life at all costs" and "death with dignity." It also explains advance-care directives and offers experts' advice for dealing with death.

Life at All Costs

Have you ever walked past a hospital morgue? Probably not. Most hospitals locate the morgue in an out-of-the-way area where people will not chance upon it. Morgue staff members may be regarded as somewhat weird and eccentric based on their choice of occupation. This may seem perfectly understandable if you grew up in a society in which death was regarded as gross and ghoulish.

Today's Grim Reaper is a modern-day version of Thanatos, the merciless and malicious Greek god born of "darkness" and "sleep." In Greek mythology, Thanatos is often depicted as a rival of Bios (Greek for "life"). The lessons of such tales are easy to divine: Death is the enemy of life. Life is victory, death a merciless and permanent defeat. In modern terms, medicine is associated with Bios. Health professionals are considered, quite literally, to be in *mortal* combat with the enemy, death. Hence we entertain such notions as "battling cancer" and "fighting for one's life." These conceptualizations thrive in an atmosphere in which death is considered taboo and unknown, and medicine the ultimate savior.

If you are a care provider pledged to maintain life, death may be more than creepy. It may represent failure. Caregivers have several incentives to keep patients from dying. For one, they are typically trained to preserve life, not allow it to end. Most physicians approach medicine as detectives and problem solvers—endeavors that are successful only if they solve the mystery and fix the problem (Ragan & Goldsmith, 2008). Moreover, death is frightening, even to professionals who have encountered it before (Hegedus, Zana, & Szabó, 2008). Saving a life is usually a rewarding experience, whereas a patient's death may bring feelings of guilt and grief. Finally, caregivers (doctors especially) may be harshly criticized or sued if a patient dies. Physicians' decisions are often intensely scrutinized by family members, lawyers, insurance companies, quality assurance and risk management personnel, administrators, and others. Jack McCue

(1995) attests, "It is little wonder that physicians engage in inappropriately heroic battles against dying and death, even when it may be apparent to physician, patient, and family that a rapid, good death is the best outcome" (para. 2).

Medicine's dedication to preserving life has many benefits. Caregivers' devotion and talent, along with their access to medical technology, has helped to increase the average American's life expectancy from 47.3 to 80.5 years since 1900 (World Population Review, 2019). But a "life at all costs" approach can rob people of the opportunity for a good death. Susan Block (2001) calls a good death "The Art of the Possible." The means of realizing this possibility, she says, lie in making people physically comfortable and helping them nurture caring relationships, maintain a sense of self, find meaning, feel a sense of control, and prepare for death. One man at the end of his life asserted, "What this last year has provided me with is the occasion to be deliberately open to receiving other people's love and care . . . and I'm delighted when it happens" (quoted by Block, p. 2902).

Many caregivers who become comfortable with death say it's a privilege to be with people at the end of their lives. A physician (Block, 2001) interviewed said of one dying patient:

I really like seeing him because no matter how distraught I am about that particular day or feeling overwhelmed. . . I feel so much better after each visit with him. It's almost like he's a doctor to me. (p. 2903)

Loved ones often feel the same way, that they have learned something precious by being present at the end of a cherished individual's life.

Conventional wisdom says we are likely to lose faith or be angry at God when someone close to us dies. However, this occurs mostly when death is sudden or when people have not accepted its inevitability. Participants in Maureen Keeley's (2004) study of "final conversations" say their loss was tempered by a renewed sense of comfort, meaning, and spirituality. Said one, "You can't go through this . . . witnessing death, without that awe of what life is. Where it comes from and where it goes" (quoted by Keeley, 2004, p. 95). In another episode, a survivor remembers asking a loved one, "When you get to heaven, you know, keep an eye out on my girls," and her reply, "I will, you know. I'll be their guardian angel" (p. 97). In these episodes, the dying individual was able to help others find peace and comfort.

Proponents of a good death remind us that it might not involve preserving life as long as possible. As McCue (1995) proposes, "a rapid, good death" is sometimes preferable to a prolonged, painful end. Prolonging life sometimes means prolonging death.

Caregivers and others who perceive death to be a frightening enemy are not well equipped to help with end-of-life care. Dying individuals sometimes feel forgotten and ignored because their caregivers are uncomfortable with death, reluctant to become emotionally involved with them, and uncertain how to act around dying people.

Unfortunately, the opportunity to die peacefully among loved ones is sometimes lost in a confusion of tubes, wires, monitors, and hospital restrictions. It may be comforting to have professionals on hand, but it's hard for loved ones to be present and difficult to maintain a sense of intimacy and individuality in an institutional setting such as a hospital. Communication scholar Sandra Ragan reflects on the difference between her father's death and her sister's:

Dad's death was a conflicted one: He died in a hospital, connected to various machines, and in constant fear, until his last 48 hours, when he entered a morphine-induced semi-consciousness, that his doctors would not give him adequate medication. (Ragan, Wittenberg, & Hall, 2003, p. 219)

In contrast, her sister died at home under hospice care:

Sherry died peacefully in her own home with no medical intervention other than oxygen, a catheter, and the blessing of morphine and Ativan. Her family and loved ones surrounded her, and throughout her last night, she was cradled by her daughter and her beloved cocker spaniel. (Ragan et al., 2003, pp. 219–220)

Death with Dignity

In Japan, a metaphor for the ideal death is *pokkuri shinu*, which translates roughly into "popping like a bubble." People in many cultures share the same wish, of living fully and then dying without languishing slowly away. In the United States, a good death is often described as one in which people maintain dignity and die surrounded by loved ones and familiar, comforting surroundings.

The motto of death with dignity is attributable mostly to **hospice**, an organization that provides support and care for individuals and their families. Hospice provides **palliative care**, which is designed to keep a person as comfortable and fulfilled as possible but is not designed to cure the main illness once it has been determined that medical care will not improve it. More than 4 in 10 of all dying patients in the United States now receive hospice care, mostly at home during the last three weeks of their lives, and of those, 86.6% consider their care to be "excellent" ("Hospice Care," 2012).

Central to hospice's philosophy is the belief that death is a natural part of life, thus personal and unique. People are encouraged to die as they have lived, surrounded by the people and things they love most. Hospice volunteers and professional caregivers visit with terminally ill individuals and their loved ones to talk with them about death (if they wish), to make sure the dying person is not in pain, to encourage spiritual exploration (if they wish), and to provide many forms of assistance. In this effort, hospice is more oriented toward personal expression, emotions, spirituality, and social concerns than is conventional Western medicine. Loved ones are considered important participants in the dying process.

Beth Perry, a hospice nurse, recalls an especially rewarding experience helping a dying patient. "Roman, a handsome man in his mid-50s, seemed too well to be a patient on a palliative care unit," she remembers (Perry, 2002, para. 5). But Roman *was* dying, and he was bored and tired of the process—ready for the tedium to end. Although Roman's caregivers knew his death was near, they sought a way to rekindle his sense of purpose. Someone remembered that he and his wife had bought a new home just before he became ill, and the grounds were not yet landscaped. They suggested that the couple plan the garden and grounds together. "The result was amazing," writes Perry:

> *The next time we visited the pair, gone was the stony silence, the painful watching of time tick by. Instead, we found the two of them with their noses in the same magazine, eagerly debating annuals versus perennials, tulips versus delphiniums. (para. 7)*

Although Roman did not live to plant the garden, his last days were filled with enthusiasm rather than boredom. Julie, another nurse caring for Roman, says, "People can take almost anything, but they can't take being forgotten. They want to know that something they have done will live on after they die, and sometimes it is part of my role to help them" (quoted by Perry, 2002, para. 8).

Sometimes it's difficult to know what to say during end-of-life experiences. Sandra Sanchez-Reilly, MD, coauthor of *Communication as Comfort: Multiple Voices in Palliative Care,* told a dying patient in her care, "There are five things I tell my patients to say to everyone in their last day of their lives. Please forgive me; I forgive you; I love you; I will miss you. Goodbye." When a patient told her he was not scared and wiped away a tear, Sanchez-Reilly said to him, "You have taught the team many things today, Mr. _____. The team is here to learn. What else would you like to teach them?" (Ragan, Wittenberg-Lyles, Goldsmith, & Sanchez-Reilly, 2008, p. 80).

In another instance described in the same book, a husband helped his wife accept the need for hospice. Elaine Wittenberg describes the hospital-room interaction, which she witnessed as a researcher. The patient expressed her fears about enrolling in hospice to a nurse who suggested the idea, until the patient's husband took his wife's hand in his and said to her through his tears, "I've been married to you for almost twenty-five years. I have never cheated on you. I have never lied to you. I'm not lying to you now. You need hospice. I need hospice. We need hospice" (Ragan et al., 2008, p. 146). Then the two leaned toward each other and cried.

Hospice volunteers also play a vital role in end-of-life communication. A beautiful account of this is available in Elissa Foster's (2007) book *Communicating at the End of Life: Finding Magic in the Mundane.* In the book, Foster chronicles her year as a hospice volunteer and shares the stories of other volunteers and the patients she meets along the way. Threaded throughout the narrative is Foster's relationship with Dorothy, a petite, energetic woman with "lively blue-green" eyes and white, close-cropped hair. Dorothy is under hospice care because doctors recognize that she is in the final stages of chronic obstructive pulmonary disease (COPD). Foster captures the confusion and concern she feels as Dorothy's condition seems, alternately, to deteriorate and to improve over time. She also reveals the mutuality of their relationship. Dorothy is not simply the recipient of Foster's care. The caring goes both ways. When Dorothy dies, Foster visits her family, shares hugs and tears with them, and thanks them for "sharing" their mother with her. She later reflects, "My relationship with Dorothy taught me that I could

Communication Skill Builder: Coping With Death

One positive aspect of death is that it draws people together. Loved ones who may not have seen each other in years unite again with a common concern. Death also provides an occasion for contemplating life and the purpose of living. A sense of insight and spirituality often surrounds death (McCormick & Conley, 1995). Moreover, by sharing in loved ones' deaths, people may become less fearful of death themselves. Joyce Dyer, who wrote *In a Tangled Wood* (1996) about her mother's nine-year experience with Alzheimer's disease, reflected after her death:

> I want to remember every moment I had with my mother, including every second of the last nine years. I want to remember her toothless grin, her screams, her growing fondness for sweets and then for nothing at all, the bouquets of uprooted flowers she picked for me from her unit's patio, the way she tried to fold her bib, the rare pats on my cheek that meant everything, her last words, her last party, her last dance. And I want to remember what I learned from aides and nurses, from volunteers and cleaning staff, from my mother's own sick friends. I don't want to forget a single thing. (Dyer, 1996, p. 136)

People may be surprised by the mixture of emotions they feel about death. Most of us are not sure what to expect, and consequently we are often uncertain how to act around dying individuals. Based on news reports and movies, people typically imagine death as violent and scary. However, the majority of deaths are nothing like that. Colin Parkes (1998) describes the typical death as a "quiet slipping away" without pain or horror.

One nurse described her initial discomfort when a young man in her care joked that he had to live quickly because he would not live long (Erdman, 1993). The nurse was eventually able to laugh with the young man when he quipped that he was watching movies on fast-forward and bathing his dog in the drive-through carwash to save time. Writes Erdman, "The nurse was at first caught off guard by the patient's comments, but the humor opened the door to further communication about death" (p. 59).

Three themes emerge in the narratives of older adults reflecting on the death of loved ones: loss, feelings, coping. The feelings are mixed, but not as negative as you might expect. In Caplan, Haslett, and Burleson's (2005) study of older adult bereavement narratives, 36% of the feelings were negative (fear, loneliness, sadness), but 43% were positive (optimism, thankfulness for time spent together, and so on). Said one woman, whose husband died in 1993, "I don't dwell on the sickness and problems of what happened then, but my thoughts and memories instead, think of all the good and wonderful life we had together with the six children" (p. 244).

In her book *On Death and Dying*, Elisabeth Kübler-Ross (1969) describes the process of coping with death in five stages: denial and isolation, anger, bargaining, depression, and acceptance. Not everyone experiences all five stages or in the order given, but dying individuals and the people around them are likely to experience many of these phases. Although with enough time and support many people eventually feel peaceful about death, they may at times refuse to believe what is told them, or they may feel angry, overwhelmed, sad, or hopeless. Often, people feel their God has let them down, and they react by showing anger or attempting to bargain for mercy. It may be reassuring to remember that these stages are common and legitimate components of the coping process.

Advance-Care Directives

Advance-care directives describe what medical care a person wishes to receive (or not receive) if they are unable to communicate their wishes directly. These directives take some of the pressure off care providers and loved ones who might otherwise be forced to make those decisions on their own.

Despite the advantages, only about 1 in 4 adults in the United States has completed an advance-care directive (Rao, Anderson, Lin, & Laux, 2014). That leaves an overwhelming number of people without written instructions about their end-of-life care, even though communicating one's preferences is central to the idea of a good death (Borreani et al., 2008). Confusion about advance directives is particularly prevalent among people with literacy challenges (Sudore, Schillinger, Knight, & Fried, 2010).

Advance-care directives have become more specific through the years. When they were first conceptualized as "living wills" in the 1960s, they typically referred in vague terms to "heroic" life-saving measures (Emanuel & Emanuel, 1998). This presented obvious difficulties in interpretation (e.g., *Is a feeding tube heroic? Is intravenous therapy heroic?*). It is now common for advance-care directives to include a person's preferences regarding specific procedures and circumstances, to endow someone with decision-making authority, and to describe the person's philosophy of life and death to help guide decisions during unanticipated circumstances. (See Box 8.5 for a discussion of the right-to-die issue.)

Communication Skill Builder: Delivering Bad News

One of the most difficult communication challenges anyone faces is sharing devastating news with another. Bad news is never easy to give or to receive, but there are a number of communication strategies that help optimize people's coping ability. Here are some suggestions from the experts on how to share bad news compassionately.

BOX 8.5 Ethical Considerations

Do People Have a Right to Die?

Oregon made history in 1997 by legalizing physician-assisted suicide for terminally ill patients. Under the law, a physician may help a person end their life if at least two physicians verify that the person has less than six months to live and the patient requests help with suicide at least once in writing and twice verbally, with at least 15 days between requests.

Physician-assisted suicide refers to instances in which, at the request of a terminally ill person, a doctor provides the means for that person to end their own life (Krug, 1998). The doctor does not actually kill the patient. This is different from **euthanasia** (also called *mercy killing*), in which a physician or family member intentionally kills the patient to end their suffering. The distinction lies in who does the killing—the patient or another person.

The person most commonly associated with physician-assisted suicide was Jack Kevorkian, a physician who, by his own estimate, assisted in the suicides of 130 people. Kevorkian was tried for murder five times, but he was not convicted until the fifth trial, which concluded in April 1999. Kevorkian was declared guilty of second-degree murder by a Michigan jury and sentenced to 10 to 25 years in prison. The conviction was based on an assisted suicide that Kevorkian videotaped and allowed to be broadcast on *60 Minutes* (Willing, 1999). Kevorkian, who was released on parole in 2007 and died in 2011, argued that he was motivated by compassion for people dying slow, painful deaths. His opponents charged that he was a medical "hitman" operating outside the law (Robertson, 1999).

Controversy over physician-assisted suicide is likely to continue for quite some time, with people vigorously arguing both sides of the issue. Proponents of physician-assisted suicide include Dax Cowart, who was badly burned in an explosion in 1973 (Cowart & Burt, 1998). Two-thirds of Cowart's body was burned in the accident, and he lost his eyesight and his fingers. For more than a year Cowart begged doctors to let him die. Despite his pleas, medical teams continued to treat his burns. The treatment kept Cowart alive and eventually helped him regain the ability to walk. But during that time he was in nearly unbearable agony. He recalled, "The pain was excruciating, it was so far beyond any pain that I ever knew was possible, that I simply could not endure it" (para. 21). Cowart supported physician-assisted suicide. However, even if a law such as Oregon's had been in place when his accident occurred, he would not have qualified for lawful physician-assisted suicide because he was not dying.

Cowart became an attorney in Corpus Christi, Texas, and described himself as "happier than most people." But he maintained his conviction that people should not be forced to undergo treatment they do not wish, even if that treatment is needed to keep them alive (Cowart & Burt, 1998). Faced with the same ordeal again, he felt he would wish to die and should have been allowed to do so. Cowart's views

continued

are captured in his videos *Please Let Me Die* and *Dax's Case*. (Cowart died in 2019 at age 71.)

On the other side of the issue, some argue that people in intense pain and grief may not see things clearly enough to make life-ending decisions. They point out that Cowart changed his mind about living with his disabilities. Although he initially felt life would be empty, he later felt happy and was successful (Cowart & Burt, 1998). Other critics say ill (even terminally ill) patients may request death for the wrong reasons. They may be afraid about the future, feel out of control and scared, or believe they are a burden to loved ones (Muskin, 1998). For these reasons, they feel it is wrong to help someone kill themselves, even if the person requests it.

What Do You Think?

1. Under what circumstances, if any, do you feel patients should be assisted in killing themselves?
2. Should it make a difference whether a patient is terminally ill or not?
3. If you were in Dax Cowart's place, do you feel you would want to die? What would you have done if you were Cowart's caregivers and loved ones?
4. What do you think of the argument that people who are scared and in pain may be not thinking clearly enough to make life-or-death decisions?
5. What do you think of the counterargument—that people should not second-guess the patient's wishes because they cannot fully understand the extent of their personal suffering?

- *Build caring relationships from the beginning*. In a study of recently diagnosed cancer patients, Pär Salander (2002) found that patients did not describe one distinct event during which they learned of their diagnosis. They considered that it occurred within the context of ongoing relationships with the medical staff. Said one woman, "The kindness, the support, and the help I received from the entire staff when treatment started is what I appreciate the most" (p. 724).
- *Foreshadow the disclosure*. A simple statement such as "The news isn't as good as we hoped" may help prepare people for what is to come.
- *Invite the recipient to bring along supportive others*.
- *Talk in a quiet, private place*. Resist the temptation to deliver bad news in a hallway or semi-private space. Likewise, avoid delivering bad news over the phone whenever possible (Sparks, Villagran, Parker-Raley, & Cunningham, 2007).
- *Tell the truth*. People typically cope better when they know what is happening and what to expect. This is true even when death is expected. A participant in Thomas McCormick and Becky Conley's (1995) study said, "That's one of the things that I like my doctor for, because he was plain with me that I was incurable" (para. 38). She explained that people who do not know they are dying cannot prepare for it emotionally or practically. They lose the chance to settle financial affairs, communicate with loved ones, set new priorities for their limited time, and adjust emotionally to what is occurring.

- *Be clear about your meaning*. Patients often interpret hedge terms such as "possible" to mean that the news giver is attempting to soften the blow of bad news rather than convey actual uncertainty (Pighin & Bonnefon, 2011). Asked to interpret comments such as "It is possible the pain will increase," most patients felt the caregiver was really saying that the pain would probably or certainly increase (Pighin & Bonnefon, 2011, p. 171).
- *Avoid medical jargon*.
- *Acknowledge and legitimize emotions*. Emotions are a natural part of the coping process. Ignoring them may make the news recipient feel foolish or inappropriate. Instead, acknowledge emotions with statements such as "I know this is very hard to hear," "I understand this can feel overwhelming," and "It's natural to feel a range of emotions when you learn something like this."
- *Take your cues from the recipient*. Do not be surprised if people seem stoic or distant on hearing bad news, whereas others are tearful or even angry. It is hard for any of us to say how we will react in such circumstances. Patients typically say it is unhelpful when someone attempts to impose a particular agenda or set of emotions on them (Maynard & Frankel, 2006). One patient whom Salander (2002) interviewed wondered, "Why did they have to be so dramatic? Suddenly, everybody looked so grave and became so low-voiced. It gave me a feeling of unreality" (p. 725).

BOX 8.6 Career Opportunities

Social Services and Mental Health

Home health aide
Hospice/palliative care provider
Mental health counselor
Psychologist
Senior citizen services providers
Social service manager
Social worker

Career Resources and Job Listings

- American Mental Health Counselors Association: www.amhca.org
- American Psychological Association: www.apa.org
- National Association of School Psychologists: www.nasponline.org
- American Board of Professional Psychology: www.abpp.org
- National Organization for Human Services: www.nationalhumanservices.org
- Hospice: www.hospicenet.org
- Hospice careers: hospicechoices.com
- National Association for Home Care and Hospice: www.nahc.org

---

- *Show genuine caring.* As one woman put it, "A hug or supportive word in passing worked miracles" (quoted by Salander, 2002, p. 727).
- *Inform and empathize.* Research shows that, no matter how bad the news, patients want both high-quality information and empathy, and one does not compensate for the other. In other words, lots of information does not make up for a lack of emotional supportiveness or vice versa. People typically want both (Sastre, Sorum, & Mullet, 2011).
- *Be aware of personal and cultural preferences for bad-news delivery.* Some people, such as members of traditional Native American cultures, prefer that bad news be delivered indirectly through metaphors and storytelling (T. Thompson & Gillotti, 2005). In some other cultures, speaking bad news aloud is considered unlucky.
- *Offer support.* Indicate your own support and offer other resources to help people learn, adjust, and cope.
- *Be ready with options and a plan of action.* Although some people may need time to take in the bad news before they make decisions, most say that having a specified next step helped them funnel their energy and emotion in positive ways and feel less like helpless victims.
- *Schedule an informational follow-up visit.* Keep in mind that few people can absorb and remember many details when they are feeling intense emotions. Written materials may help, as will a follow-up visit to talk about the details once the news has sunk in.

For career resources relevant to mental health and coping, see Box 8.6.

Summary

Conceptual Overview

- Sometimes problem solving is the most effective coping strategy, in which case instrumental and informative support are likely to be appreciated.
- When the situation calls for emotional adjustment, nurturing support may be a useful way to help people feel better about themselves, express their emotions, and feel that others will stand by them in times of trouble.
- People often cope better when they feel they have some control over their situation.
- Dialectics describes people's ongoing efforts to negotiate seemingly opposite but interdependent factors, as when a person is more "present" with a loved one because they take some time to be alone now and then.
- To members of society viewed as abnormal, achieving a sense of normalcy can seem as impossible as it is desirable. Individuals who have disabilities or are ill don't usually benefit from being treated as if they are childlike or helpless.
- Some health events are so life-changing that things are not the same afterward, leading to the creation of a "new normal," often characterized by a focus on staying healthy and watching for warning signs.

Coping and Communication

- People usually cope more effectively when they can discuss sensitive topics than when they feel compelled to feign cheerfulness.

- Don't assume that individuals are coping well because they don't display much emotion. These people often receive less support than others, although they probably need it just as much.
- Allow distressed individuals to express themselves as they wish and to set the pace for talk and action.
- Supportive listeners are attentive, nonjudgmental, and able to help people understand their own emotions.
- Information is often useful in coping, but as the theory of problematic integration points out, information can be overwhelming.

When Social Support Goes Wrong

- Too little assistance or hurtful jests can make people feel worse.
- Too much support can cause a sense of helplessness and dependence.

Animal Companions

- For many people, pets and animal visitors are a comfort.
- Pets can also be a subject of conversation and connection between patients and care providers.

Transformative Experiences

- Transcendent experiences sometimes suggest an overarching meaning that makes sense of situations that initially seemed tragic or pointless.

Friends and Family as Caregivers

- Loved ones are an important source of social support, but they, too, need support.
- Support groups, skills-training programs, and the assistance of family and friends are key.

End-of-Life Experiences

- Medicine has traditionally considered death a failure, to be avoided at all costs, but groups such as hospice promote the philosophy that there is such a thing as a good death.
- When people are able to cope effectively, death may bring people together and help them overcome their fears.

Advance-Care Directives

- Stipulating in writing what care you do and don't want can save loved ones the difficult task of deciding on your behalf and help assure that your wishes are carried out.

Communication Skill Builder: Delivering Bad News

- Build caring relationships in advance, if possible.
- Let listeners know in advance that the news isn't good.
- Invite supportive others.
- Talk in a quiet, private place.
- Tell the truth and avoid hedge words and medical jargon.
- Acknowledge and legitimize listeners' emotions, and take your cues from them.
- Show genuine caring and empathy.
- Be aware of personal and cultural preferences.
- Offer support.
- Be ready with options and a plan of action.
- Schedule a follow-up visit or conversation.

Glossary

action-facilitating A form of social support that involves performing tasks and collecting information. *See page 165.*

advance-care directive A document that describes the medical care a person wishes to receive (or not receive) if they are unable to communicate their wishes directly. *See page 181.*

buffering hypothesis The idea that social support is most important when people encounter potentially stressful experiences, in which case knowing that other people are there for them can cushion (buffer) them from feeling overwhelmed or helpless. *See page 160.*

coping The process of managing difficult situations. *See page 161.*

crisis An occurrence that exceeds a person's normal coping ability. *See page 163.*

dialectics An ongoing tension of meaning between coexisting but contradictory constructs such as hopeless and hopeful. *See page 163.*

direct-effect model (also known as the *main-effect model*) The proposition that social support is beneficial even when people are not encountering notable stressors. *See page 159.*

emotional adjustment A form of coping that involves adapting to what cannot be changed. *See page 161.*

emotional contagion Feeling emotions similar to another person's. *See page 171.*

emotional support A form of nurturing social support that includes efforts to acknowledge and understand what another person is feeling. *See page 166.*

empathic concern An intellectual appreciation of someone's feelings. *See page 171.*

empathy The ability to show that you understand how someone else is feeling. *See page 171.*

esteem support A form of nurturing social support that involves efforts to make another person feel valued and competent. *See page 166.*

euthanasia (also called *mercy killing*) An instance in which someone intentionally kills someone to end their suffering. *See page 182.*

external locus of control The belief that events are controlled mostly by outside forces. *See page 162.*

Family and Medical Leave Act of 1993 Legislation that guarantees that people can take up to 12 weeks off work to care for ailing family members, seek medical care themselves, or bring new children into their families under certain circumstances. *See page 176.*

fatalistic The belief that things happen because of fate. *See page 162.*

health self-efficacy The sense that one is in control of one's own health. *See page 162.*

hospice An organization that provides support and care for individuals and their families. *See page 179.*

informational support A form of action-facilitating social support that involves finding and sharing information. *See page 165.*

instrumental support A form of action-facilitating social support that involves doing tasks and favors for another person. *See page 165.*

internal locus of control The belief that people control their own destinies. *See page 162.*

normalcy The sense that things are comfortable, predictable, and familiar. *See page 164.*

nurturing A form of social support that involves building self-esteem, acknowledging and expressing emotions, and providing companionship. *See page 165.*

overempathizing Feeling the emotions of another person to such an extent that it is not helpful. *See page 171.*

overhelping Providing too much instrumental assistance. *See page 171.*

overinforming Forcing information on people when they are too distraught to understand it or accept it. *See page 171.*

oversupport Excessive and unnecessary help. *See page 171.*

palliative care Care and support designed to keep a person as comfortable and fulfilled as possible but not designed to cure an illness once it has been determined that medical care will not improve it. *See page 180.*

physician-assisted suicide Instances in which, at the request of a terminally ill person, a doctor provides the means for that person to end their own life. *See page 182.*

problem solving A form of coping that involves taking effective action. *See page 161.*

social support Behaviors that communicate to an individual that they are valued and cared for by others. *See page 159.*

support groups Collections of people with similar concerns who meet regularly to discuss their feelings and experiences. *See page 169.*

theory of problematic integration The idea that we orient to life in terms of *expectations* (what we think will probably happen) and *evaluations* (whether occurrences are good or bad). We use communication to adjust as our expectations and values are challenged in large and small ways. *See page 167.*

transcendent experiences Episodes in which people come to perceive an overarching meaning, or supra-meaning, within experiences that might otherwise seem senseless or unthinkable. *See page 173.*

Discussion Questions

1. On a scale of 1 to 10, how would you rate your social support network in terms of the number of people you know? In terms of the quality of your interactions? Do you think relationships have an impact on your health? If so, how? Is the quantity or quality of your social ties more important to your well-being? Why?

2. Describe an instance in which you offered someone action-facilitating support and an instance in which you offered someone nurturing support. Now describe instances in which you received these forms of support. What was the outcome in each instance? Were the supportive efforts mostly effective or ineffective? Why?

3. Divide a paper into two columns. In the left hand, write specific expectations for your future. In the right column, evaluate each expectation in terms of whether it is likely to be good or bad, easy or difficult, likely or unlikely. The theory of problematic integration suggests that some of these expectations are likely to come true and some are not. What role is communication likely to play in pursuing the expectations you value? In coping with unforeseen circumstances along the way?

4. In what ways can people be oversupportive? What are the likely outcomes of different types of oversupport? Name five tips for ensuring that social support efforts are effective.

5. Have you ever felt that an animal was a good friend? Why or why not? Do you think animal companionship affects your coping ability?

6. Compare the birth experiences of Carol Bishop Mills and her husband with those of Kate and Chris (pages 172-173). What do you learn from these examples?

7. What does the term *transcendent experience* mean? Can you think of examples from movies or your own experiences?

8. In your opinion, is there such a thing as a good death? If so, how would you describe it?

9. Do you have an advance-care directive? Why or why not?

10. What is your opinion of the right-to-die issue (Box 8.5)? Why?

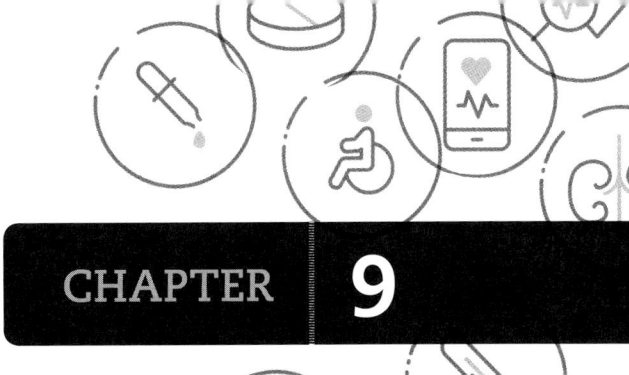

CHAPTER 9

eHealth, mHealth, and Telehealth

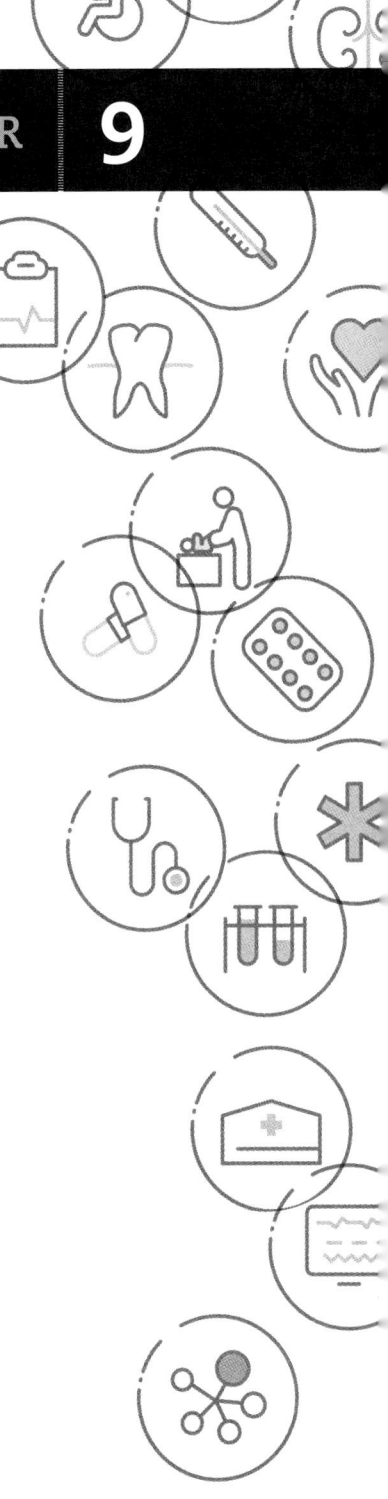

Deanna Recktenwald had a headache in April 2018, but she felt fine otherwise. The healthy 18-year-old athlete was sitting in church with her family, but something was decidedly wrong. Although she did not know it, Deanna's heart rate was an alarming 190 beats per minute. According to the American Heart Association (2019), most healthy adults have a resting heart rate of about 60 to 70 beats per minute.

Adam Love was tired after only six hours of sleep, but he felt okay. Like most college students, Adam, 24, could have done with a little more sleep. Unlike most college students, however, when Adam slept something strange happened—his heart beat abnormally fast. Adam's average resting heart rate was 140 beats per minute.

Neither Deanna nor Adam knew they had life-threatening health conditions. Deanna was in kidney failure and Adam had a hole in his heart. Because they felt okay, neither Deanna nor Adam thought that they should see a doctor—but an everyday device they wear on their wrist told them to do just that! If Deanna and Adam had ignored the advice to get help, they could have died.

In an interview with a reporter, Deanna explained that her watch advised her to "seek medical attention." Looking back, she says, "I didn't know what was going on at all and it was just out of the blue" (Smith, 2018, para. 2). Deanna's mother exclaimed to the reporter, "I didn't even know that it [the watch] had the capability of giving us that alert" (Smith, 2018, para. 4). Adam shared a similar story with a television news reporter, saying, "My Apple Watch started to notify me that I had an elevated heart rate while I was sleeping . . . it picked up something medically that I had no idea about" (Walsh, 2018, para. 12). Deanna and Adam credit their Apple Watches with saving their lives.

Heeding their watches' advice, both Deanna and Adam saw physicians right away. Deanna's kidneys were operating at 20% capacity. If she had not

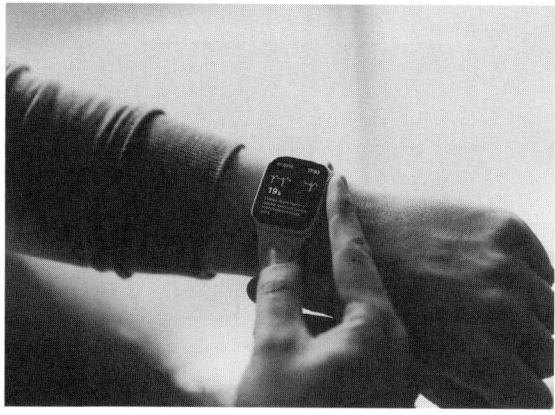

Apple Watches have become an important source of health information. Dennis Anselmo, 62, thought he had the flu, but when his watch indicated that he had a heart rate of 210 beats per minute, he realized he was having a heart attack and called for an ambulance (Snowden, 2016).

gone to the emergency room when she did, Deanna might have required a kidney transplant. Adam underwent surgery in July 2018 to fix the hole in his heart. Although he had been born with the defect, it was not detected until he got an Apple Watch.

Deanna's and Adam's stories are not unique. Apple Watches are credited with saving dozens of lives. For instance, David Gilley, 61, was enjoying Chinese takeout with his wife when his Apple Watch beeped. "I got a message on my watch that said I needed to check my heart rate," David explained (Shortsleeve, 2018, para. 10). By the time he reached the hospital, his heart was failing. He told a reporter, "If it hadn't been for the watch, I would have gone to bed that night and I probably wouldn't have woken up" (Shortsleeve, 2018, para. 11).

In this chapter we explore **eHealth**, which involves the use of technology to transcend geographical distance in promoting good health. Some people use the term "eHealth" to refer to online health resources and websites, but eHealth actually encompasses all sorts of information and communication technologies, ranging from websites and electronic medical records to social media and smartphone apps. People use eHealth for many reasons, including education, health promotion, assessment, self-monitoring, fitness tracking, and social support (Stevens, van der Sande, Beijer, Gerritsen, & Assendelft, 2019). Health care providers use eHealth to communicate with other health care providers and with patients, and eHealth is an important educational resource for doctors and nurses in training. As this chapter demonstrates, eHealth impacts many aspects of health care delivery and affects patients and providers alike.

We will learn about a number of efforts that fall within the rubric of eHealth, such as mHealth, telehealth, and telemedicine. Here is a quick primer on the terminology:

- **mHealth** involves the use of devices such as smartwatches, mobile phones, tablet computers, and personal digital assistants.
- **Telehealth** utilizes technology to facilitate long-distance health care, education, administrative teamwork, and disaster responses (WHO, 2010a, 2010b).
  - **Telemedicine** is a subset of telehealth that specifically involves offering clinical services to patients at a distance, usually through the use of teleconference exams and shared diagnostic data, but also via phone and computer-mediated conversations.

The overarching category of eHealth also includes a variety of other activities, such as communication between everyday people via blogs, tweets, text messages, and other electronic means. Our increasing reliance on these technologies as both health citizens and professionals underscores the central role communication plays in health.

Let's begin by taking a closer look at people who utilize eHealth resources.

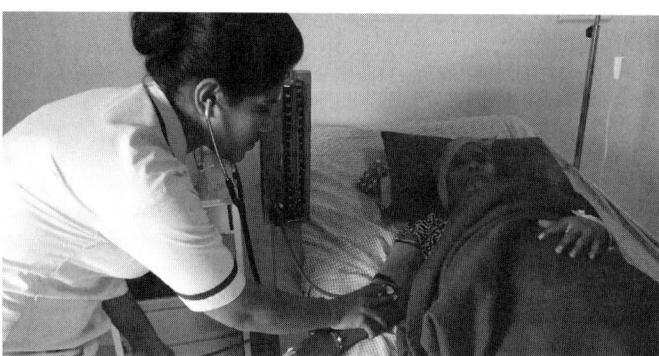

One promise of eHealth is assistance to regions of the world in which conventional care is scarce. Information about the use of medical technology in remote regions is available through the Praekelt Foundation and its Health eVillages (pronounced Healthy Villages), mHealth Alliance, and Medic Mobile programs.

Health Information Haves and Have Nots

I had a question, you know? I didn't really feel comfortable asking my mom, 'cause she was the only one around. You know, I was like, I went on the Internet and I was like, "Can a girl get pregnant during her period?"

This statement by a 17-year-old high school student in Rachel Jones and Ann Biddlecom's (2011, p. 115) study of teens' online communication illustrates one role the internet plays in health-related behavior. Sometimes eHealth is an alternative to talking about topics that are embarrassing to discuss with another person. For this and other reasons, some people use eHealth a great deal, while others do not.

ePatients

In the broadest sense, ePatients are "Internet-savvy" people who "meet their own health needs using the Internet and other information and communication technology" (Kim & Kwon, 2010, p. 712). They typically find health-related information, share it with others, investigate treatment options and more, online. They tend to be female (Magsamen-Conrad, Dillon, Bilotte Verhoff, & Faulkner, 2019a), comparatively young, well educated, and affluent, meaning they are probably already information rich (Koch-Weser et al., 2010). Even though ePatients use online resources more than other people, most of them say doctors are still their favorite source of health information. They just yearn for more detail than their physicians typically provide (Kim & Kwon, 2010). ePatients' online health information seeking does not replace face-to-face visits with doctors (Lee & Lin, 2019), but is often used to "bookend" visits: ePatients go online to research their symptoms before visits and again, afterward, to supplement what providers told them about their conditions (Magsamen-Conrad et al., 2019a).

The term *ePatient* is still evolving. Many people who look up health information online and share it with others are not patients at all. For example, nearly 7 in 10 people who seek cancer information online do not have cancer (Kim & Kwon, 2010), and teens whose family members have conditions such as diabetes and Alzheimer's often use the internet to become more knowledgeable about ways to help (Wartella, Rideout, Montague, Beaudoin-Ryan, Lauricella, 2016, p. 19).

Kyunghye Kim and Nahyun Kwon (2010) advocate a finer distinction by defining **ePatients** as "people with illness seeking information or help from the Internet to make informed health decisions" (p. 712).

Online health information seeking among patients is associated with positive health outcomes, but it "might be perceived as a double-edged sword among health care professionals" (Wernhart, Gahbauer, & Haluza, 2019, p. 9). Providers surveyed by Anna Wernhart and colleagues expressed low opinions of "Dr. Google" because they felt that "distorted and inappropriate health information retrieved online" can interfere with clinical decision making and provider–patient relationships (Wernhart et al., 2019, p. 9).

No matter how you define the concept, electronic health information and ePatients are here to stay in some form. At the same time, some people are largely left out.

Digital Divide

The irony is that people most in need of health information are least likely to have access to information online. Here we consider some of the factors that contribute to a digital divide.

SOCIODEMOGRAPHICS

In the United States, older adults and those with lower-than-average income and education levels are least likely to have access to the internet, where such information is most plentiful.

- Individuals ages 18 to 29 are three times more likely than those 60 and older to learn about health online (Smith, 2011), whereas nearly a third of adults over age 65 *never* go online (Anderson, Perrin, Jiang, & Kumar, 2019).
- Nearly 9 in 10 people ages 14 to 22 go online for health information (Rideout & Fox, 2018), but older adults are less likely to search for health information online, and they often have lower levels of eHealth literacy than younger adults (Chesser et al., 2016).
- People who are college educated, live in suburban or urban areas, and earn more than $75,000 a year are much more likely to have high-speed internet access at home than adults who have less education and/or live in rural areas (Perrin, 2019; Pew Research Center, 2019).

All of these factors point to a digital divide that privileges some people and systematically excludes others.

VISION CHALLENGES

Imagine trying to navigate the Web without using a mouse or a keyboard or without seeing the screen. Try operating a smartphone without using your hands or with your eyes closed. These challenges quickly reveal why people with physical challenges and visual impairments are less likely than others to own computers or find online information accessible (Sachdeva, Tuikka, Kimppa, & Suomi, 2015).

Software has been available for some time to convert text into audio messages and to allow people to speak rather than type messages. However, funding and training for these systems has lagged. Closed captioning, when it is available, is often inaccurate. And programmers still struggle to capture the visually complex and nonlinear character of web information (Hong, Kim, Trimi, & Hyun, 2015). John Hermann, who is blind, describes the dilemma. If you are a sighted person using the Web, he says,

> your eyes fly around, sometimes randomly and sometimes in response to cues onscreen. You hunt for links and cherrypick from galleries. The word you're looking for catches your eye, so you click it. Consciously or subconsciously, you usually know where to look. (Hermann, 2010, para. 8)

By contrast, for people with visual impairments, "there is no 'looking'" (Hermann, para. 9). Hearing the content instead means listening to a lot of information you would not have chosen and trying to mentally organize information that was designed to be seen as a whole rather than heard in a linear fashion. Hermann and others applaud emerging software that not only narrates information but describes the screen ("three menu buttons at the top that read . . . four vertical columns have the headings . . ." and so on). However, everyone agrees there is a long way to go.

There are promising solutions on the horizon. For example, Be My Eyes is a free app that partners blind and low-vision people with sighted volunteers. Through a live video call, a volunteer reads aloud to visually impaired callers things like expiration dates on food packages and printed instructions on medicine bottles. The app is available for Apple and Android devices. You can learn more at www.bemyeyes.com. Around the globe, the World Wide Web Consortium brings together people who hope eventually to make online resources accessible to everyone, regardless of reading ability, native language, physical limitations, and other factors. You can follow their efforts at www.w3.org.

CONFIDENCE

Apart from internet access and accessibility, there is something else that divides information seekers—**health information efficacy**, how confident a person is that they can find and understand health information. Health information efficacy is highest among people who are well educated and who have experience in health care situations (Hall, Bernhardt, Dodd, & Vollrath, 2015). Women are typically more likely than men—and older adults more likely than younger ones—to have high health information efficacy and to actively seek health and prevention information (Basu & Dutta, 2008). These comparisons are important because confidence and health information seeking can help people more effectively cope with health concerns and make decisions about them.

Why and When Do People Seek ehealth Information?

My alarm clock went off hours before the sun began rising. I silenced it, slowly got out of bed and began getting ready for my morning gym session. Sill half-asleep, I turned on the bright

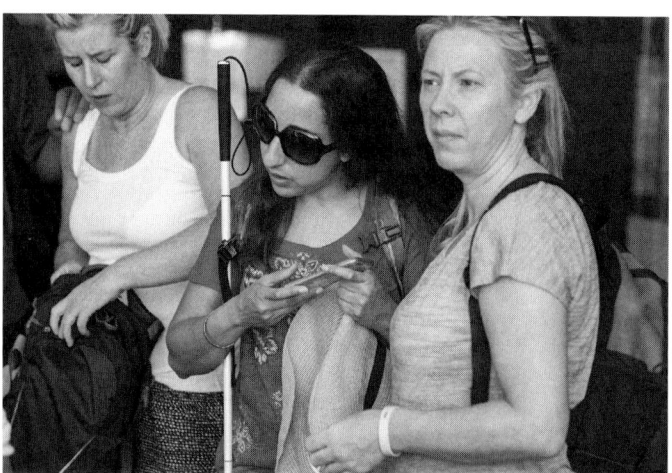

Smartphone apps like Be My Eyes help visually impaired people to lead more independent lives.

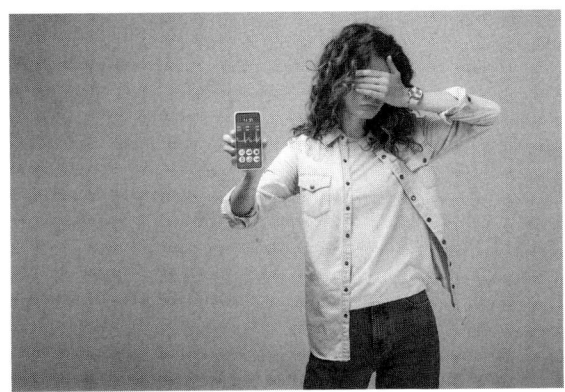

Availability is not everything. We are likely to avoid or ignore eHealth information we perceive to be overwhelming, irrelevant, or untrustworthy.

lights of the bathroom and began brushing my teeth. What happened next is something I never imagined could happen and something I will remember for the rest of my life.

Health events, such as this one described by a university student, sometimes sneak up on us when expert care is not readily available. Here, in her words, is what happened next:

I had somehow managed to open my mouth too wide while brushing my teeth and it was stuck open. My poor jaw was stuck open with toothpaste dripping from the corners of my lips. At that moment, panic set in. Tears were rolling down my cheeks. I felt so helpless. I frantically got online and tried to find solutions.

In this case, the woman's first impulse was to seek information online. "It was so early I didn't want to wake up my roommate," she explains. "So I'm standing there with my mouth hanging open trying to Google 'how to fix your jaw' in my cell phone."

In this section we examine the reasons people seek health information electronically. Earlier in the chapter we heard the perspective of a teenager who searched for sex education online because she didn't want to ask her mother. The woman with the dislocated jaw was motivated by different goals—namely, to find information quickly, to avoid inconveniencing others, and hopefully, to solve an unexpected and urgent dilemma. As we explore theories of eHealth information seeking, consider how well they describe your experiences.

Information Sufficiency Threshold

One perspective is that uncertainty motivates information seeking, especially if individuals perceive an urgent need or risk. Theorists call it **information sufficiency threshold**—the amount of information a person needs in order to feel capable of coping with and understanding a threatening issue (Chaiken, 1980; Chaiken, Giner-Sorolla, & Chen, 1996; Griffin, Dunwoody, & Neuwirth, 1999). In the story of the dislocated jaw, the young woman said her first reaction was thinking, "I don't know what to do!" That sent her scrambling for information in the quickest way she could think of—an internet search on her phone. It was a clear case of information *in*sufficiency, and she was highly motivated to learn quickly.

Health Information Acquisition Model

However, uncertainty is not always the singular or deciding factor. For a variety of reasons, people might *not* seek information, even if they acknowledge that they do not know much about an important issue. Maybe they don't believe more knowledge will make a difference. The **health information acquisition model** established the basis for many theories that have followed it. The model proposes that people are motivated to seek information under the following conditions:

- when something calls their attention to a concern,
- they do not perceive that they are well informed about it,
- it seems important to find out soon,
- and they think they will be able to find trustworthy and useful information (Freimuth, Stein, & Kean, 1989).

Central to this theory is the idea that people first consider how much they already know and then weigh the costs and rewards of seeking additional information. The woman with the dislocated jaw said she felt sure she could fix the problem if she learned how to do it online. She had high self-efficacy (a term you may remember from Chapter 8 that describes the belief that we can make a difference in managing our own health).

Theory of Motivated Information Management

Let's add some additional dimensions to the information-seeking equation. The **Theory of Motivated Information Management** (TMIM) by Walid Afifi and

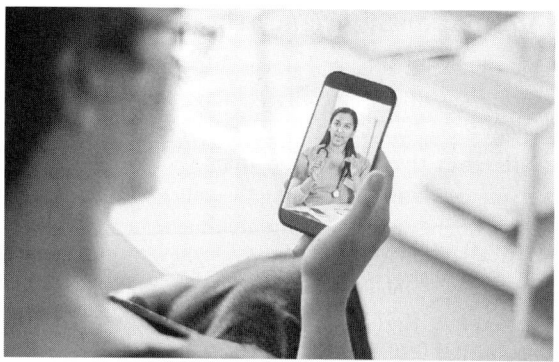

How would you like to receive bad news about your health? Would an email or an instant message be as effective as a phone call? Would a phone call be as effective as a face-to-face conversation? Why?

Judith Weiner (2004) has several aspects in common with the health information acquisition model in that both presume people seek information when they are anxious about something and feel it would be helpful to learn more about it. TMIM, however, also addresses coping confidence (*Am I ready to deal with what I might learn?*) and people's choice of information channels (*How might I get this information?*). According to TMIM, the likelihood that people will seek information depends on their perceived need for it, their coping ability, and the way in which the information is conveyed. Regarding information channels, TMIM addresses not just why people want information and what they hope to learn, but *how* they pursue that information. Afifi and Weiner propose that people seek information most readily from sources they believe to be relevant, accurate, and trustworthy.

Most people prefer that sensitive and important information be conveyed in emotionally immediate, information-rich ways—for example, in person rather than via a text or phone call (Brown, Parker, Furber, & Thomas, 2011). Especially when the stakes are high, people typically appreciate the presence of both verbal and nonverbal cues and indications that the other person cares and is willing to listen. (The exception is that some people prefer to receive emotional news at a distance so that they can avoid "flooding out" emotionally in front of other people; Beach, 2002.) Most people also prefer to hear serious news directly from an expert. In short, the source matters, and it affects how likely people are to believe what they read and hear.

It follows from TMIM that, when the stakes are high, people typically prefer interpersonal communication with individuals they trust. Partly for this reason, patients who do not feel that care providers are empathic and patient centered are more likely than satisfied patients to seek health information on the internet (Tustin, 2010). Dissatisfaction with physicians' performance is the second most popular reason for seeking health information online, second only to satisfying curiosity (Li, Orrange, Kravitz, & Bell, 2014). One lesson is that satisfied patients may already feel their needs have been met, whereas dissatisfied ones do not.

Integrative Model of Online Health Information Seeking

Yet another dimension is added by the **Integrative Model of Online Health Information Seeking**, which posits that social structures and inequities manifest in individual differences that, in turn, influence how able and motivated people are to seek eHealth information (Dutta, Bodie, & Basu, 2008). About 9% of adults in the United States have difficulty reading or understanding English, and the percentages are even higher in many parts of the world (United States Census Bureau, 2017). An increased reliance on computer-mediated information may create an even larger gap between them and people who are already rich in health information. (We'll return to this topic in a moment.)

Literacy is not the only factor. If individuals believe health authorities don't care about people like them, they are unlikely to put much stock in their advice or to actively seek health information from them. Other barriers include limited access to technology and the perception that other concerns—such as hunger or day-to-day survival in a violent neighborhood—are higher priorities than long-term health. An important aspect of this theory is that it focuses on individual differences, but it recognizes that differences don't happen by chance. Discrimination, education, hunger, violence, and other factors are often rooted in macro-level issues that benefit some groups of people and disadvantage others. Dutta, Bodie, and Basu (2008) explain:

> *In the absence of health-enhancing structures within the minority community, young people are less likely to learn about the relevance of health behaviors, to have role models promoting health behaviors, and to value health-promoting behaviors owing to the lack of*

resources that would support such behaviors. As a consequence, they are more likely to focus on the daily struggles of survival. (p. 184)

From this perspective, eHealth is not simply a matter of making information available. On a deeper level, issues such as trust and access influence how likely people are to seek out and to believe health information.

In contrast to the youth whom Dutta and colleagues describe, people who feel they are proficient at finding health information online are more likely than others to be active internet users (Duplaga, 2015). In this way, one set of advantages (skill and confidence) heightens others (knowledge and its benefits). This is noteworthy because, compared to television, internet navigation requires a higher level of confidence and a more sophisticated set of skills. There is also a degree of social expectation. The chance of going online is heightened when people perceive that (a) loved ones expect to them do so and (b) online information is valued by peers as useful and appropriate (Smith-McLallen, Fishbein, & Hornik, 2011). This points to another factor that may be lacking in underprivileged populations—the social expectation that people can use technology to improve their lives.

Not only are some people expected to go online, but, more and more, they are *required* to go online to accomplish such tasks as making appointments and paying medical bills (Magsamen-Conrad, Dillon, Verhoff, & Joa, 2019a, p. 9). Some doctors' offices send patients important health information and laboratory test results through email and confirm medical appointments via text messages. Unless patients have access to and can effectively use the internet and smartphones or tablets, they may not be able to participate fully in an increasingly digital health care system.

Age is often a factor that influences technology use. Kate Magsamen-Conrad and colleagues (2019a) found that older adults often have difficulty adopting and using communication technologies such as smartphones and tablets. Although more middle-aged and older adults use online resources than in years past (Pew Research Center, 2019), many of the older adults interviewed by Magsamen-Conrad's team (2019a) said they are unable to access email and text messages. The researchers concluded that, even when older adults use smartphones daily, their use of them is often limited "to the functionality of a land line telephone" (Magsamen-Conrad et al., 2019a, p. 9). This reflects "a serious eHealth digital divide" (p. 8) between older and younger adults, which is particularly regrettable because older adults generally have more health burdens than younger ones do (Magsamen-Conrad, Wang, Tetteh, & Lee, 2019b).

Unified Theory of Acceptance and Use of Technology

Apart from age and access (which is often determined by a person's socioeconomic status), other factors also shape how people think about and use new technologies. As it has evolved, the **Unified Theory of Acceptance and Use of Technology** (UTAUT) identifies five key factors that influence people's intention to use new technology (Venkatesh, Morris, Davis, & Davis, 2003; Venkatesh, Thong, & Xu, 2012):

- *Social influence*, in this context, is the degree to which people believe close others (such as family members or friends) value their technology use.
- *Performance expectancy* is a measure of how useful people think a technology will be in helping them complete tasks, such as looking for health information online or scheduling an appointment with a doctor.
- *Effort expectancy* refers to how hard or easy it is to use a new technology.
- *Facilitating conditions* reflect the availability of helpful resources and/or support.
- *Hedonic motivation* is the pleasure associated with using a technology. Overall, this is the single best predictor of technology use outside of settings such as work and school (Venkatesh et al., 2003).

When combined, these factors fairly accurately predict people's intention to use a particular technology (e.g., smartphone or tablet) and their subsequent behavior (Venkatesh et al., 2003). Moderating variables include gender, age, and experience (Venkatesh et al., 2012). For example, facilitating conditions and price were the most important determinants for older women, whereas hedonic motivation was the most important determinant for young, technologically inexperienced men (Venkatesh et al., 2012).

Understanding how UTAUT determinants differ among user types can help researchers and public health officials design targeted eHealth literacy campaigns. Magsamen-Conrad et al. (2019b) found that generational differences in UTAUT determinants explain (and may even predict) disparities in eHealth literacy. For example, baby boomers and generation Xers are usually less affected by social influence than are millennials (Magsamen-Conrad et al., 2019b). The implication is that eHealth campaigns that target boomers and gen Xers may be more successful if they downplay social expectations while addressing more salient determinants such as effort expectancy and facilitating conditions.

As you can see, theories about information seeking and technology use naturally overlap because they reflect similar phenomena, but theorists add various nuances to the picture. Most scholars suggest (and research supports) that people are most likely to seek health information if they are confident that they can find it and use it effectively, they feel emotionally capable of dealing with what they find, and they expect that the results will be worth the effort. The Theory of Motivated Information Management focuses a great deal on interpersonal sources of information and reminds us that the source and channel sometimes matter as much as the content. As one of the first models to focus specifically on electronic modalities, the Integrative Model of Online Health Information Seeking calls attention to social structures and opportunities that constrain individual action. The Unified Theory of Acceptance and Use of Technology explains what people take into account when deciding whether they will use new technologies.

Is eHealth Information Useful to Everyday People?

eHealth information usually comes to people's attention in one of two ways—through active searches for information on trustworthy websites or via pop-up advertisements and tangential hits. As you might imagine, these two sources of information are often contradictory. We discuss this topic in more detail later in this chapter, but, first, let's focus on the advantages of trustworthy eHealth information.

Advantages

Online sources offer plentiful opportunities for people to learn about health and connect with others on health topics. About 80% of internet users have searched for health information, which brings them many benefits (Weaver, 2013).

RICH ARRAY OF INFORMATION

The internet is typically deeply engaging, which gives it a leg up on brief TV news spots. For example, people who rely on newspapers and the internet for cancer information are typically better informed than people who rely on local TV news, probably because information in writing is usually more detailed and precise than televised content (Kealey & Berkman, 2010). Furthermore, people who rely on TV news for cancer information often underestimate their cancer risk because such programming often focuses on ways to prevent cancer, which makes cancer seem more avoidable than it sometimes is (Kealey & Berkman, 2010).

SOURCE OF PRACTICAL ADVICE

The internet offers health-related guidance 24 hours a day, making it a convenient and accessible source. Here are some of the main ways people use online health resources:

- People often go online to learn about particular conditions and treatments (Lee & Lin, 2019). These searches are typically most satisfying when they help people meet targeted goals, such as learning how to treat a minor injury or cure a headache (Lee, Park, & Widdows, 2009).
- Many people, older adults especially, use the internet to help them decide if they should see a doctor (Magsamen-Conrad et al., 2019a). Forty-six percent of the people who use the internet for this reason end up seeking medical care (Weaver, 2013).
- Health care providers and medical students often use the internet to search for the meanings of medical terms and details related to specific diseases, treatments, and medication side effects (Wernhart et al., 2019).

Of course, online advice is only useful if it is trustworthy. As we will discuss in a moment, that is sometimes a shaky supposition.

SOCIAL SUPPORT

Online resources help people share information and social support. This opportunity is particularly beneficial for people who are short on time or transportation, find comfort in the relative anonymity of technology-mediated conversations, or have disabilities or responsibilities that prevent them from leaving home. H. Erin Lee and Jaehee Cho (2019) found that among people with mobility disabilities, those who reported higher levels of social media use and participation in online support communities had lower levels of depression.

Social media plays an important role when it comes to online support, but evidence is mixed. Typically, the more "likes" and comments people receive on their social media posts, the more support they believe is available to them (Seo, Kim, & Yang, 2016). But there is evidence that too much online feedback can be overwhelming, and too little feedback on health-related posts can be hurtful (Oeldorf-Hirsch, High, & Christensen, 2019). Although researchers have drawn different conclusions, the consensus is that receiving online support is beneficial for many people.

Disadvantages

Despite the potential advantages of online communication, eHealth offerings fall short in some ways.

UNRELIABLE INFORMATION

Online information is sometimes incomplete or inaccurate (Chesser, Burke, Reyes, & Rohrberg, 2016). For example, only 1 in 5 weight loss websites studied by researchers provided consistently accurate information (Modave, Shokar, Peñaranda, & Nguyen, 2014). Misleading and inaccurate health information can cause serious harm, emotional distress, and even death (Chesser et al., 2016).

Health care providers worry that patients will use inaccurate information they find online to self-diagnose (Wernhart et al., 2019). Only 40% of "online diagnosers" have their diagnoses confirmed by medical professionals (Weaver, 2013, para. 2). This means that the majority of online diagnosers get it wrong. People sometimes avoid seeking medical care, even for very serious conditions, because they erroneously conclude that their symptoms are minor based on faulty information. To make matters worse, even when health information is wrong or incomplete, it tends to circulate quickly through social media.

Researchers led by Brittany Seymour studied the way information about fluoride proliferated among members of an online community who oppose adding it to public water supplies. The researchers traced thousands of online engagements to two highly influential Facebook posts presented as summaries of scientific research. The original posts were viewed, liked, shared, and/or commented on 4,500 times, representing what Seymour and colleagues call a "digital pandemic" of information. In this case, it was equally a pandemic of misinformation. About half of the posts misrepresented the research they purported to summarize. The discrepancies were difficult to detect, however, because 60% of hyperlinks to the original studies required viewers to sift through multiple web layers to find them, and about 12% of the links were dead ends. The researchers reflect that rampant transfer of misinformation is fed by the ease of social media use compared to in-depth data searches and by people's tendency to follow and "friend" people whose attitudes are similar to their own (Seymour, Getman, Saraf, Zhang, & Kalenderian, 2015).

In light of how much unreliable information is available, media literacy is critical. However, when researchers asked university students to rate the quality of medical information from two different sources—the U.S. National Institutes of Health and a pharmaceutical company—the students rated information from both sources about the same, although one was an independent, science-based source and the other a commercial enterprise with an interest in selling products (Kim, 2011). On the other hand, Twitter users in another study trusted original tweets from health experts more than they trusted tweets from nonprofessionals (Lee & Sundar, 2013). Even among people who reported being eHealth literate, their "skills, when put into practice, were often inadequate to appropriately locate,

Although people over age 60 are more likely than young adults to have health concerns, they are only one-third as likely to learn about health online (Smith, 2011).

understand and evaluate quality health information" (Chesser et al., 2016, p. 14). Clearly, the issue is complex. As you will see in Chapter 11, one of the keys to media literacy is considering the sender's motive and whether the sponsor is likely to be biased.

One aspect of media literacy involves the type and amount of information people seek and remember. Jeff Niederdeppe and colleagues (2007) differentiate between **health information seeking**, which involves an active search for information, and **health information scanning**, which includes information that comes up in conversation or in the media and sticks in the memory. They have found that information gained while health *seeking* is usually of greater depth and of more direct assistance in making medical decisions. However, people are exposed to far more information incidentally than purposefully, making health *scanning* important as well.

CONFLICTING INFORMATION

A second drawback concerns information that is contradictory or counterproductive. Jones and Biddlecom (2011) point out that the internet is not great at providing sex education, but research shows that 84% of teens report getting information about health, including information about sex, from the internet (Wartella et al., 2016). As one teenager put it, you can find information about safer sex and abstinence online if you look for it, but along the way you are likely to find a lot more information leading you in the opposite direction:

> *The Internet, it's pretty much just like a giant billboard for sex. It's really, it's not a good place to go if you are young, because being on Internet, because all the pop ups and things you could type in kind of makes you want to have sex. So it really doesn't enforce the abstinence rule and birth control, safe sex anything.* (quoted by Jones & Biddlecom, 2011, p. 118)

Like this teen, most of those in Jones and Biddlecom's study felt that the internet was not a helpful source of information about abstinence or contraception.

OVERWHELMING AMOUNTS OF INFORMATION

A third drawback is the sheer volume of information provided online, which can be especially baffling when it is new to the reader, complex, or far outside the realm of common knowledge. A recent Google search for "breast cancer" yielded more than 300 million hits. For most people—80%, according to Weaver (2013)—health information seeking starts with a search engine, such as Google or Yahoo, but most people are unwilling or unable to wade through millions of search results to find the best or most accurate information. For example, Wartella et al. (2016) found that half of teenagers who look for health information online click on the first Google result and only visit additional websites if they still have unanswered questions.

In a study of online resources for people with HIV or AIDS, Keith J. Horvath and colleagues (2010) found an extensive but potentially bewildering amount of information. Information overload can be especially distressing for people who are newly diagnosed and may not yet have a good idea what to expect or how to judge the timeliness and quality of the information they find. Horvath and his team suggest that website developers create a framework that begins with a general overview and allows readers to move in stages to more complex and varied information. Otherwise, they say, rather than serving as a source of comfort, online information can be frightening, confusing, and overwhelming.

PRIVACY CONCERNS

Some people are hesitant to use online health resources and health apps because of privacy concerns. This is particularly true of older adults, but among people of all ages there is heightened worry about data privacy when it comes to health (Magsamen-Conrad et al., 2019b). Health care professionals also worry about data privacy and security (Wernhart et al., 2019), especially with respect to electronic medical records (Overton, 2020). Electronic records, like records in financial and banking industries, are vulnerable to hackers. Over 113 million people—about one-third of the U.S. population—had their health records "breached" in 2015 (Office of the National Coordinator for Health Information Technology [ONCHIT], 2018).

Communication Skill Builder: Using the Internet Effectively

To distinguish between trustworthy and unreliable information online, experts offer the following suggestions:

- Don't trust information if there is no author or sponsor or if the source given is not well known.

- Look for another source if the sponsors are trying to sell a product rather than offer free information. Plenty of websites make reliable health information available free.
- Don't rely on information if it is dated or its references are missing or don't seem legitimate.
- Keep in mind that legitimate health practitioners don't speak in terms of "secret formulas" or "miraculous cures." Only con artists use such language (Kowalski, 1997). Other red-flag claims include such wording as "Treats all forms of cancer," "Cancer disappears," and "Nontoxic" (U.S. Food & Drug Administration, 2008).
- Don't be convinced by case studies of "actual" satisfied customers. An isolated case does not prove a product's effectiveness, and this may not be an actual customer.
- Do your own research. Read medical journal articles. Ask health professionals.
- Read the fine print carefully. Look for disclaimers and vague wording.
- Report suspicious claims to the Federal Trade Commission, Better Business Bureau, or state attorney general's office.

In case you are wondering what happened to the student whose jaw got stuck open: She eventually woke her roommate and the two of them conducted a more thorough search on their computer. "I had to put a washcloth in my mouth because I was drooling," the student now says, laughing. "We *had* to fix it!" But when nothing they read online worked, they went to a hospital emergency room, where a doctor was able to get her jaw in place again.

Interestingly, when the same thing happened to the student several weeks later, she did not go online. Instead, she went straight to the ER. Her sense of self-efficacy had vanished during the first experience. "I tried. It's too hard," she says. Her experience bears out the conclusion that online information can be immensely valuable, but it is not always enough.

Is eHealth Information Useful to Care Providers?

Health care providers in general, and physicians in particular, are often skeptical when it comes to new health information technologies. Numerous studies show that physicians tend to focus on eHealth's disadvantages rather than on potential benefits (Overton, 2020; Wernhart et al., 2019). A meta-analysis of 221 research articles conducted by Conceição Granja and colleagues revealed that providers' skepticism is justified in many instances because nearly half of all eHealth initiatives fail (Granja, Janssen, & Johansen, 2018). Their analysis showed that eHealth programs (e.g., electronic medical records, health apps, email, online recourses, and telehealth) most often failed for the following reasons:

- eHealth harmed provider–patient relationships and reduced face-to-face communication between the parties.
- Providers' workload increased after eHealth initiatives were implemented, as did the amount of time required to complete clinical tasks.
- Initiatives were expensive to adopt and costly to maintain.
- Initiatives were hard to integrate into existing clinic practices.
- Certain initiatives, such as electronic medical records, produced too much data for providers to reasonably sort through and effectively use during the course of regular patient care.
- Initiatives were poorly designed and thus hard to use. In fact, design and usability are among the biggest challenges eHealth developers face (Farahani et al., 2018; Moore, Wilding, Gray, & Castle, 2019; Overton, 2020; Palokangas, 2017).

To combat usability problems, scholars advocate *participatory design*—an approach that actively involves a technology's intended users from product conception to completion. The Center for eHealth Research

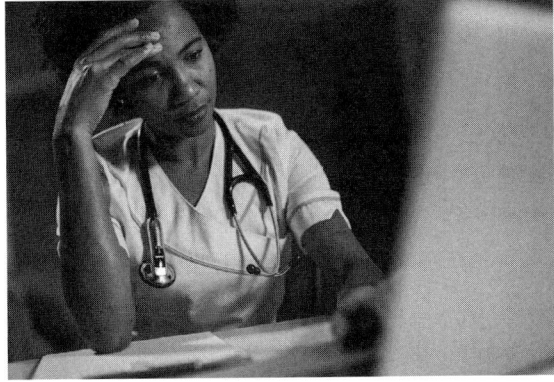

Many health care providers are frustrated by hard-to-use electronic medical records systems. Scholars believe a participatory design approach that includes providers' perspectives and ideas will alleviate some of the problems that derail many eHealth initiatives.

and Disease Management proposed a design "roadmap" to help guide eHealth developers in participatory design practices. The roadmap (van Gemert-Pijnen et al., 2011) is based on several factors: the involvement of end users, continuous evaluation and feedback, a focus on every stage of technology integration, and a commitment to improving health care. However, the roadmap is underutilized (Moore et al., 2019), and few eHealth designs—especially those involving data management and electronic medical records—incorporate users' perspectives.

Another disadvantage for providers has to do with *interoperability*, the ability to share and use data across multiple platforms (similar to the way Mac users and PC users can exchange images and documents). Unfortunately, most electronic medical records systems used in U.S. hospitals are *not* interoperable (Overton, 2020). To use an analogy, imagine you have a video game on two DVDs, one programmed for Xbox and the other for PlayStation, but you only have a desktop computer. Although both discs have the same game, you cannot play it on the computer from either disc. Because of this disconnect, patients' health records cannot be easily transferred between health care providers or hospitals. For many providers, this is the biggest eHealth disadvantage they face.

Impact of eHealth

> *With the best will in the world, unless your friends and family have been through it they just won't get it.... They won't understand the raw pain of not being able to have your own children. The only people who will understand that are other people who are in your place. And now the Internet is here, I mean what people did before the Internet I don't know.*

This statement by a participant in Lisa Hinton et al.'s (Hinton, Kurinczuk, & Ziebland, 2010, p. 439) study of people undergoing fertility treatment brings up a good question: *How are things different since the internet?*

Some analysts worry that, whereas before the internet people relied almost exclusively on health professionals and loved ones for medical information and

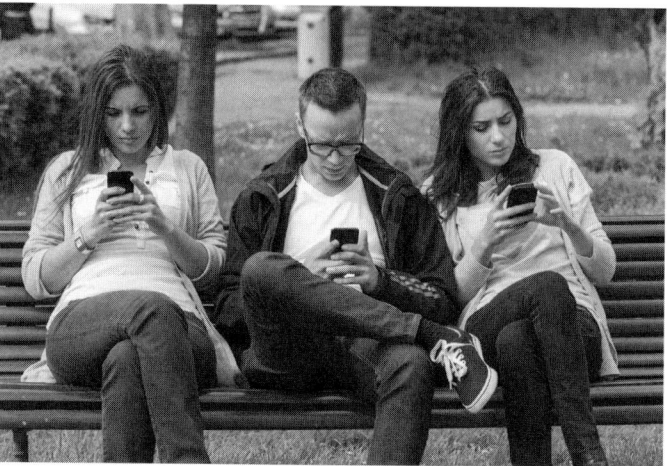

Almost half of young adults say they are online "almost constantly" (Perrin & Kumar, 2019). Uses and gratifications theory suggests that they use mobile media to meet social, information, and cognitive needs.

advice, they may now rely on internet sources instead. So far, the evidence is reassuring. People do not seem to pick only one source of information. In fact, cancer survivors who seek information both online and from health professionals often find that one source reinforces the other, adding a sense of depth and validity to what they learn from both (Moldovan-Johnson, Tan, & Hornik, 2014). Several studies show that while people value the internet as an important source of supplemental information, they rely primarily on their health care providers for health information (Jiang, 2018; Lee & Lin, 2019; Magsamen-Conrad et al., 2019a).

Overall, evidence suggests that people use online and interpersonal communication to varying degrees based on how accessible each form of communication is and how well it meets their needs. In some ways, the internet has become a means to meet social and informational needs that face-to-face communication does not satisfy (Hou & Shim, 2010). This phenomenon is well expressed in **uses and gratifications theory**, which suggests that people engage with mediated messages in an active, goal-oriented way. The implication is that, far from being passive recipients of whatever comes their way, people are motivated to engage with media when doing so satisfies their need for information, cognitive exercise, social stimulation, escape, entertainment, or some other need (Katz, Blumler, & Gurevitch, 1974).

Consider the reasons you turn on the TV, boot up your computer, or check your mobile device after a long day. Maybe you hope to catch up on the day's news (information needs), relax and forget about your worries (escape and entertainment), watch a show about the history of the solar system (cognitive exercise), enjoy the familiar personalities of characters in your favorite sitcom (social stimulation), or catch up with friends via Facebook or other social media (social interaction).

As media have changed, so have people's habits. Nearly half of adults ages 18 to 29 say they are online "almost constantly" (Perrin & Kumar, 2019) and about 60% of college students say they probably qualify as addicted to their cell phones (Roberts, Luc Honore Petnji, & Manolis, 2014). Experts agree, considering that college students spend an average of 7 to 10 hours a day on their phones (sometimes while doing other things), mostly interfacing with friends via texts, emails, and Facebook (Roberts et al., 2014).

Conversely, perhaps you had a great day and just want to sit outside and watch the sun set in peace and quiet. This may be a sign that, today at least, you do not need electronic media to satisfy needs. They have been met in other ways.

The same premises apply to health needs. As mentioned, people use the internet to expand their knowledge. They also use it to meet needs they have not been able to fulfill otherwise. For example, women newly diagnosed with breast cancer who have unmet needs for information or emotional support are more likely than others to use internet sources and to gravitate to the type of online information that best meets their needs (Lee & Hawkins, 2010).

By the same token, online interactions may help people satisfy their need for comfort and belonging. When Hinton et al. (2010) interviewed people undergoing treatment for infertility, they discovered a pervasive sense of social isolation among them. Because conceiving a baby is an intimate and emotional matter and people sometimes feel they have personally failed when they cannot conceive, many of those interviewed felt separate from the people around them—as if they were the "odd one out" or even a "leper" or "pariah" (Hinton et al., 2010, p. 438). Many said the internet was a "friend," a "lifeline," or their "only friend" during the experience (p. 438). One woman interviewed for the study described her experience with an online forum this way:

> *And you suddenly feel normal. You feel accepted. You can go on the forum and say, you know, "I've just walked past a pregnant woman in Sainsbury's and I found myself standing in the fruit and veg aisle bawling my eyes out." And everyone else would think, "Oh, that's a bit of an overreaction." The girls in the forum were just like, "No I'm with you, I've done that, I've been there." (p. 438)*

In this way, internet conversations were often a source of simultaneously personal and anonymous support. This was true both when people merely "lurked" (read without commenting) on sites and when they took an active role.

Another link between eHealth and patient–caregiver relationships is that patients do not always disclose to their doctors that they use online resources. Forty-seven percent of people do not discuss what they find online with their health care providers (Weaver, 2013), and this can often lead to misunderstandings and confusion. Rebecca Imes and colleagues found that patients are likely to stay quiet about online searches if (a) they feel confident that they can judge the quality of online information for themselves, (b) they are afraid their caregivers would think less of them, (c) they do not feel there is enough time to work the topic into a conversation, and/or (d) they do not want to give the impression of encroaching on the care provider's "turf" (Imes, Bylund, Sabee, Routsong, & Sanford, 2008, p. 545). Imes et al.

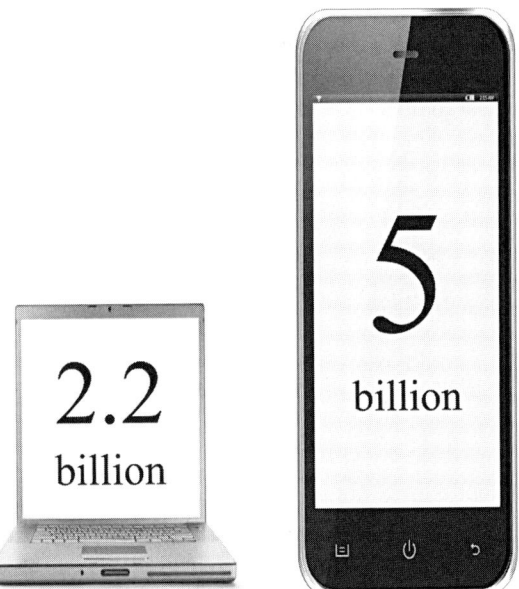

Worldwide, mobile technology is more than twice as prevalent as computer-based Internet usage, especially in developing countries, where people are more likely to have mobile technology than electricity in their homes.

caution that patient satisfaction and quality of care may be compromised if patients do not feel comfortable disclosing what they are thinking to their doctors or checking the veracity of information they have seen online.

All in all, it seems that the internet has provided people with another option for serving their information and relational needs. Like most options, it can be taken too far. However, people largely use online information as a complement to, not a substitute for, face-to-face health communication. Let's shift now to a particular type of eHealth that relies on mobile technology.

mHealth

Toralv Østvang, 67, was wearing his Apple Watch when he fell at home and fractured his skull. The watch's fall detection feature called emergency services and alerted Toralv's family via text message. The ambulance crew found Toralv "bloody and unconscious" (quoted in Thubron, 2019, para. 3). It's unlikely that Toralv would have survived the night if his watch had not summoned help.

Ed Dentel, 46, was playing with his Apple Watch's electrocardiogram feature when an alert indicated he had an abnormal heart rhythm. A trip to the doctor the next day confirmed Ed had atrial fibrillation, or AFib (Youn, 2018), a leading cause of strokes and hospitalizations in the United States (Stanford University, 2019). With a heads-up from his watch, Ed was able to get ahead of a potentially deadly condition. Now he's seeing a cardiologist regularly and taking medication to keep his AFib in check.

The Apple Watch's ability to safely and accurately detect AFib was the subject of a study involving more than 400,000 participants. Researchers at Stanford University School of Medicine found that the watch correctly identified AFib 84% of the time (Stanford University, 2019). The dean of Stanford's medical school, Lloyd Minor, says that the results "highlight the potential role that innovative digital technology can play in creating more predictive and preventive health care" (Stanford University, 2019, para. 5). He added, "Atrial fibrillation is just the beginning, as this study opens the door to further research into wearable technologies and how they might be used to prevent disease before it strikes" (Stanford University, 2019, para. 5).

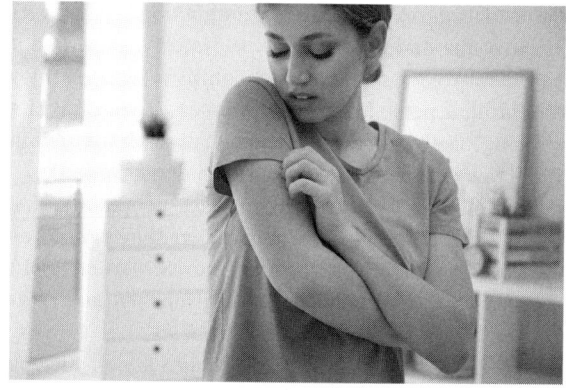

Worried about a skin rash or a suspicious mole? Smartphone apps now allow you to take a picture of it and submit it for computer analysis. Within minutes, you will receive a diagnosis and suggestions about what to do next, whether that involves treating a minor condition yourself or seeing a doctor for a more serious concern.

In addition to wearable technologies, such as Apple Watches, more than 267,000 mobile health apps are available on platforms such as iOS, Android, and Windows Phone (Research 2 Guidance, 2018). Some apps use computer algorithms to diagnose conditions and offer recommendations in minutes. For example, a person with a suspicious mole can use an app to help determine if medical attention is advised and what to do next. The process is as easy as uploading a photo, and most of the results are written so that even children can understand them (Topol, 2015). The result, according to cardiologist Eric Topol, is a rise not only in smartphones, but of increasingly smart *patients*.

In the future, Topol (2015) predicts, technology will figuratively promote people to the executive boardroom in terms of their own health. Whereas previously they may have seen themselves as low-level employees at best, with technology patients may function more as chief operating officers (COOs). "The COO monitors *all* the operations of the body. [They are] fully in charge," Topol says (p. 12). If people function as COOs of their own health, then smartphones are their crackerjack information technology departments that provide up-to-the-minute, easy-to-understand data and visuals so they can make well-informed decisions. Topol compares that process to the traditional medical model, in which people have often waited weeks for medical appointments, seen doctors for only about 10 minutes at a time, waited even longer for diagnostic tests and analysis, and then rarely had full access to their own medical charts or test results.

Within the model that Topol (2015) envisions, technology does not replace communication with one's physician; it *enhances* it. Physicians will function as chief executive officers, meaning they will not try to do everything themselves. Instead, they will help prepare patients and other members of the care team to manage day-to-day operations, which will free doctors to spend more time with patients when serious issues emerge.

Not everyone is optimistic about the move toward more virtual interactions and patient autonomy. Larry Huston, a medical journalist, worries that false positives (like Apple Watches erroneously alerting wearers that they are in AFib) will overwhelm health care systems with droves of healthy, young adults seeking medical care for conditions they do not have. Huston (2019) wrote, "There's a lot of enthusiasm out there for new, high-tech devices like the Apple Watch, but it is extremely difficult to find thoughtful perspectives on the complex medical issues they raise" (para. 17). Daniel Yazdi (2019) wrote, "As a physician, I'm excited about this new frontier in digital health. But I'm also cautious about its implications" (para. 3).

For his part, Topol (2015) is excited about a possible future in which patients understand very well what is wrong with them, and know when to manage issues on their own and when to seek help. He got a taste of that when a patient emailed him an electrocardiogram pattern with the message, "I'm in atrial fib, now what do I do?" Topol reflects:

> I knew the world had changed. The patient's phone hadn't just recorded the data—it had interpreted it! A smart algorithm was now trumping my skills as a cardiologist. Putting this power in everyone's pocket could preempt an emergency room visit or an urgent clinic appointment. (p. 6)

Whereas some health professionals might be threatened by this sea change, Topol considers it to be a "democratization of medicine" that may support good health and lower health care costs. (See Box 9.1 for more on the issue.)

We have seen that smartwatches and smartphones can detect and help monitor conditions like AFib. But what if data extracted from smartphones and tablets could be used to *predict* disease? According to cutting-edge research presented at a conference in August 2019, such a thing is possible! A team of researchers led by Richard Chen wondered if data mined from mobile devices could detect subtle signs of early cognitive impairment and/or Alzheimer's in older adults. Chen and his colleagues (2019) noted that although more than 47 million people worldwide have dementia, early diagnosis remains clinically very difficult because initial symptoms are hard to detect and many symptoms (e.g., memory problems and misplacing items) are often attributed to "normal aging." Consequently, therapeutic interventions are delayed and medications—which can slow the progression of Alzheimer's if given early (National Institute on Aging, 2018)—are not administered in time.

When comparing data extracted from the mobile devices of persons with and without cognitive impairment, Chen and his colleagues (2019) identified certain key patterns. People with cognitive impairment typed more slowly, had less structured routines and movements, picked up and used their devices for the first time later in the day, sent and received fewer text messages, used the clock app more often, and used primarily only apps that Siri suggested. Someday in the near future, physicians may be able to monitor patient's mHealth data and detect Alzheimer's before symptoms are discernable.

mHealth, broadly speaking, is any health intervention that involves a mobile device. Advances made possible by mobile technology have worldwide implications. By 2025, it is estimated that 73% of all internet users will go online using only their smartphones (Handley, 2019). This reflects a general shift toward mobile technologies. In the U.S., as well as in emerging economies, more people own smartphones than computers (Anderson, 2019; Holst, 2019; Taylor & Silver, 2019). As a result, smartphones are helping narrow the digital divide. Sixty percent of smartphone users in emerging economies use their phones to look up health information online (Silver, Huang, & Taylor, 2019). Wireless signals now cover 85% of the world. Indeed, more people now—about five billion, according to Taylor and Silver (2019)—have mobile devices than have electricity in their homes. It's easy to see why mHealth has emerged as a particularly powerful means of sharing and recording health information. In this section, we look at two areas of mHealth: health apps and text-based health interventions.

Health Apps

Already there are hundreds of thousands of mobile phone apps that function as easy-to-use, low-cost versions of equipment usually found only in hospitals. You can use an app to monitor the heart rate of

> **BOX 9.1** Ethical Considerations

The Pros and Cons of Telemedicine

Earlier, you read about how Eric Topol (2015) envisions a medical system in which everyday people use technology to assess their health and learn about their options. In what he calls "the democratization of medicine," patients are empowered to manage their health and to consult health professionals when they need assistance.

Topol proposes that doctor visits and hospital stays will be less necessary in the future because patients and caregivers will be able to communicate in real time via audiovisual technology and because a great deal of diagnostic data will be collected and shared electronically. As Topol puts it:

> *Since 2600 BC, doctors ruled the roost. Now patients increasingly will be generating their own data—by doing the physical exam through smartphone sensors, for example—and driving their own care. They'll be able to video chat with a doctor at any moment, 24/7, for the same costs as a co-pay to see a doctor in person.* (Larkin, 2014, para. 4)

A contrasting view is presented by people who fear that eHealth will compromise doctor–patient relationships and lead physicians to offer medical advice to patients they have not met or examined but have only communicated with via phone calls, emails, online chats, or text messages. In 2015, Texas set some of the strictest limits on telemedicine to date, requiring that patients who consult with a health professional via telemedicine must be physically present at a satellite medical center at the time (Definitive Healthcare. 2015). Physicians who would like to communicate with local patients via technology must meet with them in person before offering them advice over a phone, computer, or mobile device. As one doctor puts it, "What can the quality of service be when it's sight unseen and you have no relationship to the patient?" (Walters, 2015, para. 14).

What Do You Think?

1. Are there situations in which you would prefer to consult with a health professional on the phone or via a video chat rather than visiting a doctor's office or emergency room? If so, when?
2. Are there circumstances in which a virtual medical visit or hospital stay would be inferior to an in-person interaction? If so, when?
3. Consider Topol's scenario in which a patient notices an unusual mole and is able to upload a photo of the mole via a smartphone app and find out in minutes (based on computer algorithms) if it appears to be harmless or if he or she should seek medical attention for it. What are the advantages of quick access to medical information of this nature? What are the disadvantages?
4. How might your life and health be affected by easy-to-use mobile health evaluators that could instantly tell you your blood alcohol level, heart rate, blood sugar level, sleeping patterns, and so on, and provide advice on responding effectively?
5. How might your life be affected if medical visits more often occur via telemedicine than in person?

an unborn child and share that information instantly with medical professionals (WHO, 2011). Such an app can facilitate prenatal care for women in remote regions and for those with high-risk pregnancies. Other remote monitoring apps can track diabetes, hypertension, and depression symptoms without patients having to see health care providers in person. These apps are especially helpful for people living in remote areas who would otherwise have to travel long distances for medical care and monitoring.

Health-related apps are generally easy to use. Many involve little more than a smartphone camera, with which you might instantly submit photos or video to learn, for example, if the bite on your arm is from a poisonous spider or if a person is exhibiting signs of a stroke (WHO, 2011). Or you might use an app to measure your blood alcohol level before driving; get instant guidance on how to perform CPR or help someone who is choking; or track weight changes, drug reactions, and other health issues.

Health apps are increasingly popular and lucrative. According to Research 2 Guidance (2016), a market research firm, there are 267,000 health apps and counting; health apps were downloaded 3.2

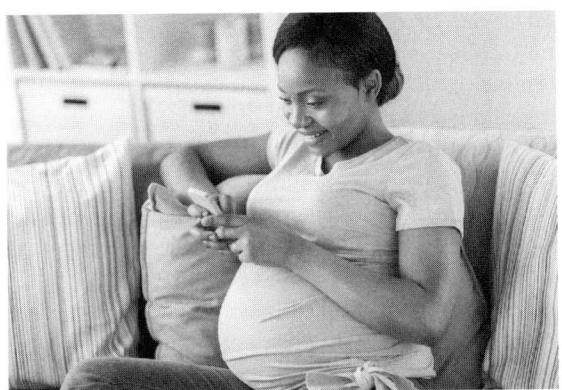

With new smartphone apps and attachable equipment, pregnant women can now monitor the movement and heart rate of their unborn babies and send the information instantly to a monitored database if they wish.

billion times in 2016 and used regularly by 551 million people; and by 2020, health apps were projected to generate $31 billion in yearly revenue. In terms of users, health apps are more popular with adults than with teens. Only a third of teens actively use health apps and they tend to focus on apps related to diet and exercise (Goodyear, Armour, & Wood, 2019). Among adult users, remote monitoring and diagnostic apps are the most widely used; about 56% of health apps are for patients with chronic conditions, like diabetes and hypertension (Research 2 Guidance, 2016).

Although most health apps are intended for patients, about a third are meant to be used by medical professionals (e.g., medical dictionaries and pharmacological encyclopedias). More than 80% of physicians and medical students surveyed reported using smartphones and medical apps regularly (Wallace, Clark, & White, 2012). Among those interviewed, many believed smartphones and apps helped improve their medical acumen, and some even predicted that apps would one day replace medical textbooks, but others worried that students' overreliance on apps could hinder their learning. As one physician said, "I think it might be promoting a more superficial knowledge of things as opposed to an in-depth knowledge of things" (Wallace et al., 2012, p. 4). One medical student admitted, "You can end up relying on it rather than memorizing" (Wallace et al., 2012, p. 4).

In another study involving medical students and apps, researchers also found that attitudes were mixed. A team led by Cara Quant that surveyed 731 medical students learned that the majority of them used medical apps daily and believed the apps enhanced their clinical knowledge, improved diagnostic accuracy, and improved patient care. Quant and colleagues also discovered that, despite medical apps being seen as useful, students were hesitant to use them in front of others. Fifty-three percent of students feared they would appear less competent if they used apps, and 54% worried that using apps while with patients would make them seem less engaged (Quant, Altieri, Torres, & Craft, 2016).

To date, it appears that mobile technologies have not been fully incorporated into medical education and clinical practice. Quant et al. (2016) concluded that "more studies are needed to better understand the impact of mobile technology in medical education and as a tool for medical professionals" (p. 5). Because mHealth is an evolving field, there is a lot we don't know. This is especially true when it comes to health apps. Little research has empirically demonstrated that health apps change people's health behaviors, and evidence is mixed as to whether apps improve health outcomes (Karcher & Presser, 2016; Oeldorf-Hirsch et al., 2019).

To better understand how apps affect health behavior, Sheana Bull and Nnamdi Ezeanochie (2016) proposed the **Integrated Theory of mHealth**. The theory posits that effective health apps are rich in content and actively engage users, thus compelling them to share their newfound health knowledge with others. Sharing that knowledge on social media leads to support, feelings of self-efficacy, and social norms that facilitate healthy behavior and better health. As Oeldorf-Hirsch et al. (2019) found, it all depends on the type of support people receive—network support, but not information support, improved people's health behaviors. The evidence on health apps is inconclusive, but other mHealth interventions have been studied more extensively and the findings, described next, are encouraging.

Texting for Health

Another area of mobile health is the use of **short message services** (**SMS**), such as texts and tweets. Many text-based health interventions are educational. For example, Kaprea Johnson and Michael Kalkbrenner (2017) analyzed several mHealth studies and found that text-based programs were popular on college campuses and were used to inform students about a wide range of topics, including nutrition, smoking cessation, alcohol abuse, sexual health, campus wellness resources, and mental health services.

Other text-based interventions have been used to effectively treat patients with eating disorders, depression, anxiety, schizophrenia, and substance use disorders (Karcher & Presser, 2016). Some text interventions are preferred by patients over more traditional interventions, like face-to-face counseling. For instance, 75% of smokers who participated in a text-based smoking cessation program reported they preferred receiving text messages to meeting with counselors (Kulhánek, Gabrhelík, Novák, Burda, & Brendryen, 2018).

Another program, Text2Quit, sends free emails and texts to people who are trying to quit smoking. In a study of university students who signed up for the program, three-quarters said they read all or most of every text (emails were less popular), and many used an online component of the program that allowed them to track how many cigarettes they smoked per day (Abroms et al., 2012). Far from being passive recipients, each student interfaced with the program an average of 12 times over three months, responding to text questions such as "Please be honest, did you quit today?" and requesting specialized messages, as when they texted CRAVE for help avoiding temptation.

Disadvantages

mHealth has many advantages, but there are some disadvantages too. Whether we're talking about apps or text messaging, privacy concerns top the list. Consider that when a health care provider texts a patient, there is no way for the provider to be certain that the person receiving the text message is the patient! Moreover, text messages can be read by anyone with access to providers' or patients' phones, and, like health apps, phones can be hacked. Patient privacy laws require providers to safeguard their patients' data, and failures to do so, even accidental failures, "can lead to civil and criminal penalties" for providers (Karcher & Presser, 2016, p. 13).

There are other potential disadvantages for providers who text their patients. First, some providers worry that texting blurs professional boundaries between themselves and patients. Second is the issue of compensation: there are no rules or laws governing how providers should charge or be paid for providing mHealth services (Karcher & Presser, 2016). Finally, interjurisdictional concerns mean some providers could be guilty of practicing medicine without a license. For instance, if a provider who is licensed in New York texts a patient who has traveled to Oregon where the provider is not licensed, is the provider breaking any laws? The answer is not always clear.

When it comes to health apps, data security is a big concern, but so too is the lack of government oversight. Because health apps are not regulated by the Food and Drug Administration, app developers are not held accountable for any false claims they make (Palmer, 2017). As a result, providers "face concerns regarding medical licensure and liability and making the choice of what apps may be best for their patients" (Palmer, 2017, p. 250). Additionally, patients have no way to know if the medical apps they use are safe. Until health apps are regulated, users should take caution when deciding which apps to use.

So far we have talked mostly about the interface between information consumers and creators. Let's move to a different component of eHealth.

Telehealth

It's common for residents in rural areas of Mississippi to drive 40 minutes or more to be seen by medical specialists. But a telehealth program offered through the University of Mississippi Medical Center has brought medicine closer to home. Since it was launched in 2003, the program has offered long-distance care, health education, disaster response, and other services to more than 500,000 residents of the state via more than 100 health centers ("Health Care Delivery," 2015).

The university's telehealth program allows patients and caregivers to interact in real time via two-way teleconferencing (Barnes, 2015). Medical personnel at the university work with staff members at medical centers throughout the state to conduct exams and discuss medical information. Digital cameras and stethoscopes transmit detailed information to everyone involved. The program was recognized by the American Telehealth Association as one of the best in the country.

Telemedicine and the broader term "telehealth" are derived from the Greek word *tele*, which means "far." As the World Health Organization (WHO) puts it, telemedicine is "healing at a distance" (WHO, 2010a, p. 8). Here are a few examples of how telehealth works, as well as the advantages and challenges it presents.

Telemedicine

Elsebeth and Ian have chronic obstructive pulmonary disease (COPD), a lung condition that affects about 65 million people worldwide and makes breathing difficult (COPD Foundation, n.d.). When they both experience a flare-up of symptoms, Elsebeth is hospitalized in the conventional sense, whereas Ian is admitted to a virtual hospital. Both see their doctors during daily

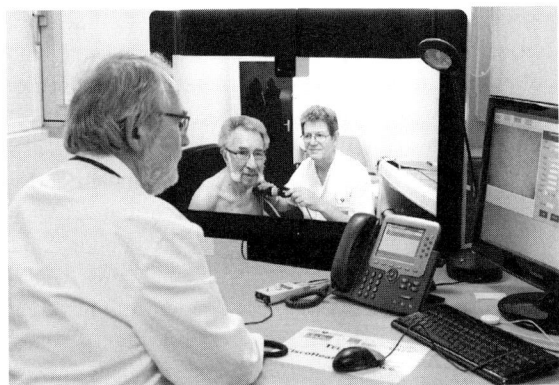

Health professionals in two locations collaborate to care for a patient using telemedicine technology.

rounds, but Elsebeth sees them in person, whereas Ian communicates via a two-way video chat. In addition, a care team visits Ian's home to provide medication, monitoring equipment, and a mobile tablet with which he can contact health professionals 24 hours a day to communicate with them in real time. Which situation would you prefer?

A team of researchers in Denmark addressed that question based on the impressions of actual COPD patients admitted to physical and virtual hospitals (Emme et al., 2014). They found that patients' impressions varied depending on the severity of their symptoms. Those who were frightened and felt their symptoms were out of control appreciated being in a conventional medical setting. However, those who were able to manage their symptoms fairly well valued the sense of being more in control of their care at home. Because patients of the virtual hospital were trained to use the medical equipment themselves, they were able to monitor their conditions and make minor adjustments to treatment regimens without seeking help or permission. Indeed, many of them were reluctant to return medical and communication equipment when they were discharged. Patients of the virtual hospital also appreciated the comforts of home and the relative ease with which loved ones could visit them. (Experts point out that there is also less exposure to contagion at home.) All in all, the researchers concluded that both brick-and-mortar hospitals and virtual care have their place.

So far, telemedicine is most popular among young and affluent patients who are most likely to be comfortable with technology. They most often use telemedicine (usually via telephone) for occasional and seasonal concerns, such as getting prescriptions refilled or treating urinary tract infections (Uscher-Pines & Mehrotra, 2014). Telemedicine may also gain footing with people who have chronic conditions such as Parkinson's disease. For them, long-distance consultations, coupled with regular in-person visits, may provide more contact with medical professionals than they would normally have, as long as the technology is readily available and people on both sides are trained to use it (Qiang & Marras, 2015).

Despite the obvious advantages telemedicine offers—especially for people living in remote areas and those who cannot travel easily to a doctor's office—demand for telemedicine services is lower than one might expect. A survey of more than 4,000 patients showed that only 20% of them felt it was important for their health care providers to offer telemedicine services (Welch, Harvey, O'Connell, & McElligott, 2017). But the Coronavirus pandemic in 2020 changed how many people viewed telemedicine. As this book was released, health care providers were offering—and patients were utilizing—telemedicine services in record numbers. Social distancing measures to combat the spread of the virus meant that telemedicine was oftentimes a safer alternative to in-office visits. It will be interesting to see if telemedicine's increasing popularity persists after the pandemic.

Patient Portals

If you have not already been granted access to a **patient portal**, you probably will be soon. These are password-protected websites, usually sponsored by people's physicians or hospitals, where patients can view lab results, schedule appointments, see their medical records and immunization history, view information and educational videos, email health professionals, make payments, and more.

Since 2011, the federal government has given financial incentives to health care providers and hospitals for adopting and meaningfully using health information technologies that can, among other things, allow patients to view, download, and share their health data electronically (Overton, 2020). Only 10% of hospitals had the technological infrastructure in place to allow patients to access or share their health records in 2010, but that percentage rose to 69% in 2015 (Office of the National Coordinator for Health Information Technology, 2018).

Despite patient portals becoming increasingly available, fewer than 20% of people use them (Pratt, 2018). Some researchers suggest that portals are underutilized because of their limited functionality and hard-to-use designs (Pratt, 2018). Others believe poor health literacy is the reason people steer clear (Coughlin, Stewart, Young, Heboyan, & Da Leo, 2018), and there is some evidence to support this.

In a study involving over 20,000 patients, Jennifer Lafata and colleagues (2018) found that only a third of the study's participants reported using patient portals. Patients with multiple chronic conditions (e.g., diabetes and hypertension) were more likely to use portals than healthier patients. Those less likely to use patient portals included African Americans, Hispanics, adults 70 years and older, and patients who preferred languages other than English—in other words, people who, traditionally, have been shown to have lower levels of health literacy. Although the study did not measure health literacy's direct impact on portal use, Lafata and colleagues maintained that it certainly played a part, along with patients' technology literacy and access to the internet.

Patient portals are designed to put patients in the driver's seat concerning their own care and to reduce busy work for health professionals. If portals are to be effective, however, they have to be easy to use and need to display data in ways that allow users—especially those with limited health literacy—to understand and manage their health data.

Telemonitoring

We have already discussed the leaps being made in mHealth monitoring, but in 2008, Glenn Forbes of Mayo Clinic envisioned an even more futuristic image of telehealth, in which people have small microchips inserted under their skin or carry digitized medical information cards that allow them—and, if they wish, medical personnel anywhere in the world—to monitor their health. Forbes imagined how the process would work if he were traveling in another country:

> *I feel fine, but I check in every once in a while. If I have a chip embedded, I might even be unknowingly "checking in." Every seven days Mayo checks my blood sugar and could send me a message about needing to cut back on the cookies because my sugar level went up from 116 to 124. This information and advice is part of my partnership—part of what I have decided to purchase for my personal benefit.* (quoted by Berry & Seltman, 2008, p. 239)

Health-monitoring chips have not yet become commonplace, but many analysts predict they will be available soon. Less invasive devices are on the horizon as well. Mayo Clinic has teamed up with a technology firm to develop disposable, stick-on biosensor patches that will help transmit information about diabetes, obesity, and other factors to people's smartphones, and with their permission, to their doctors and/or researchers (Pennic, 2015). Wearable technology, such as Apple Watches, Jawbone, Pebble Time, and Fitbit allow people to monitor their own health behaviors and may facilitate sharing that information with health professionals.

The majority of telemonitoring systems, however, require patients to do more than simply put on biosensor patches or wear smartwatches. According to a review of telemonitoring studies by Nazish Saeed et al. (2019), some users, particularly older adults, struggle with hooking up sensors and have difficulty reading data displayed on monitors. At present, the most widely used systems monitor patients with obstructive pulmonary disease, heart failure, and other chronic diseases—and mistakes that these patients or their caregivers make while using telemonitoring equipment "can lead to serious health consequences" (Saeed, Manzoor, & Khosravi, 2019, p. 2). Calls for more user-friendly technology will undoubtedly be met in coming years, bringing us closer to Forbes's vision of telemonitoring.

Forbes says this futuristic model will not alleviate the need for face-to-face health communication, good listening skills, and sensitivity. Indeed, because patients' information will be so readily available, he says, patients and caregivers might have *more* time to talk about their concerns (quoted by Berry & Seltman, 2008).

Potential Advantages of Telehealth for Consumers

The World Health Organization lists the main advantages of telemedicine as "access, equity, quality, and cost-effectiveness" (WHO, 2010a, p. 8). At this point, the pros and cons are largely speculative, but many people are optimistic that telehealth will conserve money and resources without sacrificing quality. Here are a few of the reasons why.

PATIENT-CENTERED COMMUNICATION

eHealth, including telehealth, is helping reshape our health care system by moving us away from a hospital- and physician-centered "sick care" system (which does not prioritize patient involvement) and nudging us closer to a patient-centered wellness care model (Farahani et al., 2018). Telehealth does that partly by enabling patients' increased access to care providers and more options for talking about a wider range of topics. For example, MyCareTeam.com allows people with diabetes to learn information, log their blood sugar levels, and talk to health care providers online. When James D. Robinson and colleagues (2011) studied nearly 1,000 emails exchanged by patients and providers in the program, they found that social integration messages (e.g., "Stop by next time you are in") were most common, followed by information giving and requests for information. They concluded that the interactions were "in some ways more patient-centered than a traditional office visit" (Robinson et al., p. 132).

Other researchers have also identified a patient-centered advantage. Shaohai Jiang (2018) discovered a positive association between health outcomes and patients communicating with their physicians online. Patients' general and emotional health was improved following satisfying online communication with providers, which, according to Jiang, highlights communication's curative properties.

Another study of patient–caregiver emails revealed that—in contrast to in-person visits where doctors do most of the talking—in emails, patients do most of the "talking," outnumbering physicians' comments 2 to 1 (Roter, Larson, Sands, Ford, & Houston, 2008). Patients also seemed more comfortable disclosing emotions and praising or thanking their doctors in emails than in person, perhaps because email communication is less intimidating and less constrained by time limits. Physician responses, although briefer than patients,' were usually informative, confirming, and reassuring. Doctors displayed empathy and reassurance in 53% of the emails Roter and colleagues studied. For example, one doctor told a patient via email, "Please don't ever think of doing so [emailing me] as bothering me—I welcome your participation in these decisions!" (Roter et al., 2008, p. 83). Overall, coders rated physicians' emails to be equally as friendly, respectful, and responsive as patients'.

ACCESS TO SERVICES

Telehealth may allow people in underserved communities access to care providers and services usually reserved for big-city dwellers. Doctors, particularly specialists, are disproportionately located in densely populated areas and are relatively scarce in rural ones.

With telemedicine, a person can conceivably contact a health professional anywhere in the world by phone, email, voice mail, or computer.

COST SAVINGS

Telehealth may save organizations and individuals money. For one thing, it reduces the need for each small town to have its own set of medical specialists. At an individual level, patients in smaller markets can stay close to home rather than transferring to major medical centers. Additionally, easier access may mean identifying and treating illnesses before they become severe and more costly to treat.

Potential Advantages of Telehealth for Health Professionals

Caregivers can benefit from telehealth as well. Telehealth expands health care systems' capabilities, hastens data exchange and diagnosis, improves communication, and optimizes providers' resources and time (Morozov & Vladzymyrsky, 2019). Let's focus on a few of these advantages.

EFFICIENCY

Being able to communicate with patients and colleagues in remote locations via teleconferencing, Skype, or FaceTime reduces providers' travel time and the need for office space and staff. Email also facilitates efficient communication (some scholars consider email an extension of telehealth and others classify it as mHealth). "Email is a timesaver," declares Shelly Reese (2008, para. 5). Rather than playing phone tag, health professionals can email colleagues and patients when time permits. Email also allows caregivers time to think through patients' questions and to research them before replying.

Furthermore, emails can reduce the number of unnecessary office visits and after-hours phone calls. Patients who are able to access their physicians via secure email require 7% to 10% fewer office visits and make 14% fewer after-hours calls to their doctors ("The Email Advantage," 2007; Reese, 2008). Texts and emails are also time savers for office staff members, who can use software to send out appointment reminders (Reese, 2008).

If health professionals are worried about receiving numerous and rambling emails from their patients, the evidence suggests they can rest easy most of the time. In a review of 24 studies about emails between patients and health professionals, Jiali Ye et al. (2010) found that the emails were usually concise and medically relevant. This was true of both patients' and doctors' emails. Patients typically addressed only one concern per email and avoided making urgent or inappropriate requests. In sum, patients who were invited to email seldom abused the privilege, but the knowledge that they *could* email their doctors made them feel significantly more satisfied about their care than patients without email access (Ye, Rust, Fry-Johnson, & Strothers, 2010).

TEAMWORK

Vital patient information can sometimes be transmitted from one location to another, amplifying opportunities for immediate response and medical teamwork. A cardiologist, for example, can monitor a patient's heart activity and direct paramedics' efforts even before the patient arrives at the hospital. At least 64% of the caregivers at one telemedicine site said they learned valuable skills and information while participating in exams with other doctors and specialists (Whitten, Sypher, & Patterson, 2000).

ACCESSIBLE INFORMATION

Diagnostic images and patient records can be electronically stored, retrieved, and—depending on the interoperability of different medical-records systems—shared. Caregivers thus may be able to review medical charts of patients they are seeing for the first time. This could save time in emergencies and allow medical teams to coordinate patient care more effectively. The ability to quickly and consistently share information also helps with routine decision making and teamwork. Says a radiology manager:

> *The biggest advantage is having images available all the time to everyone. So as soon as I take a picture of you, somebody can see it. In fact, everybody can see it. So where, if you were to come in . . . and you've broken an arm and you have to be referred to the orthopaedic surgeons, there is no backwards and forwards of one piece of film following you around or not as the case may be. (Murray et al., 2011, p. 6)*

Another advantage of electronic records is that a patient's records will not be destroyed in a fire or natural disaster.

Potential Disadvantages of Telehealth

With so many advantages, it may seem puzzling that telemedicine is not more prevalent. A few reasons have already been mentioned—lack of consumer demand, poorly designed patient portals, and difficult-to-use telemonitoring systems—but several other factors have stymied widespread telehealth adoption.

SCHEDULING CHALLENGES

One concern involves scheduling. Nearly half of the participants in one telemedicine center said it is a challenge to schedule two teams of medical providers (one on-site and one remote) to take part in telemedicine consultations (Whitten et al., 2000).

WORKFLOW DISRUPTIONS

Some telehealth systems have steep learning curves, so providers have to carve out time for training sessions, which means time away from treating patients. Once systems are integrated into the workflow, providers sometimes find that their workloads increase and tasks take longer to complete (Granja et al., 2018).

COST

Telemedicine is costly for providers to implement, primarily because of the expensive technology required (e.g., cameras, microphones, and remote sensors). Many smaller medical practices cannot afford the high startup costs, whereas larger, resource-rich practices are more likely to offer telemedicine services (Kane & Gillis, 2018). Smaller practices, particularly those in rural areas, have the greatest need for telemedicine yet are least able to afford it.

The issue of jurisdiction also affects cost. Many state medical boards require providers to be licensed in the state where telehealth services are provided (i.e., wherever the patient is). This increases costs for providers who acquire and pay for the medical licenses necessary to practice in multiple states.

COMPENSATION QUESTIONS

It is still somewhat unclear how caregivers can or should be compensated for services rendered long distance. Should they charge for phone conversations, email correspondence, and the like? If so, how should those rates compare to the cost of face-to-face visits? Reservations about this issue have made some caregivers leery of opening up new lines of communication.

The issue is becoming clearer, however, as health insurance agencies—mindful that a phone call or email can prevent a more expensive outcome—are increasingly willing to reimburse providers for technology-mediated communication. Some states have legislation in place that requires insurance agencies to reimburse in-person and telehealth service at the same rate. Medicare and Medicaid pay for some telemedicine services, as long as the services provided to patients are synchronous (e.g., a live video call) and take place in designated rural or underserved areas (Fathi, Modin, & Scott, 2017).

LIABILITY

There are also concerns about legal liability, especially concerning advice given online without the benefit of a full medical exam. In a study of more than 4,000 U.S. physicians, 73% said they worry they will be sued for malpractice if they offer medical advice online (Modahl et al., 2011). Legal experts caution doctors offering guidance or assistance online, especially if they have not treated the patient personally, to include disclaimers such as the following: "This is not an official medical opinion because I haven't performed an examination. If you need specific medical advice, make an appointment with me or with a physician in the appropriate specialty in your area" (Johnson, 2007, p. 30).

THREATS TO PRIVACY

Some people worry about electronic eavesdropping and the possibility that hackers could gain access to confidential patient records. Some 71% of physicians surveyed said they are worried about privacy violations (Modahl et al., 2011). To restrict access, medical networks rely on encryption (secret coding) and electronic "firewalls" designed to stop unauthorized users from reaching confidential data. Secure email systems endorsed by the American Medical Association and many private insurers are also available. By most accounts, these systems are good, although not perfect. As mentioned earlier in this chapter, 113 million people had their health records breached in 2015 (ONCHIT, 2018). Data privacy fears deter many patients from allowing their medical records to be uploaded to health information exchanges and shared among health care organizations (Esmaeilzadeh, 2019). Patients worry that sensitive information about their mental health, sexual health, and/or substance abuse could be leaked.

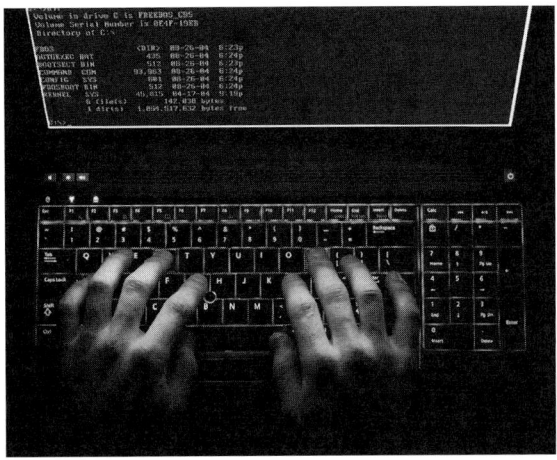

Even though electronic medical records systems have firewalls in place to prevent unauthorized access, about one third of the U.S. population has had their medical data breached.

Do you worry about the security of your health data?

UNORGANIZED INFORMATION IN ELECTRONIC MEDICAL RECORDS

Information in patients' electronic health records can be restrictive and hard to use if the platforms are not well designed and if physicians are not careful about what they include. Some electronic records systems require caregivers to document lengthy—and sometimes unnecessary—amounts of information. For example, an emergency medicine physician may have to document a male patient's last menstrual cycle (Overton, 2020), or a pediatrician may be required to ask every patient a time-consuming list of safety questions (use of bike helmets, seatbelts, etc.). Some electronic medical records systems will not allow providers to simply skip over irrelevant questions because each text box requires a response of some kind (Overton, 2020). Even typing "not applicable" (or the shorter form, "n/a") takes time, which leaves less time for providers to focus on the patient's immediate health concerns (Hartzband & Groopman, 2008).

Physicians Pamela Hartzband and Jerome Groopman (2008) describe an additional concern—namely, their frustration with doctors who include inappropriate or too much information in patients' electronic health records. In some cases, doctors copy and paste what other providers have previously documented. "We have seen portions of our own notes inserted verbatim into another doctor's note," say Hartzband and Groopman (p. 1656). In addition to being unethical, this "time-saving" practice results in repetitive, lengthy medical records that fail to present each physician's thoughtful analysis of the patient's condition.

Another factor that bogs down medical records is a lengthy hodgepodge of test results. If such information is not well organized, more is not better—it is just overwhelming. As physician Peter Viccellio explained in an interview with Overton (2020), when one of his emergency room patients was admitted to the hospital and discharged two weeks later, the patient's medical record contained over "8,000 pages of garbage [and] about 10 pages of useful data" (p. 114). Viccellio added:

> *One of the biggest disadvantages to electronic medical records is that these remain data systems, not information systems. In other words, it doesn't display information to me in an intelligent way. I have to hunt and hunt and hunt. New critical information may be in there, but there's no signal to me that it's there. I have to be lucky enough to find it. (Overton, 2020, p. 115)*

COMPROMISED QUALITY OF CARE

Stevens et al. (2019) found that some physicians—likely unsure where to look for important information in lengthy files— did not review patients' records before examinations. This is just one side effect of too-long medical records, but not reviewing patients' data can have serious consequences. For instance, providers might prescribe patients medicines that they are allergic to!

When looking at telehealth as a whole, there are other consequences to consider as well. Stevens and colleagues (2019) identified several threats telehealth posed for quality of care, chief among them being providers ordering fewer diagnostic tests and overprescribing antibiotics. Of course, these things happen during in-person medical exams too, but scholars note that the added strain of telehealth on patient–provider communication regularly compromises quality.

EFFECTS ON PATIENT–PROVIDER COMMUNICATION AND THERAPEUTIC RELATIONSHIPS

Finally, some worry that telemedicine will become a less effective substitute for face-to-face communication. No one expects (or even wants) telemedicine to replace face-to-face medical visits entirely. Still, technology changes how a patient and provider communicate, which, in turn, affects the therapeutic relationship they share.

Researchers in Japan found that patients who took part in both face-to-face interactions and telemedicine visits were equally satisfied with both formats, but doctors were less satisfied with the telemedicine visits, feeling that the technology limited communication (Lui et al., 2007). More than a decade later, Granja and associates (2018) found that providers still harbored fears about technology undermining face-to-face communication. Disrupting patient–provider relationships is one of the main reasons nearly half of all eHealth initiatives fail (Granja et al., 2018). A quarter of eHealth studies reviewed by Stevens et al. (2019) mentioned that providers felt the lack of face-to-face communication and the impossibility of physical examinations associated with telehealth created distance (physical as well as emotional) between themselves and patients.

One extreme case of telehealth going horribly wrong appears to validate providers' worst fears and poses some serious ethical questions. As told to a reporter for *The New York Times*, Annalisia Wilharm, 33, was visiting her grandfather in the hospital when "a tall machine on wheels . . . rolled into the room" (Jacobs, 2019, para. 4). The machine held a monitor which broadcast a live image of a physician wearing a headset. What happened next horrified Annalisia.

Annalisia and her family knew her grandfather's prognosis was very poor, but she "didn't think he'd get his death sentence" from a machine (Jacobs, 2019, para. 5). With the machine positioned near her grandfather's deaf ear, the telehealth physician onscreen explained that Annalisia's grandfather would not live long enough to be discharged from the hospital and admitted to hospice care. Because her grandfather could not hear the physician clearly, Annalisia had to repeat the news to him. "I wanted to throw up. It felt like someone took the air out of me," she recounted later (Jacobs, 2019, para. 5).

Annalisia's family and hospital administrators agree that the situation should have been handled differently. A spokesperson for the hospital pointed out that the telehealth visit was a follow-up to earlier in-person visits made by other members of the medical staff and emphasized that the patient's initial diagnosis was not delivered over video (Jacobs, 2019). But Annalisia was angry. "I just don't think that critically ill patients should see a screen . . . It should be a human being with compassion" (Jacobs, 2019, para. 27). Her grandfather died the next day.

> **BOX 9.2 Career Opportunities**
>
> ## Health Information Technology
>
> Computer and information systems manager
> Health information administrator or technician
> Software developer
>
> ### Career Resources and Job Listings
>
> - American Health Information Management Association: http://www.ahima.org
> - Association for Computing Machinery: http://www.acm.org
> - Commission on Accreditation for Health Informatics and Information Management Education: http://www.cahiim.org
> - Health Buzz by the U.S. Department of Health and Human Services: http://www.healthit.gov/buzz-blog/university-based-training/helping-students-launch-health-information-technology-careers-oregon-health-science-universitybased-training-program
> - U.S. Bureau of Labor Statistics Occupational Outlook Handbook: http://www.bls.gov/ooh

As Michael Chamberlain (1994) cautioned, high-tech methods cannot make up for poor communication: "No amount of technology is going to compensate for an ill-conceived or ill-designed message. The buck stops there . . . with the communicator" (para. 4).

All in all, WHO urges the creation of international guidelines in regard to privacy, access, and liability (WHO, 2010a). The authors of the Global Observatory for eHealth report write:

> *It is imperative that telemedicine be implemented equitably and to the highest ethical standards, to maintain the dignity of all individuals and ensure that differences in education, language, geographic location, physical and mental ability, age, and sex will not lead to marginalization of care.* (WHO, 2010b, p. 11)

If you are interested in the changes and opportunities involved with health information technology, see the career resources in Box 9.2.

Summary

Health Information Haves and Have Nots

- Communication technology has the capacity to revolutionize medicine.
- Some people feel communication technology will give everyday people more information and power than ever before, whereas others worry that it will affect patient–caregiver relationships for the worse.
- The internet has the potential to educate people in the greatest need of health information, but, overwhelmingly, the people who have internet access and the ability to use it are already information rich.
- A knowledge gap exists because of access, information preference, perceived relevance, ability, and health information efficacy.

Why and When People Seek eHealth Information

- Most people tend to be relatively proactive in seeking information they believe will reduce their health risk and help manage their anxiety.
- Health-seeking behaviors may be muted by distrust, lack of confidence, and the belief that some health messages do not apply to us.
- Several theories explain why people seek information. In most cases, people first consider how much they already know and then weigh the costs and rewards of seeking additional information.
- When the stakes are high, people typically prefer interpersonal communication with individuals they trust.
- The Integrative Model of Online Health Information Seeking proposes that social structures and inequities manifest in individual differences that influence how able and motivated people are to seek eHealth information.
- More and more, people are required to go online to accomplish such tasks as making appointments and paying medical bills.

Is eHealth Information Useful to Everyday People?

- About 80% of internet users have searched for health information online, and scholars recognize several advantages of trustworthy eHealth information.
- One advantage is that the internet offers a rich array of information compared with other sources (e.g., television news stories).
- Practical advice is readily available online 24 hours a day.
- The internet is also an important source of social support.
- There are several disadvantages of online communication, and eHealth attempts fall short in some ways.
- One major disadvantage is that information found online is not always reliable.
- Sometimes, eHealth information is contradictory or counterproductive.
- Another disadvantage is that there is often too much information online, which can be overwhelming.
- Privacy concerns and data security explain why some people are hesitant to search for health information online or use health apps.

Is eHealth Information Useful to Care Providers?

- Studies show that physicians tend to focus on eHealth's disadvantages rather than on potential benefits.
- Nearly half of eHealth initiatives fail for various reasons.
- One of the biggest disadvantages of eHealth is that it reduces face-to-face communication between providers and patients.
- eHealth initiatives, like electronic medical records, are costly to implement and increase providers' workload.
- Poorly designed initiatives are hard to use.
- Interoperability problems mean that providers often cannot share health information across multiple platforms. Many providers believe this to be the biggest eHealth disadvantage they face.
- Participatory design can help eliminate some of the disadvantages by incorporating providers' opinions, ideas, and preferences.

Impact of eHealth

- Studies show that while people value the internet as an important source of supplemental information, they rely primarily on their health care providers for health information.
- Evidence suggests that people use online and interpersonal communication to varying degrees based on how accessible each form of communication is and how well it meets their needs.
- Forty-seven percent of online-health-information seekers do not discuss what they find online with their health care providers. This can often lead to misunderstandings and confusion.

mHealth

- The proliferation of mobile devices represents a promising avenue. Mobile apps now allow people around the globe to capture and share data and advice about many health conditions and to monitor their activity levels, fitness goals, vital signs, and more.
- Smartwatches and smartphones can detect and help monitor conditions like AFib. Someday soon, data extracted from smart devices will be used to predict diseases.
- Health care providers also use medical apps. Many providers believe apps enhance their clinical knowledge, improve diagnostic accuracy, and improve patient care. Some providers, however, fear that using apps in front of colleagues or patients makes them appear less competent.
- mHealth carries privacy and data security concerns.

Telehealth

- Telemedicine offers many opportunities, but issues of cost, access, privacy, and legal liability continue to hamper full-scale implementation.
- Patient portals are password-protected websites where patients can view lab results, schedule appointments, see their medical records, and more. To date, many portals are hard to use and underutilized.
- There are several advantages of telehealth for patients, including better communication with providers, greater access to services, and cost savings.

- Health professionals can also benefit from telehealth initiatives, which can improve efficiency, facilitate teamwork, and improve access to patients' health information.
- Disadvantages for providers include scheduling conflicts, workflow disruptions, cost, compensation questions, medical liability risks, privacy concerns, unorganized information in electronic health records, and compromised quality of care.
- Overall, technology expands the options and the challenges for health communication. Patients and caregivers may have access to more information and more means of message transmission than ever before. The most optimistic possibility is that it will allow for higher quality and more inclusive communication at all levels.

Glossary

eHealth The use of technology to transcend geographical distance in promoting good health. *See page 118.*

ePatients People with illnesses who seek information or help from the internet to make informed health decisions. *See page 189.*

health information acquisition model The notion that people are motivated to seek information under specific conditions: when something calls their attention to a concern, they do not think that they are well informed, it seems important to find out soon, and they think they will be able to find trustworthy and useful information. *See page 191.*

health information efficacy How confident a person is that they can find and understand health information. *See page 190.*

health information scanning Information that comes up in conversation or in the media and sticks in the memory. *See page 196.*

health information seeking An active search for health information. *See page 196.*

information sufficiency threshold The amount of information a person needs in order to feel capable of coping with and understanding a threatening issue. *See page 191.*

Integrated Theory of mHealth The belief that effective health apps are rich in content and actively engage users, compelling them to share health knowledge with others. Sharing leads to support, feelings of self-efficacy, and social norms that facilitate healthy behavior and better health. *See page 203.*

Integrative Model of Online Health Information Seeking The belief that social structures and inequities manifest in individual differences that influence how able and motivated people are to seek eHealth information. *See page 192.*

mHealth The use of devices such as smartwatches, mobile phones, tablet computers, and personal digital assistants for health purposes. *See page 188.*

patient portal Password-protected websites, usually sponsored by people's physicians or hospitals, where patients can view their medical records, make appointments, and more. *See page 205.*

short message services (SMS) Text messaging service component of most telephone, internet, and mobile device systems. *See page 203.*

telehealth Using technology to facilitate long-distance health care, education, administrative teamwork, and disaster responses. *See page 188.*

telemedicine Subset of telehealth that specifically involves offering clinical services to patients at a distance, usually through the use of teleconference exams and shared diagnostic data, but also via phone and computer-mediated conversations. *See page 188.*

Theory of Motivated Information Management (TMIM) The idea that people seek information depending on their perceived need for it, their coping ability, and the channel in which the information is conveyed. *See page 191.*

Unified Theory of Acceptance and Use of Technology (UTAUT) The idea that five main variables influence people's intentions to use a new technology: social influence, how useful the technology is, how hard or easy it is to use, availability of helpful resources and support, and how pleasurable it is to use. *See page 193.*

uses and gratifications theory The idea that people engage with mediated messages in an active, goal-oriented way. *See page 198.*

Discussion Questions

1. How likely are you to sign up for texts and/or email services designed to help you reach particular health goals, such as eating better, working out more, or quitting smoking? Why? What aspects of these programs do you find most appealing (e.g., encouraging messages, online options to track your improvement, personal coaching, helpful hints, and so on)? What aspects, if any, do you find unappealing?

2. Do you think it is mostly a good idea or a bad idea for people to use mobile apps that diagnose their health conditions and suggest a course of action? Why?

3. Describe some of the most common reasons people seek health information online and the factors that might discourage them from doing so. Your answer should integrate the following terms and theories: information sufficiency threshold, the health information acquisition model, the Theory

of Motivated Information Management, and the Integrative Model of Online Health Information Seeking.

4. How does uses and gratifications theory help to explain eHealth behavior? Give an example from your own experience.

5. Imagine that you are miserable with a head cold. For what reasons, if any, might you seek information online? If you have the option, would you like to have a phone conversation or an email exchange with a health care provider, or would you rather meet with that person face to face? Why?

6. Have you ever used a patient portal? If so, what was your experience like? Did you find it easy or hard to use? Why? If you could design a patient portal, what features would it include?

7. How concerned are you about your medical records being breached? Are you worried about health information stored on your mobile devices being compromised? List some of the ramifications of your health information being made public. What steps can you take to help safeguard your health information?

8. Imagine that you are the manager of a small, suburban medical practice. Your staff is considering adopting an electronic medical record system as well as offering telehealth services. Are you for or against an electronic medical records system? What, if any, telehealth services do you believe a small medical practice like yours should offer patients? Prepare a list of pros and cons of electronic records and telehealth to share with the staff.

Communication in Health Organizations

PART V

People who devote their lives to serving others deserve excellent leaders who support their efforts and remove obstacles that might limit their effectiveness. In this section, which consists of one very important chapter, we look at what it takes to be a great leader in health care. As you will see, leaders have the potential to transform how health care is provided. They don't call all the shots. Instead, they bring out the best in people and enable them to create powerful systems designed to succeed. Leadership involves health care administrators, but also the work of human resources, marketing, and public relations professionals, whose job it is to build great teams, support outstanding service, and serve the community. Ultimately, the communication abilities of people in these diverse roles help to determine how health care happens, who is involved, how people regard health care organizations, and whether work is a joy or a daily exercise in frustration.

Good leaders make people feel that they're at the very heart of things, not at the periphery. Everyone feels that he or she makes a difference to the success of the organization. When that happens people feel centered and that gives their work meaning.

—WARREN BENNIS

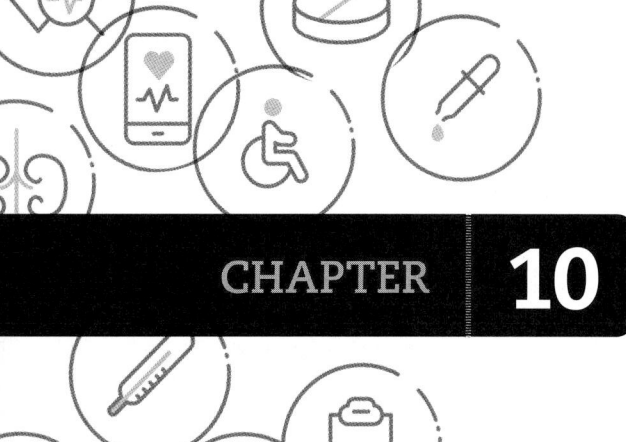

CHAPTER 10

Health Care Administration, Human Resources, Marketing, and PR

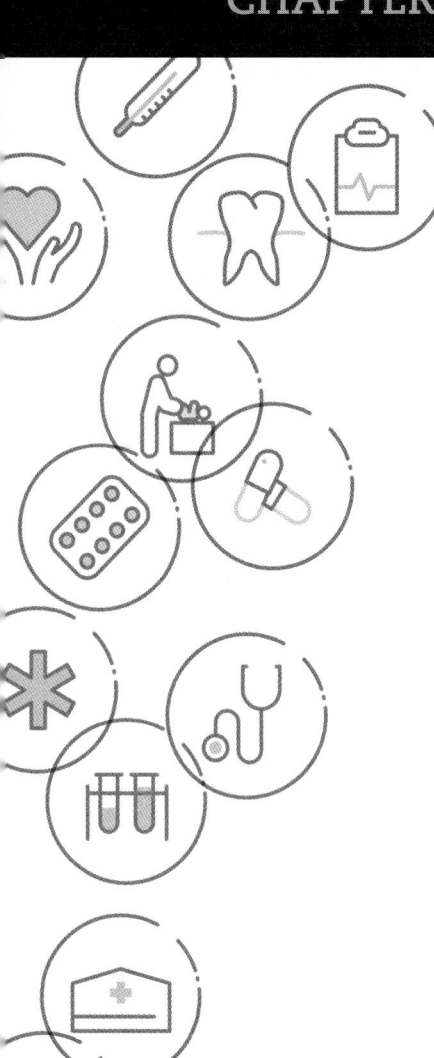

"In a nutshell, my job is to help our doctors, staff and patient families tell their stories. My job is about building relationships, working with the news media, strategic planning, crisis communication, and more. The best thing about my job is that no day is the same."

This statement by hospital public relations specialist Veronika illustrates some of the contributions made by communication specialists in health care ("All About My Job," 2016, para. 3). As you will see here, a variety of careers in the industry call for expertise in public speaking, media relations, leadership, organizational communication, crisis communication, interpersonal communication, and other functions that do not involve direct patient care.

Veronika's position mostly involves media relations, strategic communication, and relationship building in the hospital and the community. "Some days, I have a lot of desk time and can focus on pitching and writing," she says, but "other days I'm thankful I carry a cell phone charger because I'm at the hospital all day meeting with families, working with media outlets and overseeing interviews and meeting with different care teams" ("All About My Job," 2016, para. 11). Any given day might include observing a surgery, meeting with journalists, assisting a film crew, or writing educational features about health issues.

We'll hear more about Veronika's experiences as well as those of other communication specialists as we explore key issues and goals. We can't cover the full range of activities these professionals accomplish, but hopefully your curiosity will be piqued to learn more. (See Box 10.1 for information about career opportunities.)

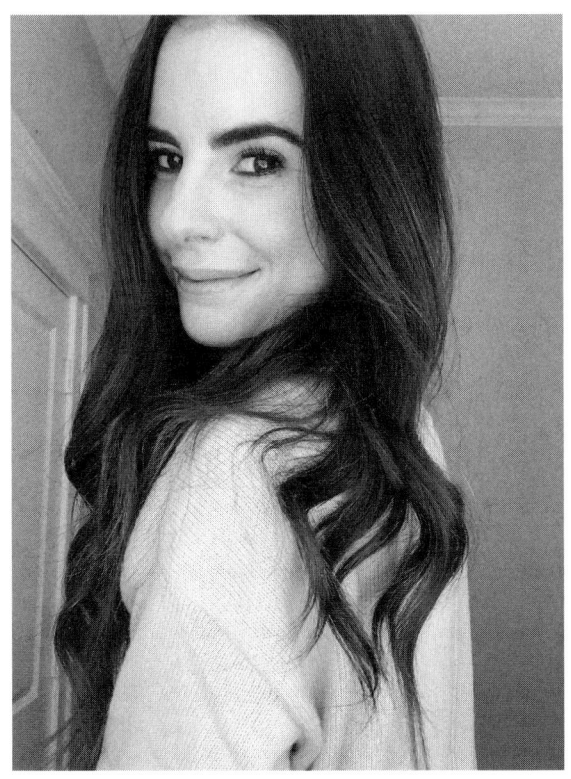

Veronika, a senior public relations specialist at a children's hospital, was honored by the Public Relations Society of America for coordinating publicity surrounding a successful surgery to separate conjoined twins Knatalye and Adeline Mata.

How might your communication skills apply to a job in health communication?

As you read, notice how central communication is in each profession. Also keep in mind the overlap between job responsibilities. Some people serve as specialists in these areas, but everyone in health care is involved with them. As we discussed in Chapter 5, systems are interrelated collections of people and ideas. What happens in one part of the system affects what happens everywhere else within it. In health care especially, leadership, human resources, public relations, and crisis management are part of everyone's job.

Health Care Administration

Since Sarah Schuyler was a child, she has dreamed of a career that would allow her to improve patient care, interact with a wide array of people, and engage in teamwork and leadership. As population health director for the New York City Hospital System, she does all of those things. Schuyler began her career working in nonprofit organizations and a consulting firm. Those were great places to build her communication skills, she says, key among them the ability to make presentations, collaborate with others, take part in projects, and provide leadership (Schuyler, n.d.).

Health care administrators range from CEOs and vice presidents to department-level managers and directors. They work in nonprofit organizations,

BOX 10.1 Career Opportunities

Health Communication Specialists

Health Care Administration
President or CEO
Chief operating officer
Chief financial officer
Health information manager
Director of human resources
Strategic planning director
Medical director
Nursing director
Departmental director (e.g., departments such as nursing, surgery, medical records, human resources, marketing, public relations, education, information technology, billing, and risk management)
Medical office manager

Career Resources and Job Listings
- U.S. Bureau of Labor Statistics: http://www.bls.gov/ooh/Management/Medical-and-health-services-managers.htm
- Association of University Programs in Health Administration: www.aupha.org

- American College of Health Care Administrators: www.achca.org
- American College of Health Care Executives: www.healthmanagementcareers.org

Health Care Human Resources

Human resource manager
Recruiter
Training and development specialist
Compensation and benefits manager
Customer service representative

Career Resources and Job Listings
- American Society for Healthcare Human Resources Administration: http://www.ashhra.org/
- Society of Human Resource Management: http://www.shrm.org/Pages/default.aspx
- U.S. Bureau of Labor Statistics: http://www.bls.gov/ooh/Business-and-Financial/Human-resources-specialists.htm

Health Care Marketing and Public Relations

Public relations professional
Strategic planning manager
Marketing professional
Advertising designer
Physician marketing coordinator
Community services director
In-house communication director
Pharmaceutical sales representative

Career Resources and Job Listings
- Society for Health Care Strategy & Market Development: www.shsmd.org
- International Association of Business Communicators: www.iabc.com
- Public Relations Society of America: www.prsa.org
- American Association of Advertising Agencies: www.aaaa.org
- American Advertising Federation: www.aaf.org
- U.S. Bureau of Labor Statistics: https://www.bls.gov/ooh/management/public-relations-managers.htm

---

hospitals, clinics, health departments, government agencies, and sometimes, in private businesses that offer health-related services to employees. Upper-level positions usually require a graduate degree in a field such as health care administration, public health, business administration, or health communication. Most health care administrators work their way up the ladder as Schuyler has (U.S. Bureau of Labor Statistics, 2019a).

On-the-job experiences vary widely. Kendrick Doidge, who is vice president of business and public relations at a hospital, spends a great deal of his time focusing on strategic communication and service excellence. After college, he worked at a visitor information and convention center and a Chamber of Commerce. He then entered health care as a specialist in hospital marketing and public relations, completing a graduate program in health communication along the way. "Never assume you know it all," he advises others. "You have to keep learning."

Part of the learning curve involves understanding current issues and collaborating with others. From an organizational perspective, the goals are threefold: to enhance the quality of health care experiences, to improve people's health across the board, and to lower costs. We take a closer look at these goals here.

Enhancing Health Care Experiences

"Being a patient is about the least amount of fun anyone can have as a consumer," point out Leonard Berry and Kent Seltman (2008, p. 167). Even more than in other industries, every customer/patient in health care wants to be treated as an individual with unique needs and perceptions. People in health organizations realize like never before the value of consumer satisfaction. Here are some of the reasons why.

First, in today's health care marketplace, patients have choices—a reality underlined by highly visible advertising and marketing efforts and by an unprecedented amount of health information available in the news media and on the internet. In this context, patients are well-informed consumers who choose between different health services vying for their business. Consumers usually form their first impression of an organization based on online reviews, friends' recommendations, and the organization's online presence ("5 Statistics," 2018). Bad experiences shared

BOX 10.2

Journals in the Field

Health Care Administration

Advances in Developing Human Resources
Health Care Management Review
Health Care Management Science
The Health Care Manager
Health Sciences Management Research
International Journal for Quality in Health Care
International Journal of Integrated Care
Journal of the American Medical Directors Association
Journal of Health Administration Education
Journal of Health Management
Journal of Health, Organisation and Management
Journal of Healthcare Management
Journal for Healthcare Quality
Journal of Public Health Management & Practice
Managed Health Care Executive

Health Care Human Resources

Human Resources Development Journal
Human Resources for Health
Journal of Health & Human Resources
Journal of Health & Human Services Administration

Health Care Marketing and Public Relations

Cases in Public Health Communication & Marketing
Health Marketing Quarterly
International Journal of Pharmaceutical and Healthcare Marketing
Journal of Health Care Marketing
Journal of Hospital Marketing and Public Relations
Journal of Management and Marketing in Healthcare
Marketing Health Services
Public Relations Journal
Public Relations Review

---

online can harm an organization's chance of success in "today's hyper-connected digital world" ("Engaging with Tomorrow's Patients," n.d., para. 2).

Second, communication correlates with health outcomes. The likelihood of timely and accurate diagnoses decreases when patients and providers don't engage in open communication and active listening (Amelung et al., 2019). Good communication also enhances shared decision-making and comprehension (Kaldjian, 2017). Patients who report that health care providers communicate effectively with them are more likely to accurately understand information, agree with treatment decisions, and follow medical advice (Okunrintemi et al., 2017).

Money is a third factor. For one, Medicare and Medicaid base nearly one-third of their reimbursement amounts on patients' assessments of care (Zusman, 2012). On the survey used to gauge patient experiences, about 75% of the questions focus on how well providers communicate with patients and their loved ones (Stamp, 2019). The upshot is that health organizations whose patients are highly satisfied receive significantly higher reimbursement payments than others.

A fourth factor involves the cost of care. Health organizations save money by minimizing mistakes, treatment duplications, and avoidable care. Poor communication (with patients and between staff members) is at the root of nearly half of serious medical errors in the United States ("Americans' Experience," 2017). And dissatisfied patients (especially those who feel that providers haven't listened to their concerns) are more likely than others to require additional hospital stays, which drives up costs (Carter, Ward, Wexler, & Donelan, 2018).

Communication Skill Builder: Servant Leadership and Empowerment

Leaders play a key role in rewarding effective behavior and cultivating communication-friendly environments. Following are experts' suggestions for bringing out the best in people.

INVERT THE PYRAMID

In a classic bureaucratic hierarchy, the people at the top make most of the decisions, get the biggest perks, reap the greatest financial rewards—and seldom see or talk to service-line employees or clients. The inherent tension and lack of communication are problematic. Moreover, whereas everyone in the organization typically tries to please the bosses, patients are not even in the hierarchy.

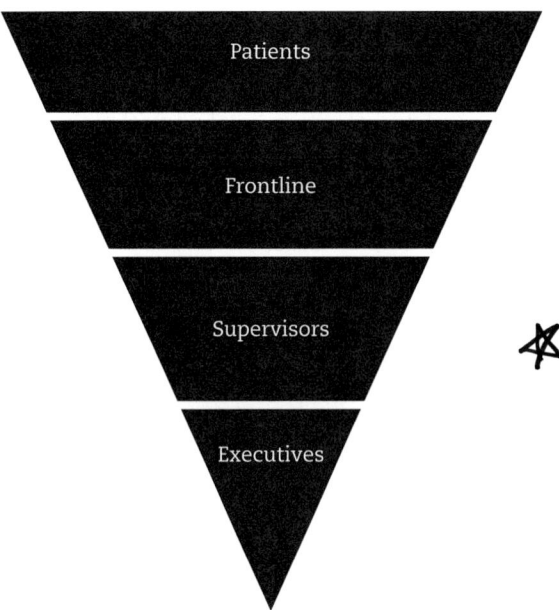

FIGURE 10.1 When the classic hierarchy is inverted, executives act as servant leaders by listening to and supporting the frontline and holding everyone accountable for excellence.

Some theorists advocate turning the pyramid upside down. Figure 10.1 In a health care organization, the largest and highest tier is then devoted to patients. Everyone in the organization is oriented to serving *them*, either directly or indirectly. The next-highest tier is made up of frontline service providers—a diverse assortment of everyone who has direct contact with people the organization is designed to serve (patients, families, community members, and so on). In health care, the frontline includes clinicians, volunteers, cafeteria staff, housekeepers, valets, event coordinators, and so on. Subsequent layers are devoted to mid-level supervisors.

In servant-leadership style, CEOs and other executives are on the bottom. From this perspective, their job is to listen, encourage, support, and remove barriers so that people throughout the organization can do what they do best. An inverted pyramid serves executive-level leaders well, too. They hold people accountable for extraordinary results, but they are spared the burden of making all the decisions. Instead, team members at every level are empowered to uphold the mission within an overall framework that upholds the vision and mission.

Empowerment allows teams to create systems and work environments that are tailor made for success. People with adequate training, authority, and resources do not usually need close supervision, particularly if everyone is responsible for meeting clear goals. The typical result is lower employee turnover and higher morale (Brohi et al., 2018). Researchers who studied hospital personnel found that those who felt highly empowered by their supervisors performed better and were more highly motivated than others (D'Innocenzo, Luciano, Mathieu, Maynard, & Chen, 2016).

BUILD RELATIONSHIPS BY LISTENING

Health care leadership expert Quint Studer (2003) maintains that feedback is as crucial as oxygen. As a hospital administrator, he borrowed a technique from physicians and began "rounding" every day—visiting units throughout the hospital to talk to patients, families, and employees. He typically introduced himself to employees this way: "Hi, I'm Quint Studer. I work for you." After a few questions about the person's experiences and the positive things going on in their unit, Studer made it a point to ask, "Do you have the tools and equipment to do your job?" and "What can I do to make your job easier?" Even more remarkably, he followed through. At one hospital, stories are still told about Studer's influence more than 15 years ago. He made hot water reliably available in the ICU, had lights added in the parking lot, provided cleaning supplies in nursing units, and much more—usually within 24 hours of learning about a need. Even changes that seem small on the surface resulted in greater efficiency and happier employees and patients (du Pré, 2005).

Kenrick Doidge, the hospital vice president we mentioned earlier, adopted a similar strategy. He set out to meet everyone he could. "It would sort of surprise people at first when I asked if I could sit with them in the hospital cafeteria," he says. But people soon got used to his friendly manner and willingness to listen. Doidge recalls one nurse who said:

> Here's what you can do to make my job easier: You can get us different printer paper. The holes in the paper don't match up to the prongs in our patient binders, so we have to fold and bend every page we add to a patient's chart.

It turned out that the same problem was plaguing staff members throughout the hospital. The misaligned holes were frustrating everyone, and had been for some time. With a quick visit to the supply-chain office, Doidge identified the problem. "Who knows how long ago, someone had apparently bumped the hole-puncher by accident and changed the alignment," says Doidge. With a simple adjustment, a long-standing problem was solved. "You wouldn't believe the response," Doidge recalls, describing the scene:

> It was the same week we announced a pay raise, but everyone was talking about the hole punches. *The nurse who suggested it was a hero. That just shows you, our job is to listen to the people caring for our patients. They'll tell you if you ask. But they don't have time to go looking for the source of problems like that.*

When leaders listen, they send the message that team members matter and are valued. And listening yields valuable information. Frontline employees are typically more familiar than anyone about clients' wishes and the organization's daily routines. Steve Miller, a worldwide manager at Shell Oil Company, emphasizes the need to treat members at every level as intelligent change agents:

> In the past, the leader was the guy with the answers. Today if you're going to have a successful company, you have to recognize that no leader can possibly have all the answers. The leader may have a vision. But the actual solutions about how best to meet the challenges of the moment have to be made by the people closest to the action. (quoted by Pascale, 1999, p. 210)

With a similar belief, Mayo Clinic staff members attribute a great deal of their success to team spirit and their respect for each other. "I know by name the custodians that work in the emergency department, and I appreciate them as much as I appreciate my physician colleagues," says Anne Sadosty, an emergency care physician with Mayo (quoted by Berry & Seltman, 2008, p. 58).

PUSH DECISION MAKING TO THE LOWEST LEVEL POSSIBLE

Determining who should be involved in decisions can be tricky. Leadership theorist Wayne Hoy observes that, if you ask human relations theorists if team members should be involved in decision making, they say, "Of course!" Ask people from the scientific management camp and they answer, "Only if they have expertise." Open-systems social scientists usually say, "It depends" (Hoy, 2003, slide 2). The **Hoy-Tarter Model of Shared Decision Making** (Hoy & Tarter, 2008) proposes that leaders consider two main questions when determining whom to include in decision making: *Does the team member have a personal stake in the outcome?* (In other words, is the topic relevant to them?) and *Does the team member have expertise on the topic?* If the answer is yes to both, the basic foundations are present for shared decision making. Layered on top of that are other considerations such as: *Is it likely that this person will agree with the decision even without being personally involved in it? Does this person have the skills to participate effectively in decision making?* and *Do the people involved trust each other?*

We can apply the Hoy-Tarter model to leaders as well as to frontline team members. Compared to the frontline, executive-level leaders often have less personal stake in workplace procedures and less personal knowledge about them, partly because they are not on the frontline as much and partly because people are typically hesitant to be candid with leaders they don't know well. The result, says health care satisfaction expert Irwin Press (2002), can be a lot of top-down rules that don't serve anyone very well.

When assessing employee satisfaction in health care organizations, Press begins by asking employees to list the "really stupid rules" that hamper them from doing a good job. "This is fun and focuses analytical attention on the often arbitrary nature of regulations," says Press (2002, p. 42). Next, he asks people to examine rules that serve a purpose but don't work well. For example, Press asks, is it necessary that nurses deliver meal trays? Could other staff members perform this task and free nurses to respond more quickly to patients' requests?

Press (2002) also advises that, if the rules and paperwork are important, leaders must allow team members the time and space to complete them. For example, it's unrealistic to expect an employee to answer the phone, file reports, and respond to others' needs in the same small space or in brief amounts of time. Frustration and poor service are likely to result. If the regulations are important, Press declares, make fulfilling them part of the job.

One drawback of centralized decision making is the time it takes. Opportunities for change are often lost or delayed before top-level leaders know about them or can act upon them. This can be fatal in today's fast-moving market. And when service breakdowns occur, frontline team members may have to wait for authorization from "higher-ups" before they can resolve the issues. The result is often a delay on top of an already disappointing situation.

Health care consultant Fred Lee (2004) offered a frustrating example of centralized decision making.

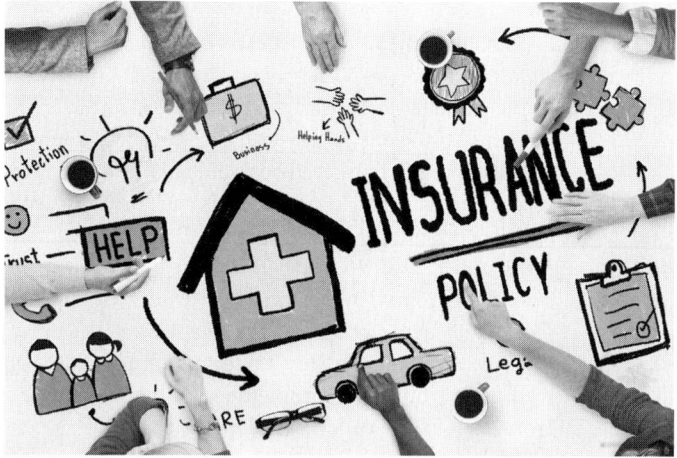

"Make creativity a habit," encourages one health care consultant, who suggests that health organizations invest in communication-friendly meetings spaces, bulletin boards, white boards, and "sticky" areas where patients and health care associates can post ideas and suggestions.

If you were to design a work space to encourage communication and group meetings, what features would you include?

He arrived at a hospital one morning to conduct a training session, only to find that the classroom was locked. A security officer arrived, but even though he had a key, he was required to get permission from his supervisors across town to open the door, and they were not available. "I'm really sorry," said the security officer while the entire class waited in the hall. Lee reflects, "How could central dispatch, 20 miles away, have a better understanding of the situation than the officer at the scene? Any information about the problem would be coming from the officer anyway." Lee sympathizes with the employee who was rendered powerless (and no doubt embarrassed) because supervisors did not trust employees to act on their own judgment.

Considerations such as these have led health care experts Thom Mayer and Robert Cates (2004) to advise, "Make no decision at a higher level that can be made at a lower level" (p. 58). They point out that health care is a personal service offered at an individual level, therefore "the people responsible for the service delivery must be entrusted with the power to make service meaningful" (p. 58).

HOLD PEOPLE ACCOUNTABLE

A key component of empowerment is holding people at every level of the organization responsible for goals they help to set and regularly measuring progress to help team members gauge what is working and what is not (Chang, Shih, & Lin, 2010; Donahue, Piazza, Griffin, Dykes, & Fitzpatrick, 2008).

To make the process effective, experts suggest that measurement not be used to punish team members. If so, they will have an incentive to set goals too low and to enhance the results artificially, as in asking patients to give them perfect scores rather than constructive ideas. Feedback mechanisms should be based on what team members *themselves* want to know in the interest of continual self-improvement. In Mayer and Cates's (2004) terms, measurement should be a tool, not a club.

Here's a great example. Lynn Pierce was a nurse manager in a hospital where the staff decided to post the results of weekly patient satisfaction surveys on bulletin boards. That meant that everyone (staff members, patients, visitors, VIPs, and anyone else) could see the scores, as well as charts that compared patient satisfaction scores in various departments.

There was no punishment involved, but the numbers were hard to ignore. Pierce says that, although she frequently made excuses for her unit's scores when they were kept private, seeing them publicly posted changed her point of view. "I started thinking, 'My numbers are going to come up! I won't be left behind,'" she says. Pierce says she began seeing patient requests not as time-consuming chores, but as opportunities. She laughs, "'You want a Coke?' I'd call Dietary and say, 'Send 'em a six-pack!'" (quoted by du Pré, 2005, p. 317).

CELEBRATE SUCCESSES [making it personable]

One benefit of measuring performance is the opportunity to celebrate when things go well. Experts suggest sending handwritten thank-you letters to employees and their families, posting thank-you letters from patients, holding celebrations when the organization reaches key goals, informally praising people who do good work, and developing formal recognition programs to honor heroic efforts.

In closing this section, it bears emphasizing that leaders are not obsolete once they empower team members. As James Pepicello and Emmett Murphy (1996) point out, empowerment "does not relieve leadership of its responsibility to lead" (para. 17). It does mean that leaders' roles are more supportive than autocratic. Key to success are interpersonal skills, including the ability to inspire, recognize, and reward others (Jobes & Steinbinder, 1996, para. 23).

If it seems overwhelming to contemplate all that health care administrators do, keep in mind that they don't do it alone. Success relies on the integrated efforts of many people. In the next section we will explore how human resources specialists contribute.

Human Resources

Nothing beats being part of a team that is expected to produce great results. . . . If you have the wrong people on the bus, nothing else matters. You may be headed in the right direction, but you still won't achieve greatness. Great vision with mediocre people still produces mediocre results.
—Jim Collins (2001a, *Disciplined People*, para. 7)

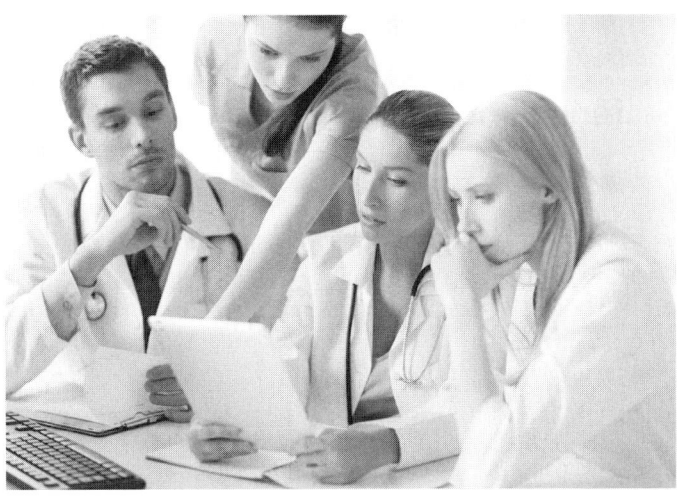

Effective teamwork and well-designed systems ease the burden on professionals and help them avoid tragic and costly mistakes.

How might a team approach help you with some of your toughest challenges?

After studying consistently top-performing companies in the United States, Collins (2001b) debunked the idea that people are a company's most important asset. "People are *not* your most important asset," he clarified, "the *right* people are" (p. 13). Indeed, as we all know, the wrong people, or people who are not well prepared, can be your worst nightmare—damaging trust, running off great team members, causing mistakes, and damaging morale.

In a book with the provocative title *The No Asshole Rule*, Stanford University professor Robert Sutton (R. L. Sutton, 2007) presents empirical evidence that people who treat others badly are bad for business, no matter how good they seem to be at some aspects of the job. Sutton calculated what he dubs the TCA (total cost per asshole) of workers in a wide variety of fields and concluded that the disadvantages of people who insult, belittle, and bully others far outweigh the advantages. Even bullies considered to be "top" salespeople, he says, cost companies more than they bring in because of lawsuits, staff turnover, angry clients, and so on. Moreover, their attitudes tend to be contagious, such that the people around them offer poorer service as well. Sutton advises, "Avoid pompous jerks whenever possible. They not only can make you feel bad about yourself, chances are you will eventually start acting like them" (B. Sutton, 2007).

The odds are you have worked with people who evoke fear and anxiety in the people around them. Typically, even their bosses would rather not deal with them, so the bullies often remain where they are, running off clients and colleagues. The challenge of working with hostile team members is unacceptable anywhere, but particularly in health care organizations, where leaders struggle to attract and keep qualified personnel in already stressful environments. Health care staffing shortages (see Box 10.3) make it imperative for leaders to do whatever they can to attract and keep qualified personnel. This includes listening closely to employees' needs, responding to their ideas, and involving them in collaborative efforts to create satisfying environments.

In this section, we look at the contributions of human resource personnel and others who cultivate talent and vision and, ideally, give us the luxury of working with ethical, dedicated people. Human resource specialists are involved in recruiting, hiring, and training staff members; overseeing employee benefits and compensation; mediating employee concerns; providing for mentoring, counseling, and assistance; recognizing outstanding achievements; and monitoring team member satisfaction and retention. Qualifications typically include at least a bachelor's degree in human resources, personnel, communication, psychology, or another field related to human dynamics ("Becoming," 2011).

Theoretical Foundations

Before exploring the research and strategies relevant to human resources, let's consider some of the foundational theories in the field. As you will see, theorists

BOX 10.3

Staffing Shortages in Health Care

Experts estimate that the United States will be short-staffed by nearly 1 million nurses, 124,000 physicians, and 706,000 home health aides by the year 2025 (AHA, 2008; Dill & Salsberg, 2008; U.S. Bureau of Labor Statistics, 2012a, 2012b, 2019b). There are numerous reasons for the shortfall.

One involves population shifts. A growing elderly population is placing increasing demands on the health care system. Indications are that the number of people over age 85 in the year 2050 will be triple what it was in 2008, reaching an unprecedented 19 million, and increasing the overall need for health services by at least 40% (U.S. Census Bureau News, 2008).

A second factor is the Affordable Care Act, passed in 2010. Although the future of the ACA is uncertain, it has led to a dramatic increase in the number of Americans who are insured and receive regular health care, increasing the need for qualified care providers. (The act also includes billions of dollars in grants and training opportunities to prepare new caregivers.)

Third, at the same time health care needs are increasing, the number of trained caregivers, which is already insufficient, is expected to *decrease*. This is partly because many caregivers are at retirement age themselves. Experts predict that about one-half of registered nurses and one-third of physicians currently practicing in the United States will retire by the year 2025 (Budden, Zhong, Moulton, & Cimiotti, 2013; Dall & West, 2015).

The physician shortage is slightly less extensive than the nursing shortage, partly because some women who might previously have pursued nursing careers are now going to medical school instead (Green, 1988). As a result of that fairly recent shift, female physicians are younger, on average, than their male counterparts. However, men have not joined nursing at the rate once expected. Today, only about 9% of registered nurses in the United States are male ("National Nursing," 2018).

A fourth factor is insufficient funding for colleges and universities. U.S. nursing schools turn away nearly 69,000 qualified applicants a year because they do not have the budgets or faculty necessary to accept more students (American Association of Colleges of Nursing, 2015).

Finally, many health professionals are changing careers. One survey showed that 49% of nurses in the United States have considered leaving the field, mostly because of intense workloads, stress, and poor treatment by patients, administrations, and physicians (Cornwall, 2018). At the same time, about 12% of physicians say they plan to stop seeing patients, mostly because of frustrations over excessive paperwork and bureaucratic oversight (Physicians Foundation, 2018).

Staffing shortages hurt care and drive up avoidable costs. Patients in understaffed units are significantly more likely than others to have urinary tract infections, pneumonia, shock, and upper gastrointestinal bleeding—conditions that can often be averted or minimized with careful attention ("HHS Study Finds," 2001). Patients in understaffed units are also more likely to have extended hospital stays and less likely to be successfully resuscitated after cardiac arrest. Jack Needleman and associates (2006) found that hospitals can actually save money by hiring more RNs because nurses in well-staffed units have fewer emergencies, patient deaths, and mistakes to manage.

---

have examined issues such as: *What ethical principles should we consider concerning the treatment of people on our teams? How are people different from other types of resources?* and *What brings out the best in team members so that, together, we have the greatest chance of success?*

Richard de Charms laid the groundwork for many current theories of motivation and workplace dynamics. His (1968) **theory of personal causation** proposes that people naturally resist being treated as *pawns* who are required to relinquish control and unthinkingly follow orders, but people typically respond enthusiastically and with dedication when they are treated as *origins*—active participants in designing and carrying out worthwhile tasks. de Charms's work was as much about ethics as productivity. He felt that people deserve to be treated as something more than cogs in a machine, and he observed that associates make their greatest contributions when they are actively engaged. Consequently, de Charms (1977) advocated a participatory model that he called "plan-choose-act-take responsibility" in which people work together to make decisions, carry them out, and then continually analyze and improve their own performance.

A similar idea is available in Douglas McGregor's (1960) **Theory X and Theory Y** model, which proposes that managers tend to fall into one of two basic camps—those who believe people are naturally lazy and must be prodded and supervised to be productive (Theory X managers) and those who believe people enjoy the inherent rewards of work and are motivated to make a positive difference (Theory Y managers). McGregor observed that managers' attitudes are influential in bringing out either the worst or the best in people. People treated as if they are lazy and untrustworthy are likely to act that way. On the other hand, Theory Y managers tend to take a human relations approach, recognizing that people are most effective when they feel appreciated, satisfied, and proud of the work they do. McGregor's theory and relevant research lend further credence to the notion that it is both ethical and expedient to empower team members.

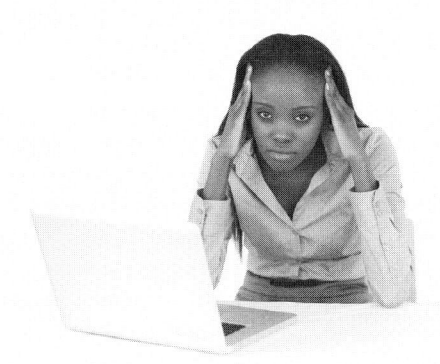

According to the theory of personal causation, people resist being treated as *pawns* who are required to relinquish control and unthinkingly follow orders, but they typically respond enthusiastically and with dedication when they are treated as *origins*, that is, active participants in designing and carrying out worthwhile tasks.

Under what circumstances do you like someone to tell you what to do? When do you prefer to have a voice in making decisions and coming up with solutions?

Frederick Herzberg conceived of a more complicated interplay between factors. His **motivation-hygiene theory** suggests that a different set of issues engender satisfaction versus dissatisfaction (Herzberg, 1968; Herzberg, Mausner, & Snyderman, 1959). According to the theory, people are typically satisfied with their work if they believe they are making an important difference, are respected, and are learning and improving. Herzberg called these factors *motivators*. However, dissatisfaction typically arises over a different set of issues, which he called *hygiene factors*. These include feeling underpaid, being forced to work in unhealthy or unproductive conditions, and perceiving that rules and policies are unfair. Herzberg found that, in the absence of such factors, people are typically not dissatisfied. However, it does not follow that they are satisfied, either. To be satisfied, if you recall, we must feel that our work is important and we are respected. The lesson here is that dissatisfaction typically arises from factors (such as pay) that are extrinsic to our work, and motivation arises from the inherent satisfaction of making a difference. Managers who focus on only one or the other are unlikely to create the conditions in which people are both satisfied and highly motivated.

In health care, it is particularly important to recruit outstanding people and to make sure they feel rewarded and valued. Although human resource personnel typically do not work directly with patients, they have immense influence on the quality of those interactions.

Communication Skill Builder: Building Great Teams

When a very ill patient was admitted to a Mayo Clinic hospital, her daughter told the care team that she was worried her mother would not live long enough to be present at her upcoming wedding. Sensing that this was important to both mother and daughter, the Mayo team sprang into action. Within hours, they transformed the hospital atrium into a flower- and balloon-filled wedding venue. Personnel from many units volunteered to help out:

> *Staff members provided a cake and a pianist, and nurses arranged the patient's hair and makeup, dressed her, and wheeled her bed to the atrium. The chaplain performed the service. On every floor, hospital staff members, other patients, and visiting family and friends ringed the atrium balconies "like*

angels from above," to quote the bride. (Berry & Seltman, 2008, p. 57)

This moving story is evidence of Mayo's simple vision, known to every employee and used as the basis for all decisions: *The needs of the patient come first* (Berry & Seltman, 2008, p. 24). Within that culture, the term *volunteerism* refers to employees' willingness to do more than they have to do because they want to make a difference and they know organizational leaders will back them up.

This level of commitment and compassion does not happen automatically, but results from a concerted effort on many levels. The process begins with selecting the right people, then training them well and weaving the mission into every aspect of daily work. Following are strategies for creating and building outstanding teams from a human resources perspective.

HIRE CAREFULLY

The first step toward success, says Collins (2001b), is getting the "right people on the bus." Mayer and Cates (2004) wholeheartedly concur. They ask, "Are there days when you come to work and see the people you are working with and think to yourself, 'Bring it on! Whatever we've got to do today, this team of people can make it happen!'?" (p. 7). If so, they say, you are surrounded by **A-team players**, the type who love a challenge, have a positive attitude, and inspire everyone around them. But if you said no, you understand the concept of **B-team players**. They inspire a different internal dialogue on the way to work, one that sounds more like this: "Shoot me, shoot me, shoot me! I can't work with him—I worked with him yesterday!" (Mayer & Cates, p. 7).

Mayer and Cates describe **B-team players** as negative, lazy, late, and confused. B-team players are "fundamentally toxic" and quite potent, in that it just takes one to poison things for everyone. A major part of a leader's job, maintain Mayer and Cates, is getting B-team members either to reform (which might involve moving them to positions more in line with their talents and passions) or to leave. An even better strategy, they say, is to hire the right people in the first place.

Linda Minton of Parkwest Medical Center in Knoxville, Tennessee, describes how she knew that a new nurse, Paul, would be an A-team member. A woman in her eighties with Alzheimer's was admitted for a blood transfusion under Paul's supervision. When the woman became afraid and pulled out her IVs, her daughter was tearful and distraught. The patient repeatedly requested to be left alone and allowed to go home, but Paul knew that she needed the life-saving treatment. Minton recalls:

> *Paul again quietly explained that she could not go home, but he also asked if there were anything else she might like to do. Quickly she responded, with a big smile on her face, "I would like to dance." Paul, who is not a dancer, said, "You will have to lead." She agreed, and so—they danced. What a wonderful sight, seeing this lovely lady calmed by the impromptu dance. It was at that moment that we all knew Paul had a place at Parkwest Medical Center.* (What's Right in Health Care, 2007, p. 666)

Human resource personnel can be influential in recruiting and selecting A-team players. Experts remind us that it's important to find people with the right attitude and passion as well as the right credentials. Before making hiring decisions, members of highly successful organizations typically conduct multiple interviews with candidates, invite input from people with whom they would work, and consider candidates' intangible qualifications such as patience, appreciation for diversity, and interpersonal skills.

TEACH THE CULTURE AND VALUES

This section began with an example of the volunteer spirit of Mayo Clinic. By helping to teach the organization's culture and values, human resource personnel are involved in making such remarkable encounters possible. At Mayo, employees hear the clinic's motto, *The needs of the patient come first*, within the first five minutes of new-employee orientation and several times a day ever after. As one employee said, "Mayo becomes part of your DNA" (quoted by Berry & Seltman, 2008, p. 26). Having a strong, clear purpose provides unity, even among diverse people and departments. Team members contribute in different ways, but because they are united by a clear mission, they all know and agree on what they are trying to achieve together.

CONTINUALLY RECRUIT INTERNAL TALENT

By most estimates, it costs about $75,000 to replace an employee who earns $50,000, and even more for people in higher pay grades (Bliss, 2012). Expenses involve lost productivity and the cost of recruiting, interviewing, and training new employees. That doesn't even include the frustration of disrupted relationships and being short-staffed in the meantime. It's in everyone's best interest to keep great team members on board. Human resources personnel can help retain talented people in the following ways:

- *Provide ongoing leadership training.* Ideally, leadership training and development don't begin or end when people become designated leaders. The process begins long before that and continues throughout a person's career.
- *Keep no secrets.* If people are to be accountable, they must know where they stand and how the organization is performing. One strategy is to make financial records and satisfaction survey reports available to all employees so they can chart their success and receive immediate market feedback on what works well and what does not (Studer, 2003).
- *Make organizational leaders accessible.* Avoid placing administrative officers in far-off or segregated areas. Encourage leaders to interact freely throughout the organization and to share conversations, praise, and ideas.
- *Reward people for sharing ideas.* Develop a program that invites employees' suggestions and rewards them for submitting workable ideas that improve services, save money, and increase employee morale.
- *Respond to ideas.* Even when the ideas can't be implemented, people want to know they have been heard. Designate committees to review ideas, respond to them all, and initiate implementation whenever possible.
- *Prepare people to participate actively.* In the previous section, we explored reasons to invest in dispersed leadership. Empowered team members typically perform at higher levels, are more creative, and more satisfied than others (Fernandez & Moldogaziev, 2013). Human resource personnel can help people build the skills to effectively engage in shared governance.

Based on the theories we have reviewed, encouraging people to use and develop their talents is productive for health care organizations and enriching for the people who comprise them. Recruitment is the first step, but it also pays to continually re-recruit talented team members and hire from within when the talent is available. In a way, point out Berry and Seltman (2008), employment is a job interview "that lasts for years" (p. 29).

Now let's look at the contributions of marketing and public relations professionals, who work both internally and externally to help health care organizations succeed.

Marketing and Public Relations

We began this chapter with Veronika, a senior public relations specialist, who says that every day is different. "We work regularly with families, experiencing the environment and culture in which our patients are cared for," she says ("All About," 2016, para. 19). PR specialists perform a range of functions. Her job primarily involves educating the public about health news—everything from surgical breakthroughs to infertility treatments—and sharing stories that touch people's lives. For example, Veronika was present when a local news station visited the hospital to feature a boy who was celebrating his last chemotherapy treatment. Veronika remembers what happened later:

> *A year or so later at a fundraising event for the hospital I ran into his parents and his mom showed me a picture of him on her iPhone and I became quite emotional. It was the little boy with a full head of hair—and he was kicking a soccer ball. It was one of the best photos I saw that year.* ("All About," 2016, para. 15)

In this section we talk more about health care marketing and public relations, two career fields that, while not the same, are often interrelated.

Traditionally, health care *marketing* has been concerned mostly with promoting business and profitability, and *public relations* has focused on enhancing an organization's image and larger mission. Marketing professionals are likely to be involved with stakeholder groups who are central to business development. This may include marketing directly to physicians who might make patient referrals, conducting market research, helping develop new services to meet market needs, branding and promoting an organization through advertising and other means, communicating internally, and engaging in strategic planning. Results are often measured in terms of financial success and organizational growth.

Public relations professionals in health care are usually involved in such activities as media relations and publicity, publication design, internal communication, strategic planning, special events, health education and promotion, fundraising, volunteer recruitment, and crisis management. The most coveted public relations professionals are those who work in an integrated fashion both within an organization and with external stakeholders. "Long gone are the days when public relations practitioners could claim they were successful after getting their organization positive publicity in the local newspaper," says PR theorist and researcher Kurt Wise (2007), pointing out that "CEOs now expect public relations professionals to demonstrate they can contribute to the bottom-line success of an organization" (p. 162).

Although marketing and public relations are not the same, if they are done well they complement each other. An organization that is not financially sustainable will accomplish very little. At the same time, an organization without a strong reputation and mission is unlikely to be financially successful. It is common in health care for marketing and public relations professionals to work closely together. And sometimes people do both.

Foundations for Theory and Practice

Following are communication best practices from marketing and public relations experts, as well as the theories behind them. As a foundation for the rest, we will spend the most time on cultivating mutually beneficial relationships.

FOCUS ON RELATIONSHIPS

Relationship management and relationship marketing emerged in the late 1980s and have been received with particular enthusiasm in health care. They reflect the idea that transactions do not always (or even, usually) have a distinct beginning, middle, and end (Dwyer, Schurr, & Oh, 1987). For example, if you undergo surgery, your impression of the hospital probably doesn't begin when you walk in the door. It begins much earlier, perhaps with friends' stories about their experiences there, the hospital's generosity in sponsoring your niece's softball team, the general friendliness of people you know who work there, and so on. And what happens while you are a patient is likely to influence your willingness to seek care there in the future. Considering these factors, marketing and public relations professionals who focus on ongoing relationships are more effective than others in attracting and sustaining not only consumers and partners, but loyal fans of the organization.

Relationships of all types matter. Coworker relationships influence organizational culture and set the tone for consumer interactions. Relationships with external stakeholders play a powerful role as well. Their support (or lack of it) can be the difference between building a new wing and going without. As Berkowitz (2007) points out, "it is extremely difficult to seek donations to build a cancer center, heart center, or women's health program, and ask for a donation from any individual before the organization has a relationship with that donor" (p. 128). In health care, even supposed competitors often team up to fund community clinics for the uninsured, host health fairs, coordinate care in crisis situations, and more. "The demands on and responsibilities of today's health care organizations are too difficult and overwhelming to accomplish without the assistance of strategic partners and other publics," attest Guy, Williams, Aldridge, and Roggenkamp (2007, p. 2).

Many people feel that relationship development is not only good business but is also the key to improving health care and lowering costs. As marketing theorist Lawrence Crosby (2011) puts it:

> *Quality and cost issues are not about healthy individuals collapsing on the street and being rushed to the hospital for a sophisticated diagnosis by TV's Dr. House. They are about chronic problems that have been simmering for years that eventually boil over into far bigger problems. Managing the prevention/treatment/follow-up life cycle requires a relationship approach.* (p. 13)

Crosby posits that today's often-fragmented approach to health care encourages treatment overlaps, inconsistencies, distrust, and neglect that could be overcome with stronger, more trusting relationships.

Robert Morgan and Shelby Hunt's (1994) **commitment-trust theory of relationships** proposes that people make relatively enduring judgments between alternatives based on trust, shared values, loyalty, and commitment—and that, of these, *commitment* and *trust* are the greatest predictors of relationship strength. The theory further posits that, once enduring relationships are formed, we (as consumers, providers, or colleagues) benefit from a sense of stability, uncertainty reduction, and enhanced identity, and we are likely to remain invested in those relationships as long as the benefits outweigh the relational costs, which may include conflict and a sense that other alternatives have emerged that are even more rewarding. This means it's important to foster relationships, to continually nurture them, and to work through relationship threats.

Relationship management has dispelled the notion that marketing and public relations professionals can be effective engaging in only one-way communication with the public. Actually, that notion was never very satisfying, particularly in health care. As early as 1939, Alden Brewster Mills prescribed that health care public relations should be, more than anything else, an effort to develop "mutual understanding, good will and respect" (Mills, 1939, p. 3).

With the same conviction, James Grunig and colleagues advocate **two-way symmetrical communication**, meaning ongoing, open dialogue between members of an organization and the larger publics it serves (Grunig, 1992; Grunig, Grunig, & Dozier, 2002). The lesson is that, as in any relationship, listening is as important as talking.

In sum, many people believe that relationship management—with its focus on enduring, mutual benefits for everyone involved—is the most important focus of public relations and marketing. As you might imagine, communication is central to relationship management, being the mechanism by which we convey trust and commitment and manage conflict. And it's not enough for only marketing and public relations professionals to engage in relationship development. Everyone must be involved. We focus next on efforts to integrate marketing and public relations throughout an organization.

INTEGRATE

"Selling is trying to get people to want what you have. Marketing is trying to have what people want," says health care consultant Terrance Rynn (quoted by Lee, 2004. p. 5).

One mistake professionals make is trying to boost business by promoting substandard services. Not only will that not work, says Fred Lee (2004), it will make matters worse. He advises that if a service is subpar, don't promote it. "The worst thing you can do for a poorly delivered service is to get more physicians or patients to try it and find out how bad it is" (p. 6). For this reason, it's important not to consider marketing and public relations as "add-ons" to a health care system, but as integral components in strategic planning and organizational design.

Because marketing and PR professionals are continually involved in scanning the larger environment and listening to what people want and need, they can be valuable players in internal decision making. Besides, the more they know about services, the better and more authentically they can promote them to others.

An interesting example of internal public relations is provided in Trent Seltzer et al.'s (2012) article "PR in the ER" in which they describe communication in a busy, university-affiliated emergency department. The researchers observed and interviewed staff members, most of whom felt they were "under bombardment" (p. 131), unprepared for the communication challenges they faced every day and discouraged by the hostile attitudes of their coworkers. Worst of all, perhaps, the staff largely perceived that administrators were indifferent to their concerns. The researchers observed that the personnel who were confused, frustrated, and anxious were hampered in their ability to do a good job and were poor ambassadors for the organization. Based on these observations, the researchers encouraged leaders to focus on employee concerns, recognizing that public relations is as much an internal function as an external one.

DEVELOP REPUTATION, NOT ONLY IMAGE

An organization's greatest competitive advantage is not its size, location, or prices. The greatest predictor of success is its character and the constancy of its reputation (Jackson, 2004). In the book *Building Reputational Capital*, Jackson (2004) presents compelling evidence supporting a simple but powerful idea: *Organizations flourish when people are loyal to them*. The principle applies to clients as well as employees. Jackson found that the best employees—the kind with strong integrity, lasting commitment, and goodwill themselves—flock to companies that make them feel proud to work there. In appreciation of being treated well, the people served by those organizations are likely to come back again and again.

In contrast, organizations that defy public trust are often eventually toppled by scandal. These companies experience what Jackson (2004) calls "relational bankruptcy," which no amount of marketing or public relations can undo. Jackson proposes that "the things

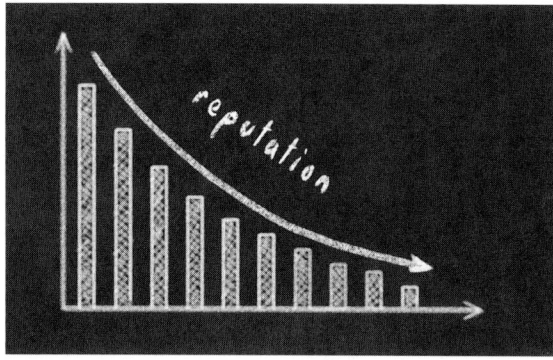

Promoting an image that does not reflect an organization's true character is likely to cause disappointment and foster a poor reputation.

Have you ever formed a poor opinion of an organization because it didn't live up to its promises? If so, what happened?

that matter most to your business, that enable it to work, to be productive—trust, integrity, fair dealing—exist beyond conventional measurements of the firm's value" (p. 2).

This is particularly true in health care. It's difficult to judge a clinic, hospital, or nonprofit organization except on the basis of its reputation. No matter how high-tech or beautiful a medical center is, it's unlikely that people will trust their lives or their donations to people they don't trust.

Jackson (2004) distinguishes between **corporate identity** (what makes an organization recognizable in comparison to others), **image** (an overall but sometimes fleeting feeling about a company based on its "personality"), and **reputation** (a long-term assessment by a range of constituencies about the "character, conscience, and credibility" of an organization; p. 43). He presents a model of three different types of companies, described here.

People in what we might call **Point-A-to-Point-B companies** are motivated primarily by profits and are willing to engage in questionable means to reach profitable ends. Although the bottom line might look healthy for a while, people in these companies usually experience short-term success at best. They engender little loyalty from customers or employees, and in the end, they may expend a great deal of time and money dealing with legal troubles and scandals, if the company survives at all.

People in the second type of company, which Jackson calls **superficially image based**, realize the value of a positive image, but they seek it through advertising campaigns and slogans that sound good but do not necessarily reflect the true nature of the company. In this company, principles are espoused, but they are not always enacted. This approach is not likely to engender long-term success.

The third company is **reputation based**, meaning that it has a positive image, but more importantly, people throughout the organization consistently embody high principles in all that they do. This is possible because people know the principles and because leaders and policies support those principles, even when it takes a little more time and money to live up to them. Jackson (2004) demonstrates that only in this type of organization can people afford to engage in transparent decision making, which is important because transparency is the key to lasting trust. His research suggests that reputation-based companies are the only ones that experience long-term success.

In summary, Jackson (2004) makes the point that image can be superficial, but an organization's reputation—good or bad—is based on how its members treat people every day in every situation.

So far we have been talking mostly about guiding principles. We will close this section with a skill-builder about one of the many communication tools marketing and public relations professionals use.

Communication Skill Builder: Two-Way Communication and Social Media

Throughout much of the past 100 years, marketing and public relations professionals have worked in concert with journalists to educate and inform the public. That is still an important part of what they do, but as you know, technologies such as the internet, Facebook, and Twitter now make it possible to disseminate messages without going through formal media channels—and relatively inexpensively. That doesn't mean social media campaigns are always easy or effective. Here are some experts' suggestions for making the most of them.

- *Be interactive.* Health journalist Carrie Vaughan (2012) describes a hospital that had only 80 "friends" (most of them employees) on Facebook until the PR and marketing staff hosted an online cute-baby contest in conjunction with an upcoming event. The number of friends quickly soared to 1,153.
- *Link messages to key services.* To make the most of high readership numbers, link social media messages to services you would like to promote.

Vaughan (2012) gives the example of a "What Do You Heart?" online contest linked to publicity about cardiac services.

- *Be educational.* Social media can allow people to watch medical procedures and receive other health-related information not previously available. The staff at Henry Ford Hospital in Detroit uses Twitter to record and broadcast some surgeries, along with the surgeons' comments. "Doing this removes a real communication barrier," says health care technology expert Charles Parks. "It helps make something scary much more comprehendable" (Cohen, 2009, para. 12).
- *Integrate a range of channels.* The most effective campaigns involve a range of social media platforms and links from one to the others (Vaughan, 2012).
- *Maintain relationships.* As we have discussed, strong relationships may enhance patient outcomes, build loyalty, and help with fundraising. Social media can help. A surgical weight loss center in Las Vegas regularly sends Facebook messages with encouraging words, online links, and healthy information to friends of the site (Patterson, 2012).
- *Develop a social media policy.* One downside of social media is that it is quick, accessible, and inexpensive for *everybody*. For example, comments an employee posts on Facebook or Instagram can violate patient confidentiality or endanger partnerships with other organizations. Consequently, many organizations are educating employees about social media practices and establishing policies such as the following: Be respectful (avoid offensive, profane, embarrassing, or slanderous statements), uphold copyright laws, obtain approval before linking to the company website, maintain confidentiality concerning patients and proprietary information about the company, and don't speak as a member of the organization without getting approval to do so.

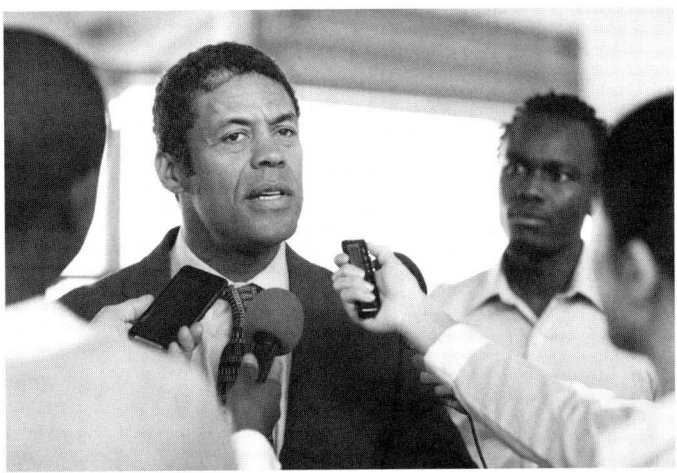

It's important to decide in advance who will speak for the organization in the event of a crisis.

What qualities would you look for in a spokesperson?

Crisis Management

By their nature, health organizations are likely to be part of crises. As Kathleen Fearn-Banks (1996) defines it, from an organizational perspective, a crisis is "a major occurrence with a potentially negative outcome affecting an organization, company, or industry, as well as its publics, products, services, or good name" (p. 1).

In health care, the crisis usually has an external origin: a natural disaster, an accident, or an outbreak of contagious disease. In such cases, members of health care organizations (especially hospitals and health departments) may be called on to explain the crisis and to keep the public informed about it. In some cases, the crisis originates within the organization—a fire, a baby kidnapped from the nursery, charges of extortion. In any case, it is important to have a well-developed plan for handling crises, collecting information, and making information available to members of the organization, the media, and the public.

In Chapter 12, we talk extensively about handling public health crises, and many of the same principles apply, so we will keep this overview brief. But it is worth mentioning that crises have implications not just for the public. There is an organizational component as well. Crisis management is a job for communication specialists, especially those in public relations. Here are some helpful tips for preparing a crisis plan and managing publicity during a crisis ("Crisis," 2014; Fearn-Banks, 1996):

- Let people within the organization know what constitutes a crisis and whom to contact at the first sign of crisis.
- Designate a primary spokesperson for the organization (usually the CEO or public relations

director), and help that person decide what information to release and how.
- Develop good relationships with media professionals before a crisis occurs, and do not play favorites during a crisis.
- Cultivate relationships with people in the community. "Emergency managers use the axiom 'all disasters are local' to emphasize that crises happen in a specific place and affect a specific community or group of communities," say analysts for the U.S. Department of Health and Human Services ("Crisis," 2014, p. 4). Knowing key people in local nonprofit organizations, schools, churches, neighborhoods, and more can be invaluable in a crisis.
- Educate people in the organization about how to handle a crisis and how to get information.
- Verify and update information before sharing it.
- Don't forget the "worried well." Nathan Huebner of the CDC urges crisis managers to consider people who are not directly affected by a crisis but are distressed by it or anxious about loved ones. The "worried well" typically outnumber the people who are directly affected, Huebner points out, and keeping them well informed prevents undue anxiety and may keep them out of harm's way themselves (Currie, 2009).
- Keep up-to-date contact information for designated spokespersons, media professionals, stakeholders, and emergency management professionals.
- Maintain supplies that will be necessary if electricity or web access is unavailable.
- Plan ahead how you will accommodate members of the media on site.

As you can see, none of the strategies outlined in this chapter occur in isolation. Public relations specialists usually head crisis management teams, but they are the first to admit that outstanding team members make it possible to offer excellent service both routinely and in extraordinary times. Leaders, human resource personnel, and others make that possible. Let's conclude the chapter with advice from service excellence experts.

Service Excellence

Many of the ideas in this chapter are oriented to service excellence. Based on decades of experience conducting patient satisfaction surveys, Irwin Press (2002) presents five reasons to focus on patient satisfaction:

- Patients are satisfied when they receive great care, even when that involves frightening and uncomfortable procedures.
- Satisfied patients experience less stress than others.
- Highly satisfied patients actually *feel* better than others and recover more quickly.
- Patients who have positive experiences become "apostles" for the organization, promoting it to others.
- There is a high correlation between satisfied employees and satisfied patients.

All of these add up to competitive strength and bottom-line gains. And there is another reason not to be overlooked. In their book *Leadership for Great Customer Service,* Mayer and Cates (2004) suggest that the number-one reason "to get customer service right in health care is . . . it makes the job easier" (p. 5). Mayer and Cates observe that team members *like* coming to work when they feel they are making a difference rather than swimming upstream, when they enjoy the work they do and are able to have creative input, and when they feel valued and supported by coworkers and supervisors.

Here are some tips from the experts on building cultures that sustain service excellence. You will see that much of the emphasis is on employee satisfaction. As many have observed, it is unlikely that dissatisfied employees will lead to happy clients, but happy employees will go far beyond the job description to do a good job.

- *Go beyond expectations.* Inspiring customer loyalty requires giving people *more* than they expect. Mayer and Cates (2004) put it this way: "How much credit do we give airlines for getting us from point A to point B and not killing us? How about *none*—we expect that. Your patients expect excellent clinical care (the destination). But they also expect excellent service (the journey)" (p. 26).
- *Recognize and create moments of truth.* Moments of truth occur any time people develop an impression of an organization based on how they are treated. The Mayo Clinic staff encountered a moment of truth when a woman seeking care in the emergency department was worried about her dog, which was outside in the 18-wheeler truck she drove for a living. Nurses got permission to park the truck at a local shopping mall and looked after the woman's dog until she was well enough to leave the hospital.

- *Use service failures as a springboard.* When employees of a large hospital were asked to think of times they had experienced outstanding customer service, their answers were inspiring. One woman was frustrated when a department store was late making alterations to a dress she had bought, until a sales clerk called her to apologize and personally delivered the dress to her at home. Another was dismayed when a car she had just bought died on her way to work, until a person from the dealership arrived 10 minutes after she had called, met her on the roadside, handed her the keys to a loaner car, and had her car fixed and waiting for her when she got home that day. These are not only stories of service; they are *service-recovery* stories. The customers were ready to walk away forever—frustrated and inclined to tell everyone they knew about the poor treatment. But in each case, an associate (who was often not to blame for the service failure) turned the situation around by apologizing and giving better-than-expected service. The moral is that service recovery is often an opportunity to turn a customer into a loyal fan.
- *Tell stories and honor heroes.* Stories such as the ones in this chapter become guiding principles for others. They portray what is best and most noble in the things we do. One of the most effective ways to support a culture is to encourage its stories. Good leaders appreciate their value and share them often.

Here is one more story, from Lafayette General Hospital in Lafayette, Louisiana. An ambulance arrived late in the evening on Christmas Eve with a woman and her two young children, who had been involved in an automobile accident. The children were okay, but the woman died soon after arriving at the hospital. Her husband was working on an offshore oil rig, and police were unable to reach him.

The emergency department staff was devastated for these two children who had just lost their mother and were stranded in a hospital with no family on Christmas Eve. The nurses, doctors, and unit receptionist tried to comfort and entertain the children as best they could until their shift change. The stores were closed, so they took turns driving to their homes to get supplies and gifts to create a makeshift holiday for the children. Sacrificing time they might have spent relaxing with their own families, the nurses worked into the night so that, when the children awoke on Christmas morning, the room was decorated with a tree surrounded by presents. Many staff members had brought their families to the hospital to share Christmas morning with the children.

"The employees' kids were amazing," remembers one nurse. "Here they were, in a hospital on Christmas morning, watching children they didn't know open gifts that had been under *their* trees with *their* names on them the day before. And they were just so happy to share. There wasn't a dry eye in the place, I can tell you!"

Summary

Health Care Administration

- Health care administrators play a key role in uniting diverse people toward a common mission and enabling team members to do their best. Well-designed systems can also reduce stress and minimize errors.
- Empowerment means that administrators are servant leaders who are open to the ideas and concerns of team members who are encouraged to be decisive and accountable.
- In many health care organizations, employees are increasingly encouraged to think of ways to please customers, solve problems, work together in teams, and come up with innovative methods to improve care and conserve resources.

Human Resources

- Appealing work environments help to retain and develop talented people in health care.
- Human resource personnel play an important role by helping to recruit, train, support, and retain outstanding team members.
- Informed by evidence that people perform best when they are actively engaged, human resource personnel can help people develop the skills and confidence to participate in decision making and leadership.
- To navigate the challenges ahead and offset staffing shortages, we must help health care professionals do their jobs without burning out. This means giving them the freedom to create pleasant work environments that foster teamwork and relieve stress, resisting the temptation to overwork staff members, and providing frequent breaks and replenishment.

Marketing and Public Relations

- With health care dollars limited and competition steep, people in health organizations are challenged to anticipate as accurately as possible what health services people are likely to want and need. Marketing and public relations professionals can help with this.
- Marketing and public relations specialists build trusting relationships with internal and external stakeholders to attract loyal patients and benefactors.

Crisis Management

- Crisis communication plans are critical for dealing with image-threatening or high-profile events, health scares, and other situations that put health care organizations in the limelight.
- Handling crises well requires communication skills, preparation, a commitment to key values, and a willingness to handle unexpected demands.

Service Excellence

- Service is everyone's job.
- People throughout health care organizations are called upon to offer legendary service, recognize moments of truth, overcome service obstacles, and honor the noble spirit of helping other people.

Glossary

A-team players Team members who love a challenge, have a positive attitude, and inspire everyone around them (as opposed to B-team players). *See page 226.*

B-team players Team members who have bad attitudes, who are often lazy or late, and who resent the demands of the job (as opposed to A-team players). *See page 226.*

commitment-trust theory of relationships The theory that people make relatively enduring judgments based on trust, shared values, loyalty, and commitment. *See page 228.*

corporate identity Enduring qualities that make an organization recognizable in comparison to others (compared to corporate image, which can be superficial and fleeting). *See page 230.*

Hoy-Tarter Model of Shared Decision Making The perspective that leaders should considering involving people in shared decision making if they have a personal stake in the outcome and expertise on the topic. *See page 221.*

image An overall but sometimes fleeting feeling about a company based on its "personality" (compared to corporate identity, which is more enduring). *See page 230.*

motivation-hygiene theory The idea that satisfaction is based on one set of factors (e.g., feeling satisfied, making an important difference, feeling respected, learning and improving) and dissatisfaction is based on a different set of factors (e.g., feeling underpaid, working in unhealthy or unproductive conditions, perceiving that rules and policies are unfair). *See page 225.*

Point-A-to-Point-B companies Organizations in which members are motivated primarily by profits and are willing to engage in questionable means in pursuit of money. *See page 230.*

reputation A long-term assessment about the "character, conscience, and credibility" of an organization. *See page 230.*

reputation based [companies] Those that have a positive image based on values consistently embodied by people through the organization. *See page 230.*

superficially image based [companies] Those that realize the value of a positive image but seek it through advertising campaigns and slogans that sound good but don't reflect the true nature of the organization. *See page 230.*

theory of personal causation The proposition that people resist being treated as pawns (required to relinquish control and unthinkingly follow orders) but respond well when they are treated as origins (active participants in designing and carrying out worthwhile tasks). *See page 224.*

Theory X and Theory Y The perspective that managers tend to fall into one of two basic camps: Theory X managers believe people are naturally lazy and must be prodded and supervised to be productive, whereas Theory Y managers believe people enjoy the inherent rewards of work and are motivated to make a positive difference. *See page 225.*

two-way symmetrical communication Ongoing, open dialogue between members of an organization and the larger publics it serves. *See page 229.*

Discussion Questions

1. Describe the best boss or teacher you have ever had. How did they communicate with others? How did they make you and other people feel? Which of the behaviors described in this chapter did that person embody?

2. Describe the significance of pawns and origins in de Charms's theory of personal causation. Give an example from your own experience in which you felt like a pawn and an example in which you were treated as an origin.

3. Imagine that you have been promoted to supervisor. If you adopt a Theory X approach, how will you treat team members? How will you treat them if you adopt a Theory Y approach? Which do you think will be more effective? Why?

4. Explain the concept of relationship marketing and relationship management. What are some of the main ideas that support a relationship approach to marketing and public relations? Include in your answer a description of the commitment-trust theory of relationships and two-way symmetrical communication.

5. What are the differences between corporate identity, image, and reputation? How do these concepts characterize Point-A-to-Point-B companies, superficially image-based companies, and reputation-based companies?

6. Identify several current examples of health-related social media messages. How effective do you think each message is? Why? How many of the tips presented in this chapter do the messages reflect?

7. Imagine that you have been asked to create a crisis management plan for an organization that doesn't yet have one. What steps would you take before a crisis arises? What would you do during a crisis? In what ways would communication be involved at each step?

8. Describe a time when you received great customer service, and a time when you received poor service. What role did communication play in each episode? How did each experience affect the way you think about the people and organization involved?

PART VI

Media, Public Policy, and Health Promotion

In this section we look at people and events that change the world. We explore the role of mass media in shaping cultural and global ideas about what it means to be healthy and successful. We also look at the efforts of public health experts and consider how we might apply the lessons from Ebola, AIDS, terrorism, and the opioid epidemic to our own efforts. In the final two chapters, we use theory and expert advice to create a hypothetical public health campaign.

As you end this unit, we hope you will feel that your understanding of health communication has deepened and broadened. Keep an eye on the news. Health care is ever changing, and perhaps with the insights and examples we have discussed, you can take an active role in shaping the future of health and health communication.

How wonderful it is that nobody need wait a single moment before starting to improve the world.

—ANNE FRANK

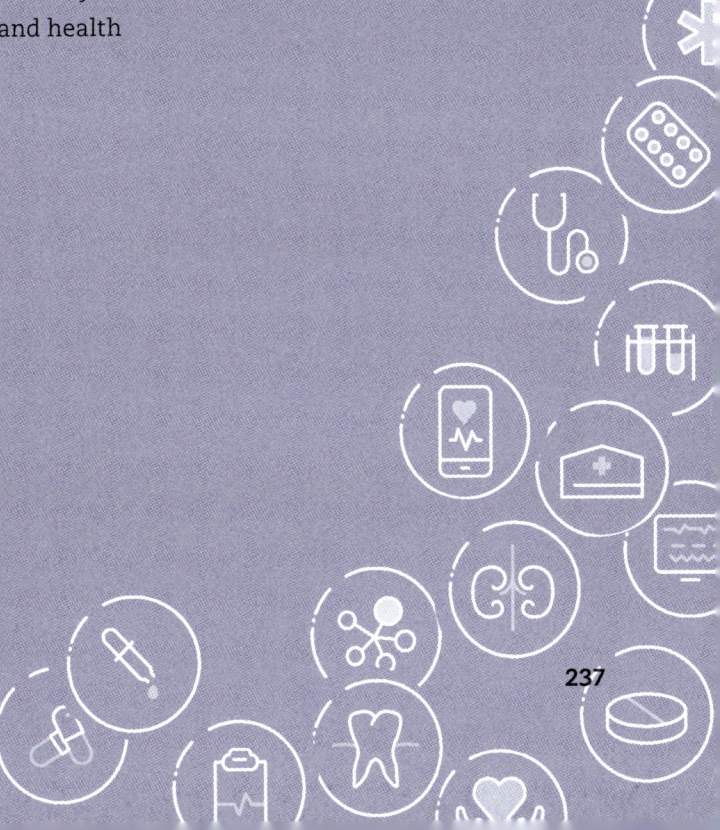

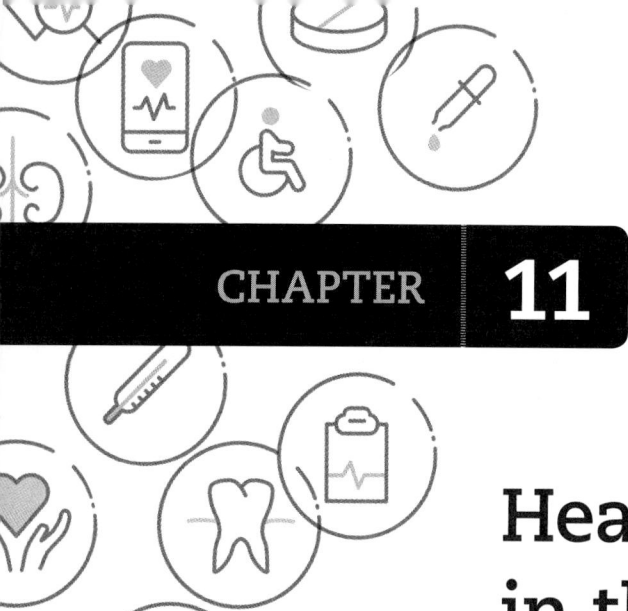

CHAPTER 11

Health Images in the Media

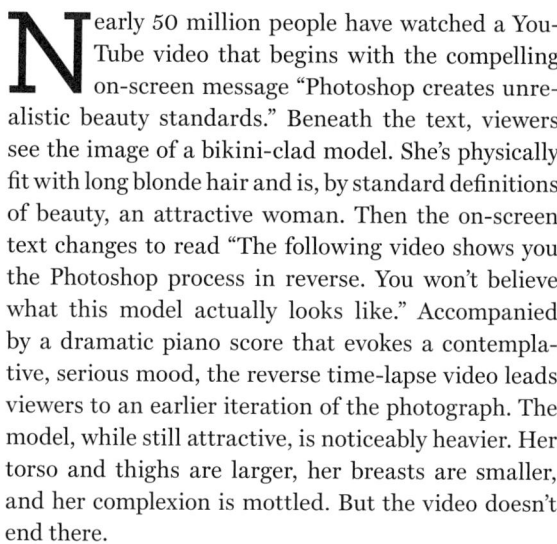

Nearly 50 million people have watched a YouTube video that begins with the compelling on-screen message "Photoshop creates unrealistic beauty standards." Beneath the text, viewers see the image of a bikini-clad model. She's physically fit with long blonde hair and is, by standard definitions of beauty, an attractive woman. Then the on-screen text changes to read "The following video shows you the Photoshop process in reverse. You won't believe what this model actually looks like." Accompanied by a dramatic piano score that evokes a contemplative, serious mood, the reverse time-lapse video leads viewers to an earlier iteration of the photograph. The model, while still attractive, is noticeably heavier. Her torso and thighs are larger, her breasts are smaller, and her complexion is mottled. But the video doesn't end there.

In the 90 seconds that follow, viewers watch as the photograph is taken all the way back to what is purported to be to its unedited, original form. The "before" image depicts a slice of pepperoni pizza! Lucia Peters (2014), in a piece for *Bustle*, wrote, "You know Photoshop has gone too far when you can use it to turn a piece of pizza into a glamorous model" (para. 2).

The video, made by CollegeHumor Media in 2014, is funny and, according to Peters (2014), uses satire to make a cogent point: "Why are we basing our standards of beauty on a piece of software that can turn a pizza into a human? When you look at it through this particular lens, it's completely and utterly absurd" (para. 3). While it may be absurd, standards of beauty are often based on unrealistic media images—most photos in popular magazines have been "airbrushed to perfection," in the words of researchers Lindsey Conlin and Kim Bissell (2014, p. 2.).

The same illusionary tactics lie behind many media images, and the result is that what *appears* to be real often is not. Even the models who appear in advertisements do not always look like themselves when compared with the stylized images that others see of them. These unrealistic depictions have an influence on health when they affect people's self-esteem, their eating patterns, and more. Eating disorders, which have the highest mortality rate of any mental illness, affect 30 million Americans (most of them female) and kill nearly 24 people every day (Alliance for Eating Disorders Awareness, 2019). There is solid evidence linking eating disorders to media consumption (Rodgers, O'Flynn, & McLean, 2019), which means that media users, including social media users, are more likely to suffer disordered eating than people who consume little to no media. Media consumption affects people's health in other ways too, as this chapter demonstrates.

In the following sections, we explore the impact of mass-communicated messages on health. **Mass communication** is defined as the dissemination of messages from one person or group to large numbers of people via media including television, radio, computers, newspapers, magazines, billboards, video games, and other means. As you will see, there is evidence that media messages prompt some people to eat too little or too much, doubt their attractiveness, drink alcohol, smoke, and neglect their health in other ways.

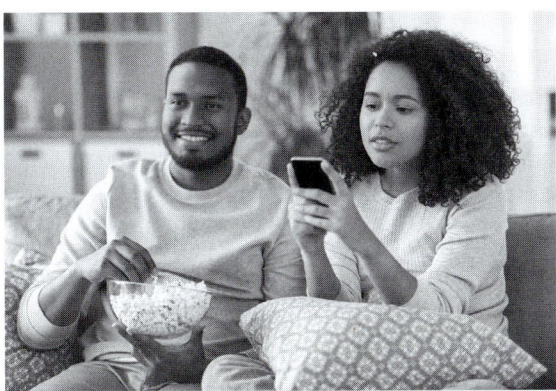

American adults spend nearly half of each day connected to media (Nielsen Company, 2019).

How much time, per day, do you spend watching television? Playing video games? Texting? Talking on the phone? Are you influenced by media messages? If so, how?

However, the outlook is not entirely grim. Although media content can have harmful effects on health, it is also a means of sharing information that can help people better understand their health and health-related behaviors.

As we explore some of the ways mass media messages shape our ideas about health and how we behave, remember that a link or an association does not prove that media, or media alone, *cause* behaviors. Mass-mediated messages are just one of many influences. Message effects are likely to be lessened or exaggerated by a range of other factors, including personal preferences, culture, social networks, health status, and media literacy. We conclude this chapter with information about media literacy—a systematic process of becoming more skeptical and better informed mass-media consumers so we don't unwittingly buy into harmful and unrealistic ideas.

Theoretical Foundations

Before considering the impact of media use on health, it's useful to get a feel for how much media people actually use. The numbers may surprise you.

Worldwide, adults spend an average of 7½ hours each day watching television, listening to the radio, surfing the web, and reading newspapers or magazines (Watson, 2018). Americans consume more media than most people around the world. According to the U.S. Bureau of Labor Statistics, 80% of Americans over age 15 watch television on any given day, making it "the choice leisure activity for many Americans" (Krantz-Kent, 2018, para. 1).

Adults in the U.S. spend an average of 11 hours and 27 minutes connected to media every day (Nielsen Company, 2019). More than half of that time is spent watching video. Most adults (especially those younger than 65) prefer streaming video over watching live television, which reflects a shift away from traditional media like broadcast television and DVDs. Adults over age 65 and African Americans tend to watch more live television than other groups.

It's hard to pin down the average daily media use of children and teens. Studies suggest that their media consumption is as little as a few hours a day all the way up to 12 or more hours a day (Nielsen Company, 2019; Wakefield, 2018). One extensive study showed that U.S. children ages 8 to 18 spend about 7½ hours a day using entertainment media devices such as smartphones, MP3 players, computer tablets, and television—sometimes several of them at once (Henry J. Kaiser Family Foundation, 2010). The average is lower (about 4½ hours per day) among children whose parents have set time limits on media use, but only about 30% of youth fall into that category. And the average is much higher (about 13 hours a day) among heavy users. Black and Hispanic children tend to fall disproportionately in the range of heavy media use, especially TV watching.

Excessive media use is associated with social and health risks. Heavy digital media use by teens is associated with symptoms of attention-deficit/hyperactivity disorder (Ra et al., 2018), and early childhood exposure to media (particularly video) is associated with delayed language development, poor reading skills, short-term memory problems, and shortened attention span (Hill, 2016). Additionally, regular exposure to advertisements for unhealthy foods (e.g., chips and sugary cereals) often makes it difficult for young children to make sensible food choices (Radesky, 2017), which increases their likelihood of becoming obese and/or developing diabetes. (We'll talk about this more in a moment.)

The theories described here—third-person effect, cultivation theory, social learning theory, and social comparison theory—consider how media messages influence our attitudes, expectations, and health.

Third-Person Effect

Most of us believe we are not personally susceptible to persuasive messages in the media, but we think other people are. W. Phillips Davison (1983) coined the term **third-person effect** to describe this perception. For example, teens often believe their peers will be more likely to smoke if they see pro-smoking messages in the media, but they tend to feel immune from that effect themselves (Gunther, Bolt, Borzekowski, Liebhart, & Dillard, 2006). In a video about sexist images in advertising, Jean Kilbourne (2000) observes that people frequently tell her they are not affected by the media. "Of course, they are usually standing there in their Gap t-shirt while they say this," she laughs. The reality is that we are all affected by media messages to varying extents, and the impact is greatest if we spend a lot of time with media and have limited personal experience with the phenomena we see depicted.

Cultivation Theory

Cultivation theory helps to explain why children may be especially vulnerable to advertising messages. According to the theory, people develop beliefs about the world based on a complex array of influences, media among them. Media's influence is not uniform or automatic, but it is likely to be most profound if (a) media images are highly consistent, (b) people are exposed to large amounts of media, and (c) people have a limited basis for evaluating what they see and hear (Gerbner, Gross, Morgan, & Signorielli, 1994). Consider that children have fewer experiences and less knowledge than adults. Because of this, they are less able to perceive that media images may be wrong or unrealistic. The same principle would hold true if you watched a documentary about a faraway land about which you knew very little. People familiar with that land might see inaccuracies in the documentary that you would be unable to identify.

The effect is compounded among high media users because not only is their exposure high, but the more time they spend tuned into mass media, the less opportunity they have to experience activities that might provide them with a basis for comparison. For example, children in the United States who watch a lot of television aimed at young audiences are inundated with depictions of heterosexual romance in which boys mostly value girls for their physical appearance and girls spend their time trying to look attractive for boys while also complimenting boys on their personalities and accomplishments (Kirsch & Murnen, 2015). Considering that children typically regard media characters as peers and role models, such consistent and gendered characterizations are likely to influence how they view themselves and those around them. Media characterizations also influence how children—and adults—behave.

Social Learning Theory

People learn social behaviors by imitating others. This is the central tenet of **social learning theory**, proposed by Albert Bandura (1977). The theory explains that people learn how to behave by (a) watching others, (b) watching media depictions of others, and (c) watching and attending to the consequences of others' behavioral choices. For example, if children observe that violent acts perpetrated by characters in cartoons and video games are rarely (if ever) met with

CHAPTER 11 HEALTH IMAGES IN THE MEDIA

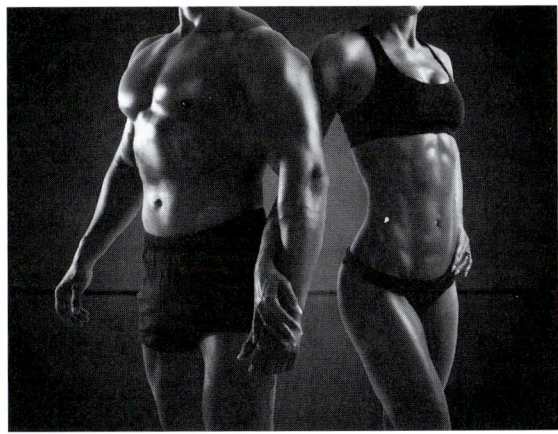

Researchers have found that some people suffer low self-esteem because they regularly compare themselves to unrealistic standards embodied by supermodels or bodybuilders.

Do you compare yourself to media images? Why or why not? How do you think we can minimize the effects of media images that establish unrealistic standards of attractiveness?

punishment or consequences, such acts may inform children's repertoire of acceptable behavioral choices. But media is just one of many factors that influence behavior.

Social Comparison Theory

Social comparison theory helps to explain why people yearn to emulate the characters, models, and celebrities they see in the media. Proposed by Leon Festinger (1957), **social comparison theory** suggests that people judge themselves largely in comparison to others. Want to know if you are attractive, popular, healthy, or smart? The answer may lie in how you stack up to the people around you. Social comparisons can be useful when they enhance self-esteem or serve as the basis for self-improvement. However, they become dysfunctional when the comparison establishes an unrealistic standard (like being supermodel thin or weightlifter strong).

Next, let's look at deliberate attempts to influence people's behavior through advertisements.

Advertising

Can you fill in the blanks to complete the following slogans?

Melts in your mouth, not in your _____.

Tastes great, less _____.

Finger-_____ good.

If you guessed *hand* (M&Ms), *filling* (Miller Lite), and *lickin'* (KFC), you are right. But perhaps you do not usually stop to think about the connection between brand-name exposure and health. In this section we explore the impact of mass media advertising in terms of nutrition, body image, alcohol and tobacco use, and prescription drugs.

Nutrition and Obesity

Heavy TV viewing is consistently linked to obesity and a "coach potato physique," characterized by soft bulges where muscle ought to be. This is partly because television is a triple threat: people usually burn few calories while watching, they tend to snack while viewing, and commercials often encourage consumption of foods that are not nutritious. In addition, commercials sometimes distort people's knowledge of nutrition and influence their food preferences for the worse. For example, teens who are heavy TV viewers tend to overestimate the nutritional value of fast food, perhaps because they see numerous commercials for it in the context of viewing mostly slim and fit people (Russell & Buhrau, 2015). As this section shows, weight and nutrition issues often begin in childhood.

EFFECTS ON CHILDREN

Children's body mass index often correlates with their ability to recognize the brand names of companies that manufacture unhealthy food products such as chips and cookies (Cornwell, McAlister, & Polmear-Swendris, 2014). This is a serious concern, considering that children are exposed to an average of 5,500 to 7,500 televised food commercials per year (Desrochers & Holt, 2007; Mazur et al., 2018), and half of all food ads target children (Barclay, 2016).

Food commercials often misrepresent foods' nutritional value, and this misleading information can prompt children to make poor health choices. For example, in a study conducted by Kristin Harrison (2005), children were asked to choose the more nutritious option between cottage cheese and fat-free ice cream and between orange juice and Diet Coke. Children who watched a lot of television were more likely to consider (incorrectly) that the heavily advertised diet products were better for them. The chances are high, Harrison concluded, that children exposed to a lot of commercials will assume that diet products are, by nature, more nutritious than other foods.

Ads not only encourage poor food choices, but also may trigger children to eat more. After analyzing 18 studies on advertising and food consumption, Emma Boyland and colleagues (2016) concluded that "exposure to unhealthy food advertising increases food intake in children" (p. 532). Interestingly, similar effects were not seen in adults. In line with cultivation theory, Boyland et al. explained that adults are more critical viewers of media, whereas "young children may be particularly vulnerable to the effects of marketing because they are unable to understand its selling or persuasive intent" (p. 531).

The numbers paint a disturbing picture. In the U.S. alone, the number of obese children has more than doubled and the number of obese adolescents has quadrupled since the 1980s (National Center for Health Statistics, 2012; Ogden et al., 2014). At least 30% of children and teens in the United States are now overweight or obese (Data Resource Center for Child and Adolescent Health, 2017). The numbers are especially high among 16- to 19-year-olds; about 42% of them are obese (Skinner, Ravanbakht, Skelton, Perrin, & Armstrong, 2018). Obesity is highest among African American and Hispanic children. In 2013 and 2014, rates of severe obesity spiked in children ages 2 to 5, and data suggest rates will continue rising.

Childhood obesity is not only an American problem. There has been a steady rise in obesity among European children over the last 25 years (Mazur et al., 2018). Across Europe, rates range from 10% to 40%, reflecting a strong link between obesity and childhood media exposure. Worldwide, children and adults are getting heavier.

There is some encouraging news. When researchers showed preschoolers in the Netherlands fresh banana slices and banana candy, the children preferred the candy. But when the fresh fruit was packaged and decorated with depictions of popular cartoon characters, the children considered the fruit to be just as appealing as the candy (de Droog, Valkenburg, & Buijzen, 2011). Pairing fruit with images that children already view favorably may increase its appeal.

EFFECTS ON ADULTS

Adults are not immune to unhealthy images, and the numbers are stacked against healthy food. Less than half of 1% of food advertisements are for fruits and vegetables (Barclay, 2016). The majority of commercials are for fatty and sugary foods—specifically, fast food, sugary beverages, and cereal—and this can have serious implications for health. Analyzing 45 studies on the subject, researchers found that seeing pictures or videos of food triggered cravings in adults that led them to make poor food choices (Boswell & Kober, 2016). Such choices can, and often do, lead to weight gain. These findings are worrisome considering that overweight people are at elevated risk for heart disease, cancer, diabetes, and sudden death.

African American women are at especially high risk for obesity and related concerns. About 55% of African American women are obese (Hales, Carroll, Fryar, & Ogden, 2017). This may be partly because of advertisements that target them. When researchers compared ads in *Essence* (aimed mostly at African American women) and *Cosmopolitan* (targeted to women in general), they found that 13% of the *Essence* ads were for fast food, compared to 1% of the *Cosmopolitan* ads (Kean & Prividera, 2007). Furthermore, *Cosmopolitan* readers were exposed to more ads for weight-loss products (mentioned in 41% of the ads) than were *Essence* readers (12% of ads). (While these messages may be helpful to *Cosmopolitan* readers trying to maintain a healthy weight, it should also be noted that many of the weight-loss claims—such as those for low-carbohydrate whiskey—were not exactly health conscious.)

The editorial content in women's magazines does little to offset themes found in advertisements. When Conlin and Bissell (2014) studied women's magazines, they found that both fashion and fitness magazines focused mostly on women's appearance rather than their health. In the fashion magazines, references to appearance outnumbered references to health nearly 19 to 1. But even in the fitness magazines, diet and physical activity were typically framed in terms of enhancing one's appearance rather than one's health. And appearance was measured mostly in terms of a "thin ideal" in all the magazines. Although many of the models appeared to be dangerously thin, they were promoted as being physically fit and appealing. The researchers concluded that women's magazines tend to frame health in terms of "thinness and glamor" (p. 12).

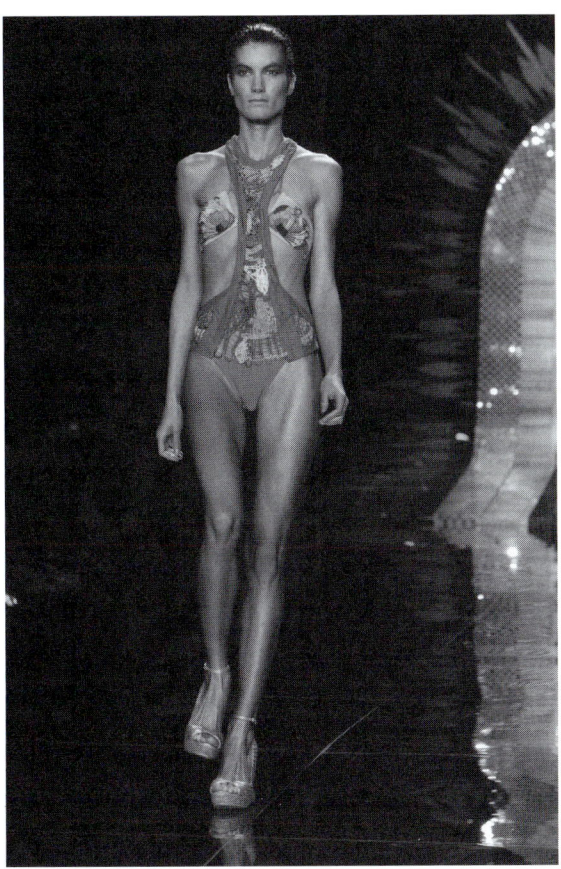

In contrast to the average woman, who wears a size 12 to 14, fashion models typically wear sizes 0 or 2 (Betts, 2002).

ACTIVITY LEVELS

Note that advertising is not entirely to blame for the obesity linked to TV viewing. Some researchers suggest that the sedentary nature of heavy viewing is just as unhealthy as the content viewed. Children and teens with televisions in their bedrooms are heavier, on average, than their peers (Rey-Lopez et al., 2012). And heavy television viewing may lead to other unhealthy behaviors. For example, youngsters with high media exposure are more likely than their peers to smoke (Yang, Salmon, Pang, & Cheng, 2015). Researchers speculate that extensive viewing substitutes for physical activities and, consequently, limits social development that might otherwise help teens avoid peer pressure.

High media use is also linked to sleep deprivation (Radesky, 2017). Children today sleep an average of two hours less per night than did children in the 1980s (Zimmerman, 2008). Authorities blame TV, video, the internet, and computer games. They say these activities sometimes cut into sleep time and leave children too excited to sleep when the lights go out. Children may also feel less sleepy because they are not getting much exercise and because the glow from TV and computer screens inhibits melatonin secretion, an important chemical in sleep functioning (Zimmerman, 2008).

Alcohol

Beer commercials often show drinkers surrounded by beautiful women and fun-loving friends in exotic locales. But the reality is not nearly so glamorous. Worldwide, alcohol is the leading cause of preventable death and disability in persons ages 15 to 49 (National Institute on Alcohol Abuse and Alcoholism [NIAAA], 2018). Heavy drinkers risk liver damage, hypertension, and strokes, and they are more likely than their peers to hurt others and to be hurt in accidents and/or violent acts (Nestle, 1997). Moreover, for adolescents who drink, alcohol interferes with their brain development and increases their chances of being sexually assaulted and/or killed in a car accident (NIAAA, 2018). In the United States, alcohol factors into one-third of driving fatalities (NIAAA, 2018). Considering these risks, it is no wonder that alcohol companies are criticized for portraying drinking as fun and sexy.

Unfortunately, health warnings tend to get lost in the sea of pro-alcohol messages. Alcoholic beverage ads outnumber responsible drinking PSAs at least 22 to 1 ("Youth Exposure," 2010). And alcohol ads have appeal. When market researchers asked teens to name their five favorite Super Bowl commercials, three of them were ads for beer ("Beer Commercials," 2009). Young people may remember and like these commercials so much because the spots are designed for them. Nearly one-third of radio ads for alcoholic beverages air when the listening audience is mostly teens rather than adults ("Youth Exposure," 2010). Promotional efforts for wine and alcopops (alcoholic beverages mixed with fruit juice or other flavoring) are most often broadcast on the radio when teenage girls, rather than women, are likely to be listening ("Youth Exposure," 2010).

This early exposure seems to make a significant difference in alcohol consumption. When researchers Gert-Jan Meerkerk and Barbara van Straaten (2019)

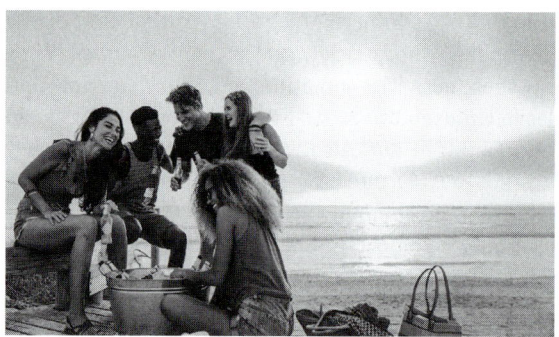

Alcohol ads often make drinking seem fun and exciting, but alcohol is the leading cause of preventable death and disability in adults worldwide (National Institute on Alcohol Abuse and Alcoholism, 2018).

studied teenagers, they found a positive association between viewing alcohol advertisements and a pattern of consuming four or more alcoholic drinks in one sitting (considered binge drinking). The association between ads and drinking was strongest among young participants in the study, which is alarming considering that the participants' average age was 13!

Statistics describing alcohol consumption among teens and young adults are sobering. About 1 in 4 eighth graders and 6 in 10 high school seniors in the United States have tried alcohol (NIDA, 2018). Consider the following figures compiled by the NIAAA (2018):

> *Thirteen percent of 12- to 29-year-olds have engaged in binge drinking and nationally an estimated 623,000 adolescents qualify as having alcohol use disorder*, defined as "a chronic relapsing brain disease characterized by an impaired ability to stop or control alcohol use despite adverse social, occupational, or health consequences." (para. 34)

- A national survey of college students found that 58% reported drinking during the previous month, 38% binged, and 13% qualified as heavy drinkers (drinking alcohol five or more days a month). About 20% met the criteria for alcohol use disorder, and 25% had suffered academic consequences as a result of drinking (e.g., earning poor grades and failing tests). On average, about 100,000 college students are victims of alcohol-related sexual assault each year.

Alcohol and sex are co-mingled in the media to such a degree that many teens and college students believe that drinking alcohol leads to sexual activity. When 70% of alcohol ads focus on sex (Rhoades & Jernigan, 2013), it is perhaps not surprising that some people equate the two. Kathleen Boyce Rogers et al. (2019) found that teens were more likely to believe that alcohol facilitates sex after they viewed sexually suggestive alcohol advertisements that objectified women. As a result, young women may see that drinking alcohol is a way to look and feel sexy, and it may embolden them to pursue sex. But the researchers concluded that young men "may use alcohol coercively to attain sexual activity" (Rodgers et al., 2019, p. 402) and doing so may qualify as sexual assault. Many states have laws that specify that sex cannot be considered consensual if either person is intoxicated (DeMatteo, Galloway, Arnold, & Patel, 2015).

Alcohol-related sexual assault, especially on college campuses, is a huge problem. One study found that most victims of college sexual assault were raped after they and their attackers consumed alcohol (Hines, Armstrong, Reed, & Cameron, 2012). In some instances, bystanders intervened, as was the case in 2016 when two Stanford students saw an unconscious woman being sexually assaulted behind a dumpster on campus. Both the victim and her attacker had been drinking earlier while at a fraternity party. The incident sparked national debate when the perpetrator, a member of Stanford's swim team, served only a few weeks of a six-month sentence (Baker, 2016; Iati, 2019). In most instances of sexual assault, however, bystanders do not step in. Researchers have found a link between viewing objectifying alcohol advertisements and young people's reluctance to intervene in situations involving sexual assault and alcohol (Hust, Rogers, Cameron, & Li, 2019).

What we see on TV and in magazines influences our behaviors in ways that can be detrimental to our health and well-being, as this chapter demonstrates, but media can also promote healthy behaviors. For instance, responsible drinking messages have had some influence. When analysts reviewed 14 years of research about the effects of campaigns to discourage underage drinking, they found that there were small but significant reductions in the number of teen drinkers over time (Kyrrestad Strøm, Adolfsen, Fossum, Kaiser, & Martinussen, 2014). Anti-drinking campaigns on college campuses have had some success as well. For example, Hannah Kang & Moon J. Lee (2017) found that students exposed to anti–binge drinking messages reported higher intentions to avoid binge drinking compared with students in a control group.

Tobacco and Nicotine

In 1994, some 46 states entered an agreement with the tobacco industry that included restrictions on the number and placement of tobacco advertisements. The Master Settlement Agreement (MSA), as it is called, bans tobacco advertising in public transit systems, on television, and in the movies, and it severely limits the placement of tobacco billboards near sports stadiums, shopping malls, arcades, and other places young people frequent. The MSA is meant to restrict tobacco marketing overall, but in particular, to shield young audiences from it. Beyond requiring a warning label, the rules do not otherwise restrict how tobacco is advertised, the content of tobacco ads, or how tobacco products are packaged.

To see how tobacco marketing has changed over time, Tae Hyun Baek and Mark Mayer (2010) compared tobacco ads in *Cosmopolitan*, *Sports Illustrated*, and *Rolling Stone* in 1994 with those that ran nearly 10 years later. They found that the ads have become more sexually suggestive since 1994—frequently featuring young, scantily clad women—and more, rather than fewer, youthful models. The researchers reflect that, while objectifying women is not a new trend, it is disappointing in light of health threats that companies continue to depict smokers as young and sexy.

Although the MSA places restrictions on ads promoting cigarettes and smokeless tobacco, it does not restrict advertisements for e-cigarettes or "vaping." Vaping has been hyped as a safe alternative to cigarette smoking, promising a "clean" nicotine delivery experience without the carcinogens associated with burning tobacco. Vaping works by heating a liquid that contains nicotine (often with flavoring compounds added to the mix); as the liquid heats up, it turns into a vapor that users inhale. Vaping, as it turns out, is just as addictive as smoking cigarettes and harder to quit (Thomas, 2019).

Vaping is popular among teens. In fact, more teens vape than smoke cigarettes and the numbers are rising. About 20% of high school students use e-cigarettes—up from 1.5% in 2011 (CDC, 2019). Some studies report that as many as 43% of high school seniors have vaped (NIDA, 2018), likely because they are targeted by e-cigarette ads that (a) tout fun flavors such as watermelon and Fruity Pebbles, and (b) highlight the advantages of vaping over smoking (e.g., there are no cigarette butts to dispose of and vaping does not stain teeth or skin). The majority of radio ads for e-cigarettes focus on the wide range of flavors available and frequently use humor, sound effects, and music that appeals to young audiences (Nicksic, Brosnan, Chowdhury, Barnes, & Cobb, 2019).

There is strong evidence that viewing e-cigarette ads is positively associated with teens' intention to vape (see Kim, Popova, Halpern-Felsher, & Ling, 2019; Thomas, 2019), and manufacturers of vaping-related products know this. E-cigarette makers quintupled their marketing budgets between 2012 and 2014 (Kim et al., 2019) and, in the same period, turned out ads with animations and sexual themes that appealed to young audiences (Padon, Maloney, & Cappella, 2017). The increase in ad spending coincided with an uptick in vaping among high schoolers and young adults. By 2019, e-cigarette ads had penetrated a sizeable majority of the youth market. Surveying more than 12,000 teens (ages 16–19) living in the United States, Canada, and England, researchers found that between 74% and 83% reported having seen ads for e-cigarettes (Cho, Thrasher, Reid, Hitchman, & Hammond, 2019).

In September 2019, U.S. president Donald Trump announced a ban (a decision, he later reversed) on flavored e-cigarettes, citing the role they played in escalating nicotine use among teens, which he linked to a spate of vaping-related illness and deaths (Fertig & Owermohl, 2019). Hundreds of people fell ill with severe lung disease and several died after using vaping products containing THC (the psychoactive compound in marijuana) and, according to CDC officials, some people fell ill after vaping only nicotine (Fertig & Owermohl, 2019; see also Carlisle, 2019). Walmart announced it would stop selling all e-cigarette products, and Amazon pulled vaping paraphernalia from its online stores (Bose, 2019). But as one 17-year-old hospitalized with vaping-related lung disease told reporters, vaping products are easily found on the illegal market (Bosman & Richtel, 2019). Regulatory efforts, thus, may do little to curb teen vaping.

Next, we examine direct-to-consumer pharmaceutical advertising.

Pharmaceutical Advertisements

This product may cause headaches, drowsiness, stomach upset, liver problems, heartbeat irregularities . . .

BOX 11.1 PERSPECTIVES

Viagra Ads Promise Male Transformation

Commercials for erectile dysfunction (ED) have varied over time. Early ads featured 75-year-old former U.S. senator and presidential candidate Bob Dole. In one ad, he explains to viewers that he had worried about potential side effects following his prostate surgery, "like erectile dysfunction, often called 'impotence.'" While the topic may be embarrassing, he says that his experience and subsequent treatment (i.e., Viagra) might help "the millions of men and their partners" affected by ED. A few years later, Pfizer switched things up with the "get things done" commercials. In one, a handsome man driving a muscle car along a country road deftly gets his wheels rolling again after the car overheats, with the implication that he is also able to "get things done" in the bedroom with help from Viagra.

In 2014, Pfizer pharmaceuticals shed innuendo with a series of commercials featuring a beautiful woman who spoke directly to men. In one, a woman lounges on a day bed in a tropical setting. "Plenty of guys have this issue—not just getting an erection, but keeping it," she says directly into the camera. "Well, Viagra helps. . . . Good to know, right?"

Jay Baglia, author of *The Viagra Ad Venture* (2005), challenges viewers to think carefully about these ads. For one thing, he says, notice the age of the actors. Although erectile dysfunction is most common among men age 65 and older, Pfizer tends to target younger men, insinuating that their sexual performance could use a pharmaceutical boost as well. Case in point, Pfizer's website for Viagra proclaims in big letters, "About 50% of men over 40 have some degree of ED" (www.viagra.com).

Apparently, the ads work. A 2010 study found that about 1 in 5 healthy men ages 18 to 30 had taken some form of erectile dysfunction drug, usually, they said, to boost their "sexual confidence" or "sexual performance" (Bechara, Casabé, De Bonis, Hellen, & Bertolino, 2010). The notion of Viagra as a recreational drug is serious, considering that the active ingredient, sildenafil, has serious side effects. Although current numbers are not available, reports have linked sildenafil to at least 1,824 deaths and 14,818 instances of serious adverse effects over a 10-year period (Lowe & Costabile, 2012).

Baglia (2005) also challenges the insinuation that men's penises reflect their worth as people. The message in Viagra ads is clear, he says: "Nothing tells a man he is masculine—not muscles, earning potential, an attractive partner, or even height—so much as his erection does" (p. 9). And if that is not reductive and intimidating enough, Pfizer has raised the bar on acceptable "male sexual performance" so high that men are nearly certain to feel inadequate. A man who scores 21 points or fewer on Pfizer's 25-point Sexual Health Inventory for Men is instructed to ask his doctor for help. In the tricky game of measuring up to social expectations, it seems Pfizer has defined *normal* and *masculine* to suit its own ends (Baglia, 2005).

Judging by the 25 million males who have secured Viagra prescriptions so far (www.viagra.com), men are buying it—literally and figuratively. "You get the 24-year-old who thinks he has erectile dysfunction if they stay up all night and can't get up and do it five times the next morning," says Thomas Jarrett, MD, head of urology at George Washington University (quoted by James, 2011, para. 19).

Baglia (2005) also points out that, in the pervasive images that Pfizer presents, masculinity is portrayed in mostly White, relentlessly heterosexual ways. In this context, "other ways of being a socio/sexual human being don't exist" he says (2005, p. 98).

Finally, the suggestion that Viagra yields virility, confidence, and sexual fulfillment is so palpable that it overshadows what Viagra does *not* do. "What happens when a man first takes a Viagra pill? Absolutely nothing," writes Tara Parker-Pope (2002, para. 10). She explains that the drug is not an aphrodisiac, adding that "the nothingness is so intense that the most common reaction is a slight panic that the drug isn't going to work" (para. 11).

Just as Viagra does not produce sexual feelings in men, neither does it create intimacy between people. True intimacy, Baglia (2005) reminds us, does not come in a pill but through communication, closeness, trust, and mutual respect. And sex comes in many forms that do not require a rigid member, served up pronto. Baglia quotes a *Newsweek* reporter who made the point that "a poor lover plus Viagra does not make a good lover, but merely a poor lover with an erection" (p. 37).

Side effects such as these probably sound familiar. But that was not always the case. Pharmaceutical companies used to only market their products to physicians, but in the early 1980s, the FDA okayed magazine ads targeting consumers. In 1985, TV and radio ads were given the green light, but the FDA's regulations on what commercials could and could not mention were so restrictive that few drug companies even bothered making ads (Angell, 2004; Silberner, 1997). But in 1997, those rules were relaxed. Now, **direct-to-consumer (DTC) advertisements**—those that encourage everyday people to ask their health care providers about and/or request particular drugs—comprise a $10-billion-a-year industry in the United States and represent one-third of all money spent on pharmaceutical advertising (Schwartz & Woloshin, 2019). (It is worth noting that drug ads targeting consumers are banned everywhere but in the United States and New Zealand.)

Because of DTC pharmaceutical ads, brand names such as Claritin, Lipitor, and Viagra are as familiar as Coca-Cola and Tide. (See Box 11.1 for more about Viagra advertising.) And along with those ads came the now-familiar list of disclaimers—so familiar that one visitor to a medical website asked, "Do *all* prescription drugs cause diarrhea and dry mouth?" These *are* common side effects, but you hear about them so much because of a rather nebulous FDA guideline known as "fair balance," which states that if advertisers present the potential benefits of a drug, they must also report some of the potentially harmful side effects. In the name of fairness, for every promise of relief you are likely to hear a list of disagreeable outcomes you might also experience. One study found that 59% of patients who were exposed to drug ads changed how they took their medicines or stopped taking them outright based on information about potential side effects contained in the ads (Green et al., 2017).

The "fair balance" guideline also explains why some prescription drug ads make no claims at all. The announcer might just say, "Ask your doctor about Zyrtec." Based on FDA guidelines, an ad that does not make a *positive* claim does not have to provide cautionary information either. In the case of no-claim ads, sponsors apparently believe that (a) you will recognize the drug and its purpose by name; (b) disclaimers, if mentioned, would scare you away; or (c) you will be curious enough to ask about the drug or research it on your own.

The fair balance guideline is only loosely and rather lopsidedly upheld. For quick evidence of this, compare the amount of information in a magazine pharmaceutical ad to the brief disclaimer you hear on a TV or radio commercial for the same drug. Enforcement is a problem, in part, because there are too few reviewers to critique the sheer volume of ads being produced. The number of drug ads tripled between 1997 and 2016 (from about 30,000 a year to nearly 100,000), and the number of violation letters issued by the FDA during that same period fell from 156 to 11 (Schwartz & Woloshin, 2019). In 2016, the FDA only reviewed 41% of new drug ads for content accuracy and fair balance (Schwartz & Woloshin, 2019).

ADVANTAGES OF DTC ADVERTISING

From one angle, advertisements for needed medications are beneficial. Without them, consumers might not know that treatment options are available for indigestion, asthma, allergies, depression, restless legs, and the like. Jessica DeFrank and colleagues (2019) looked at 38 studies conducted between 1982 and 2017 and found that between 32% and 43% of patients said they had asked about specific drugs after seeing DTC ads.

Some believe patient–provider relationships benefit when ads encourage patients to initiate conversations with their providers. For example, DeFrank et al. (2019) noted that, overall, about a quarter of patients and physicians reported improved relationships after DTC-inspired conversations, but 5% of patients in one study and 39% of physicians in another said such

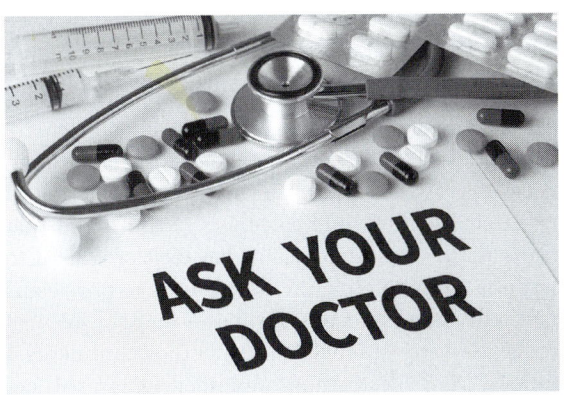

Have you ever become interested in a drug because you saw it advertised? If so, why? Have you done research or asked your doctor or pharmacist about a particular drug? Why or why not?

conversations made their relationships worse. The potential for harming patient–provider relationships is just one disadvantage of DTC advertising. Let's look at a few more.

DISADVANTAGES OF DTC ADVERTISING

Although health information about new drugs can be beneficial (to a point), expensive advertising has drawbacks. First, big drug companies spend more on advertising than they do on research and development (Swanson, 2015) and, according to physician Marcia Angell (2004), this has been the case since 1997. Because pharmaceutical companies shift advertising costs to patients, patients end up paying more for their medicines (Schwartz & Woloshin, 2019). Consider that prescription drug prices have risen by more than 26% since 2005 for the drugs used most often by older Americans (Thomas, 2012).

Second, health professionals worry that based on the dazzling scenarios in prescription-drug commercials, people may believe that high-priced designer drugs are better than their generic equivalents. In addition to curing anything that ails them, designer drugs, people might also believe, will make them happier and their lives more exciting. Consider a few examples from Rebecca Cline and Henry Young's (2004) content analysis of pharmaceutical ads:

- 93% of the models in arthritis drug ads were shown engaging in physical activity,
- 100% of the models in ads for HIV treatments appeared healthy, and
- 85.7% of models in cancer-related ads appeared healthy.

"The message is obvious," the researchers conclude. "With treatment by prescription drugs, the consumer with the associated condition can be attractively healthy looking and lively" (Cline & Young, 2004, p. 151). As a result of such unrealistic expectations, consumers may squander money on unnecessary medications, seek prescriptions for the wrong reasons, feel disappointed if their doctors do not prescribe the requested drugs, or feel discouraged when results are less dramatic than advertisements led them to expect. Critics also worry that ads promising "quick and easy" cures will dissuade people from taking care of themselves in the first place.

Third, in the interest of attracting consumers, drug companies sometimes downplay their products' risks. When Wendy Macias and colleagues studied 106 pharmaceutical TV commercials, they found that 2 violated the FDA's "fair balance" requirement and another 10 were borderline. The rest gave customary, but minimal, amounts of information about potential side effects (Macias, Pashupati, & Lewis, 2007). Even more frightening is evidence that the side effects drug companies report often come from research they have funded and overseen themselves. Researcher Sergio Sismondo (2008) concluded that pharmaceutical companies "not only fund clinical trials but also routinely design and shape them" (para. 5). He reports that these companies often have their staff statisticians perform data analyses and then hire people to write the research reports and corral them through the publication process. For example, after years of denying that its top-selling pain medication (Vioxx) posed significant health risks, Merck Pharmaceutical officials finally withdrew the drug in 2004. By that time, between 27,000 and 60,000 people had died from the drug's side effects (Lyon, 2007). In studying Merck documents and communiqués, researcher Alexander Lyon found that a pervasive "market mentality" led Merck decision makers to suppress and minimize information about Vioxx's harmful side effects.

Fourth, some experts worry that Americans are developing an unhealthy preoccupation with their own health, based largely on the amount of health care products and information now surrounding them. Some analysts have coined the term *cyberchondriacs* to describe people who are habitually fearful about their health because of how many health conditions and risk factors are brought to their attention every day (Vardigan, 2015).

Fifth, some research suggests that physicians may feel pressured to prescribe medications even when the requested drugs are not medically appropriate. This can harm physician–patient relationships, increase health care costs for patients, and expose them to unnecessary risk. While reviewing 35 years' worth of research, DeFrank and coauthors (2019) found that from 5% to 78% of physicians have felt pressured to write prescriptions. In one study, 39% of physicians granted patients' requests while in another, 55% of requests were granted. In that study, antidepressants were requested and prescribed in cases where patients' conditions did not warrant (and would not benefit from) antidepressants.

Finally, while some people are overrepresented in DTC images, others are left out of the picture, reinforcing health disparities. For example, although heart disease is the leading cause of death among both men and women, nearly two in three heart health ads show only men (Cline & Young, 2004). And African Americans and Hispanics almost always play minor roles in general-audience DTC advertising, if they are pictured at all (Ball, Liang, & Wei-Na, 2009; Cline & Young, 2004; Mastin, Andsager, Choi, & Lee, 2007).

There are exceptions to the mostly White rule, but you have to look in Black-oriented publications to find most of them. According to research by Teresa Mastin et al. (2007), about 75% of the pharmaceutical ads they analyzed in Black-oriented magazines featured only Black models. But 80% of the ads directed to Black females were for birth control pills, a bias not present in general-readership women's magazines. And even though African American women are at higher risk for heart disease than other groups, there were significantly fewer heart health ads in magazines targeted to African American women compared with general-readership women's magazines. Mastin and colleagues concluded that direct-to-consumer ads are not educating *all* consumers about health risks and treatment options (Mastin et al., 2007).

COMMUNICATION SKILL BUILDER: EVALUATING MEDICAL CLAIMS

As you have seen, consumers who rely on advertisements for health information do not always (or even often) get a clear picture. Here are some tips for evaluating the claims in medication ads.

- *Don't put too much stock in the wording.* Joel Davis (2007) found that people were most optimistic about drugs when the side effects were presented in language that downplayed their severity, such as "Side effects were mild and might include . . .", "Side effects tend to be mild and often go away," and "Few people were bothered enough to stop taking the drug." Keep in mind that reassuring word choices do not necessarily mean these drugs are safer than others.
- *Look to print sources for detailed information.* Broadcast commercials mention potential side effects only briefly. Magazine ads include a great deal more information (Boden & Diamond, 2008).
- *"Newer" does not necessarily mean better.* Pharmaceutical companies vie for the public's attention by advertising the "newest" and "latest" therapies. But the rush to the marketplace does not actually mean the medication is "improved," or even that it is safe (Lyon, 2007).

Even advertisements that seem unrelated to health care often affect our health by influencing social expectations about how we should behave, what we should eat and drink, and how we should look.

Let's turn, now, to a different type of programming that often includes health-related messages.

News Coverage

"New Study Suggests that Vaccines Don't Cause Autism"

How do you think people would respond if they saw this banner on the day's news? Christopher Clarke et al. (2015) used the headline in a study that compared readers' responses to three slightly different stories about the vaccine controversy.

The issue is an important one. Since 1998, when a medical study (later exposed to be fraudulent) proposed a link between autism and the measles–mumps–rubella (MMR) vaccine, a small but influential percentage of parents have refused MMR immunizations for their children. Since then, outbreaks of the measles virus have reached record numbers among children who have not been immunized and those with medical conditions that make them vulnerable to the measles virus even if they have been vaccinated (CDC, 2015; Fox & Connor, 2015). The World Health Organization (2019) announced that in the first six months of 2019, measles cases were the highest they had been since 2006, "with outbreaks straining health care systems, and leading to serious illness, disability, and deaths in many parts of the world" (para. 2). (See Chapter 12 for more about measles as a public health communication issue.)

Clarke et al. (2015) explored the conundrum that journalists face because they are expected to present both sides of a controversial issue. At the same time, however, they may be considered irresponsible for presenting information that is not well supported by evidence. Clarke and collaborators created three versions of a *USA Today* story about vaccines. One version included a section describing the preponderance of scientific evidence that vaccines are safe and effective. Another included, instead, a section about advocacy groups and scientists who believe there is a vaccine–autism link. The third version included both of the sections just described. Participants who read the science-only and science-and-opposition versions were more likely to believe there is scientific consensus about the safety of vaccines than those who read only about opposition to vaccines. In other words, the presence of controversy did not significantly diminish most readers' confidence in scientific evidence. Clarke and his team concluded that journalists need not choose between presenting both sides of an issue and letting readers know that the weight of scientific evidence supports one side or the other (Clarke, Dixon, Holton, & McKeever, 2015).

Health news is instrumental in educating people. However, it is not an easy topic to cover. In the rush to provide the latest information, media professionals sometimes oversell scientific findings and overlook ongoing, everyday concerns. This section examines health news in terms of accuracy and sensationalism and discusses the advantages of media coverage.

Accuracy and Fairness

Although many media professionals do an admirable job of informing the public about health issues, a sizable amount of health information available in the media is misleading and exaggerated. When researchers compared 462 press releases about health studies to the actual studies they described, they found that at least one-third of the press releases included exaggerated claims or unsupported generalizations. Media outlets often further exaggerated the claims before publishing them, resulting in health science news that was substantially inflated compared to actual results (Sumner et al., 2014).

Overgeneralizations are common. For instance, a study of older women might be reported simply as a study about women or older adults, although the health concerns of these populations may be significantly different. Such inaccuracies are particularly troubling since it is often difficult for readers to verify scientific information for themselves.

One worry is that overly optimistic news about medical research will give people false hope. As early as 1997, headlines in major publications suggested an imminent cure for AIDS—such as "When AIDS Ends" in the *New York Times Magazine* and "The End of AIDS?" in *Newsweek*. Jon Cohen (1997) cautioned, "If treatments don't live up to unrealistic expectations, researchers fear a public backlash against medical science" (para. 2). Premature reports about cures for cancer raise the same fear.

Sensationalism

Media professionals are also criticized for focusing on sensational health news rather than useful information about everyday concerns. Heart disease, which is the world's leading cause of death, typically receives less coverage than emergent issues—especially those associated with the kind of striking visuals that newspapers and TV news shows tend to prioritize (e.g., Ebola and Zika, which are characterized by depictions of uncontrolled bleeding and birth defects, respectively). Heart disease, in comparison, is less visually dynamic. A case in point is how the 2016 Zika outbreak was covered and sensationalized by news media.

A study comparing stories about Zika that ran in two major American newspapers found that about half of the stories used emotionally charged language and 80% mentioned the worst possible outcomes of Zika—birth defects, including microcephaly, and Guillain–Barré syndrome, a rare disorder causing paralysis (Jerit, Zhao, Tan, & Wheeler, 2018). The percentage of stories that included information about how readers could protect themselves from infection

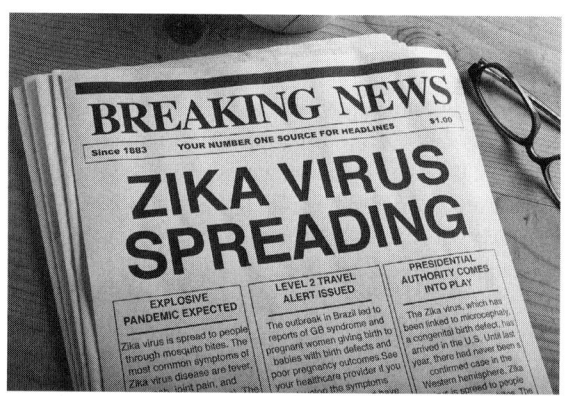

News stories about the 2016 Zika outbreak sensationalized some aspects of the epidemic while underreporting others. Stories regularly focused on mosquitos as a vector but seldom mentioned that Zika can also be sexually transmitted. As a result, people lacked important information about how to protect themselves from infection. (Ophir & Jamieson, 2018).

was smaller than one might expect—60% in one paper and 26% in the other (Jerit et al., 2018).

Additionally, certain aspects of the Zika outbreak received a disproportionate share of media coverage. For instance, stories that focused on mosquitoes and babies born with birth defects were more common than stories about Zika being sexually transmitted or being largely asymptomatic in adults (Ophir & Jamieson, 2018). This is because sexual images—apart from condoms and contraceptives—rarely appear in the news and asymptomatic conditions are hard (if not impossible) to convey using pictures. (If you were a TV news reporter, how would you show "asymptomatic" to an audience?) Consequently, the public knew more about mosquitoes as a vector and microcephaly than about Zika's other transmission route (sexual intercourse) and how to identify infected adults (Ophir & Jamieson, 2018). Thus, members of the public lacked important information about how to prevent and detect infection.

Coverage of other health issues is also skewed. Newspapers in the United States tend to overreport information on breast cancer, leukemia, and pancreatic cancer, especially when someone famous had been diagnosed with them. However, they underreport information about male reproductive cancer, lymphatic/Hodgkin's disease, and thyroid cancer (Jensen, Moriarty, Hurley, & Stryker, 2010). Likewise, although HIV and AIDS have gotten a great deal of attention, less than 1% of stories have addressed their incidence in older adults, which may be one reason that people over age 50 know less about the subject than younger people and tend to feel shocked and ashamed if they become infected (LaVail, 2010).

In some instances, snappy headlines have little to do with conclusive evidence. In the United States, news coverage (especially TV news coverage) of cancer often highlights potential causes of cancer that have not been substantiated, like dry-cleaning chemicals, excessive exercise, and deodorant (Niederdeppe, Fowler, Goldstein, & Pribble, 2010). Partly for that reason, people who rely on TV news coverage a great deal are likely to think that cancer is unavoidable (Niederdeppe et al., 2010).

Advantages of Health News

Despite the criticisms, health news does offer several advantages. Media organizations are credited with increasing people's awareness about health. And even when medical news is not what scientists would wish, its presence keeps health on the public agenda and (hopefully) garners support for medical science (Deary, Whiteman, & Fowkes, 1998). For example, coverage of breast cancer has substantially increased since the 1970s and has focused mostly on new treatment methods and scientific breakthroughs (Cho, 2006). That is good, except that some other forms of cancer receive minimal coverage by comparison.

It should also be said that news writers are not entirely to blame for misleading health coverage. The fault lies partly with the nature of news and the nature of science. News, especially TV news, is inherently brief. About 74.5% of TV news stories last less than 60 seconds (Wang & Gantz, 2010). Furthermore, it is the nature of news to be unusual and recent. The public is hungry for current and interesting information, and media professionals strive to provide it. However, it is the nature of science to be meticulous and cautious, weighing diverse evidence over long periods (Taubes, 1998). Consequently, news writers are at a disadvantage in trying to cover scientific news accurately. The latest groundbreaking study today may reach different conclusions from a study that came out last week or one that will come out next month. Science is full of reliable accounts that, for one reason or another, arrive at different conclusions, so that even experts do not agree.

Furthermore, reporters may be ill prepared to meet the extraordinary challenges that health coverage presents. Medical terminology and statistical analyses make medical science difficult to understand and interpret, and comparatively few reporters are trained to do so (Tanner, Friedman, & Zheng, 2015). On the bright side, with many sources of health news available, the chances are greater that people can evaluate and compare information, judging for themselves what is credible and useful.

Communication Skill Builder: Presenting Health News

Here are some suggestions offered by Melissa Ludtke and Cathy Trost (1998) and the Association of Health Care Journalists (2015) to help media news writers present fair and accurate coverage:

- *Favor the factual over the sensational and trendy.*
- *Don't allow ongoing issues to fade from coverage.* "Put a fresh face on coverage of long-standing

BOX 11.2 PERSPECTIVES

Barbie: Feminist Icon or Woman as Sex Object?

By Annina Dahlstrom

When Barbie debuted in 1959, the second wave of feminism was gaining momentum. The doll's long limbs, curvaceous figure, and lavish wardrobe distinguished her in what had mostly been a *baby* doll market until that time. She also represented a shift from the traditional view of women as mothers and housewives. From some perspectives, Barbie represented the new self-confident and independent woman of the future (Forman-Brunell, n.d.)—albeit with outlandishly impossible proportions and a sex-centric appearance (Alter, 2014).

In the decades since, Barbie has inspired her share of dismay and revulsion. Diane Levin and Jean Kilbourne feature her in *So Sexy So Soon* (2008), a book about the harmful effects of overexposing young children to sexuality. As Levin puts it, "when Barbie came around, play suddenly became about dressing up and looking right and it eventually played a role in how women wanted to look in real life" (quoted by Conley, 2012, para. 8). Some Barbie admirers (such as the woman pictured here) have taken that to extremes, having their faces and bodies altered to look more like the vinyl and plastic icon. Others fuel the demand for hundreds of YouTube tutorials on how to emulate Barbie's makeup and wardrobe.

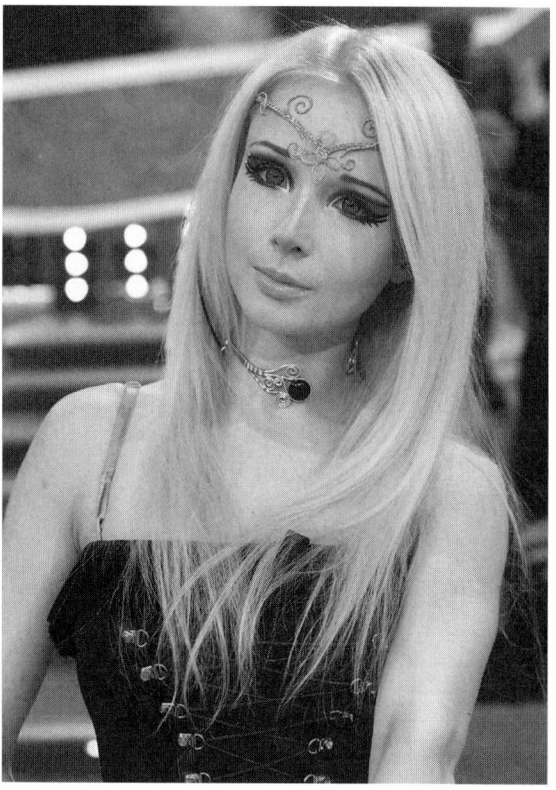

Spokespersons for Mattel, which markets Barbie, counter that detractors are being size-ist. They defend their tiny trendsetter (who in real life would be nearing retirement age) by saying that there is room—in the doll world and the people world—for bodies of all sizes. Mattel launched a Barbie Twitter campaign to declare (in glittery, pink text) *Be You. Be Bold. Be #Unapologetic* (Barbie, 2014) and an "Anything is Possible" campaign that draws attention to the 150+ careers Barbie has pursued, including Entrepreneur Barbie with her own LinkedIn account. Lisa McKnight, senior VP of marketing for Mattel North America, maintains that Barbie is a hard-working feminist icon and says "we will continue to promote Barbie in this way for many years to come" (Bulik, 2014, para. 16).

Meanwhile, Barbie's market share has been eroded by a new wave of sexed-up dolls, such as the Monster High collection, that are marketed to an even younger demographic. One cultural observer refers to the newcomers as "younger, sluttier dolls with bigger heads" who "dress like prostitutes and have the dimensions of lollipops" (Alter, 2014, paras. 2 and 3).

On the other side of the issue, Lammily dolls have realistic body proportions and come complete with optional cellulite, stretch marks, acne, tattoos, and freckles, among other features, known as "Lammily Marks." When they were introduced on a crowd-funding website, 13,621 supporters preordered 19,000 Lammily dolls. (See more at http://lammily.com/about/.)

What Do You Think?

1. Do you agree more with the idea that Barbie inspires objectification of women and unrealistic standards of beauty or that she is a symbol of feminine diversity and empowerment? Why?
2. Would you prefer that your young daughter or niece play with Barbie or a Lammily doll? Why?

health issues like asthma, lead poisoning and infant mortality" (Ludtke & Trost, 1998, para. 20).
- *Don't forget rural America.* Health issues outside the big city, such as lack of dental care and exposure to pesticides, are important although they are often distant from major news outlets.
- *Never rely on just one source.* Consult a number of experts; read a variety of reliable literature.
- *Seek training.* Seek out lectures, workshops, and conferences at which you can learn the lingo and become proficient at interpreting health science.
- *Set the record straight.* If a health news item is revealed to be untrue or misleading, update the public.

Media and Body Image

Jacob saunters in, leanly muscled and confident, armed with darts, knives, guns, and other devices ready at hand. He is a "charismatic brawler," a fearless fighter who impudently wears his top hat into battle. (Corriea, 2015, para. 18.)

Jacob is one of the main characters in the video game *Assassin's Creed Syndicate*. Some analysts suggest that Jacob and similar video heroes provide a healthy outlet for children and their imaginations. Others worry that video game characters present an unattainable version of masculinity. Male avatars tend to be both dramatically more slender and more muscular than flesh-and-blood men. One result is that while male players often report feeling especially confident and powerful when they embody these personae online, they report feeling *inadequate* in real life because their weight and muscularity do not measure up (Cacioli & Mussap, 2014).

Video games are not alone in making people feel like they don't measure up. Media consumers are consistently urged by advertisements to believe that their skin, weight, hair, breath, clothing, and teeth are "problem areas" requiring vigorous and immediate attention—at a price. Theorists call this **pathologizing the human body, making natural functions seem weird and unnatural** (Wood, 1999). In short, advertisers are accused of making people feel bad about themselves so they will considering buying products that will help them make the "necessary" fixes.

Teenagers are particularly susceptible to these kinds of ads. Along with the physical and social changes that accompany adolescence comes a heightened self-consciousness that makes it easy to escalate (and capitalize on) teens' insecurity. Media messages often encourage an obsessive concern with physical appearance, sometimes to the detriment of people's health and self-esteem. As a case in point, nearly 68,000 people, mostly tweens (ages 10–13) and teens, have posted "Am I Pretty or Ugly?" videos on YouTube, seeking reassurance in the very same mass-media environment that often feeds their insecurities in the first place. One 13-year-old, who whispered into the camera, "I could be the ugliest person that could ever be living. Be honest and tell me if I am ugly or not" inspired tens of thousands of viewings. Some people posted reassuring comments, whereas others left demeaning comments and some even suggested that she kill herself (Quenqua, 2014). As one analyst observes, teens now have the power to broadcast their feelings of insecurity to the world and, in return, they may be subjected to insults and bullying that would crumble the confidence of even the most self-assured adult (Quenqua, 2014).

Like YouTube, Instagram is popular among teens seeking validation. Seventy-two percent of teens use Instagram—as do 25 million businesses that pay billions for ads, sponsored content, and shout-outs from influencers (Aslam, 2019). Many teens find validation in the number of "likes" or comments their Instagram posts receive. Others use the social media platform to see how they measure up to their peers. It's important to note this because several theorists suggest that people compare themselves to similar others much more than they compare themselves to models or celebrities (Kleemans, Daalmans, Carbaat, & Anschütz, 2018). While it's widely known that pictures of celebrities are frequently enhanced or "Photoshopped," viewers cannot always tell if pictures posted on Instagram (some of which are ads in disguise) have been manipulated, adding to the potential for unrealistic and unfavorable comparisons to oneself (Kleemans et al., 2018).

In a study involving girls ages 14 to 18, Kleemans's team showed one group of participants pictures in which a model's legs and waist were edited to appear smaller and filters were used to perfect her complexion. A second group was shown the unedited, original photos. Despite the fact that some girls in the first group picked up on the use of filters, they found the edited photos to be "realistic" and virtually none of the girls detected that the model's body had been reshaped. Overwhelmingly, the edited images were

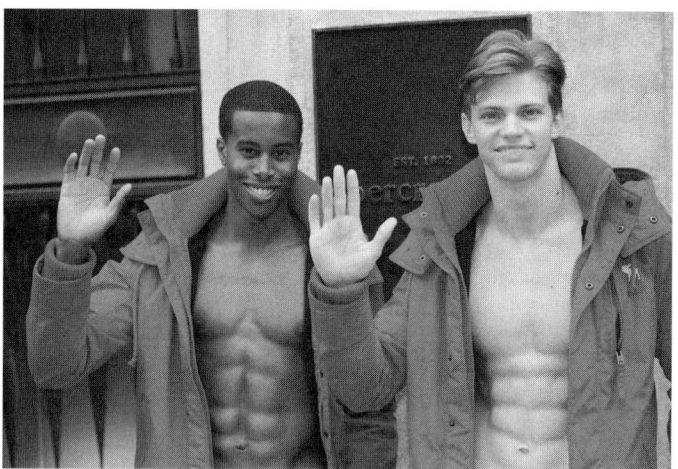

Abercrombie & Fitch models pose at the grand opening of a store in Munich, Germany, representing a trend toward what some analysts call the sanitized male, distinguished by ripped abs, a hairless body, smooth skin, and grooming so meticulous that he nearly looks plastic.

rated more positively and the model in the edited photos was deemed prettier. Even worse, the girls who saw the manipulated photos were more likely than others to report dissatisfaction with their own bodies (Kleemans et al., 2018, p. 93).

The take-away is that while teens expect to see Photoshopped images of celebrities, they do not always recognize similar photo-editing techniques that are used by their peers. Consequently, teens compare themselves to edited social media images of seemingly perfect others in the "real world" and often end up feeling worse about themselves.

Even among adults, knowing that social media images have been altered does not always mitigate their impact. For example, Jasmine Fardouly and Elise Holland (2018) found that disclaimers made no difference to women ages 18 to 25 who viewed social media photos that had been heavily edited. The women's body images were harmed by viewing the edited photos, even when disclaimers informed them that the pictures had been doctored. In another study, when women were shown news stories about digitally altered images and then shown fashion ads with disclaimers, the women reported even higher levels of body dissatisfaction (Tiggemann, Brown, & Anderberg, 2019). Ironically, brands that include disclaimers in their advertisements were rated higher by women than brands that do not disclose that their advertising images are retouched (Semaan, Kocher, & Gould, 2018).

Although women's responses to unrealistic media images have been more widely studied, men also suffer with body image concerns when they compare themselves to images they see in advertisements (Pan & Peña, 2019).

Part of the problem is that male and female cultural icons are inherently unrealistic. For example, to attain the proportions of a Barbie doll, a woman would have to be more than 7 feet tall, with a bust 5 inches larger than normal and a waist 6 inches smaller (Duewald, 2003). (See Box 11.2 for more about Barbie.) Likewise, many of today's action figures bear little resemblance to actual body types (see Box 11.3). "When did male body hair become a bad thing?" asks a reporter for *The Guardian* (Bilmes, 2014). Apparently, college women wonder the same thing. Although most female students surveyed said they like or do not mind body hair on men, most male students said they regularly remove their body hair because they believe it is sexier to be bare (Basow & O'Neil, 2014).

Health Effects

"Self-acceptance has become a movement," says fashion writer Shaun Dreisbach (2014, para. 2). Some celebrities now post bare-faced selfies, defend their cellulite, and say they love their bodies. "So our body confidence should be better, right?" asks Dreisbach (para. 2). As it turns out, progress is marginal at best for women. And for men, it has gotten worse.

Today, about 13% of women and 9% of men in the United States are dissatisfied with their overall appearance, and double or triple that many are unhappy with particular areas of their bodies (Fallon, Harris, & Johnson, 2014). One study found that an astonishing 68% to 95% of men report significant levels of body dissatisfaction (Jung, Forbes, & Chan, 2010).

Although obesity is a serious health threat, extreme efforts to change one's weight can also be dangerous or even deadly. About 30 million Americans (most of them female) will suffer from an eating disorder sometime in their lives (Alliance for Eating Disorders Awareness, 2019), which may damage their hearts and livers, make their bones brittle, and even kill them (National Eating Disorders Association, 2015). Eating disorders often start in

BOX 11.3 PERSPECTIVES

Boys' Toys on Steroids

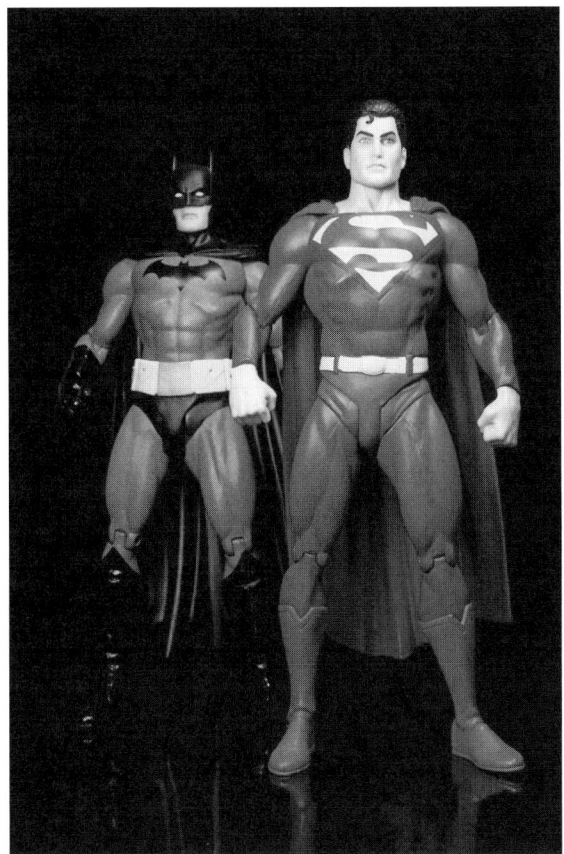

Even with starvation dieting and steroids, it would be impossible for most boys to grow up looking like popular action figures.

At the same time girls are encouraged to be thin, toys encourage boys to be both sleek and strong. Male action figures guide the male psyche toward this conclusion: Desirability involves being implausibly slim waisted, hypermuscular, and lean. "Only 1 or 2 percent of [males] actually have that body type," protests psychologist Raymond Lemberg. "We're presenting men in a way that is unnatural" (Santa Cruz, 2014, para. 8).

Take G.I. Joe as an example. In the 1960s, he had the athletic proportions of a 5-foot-10-inch man with a 32-inch waist and 12-inch biceps. However, if today's G.I. Joe Extreme figure were a real man, he would have a 29-inch waist (more than 10 inches smaller than the average American man's) and his 32-inch biceps would literally set a new bodybuilding world record (Moss, 2011).

"So here we are," says health sciences professor Tim Olds, "surrounded by images of ideal bodies: actors, sports stars, steroid-pumped bodybuilders, shop mannequins, dolls, dolled-up personal trainers, air-brushed models and digitally-enhanced video game avatars. And not one of them reflects reality" (Olds, 2014, para. 5). His advice? "I'm not G.I. Joe and you're not Barbie, but . . . there are a lot more people in this world like you and me than there are like these dolls. Aim for good health and get comfortable with your normality" (last para.).

---

adolescence, but children are at risk too. Children are likely to feel that their bodies are inferior if their parents are preoccupied with their own weight and appearance.

To help children and teens lose weight, WW (formerly "Weight Watchers") released its Kurbo app in 2019. While the app was intended to help users make sensible food choices, some dieticians and medical experts denounced it because "it could put kids at risk for developing life-threatening eating disorders, body image dissatisfaction as well as potentially interrupt their growth and development" (Sterling, 2019, para. 4).

WW officials countered, claiming Kurbo addressed "extraordinarily high" rates of obesity and subsequent "medical and psychosocial consequences" that obese children and teens endure (quoted in Landsverk, 2019, para. 5). Clearly, addressing childhood and adolescent obesity is a contentious subject and there are no clear-cut answers.

Abusing anabolic steroids is another way people try to change their bodies. More than 1 million Americans (most of them male) have abused steroids (National Institute on Drug Abuse [NIDA], 2007). Adolescents have reported using steroids as well, and some start as early as the eighth grade (NIDA, 2018). The risks include cardiovascular disease, liver damage, hair loss, sterility, acne, aggressiveness, and depression. Additionally, for men who abuse steroids, they may see a growth in breast tissue and their testicles may shrink.

Researchers observe that, for most steroid users, the goal is to measure up to Western ideals of masculine attractiveness rather than to excel at sports. Steroid use is disproportionately high among men ages 22 to 35 who are fans of bodybuilding magazines and TV programs and those who are exposed to explicit pornography (Melki, Hitti, Oghia, & Mufarrij, 2015). They are more likely than other men to think that people like men with large muscles and to feel that muscular men in the media are a realistic benchmark of masculine appearance.

The desire to appeal to women has led to an interesting evolutionary paradox for men who abuse steroids. Called the "Mossman-Pacey Paradox" by the scientists who first described it, the quandary is that for men who take steroids to look bigger and appeal to potential mates, "they are making themselves very unfit in an evolutionary sense," according to James Mossman (quoted in Gallagher, 2019, para. 8). As Allan Pacey explains, this is because 90% of steroid abusers are "likely to become sterile" (Gallagher, para. 16) and, consequently, "evolutionary duds" (para. 19).

Beauty Sells . . . Sometimes

Why do we buy what the media sells? There is evidence that people sometimes feel a vicarious sense of well-being and optimism when they see idealized models in the media. That's one reason advertisers tend to use beautiful people to sell products that have nothing to do with improving one's appearance. "Seeing a pretty person activates thoughts of 'goodness,' which extends to our evaluations of other things," says one psychology scholar ("Beautiful People," 2011, para. 8). When the advertisement *is* for a beauty enhancement, such as cosmetics or shampoo, people may react one of two ways, she says. Those who think their own appearance will not change substantially are typically skeptical and may even be angered by the unrealistic depiction. On the other hand, people who are optimistic that the product will make them attractive are usually drawn to it. (Of course, this optimism can backfire if the product does not deliver.)

Entertainment

In this section we examine how health issues and medical care are portrayed in entertainment programming. We first explore fictional portrayals of health care settings. We then switch gears to focus on depictions of mental illness and disabilities. Finally, we examine sex and violence in the media. These topics reflect the preponderance of research about entertainment programming and health.

Portrayals of Health Care Situations

> *"On one* Grey's Anatomy *episode, a patient comes in with chest pain, and two seconds later, he is rushed to open-heart surgery. That is hardly realistic."*

Prasanna Ananth said this when she was a medical student (Baker, 2007). A lot of health care providers share her sentiments. Many medical professionals "have a love–hate relationship" with medical dramas, says Mitzi Baker. "They pretty much love to hate everything the shows get wrong" (Baker, 2007, para. 3). And with good reason. Viewers who frequently watch medical dramas are more likely than other people to think the dramas are realistic (Tian & Yoo, 2018). Shows such as *Grey's Anatomy* are often regarded as valid sources of health information, but medical dramas are likely to give people mistaken impressions about the way medical work is done. For example, they often show providers successfully reviving patients with cardiopulmonary resuscitation (CPR) far more often than actually happens (Hinkelbein et al., 2014). A physician-authored study that appeared in the *Journal of the American Medical Association* found that 67% of patients in medical dramas who receive CPR survive, compared with only 2% to 30% of real patients (Diem, Lantos, & Tulsky, 1996). The authors worried that "misrepresentation of CPR on television shows undermines trust in data and fosters trust in miracles" (Diem et al., 1996, p. 1581).

In fact, people who watch a lot of medical dramas are more inclined to believe that luck and chance—maybe even miracles—decide the state of their health (Kim & Baek, 2019). Thus, heavy viewers of medical shows exhibit an external locus of control (LOC) (Chapter 8). By contrast, people with an internal LOC believe their health is shaped more by their own behaviors. Researchers speculate that the association between viewing frequency and external LOC may be a result of medical dramas focusing attention on depictions of "injuries rather than preventable diseases" (Kim & Baek, 2019, p. 398), which means preventive health measures people can take (e.g., healthy eating, exercise, and limiting alcohol) are not central to most storylines.

Of course, injuries are dramatic and help make television shows more exciting. This is why medical dramas tend to overrepresent traumatic events, especially those involving younger characters. For example, younger adults (and even teens) are often depicted suffering heart attacks when in reality, heart attacks are most common in middle-aged and older adults (Diem et al., 1996). There are other mischaracterizations too. In real life, about 40% of hospital patients are male. On TV, however, 70% are male (Hetsroni, 2009). And, whereas men are overrepresented in medical dramas, Hispanic Americans and older adults are underrepresented (Hetsroni, 2009).

Medical dramas also rely on death as a dramatic element. The mortality rate among TV patients is nearly nine times greater than the norm, prompting the researcher who discovered the disparity to quip that "if you must be hospitalized, television is not the place" (Hetsroni, 2009, p. 311). Most television deaths are quick and dramatic—overwhelmingly traumatic, in fact—but don't let that fool you. In the real world, most people die from diseases, not traumatic accidents. All in all, medical dramas "teach viewers very little about how to prepare for or create a good death" (p. 752), observe researchers Jennifer Freytag and Srividya Ramasubramanian (2019).

Entertainment programming also presents dramatic but untrue information about organ donation. In their study of network television programs, Susan Morgan et al. (2007) found numerous story lines about organs sold illegally, people murdered for their organs, doctors giving preferential treatment, and people allowed to die so that others could have their organs. All of these depictions—though the stuff of exciting drama—are grossly unrealistic. "We often wonder where members of the public get 'crazy ideas' about organ donation like the existence of the black market, the corruption of the organ allocation system, and the untrustworthiness of doctors," the authors reflect. "The answer may have been quite literally in front of us for years" (Morgan, Harrison, Chewning, Davis, & DiCorcia, 2007, p. 149).

Portrayals of Health-Related Conditions

For better or worse, even programs designed primarily to entertain can have important implications for health and identity.

MENTAL ILLNESS

Mentally ill individuals are often portrayed in the media as wild eyed, disheveled, violent, and dangerous. That characterization has never reflected the reality of most people with psychological disorders. In truth, only about 11% of them are violent, which is roughly equal to the proportion of violent people in the overall population (Hetsroni, 2009). In fact, attests Kristin Fawcett (2015), "Not only are individuals with mental illness less likely [than other people] to

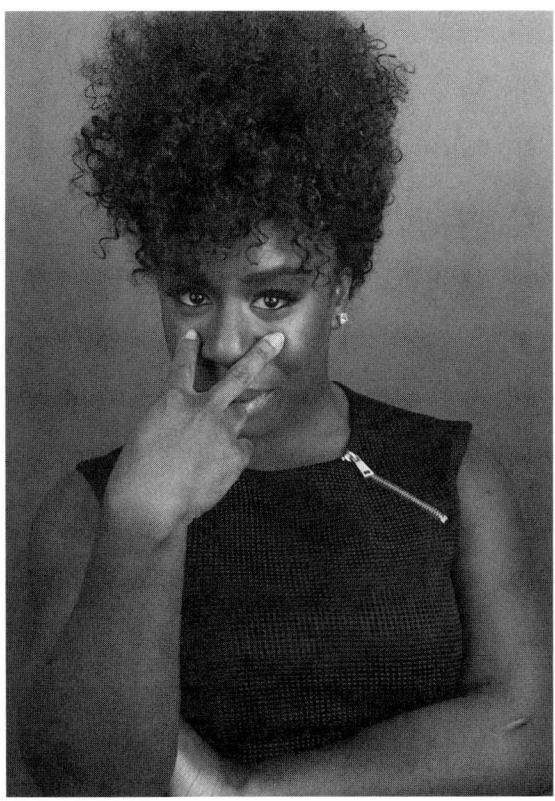

Uzo Abuda plays Suzanne "Crazy Eyes" Warren in the TV show *Orange is the New Black*. Her appearance is altered for the role to make her appear emotionally volatile and eccentric. At the same time, the character is funny and endearing, leading many observers to wonder whether she is mostly reinforcing or dispelling stereotypes about people with mental illnesses.

commit crimes, they're actually more likely to be victimized" (para. 8).

One harmful effect of stigmatizing images in the media is that people who might benefit from mental health services often consider it personally and socially unacceptable to seek help, especially if the on-screen "professionals" and "health care" situations that they see are portrayed in a negative light (Maier, Gentile, Vogel, & Kaplan, 2014).

Although entertainment programming may dramatize and demonize mental illness, as one media analyst reminds us, "getting sick is something that happens to everyone, and since our bodies and minds are linked and not separate, mental illness is no more sensational than physical sickness" (Uwujaren, 2012).

DISABILITIES

As the audience watches, a police officer apprehends and arrests a man who has just robbed a cab driver. It might be a scene from any number of television shows or movies. But this one has a twist. The officer, who is partially paralyzed, uses a wheelchair.

When researchers showed this clip (from a German television series) to people without physical disabilities, they found that people were significantly more likely than before to believe that those with disabilities can successfully serve as police officers (Reinhardt, Pennycott, & Fellinghauer, 2014). The experiment points to the media's influence in shaping popular opinion, at least some of the time.

People with disabilities are typically underrepresented and misrepresented in mainstream media (Renwick, Schormans, & Shore, 2014). When they are shown, they are typically portrayed in one of three ways—as disadvantaged, as unhealthy victims, or as so-called super crips who do everything able-bodied people can do but better (Zhang & Haller, 2013). As you might imagine, the first two characterizations are associated with stigma and discrimination. By contrast, the super crip image tends to inspire confidence; think Professor Charles Xavier from the *X-Men* comic book and movie franchise. But at the same time, many people worry that over-the-top portrayals will foster unrealistic expectations (Zhang & Haller, 2013). In the study involving the fictional cop who is partially paralyzed, viewers with physical disabilities were more likely than other viewers to doubt that people with paraplegia could successfully serve as police officers because they considered the TV actor's on-screen feats unrealistic or because they felt society at large would not accept disabled police officers (Reinhardt et al., 2014).

Regular and realistic exposure to people with disabilities is the most successful means of diminishing negative attitudes. Sensitive use of humor may also help. In one study, college students either watched a serious documentary called *Without Pity: A Film About Disabilities* or a video featuring a stand-up comedian sharing funny stories about his experiences since having a leg amputated. On the whole, students who watched the serious film did not experience a change in attitude, but those who watched the stand-up routine were significantly more willing than before to interact with people who have disabilities (Smedema, Ebener, & Grist-Gordon, 2012). Clearly, there are many circumstances in which joking about a physical challenge would be hurtful, but in this case, the researchers speculate that viewers felt they could relate to the comedian, and the humor relieved some of their tension about the topic.

As with mental illness, people with disabilities are much like everyone else, regardless of how they are portrayed in the media. "Disability is just one part of a person and one aspect of human diversity," reflect researchers Lingling Zhang and Beth Haller (2013), adding that "the best way to portray people with disabilities is to not use a sticker or label, not to focus on their disability, but to report from their perspectives" (p. 330).

We now turn our attention to another aspect of entertainment programming—the way it depicts health-related behaviors.

Portrayals of Health-Related Behaviors

Two of the most controversial elements of entertainment programming are sex and violence. Here we explore common media depictions and their implications for people's well-being and identity.

SEX

When Rachel Hills began writing a book about sex, she realized, as she puts it, that "the story I had been telling myself all those years had been wrong" (2015a, para. 16). As a college student, she had spent countless hours ironing her hair straight, applying makeup, choosing just the right clothes, walking to class in 3-inch heels, and regularly vomiting in hopes of staying slender. Even so, she never felt as sexy as the women she saw in magazines and movies. After some soul-searching, Hills realized she had "failed" as a sex object, but she had succeeded at something much more important. We will return to her story in a moment. But first, let's consider the ramifications of the way sex is portrayed in the media.

OBJECTIFICATION. Few people dispute that, under the right conditions, sex is an intimate and loving act. One concern is that media images often present it in a different way. Take music and music videos, for example. Over the last 40 years or so, about 80% of Top 40 songs have been about love and/or sexual attraction, and during that same time, an increasing number of hit songs have described casual sex without the love (Madanikia & Bartholomew, 2014). To emphasize the point, music videos, particularly those of rap and hip-hop performers, typically feature women (disproportionately women of color) who are naked or provocatively dressed (Turner, 2011). One analyst observes that many videos have devolved into "twerking competitions" in which the bodies of Black women are dehumanized (reduced to accessories) and African American men are depicted as sexually voracious (Larasi, 2013).

Additionally, young women who think music videos are realistic, and who also think sexually objectifying women is okay, have more tolerance for being physically harassed by men (Rodgers & Hust, 2018). When women are objectified in the media to such a degree that it seems "okay" or "realistic," the normalized behavior is more easily perpetuated (and tolerated) by men and women alike.

Sexual objectification occurs when an individual is treated primarily as the object of another person's desire, not as a whole and unique person with needs and desires of their own. Objectification is evident when the focus is on particular body parts rather than the whole person, when people are depicted as animals or things (as when a model is dressed to resemble a cheetah or a beer bottle), when people are treated as interchangeable (one person looks and acts so much like another that it is difficult to tell them apart), and when people are treated as commodities to be chosen and used by others (Heldman, 2014).

One result of feeling objectified is a sense of inadequacy. If one's worth is measured in terms of other people's desire—and the terms of that desire are narrow, unrealistic, and impersonal—it is difficult to feel appreciated and worthy. "I was a mess of insecurities," remembers Rachel Hills, whose narrative begins this section. "I could never trust that men were interested in me, and on occasions when they seemed to be, I would internally rebut myself with reasons that they never would be" (2015a, para. 8). The worth of an object often equates to how much it is used. Being "used" as a sex object can be demeaning, humiliating, and even dangerous.

A particularly alarming trend involves posting videos of rape on social media. Such glorifications of sexual violence contribute to what some analysts call a **rape culture**, the attitude among some people that it is acceptable, sexy, or even funny to force sex on women, men, or children. Many people feel that *Fifty Shades of Grey* and similar books and movies trivialize and normalize rape and abuse, thereby making them seem acceptable.

Rachel Hills, who went on to author the book *The Sex Myth* (2015b), proposes that she became attractive in her own mind when she stopped basing her self-worth on other people's opinion of her sex appeal and began celebrating her individuality. "An object may be beautiful, cherished, and adored," she reflects, "but by definition it cannot act; it can only be acted upon by others" (Hills, 2015a, para. 19). These days, she says, she prides herself on being a *subject*, a dynamic creator of her own life story, rather than a mere *object* in someone else's.

Another issue involves the media's treatment of safer sex practices.

SAFER SEX. A good deal of evidence suggests that people who regularly watch pornography are more likely than others to be sexually promiscuous and to engage in unsafe sexual practices (Harkness, Mullan, & Blaszczynski, 2015). This may be partly because sexually explicit programming provides a script of sorts for initiating sexual encounters but almost never includes discussion of contraception or disease barriers. Teens who are heavy porn users are more likely than their peers to send and receive sexually explicitly texts (Van Ouytsel, Ponnet, & Walrave, 2014), and college students who frequently view pornography are more likely to initiate casual sex and to engage in risky sex (Braithwaite, Coulson, Keddington, & Fincham, 2015).

Safer-sex practices, such as using condoms, are rarely included in sexual references that appear in music, magazines, and movies aimed at teen audiences. In one study, researchers found that only about 1 out of every 200 sexual references in popular media mentioned safe sex (Hust, Brown, & L'Engle, 2008). Since that study, not much has changed. Today, scripted TV shows that are popular with teens and young adults (shows like *Empire*, *Modern Family*, and *Scandal*) rarely address sexual risks and consequences. Instead, most storylines about sex highlight casual sex, unsafe sex practices (e.g., not using condoms), and sexual violence (Kinsler et al., 2019). Very few shows that Kinsler et al. (2019) analyzed touched on issues such as teen pregnancy or sexually transmitted diseases, focusing more on affairs, love triangles, and seduction.

The good news is that not all media encourage unsafe sex practices. When teens were regularly exposed to safer-sex PSAs, they were subsequently more likely than their peers to use condoms, which suggests that the media can be a role model for healthy sexual behaviors (Hennessy et al., 2013).

SEXUAL ORIENTATION. There is a double standard when it comes to depictions of sexual orientation in the media. Relationships between same-sex partners have long been depicted as less valid and less normal than relationships between heterosexuals (Bond, 2015). But things might be changing. Kinsler et al. (2019) found a great deal of "normalizing" storylines about gender identity, sexual orientation, and same-sex marriage in popular media. Many media depictions that center on gay and lesbian primary characters now tackle negative stereotypes and demonstrate "that sexual orientation does not hinder one's ability to raise a family or achieve workplace success" (Kinsler et al., p. 648).

Despite these advances, not all members of the LGBTQ+ community are featured regularly in mainstream media. In particular, the transgender community remains underrepresented. Some notable exceptions include Chaz Bono, Caitlyn Jenner, and Laverne Cox, the first transgender person to get an Emmy nomination (Gjorgievska & Rothman, 2014). Cox, who was also the first transgender person to make the cover of *Time* magazine, was nominated for her role as Sophia Burset in *Orange Is the New Black*.

Next we explore an element of entertainment programming that sometimes overlaps with depictions of sex.

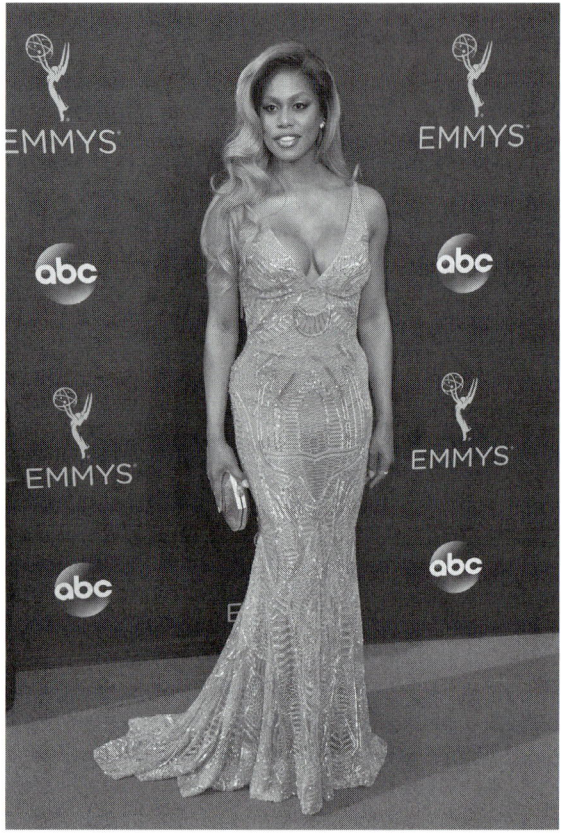

Today, storylines about gender identity, sexual orientation, and gay marriage are more common in popular media than in years' past. (Kinsler et al., 2019). Pictured here is Laverne Cox, the first transgender person nominated for an Emmy.

VIOLENCE

"Blood on" versus "blood off" is common parlance in video games. It refers to the level of gore and graphic realism players may select in games that involve killing other characters. In one study, youth who played a video game with "blood on" were slightly but significantly more likely than "blood off" players to indicate feelings of anger and to say they would react violently if someone ran into them on the sidewalk (Farrar, Krcmar, & Nowak, 2006). The evidence is mixed. In a similar study, researchers found that violence in video games did not predict aggressive behavior in male college students (Hilgard, Englehardt, Rouder, Segert, & Bartholow, 2019). However, in yet another study, researchers connected media violence with aggression, bullying, and cyberbullying (Barlett, Kowalewski, Kramer, Helmstetter, 2019). It can be confusing when studies present conflicting data, but the vast majority of researchers agree that there is an association between violence in the media and violence in real life.

When a team led by Patrick Bender reviewed research about media violence, they found that hundreds of studies present evidence that regular consumption of violent media content "increases the risk of aggressive thoughts, feelings, appraisals, and behavior" (Bender, Plante, & Gentile, 2019, p. 104). They say that "recent research is moving beyond the question of *whether* violent content effects exist to focus instead on the mechanisms explaining *how* these effects operate" (Bender et al., 2019, p. 105). Based on their review of the research, there is evidence that people (especially children and teens) who habitually play violent video games:

- Have a less emotional reaction to onscreen violence than do people who play nonviolent games.
- Have higher-than-average levels of cortisol, the body's main stress hormone.
- Experience diminished interpersonal trust.
- Tend to have more pro-violence attitudes than others.
- Can experience trigger aggression that manifests "months, years, and even decades later" (p. 105).

Of course, not everyone reacts to media violence in the same way. For some people, watching violence in the media is a substitute for acting out, but for others, watching violence triggers acting out. Still others experience something called "mean world syndrome"—a tendency among high media users to feel afraid and to overestimate the threat of violence in their environment (Gerbner, Gross, Morgan, & Signorielli, 1980; Jamieson & Romer, 2014).

Even businesses are affected by media violence. Researchers found a link between exposure to violence (including media depictions of violence) and unethical business behavior, and they also found that employees of businesses headquartered in violent areas were more likely than others to doctor their institutions' financial statements (Gubler, Herrick, Price, & Wood, 2018).

One criticism of the way media often depict violence is that the effects are unrealistic. People run through machine gun fire unscathed. They are shot or stabbed but continue performing like athletes or superheroes. Evil characters die, but heroes seldom do. George Gerbner (1996) dubbed this *happy violence*: "'Happy violence' is cool, swift, painless, and always leads to a happy ending, so as to deliver the audience to the next commercial in a receptive mood" (para. 10). In a study of PG-13 movies, Theresa Webb and colleagues (2007) report that, although violence was prevalent, enduring harm to victims was "either nonexistent or largely unrealistic" (p. e1226). In the fast-paced world of entertainment, it seems that violence is popular, but lengthy recoveries are boring. The result is an on-screen world in which violence lacks serious consequences.

Entertainment and Commercialism

It's usually easy to tell the difference between a commercial and a television program or movie. But what if a commercial looks like entertainment or commercial messages are subtly embedded in entertainment programming?

ENTERTAINOMERCIALS

Journalists have coined the term **entertainomercials** to characterize sales pitches that resemble entertainment programming ("Entertainomercials," 1996). A classic example involved Joe Camel, the former cartoon-like mascot of Camel cigarettes. R. J. Reynolds Tobacco Company introduced the colorful, sunglasses-wearing camel in 1988 advertising. Although company officials insisted that the animated character was not meant to capture children's interest, it had that effect. Sales of Camel cigarettes to children rose from $6 million per year to $476 million per year (DiFranza et al., 1991). Within a few years, children were as familiar with Joe Camel as with Mickey Mouse (Fischer, Schwartz, Richards, & Goldstein, 1991). Under public and legal pressure, Reynolds ceased using images of Joe Camel after a nine-year run (Vest, 1997).

PRODUCT PLACEMENT

The tobacco industry is also involved in another type of commercial/entertainment blend called product placement. **Product placement** means that a sponsor pays (with cash, props, services, or so on) to have a product or brand name included in a movie, a television program, a video game, or some other form of entertainment. Subtle product placements (sometimes called *stealth ads*) can be considered a form of subliminal advertising, in that the viewer may not be consciously aware of seeing items displayed but may develop an impression about them based on their association with other elements of the drama

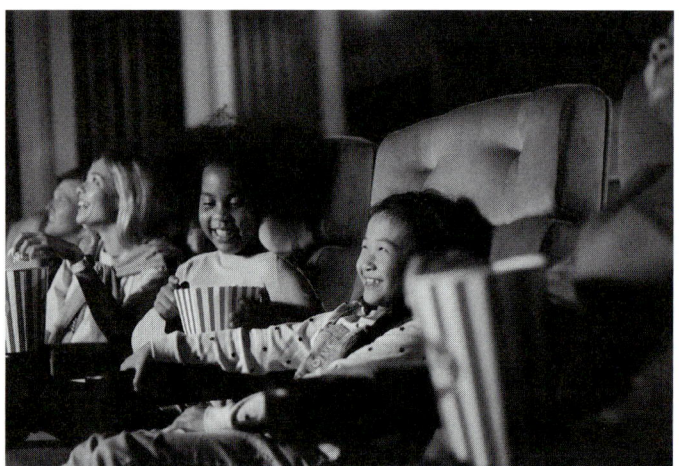

Do you think viewers are affected by product placements in the movies and on television? If so, how? Do you agree or disagree with the argument that people should be able to enjoy entertainment programming without being wary of embedded sales pitches? Why?

(Erdelyi & Zizak, 2004). Many advertisers are turning to product placements as a way to sneak their products into the public eye, realizing perhaps that four out of five TV viewers ignore commercials or fast-forward through them (Boris, 2014).

Product placements become health communication when they involve the way people think or behave concerning health issues. A particular concern arises when product placements are used to dodge restrictions on conventional advertising. Although most states forbid tobacco advertisements on radio and TV, tobacco companies have reportedly rewarded movie stars and producers for embedding them in movie scenes. Analysts expect that e-cigarettes and legalized marijuana—neither of which were addressed in the tobacco advertisement ban—may surface in product placements (D. E. Williams, 2015).

As the next section shows, some people fight fire with fire, using the product placement strategy to promote recommended health behaviors. See Box 11.4 for ethical issues related to health images in entertainment programs.

Entertainment-Education Programming

Producers may embed subtle messages in programs, not to sell products but to educate or persuade people regarding health matters. Efforts to benefit the public using an entertainment format are known as **entertainment-education** or prosocial programming. The idea, say Piotrow and colleagues, is that "no one enjoys being lectured to but everyone enjoys and often learns from entertainment, whether broadcast through radio or television, or performed in person" (Piotrow, Rimon, Merritt, & Saffitz, 2003, p. 5).

Entertainment producers today are likely to be lobbied by health advocates who urge them to incorporate health messages in their scripts, props, and storylines. Organizations such as Hollywood, Health & Society and the Entertainment Industries Council (EIC) encourage entertainment writers to portray health issues in accurate and informative ways. They provide tips, story ideas, and scripts about topics ranging from AIDS to bat bites, car seats, and suicide. For example, the EIC urges writers not to use the term *hard drugs* because it implies incorrectly that drugs that are not "hard" are relatively harmless. It also recommends that characters be shown using seatbelts and other safety devices.

Following are a few of the suggestions (quoted verbatim) from the EIC to people in the entertainment industry:

- Keep in mind that manic depression does not result from isolated personal traumas, such as the death of a loved one or the breakup of a relationship.
- Have one of your characters remind another to apply sunscreen before going outside.
- Consider reflecting the reality that homeowners often freeze up or tremble so badly when trying to use a gun in self-defense that they are unable to deploy it.

In some countries, entire programs have been created to promote healthy behaviors. For example, health promoters developed a talk show in Singapore that used edutainment techniques—like humor, learning through jokes, and personal narratives—to boost condom use from 52% to 80% in men who pay for sex (Lim, Tham, Cheung, Adaikan, & Wong, 2019).

A radio drama in Ethiopia, *Journal of Life*, depicted a main character who contracted HIV during a sexual indiscretion and then unknowingly infected his wife. Listeners who were surveyed reported that they were emotionally involved in the storyline and with each episode they heard, their resolve to engage

BOX 11.4 Ethical Considerations

Is the Entertainment Industry Responsible for Health Images?

Does the entertainment industry have a responsibility to promote healthy behaviors? Some claim that entertainment writers and producers behave irresponsibly when they consistently portray unhealthy and unrealistic images of life and health.

One way that the media distort reality is by showing unhealthy and violent behaviors without the natural consequences. People are shot with guns but continue to run and fight. Others overeat but appear to be slender and healthy nevertheless. Another way that media messages often misrepresent health is by depicting ill (especially mentally ill) individuals as dangerous, corrupt, and antisocial.

There is a gray zone where health and entertainment overlap. Even programs presented as healthy sometimes aren't. For example, *The Biggest Loser* and similar reality shows chronicle people involved in multiweek, boot-campish efforts to shed 50, 60, or even 100 pounds. Their experiences can be inspirational, but are they realistic or even healthy? Fitness guru/physician Pamela Peeke (2011) reflects on the show *Heavy*:

> *The people who were chosen are severely obese, with average weights in the range of 400–600 pounds. . . . There are frequent moments of what seems to be embarrassing over exposure of the participants, with numerous half-naked shots revealing enormous rolls of fat. If the producers wanted shock value, they achieved their goal. (para. 5)*

Even worse, she reflects, is the producers' insistence that all the participants need is discipline and sweat, prescribed in a merciless fashion by trainers (always thin) who show the participants little understanding or compassion. The people featured "repeatedly noted that they felt addicted to food, and that food had become the default for life's stresses as well as pleasures. Yet, despite their pleading for help, all they seemed to experience was a grueling workout schedule," Peeke says (para. 6). It's no wonder, she asserts, that most people regain the weight when they leave the show. The routines aren't sustainable, and "biceps curls, although integral to physical health, don't help to change eating behavior" (para. 6).

Some people argue that the entertainment industry need not offer shocking or distorted views of reality. They challenge Hollywood to create engrossing yet realistic programming. Going one step further, some people advocate prosocial programming to educate people while they are entertained.

On the other side of the issue, people argue that entertainment programming should not be harnessed to a social agenda. They feel that artistic creativity is compromised when writers and producers must adhere to social guidelines. Moreover, they say, it is difficult to know whose agenda should prevail. When health professionals disagree about specific guidelines for healthy living, is it the entertainer's job to decide which viewpoint should be represented? If the industry is held to a standard of realism, they wonder, what will become of fantasy themes and movies made famous by earlier generations, when different social expectations prevailed?

What Do You Think?

1. Do you think entertainment programming influences people's behavior? For instance, are people more likely to use condoms if they see their favorite characters talking about them in television programs and in the movies?
2. Should entertainers consider how their programs might influence audience members?
3. Do you think it is irresponsible of the entertainment industry to misrepresent the natural consequences of violent or otherwise unhealthy behavior?
4. Do you think it would diminish the entertainment value of your favorite movies and TV shows if they showed healthy behaviors or realistic consequences?
5. Do you believe programs designed specifically to promote healthy behaviors would be popular in the United States? Do you think such programs should be created? Why or why not?

in safer sex practices increased (Smith, Downs, & Witte, 2007).

In *Nunl Dhuhyo!* (Open Your Eyes!), celebrity hosts conducted moving interviews with people who were hoping for cornea transplants to restore their sight, and the number of people who signed cornea-donation cards increased from just over 1,000 to nearly 14,000 (Bae & Kang, 2008).

Impact of Persuasive Entertainment

Before you become too optimistic (or perturbed) about the prospects for embedding health messages in entertainment, it's important to ask: Beyond the effects already mentioned, do messages in entertainment programs make much difference?

Product placements seem to increase brand-name recognition. Although people are seldom motivated to go out and buy a product if they did not already want or need it, brands prominently displayed in entertaining programming have a slight edge over others when people are in the market for similar products (Moonhee & Roskos-Ewoldsen, 2007).

Entertainment-education yields mixed results. When researchers led by Jessie Quintero Johnson (2013) exposed some university students to fact sheets about a health issue and others to a storyline in which the characters experienced that health issue, the students varied in terms of information recall. In some cases, those who read the entertainment-education narrative remembered more about the health issue than those who read the fact sheets. In other cases, however, students were apparently distracted by other details of the storyline so that, even when they were highly engaged in the story, they did not remember key information about the health issue.

One cause for concern is the underlying power dynamic of some education-entertainment programs. From a critical-cultural perspective, Dutta (2006) argues that education-entertainment programs are often designed to serve the goals, values, and priorities of the funding entity, rather than those of the target community. The result can be a form of cultural hegemony in which the values of the dominant culture are imposed on members of the marginalized community, without respect for (or even awareness of) the community's own values, culture, and circumstances. Another danger is that sponsors will focus on individual aspects of a problem—such as having fewer children per family—rather than tackling larger and more systemic issues, such as the need to allocate resources fairly to all people (Dutta, 2006). (We talk more about the critical-cultural perspective in Chapter 14.)

Media Literacy

This chapter concludes where it began, with a reminder that the media's influence is by no means uniform. People are affected differently and to varying extents. Perhaps the best defense against excessive or negative media influence is the ability to analyze messages logically (Austin & Meili, 1994). That is a central tenet of media literacy.

Media literacy is defined as awareness and skills that allow a person to evaluate media content in terms of what is realistic and useful (adapted from Potter, 1998). According to Dorothy Singer and Jerome Singer's (1998) seminal overview, media-literate individuals are aware that advertisers are apt to highlight (and even exaggerate) the attractive aspects of their products and to downplay the disadvantages. They evaluate the creators' intent and try to figure out what is not being said and why. Media-literate individuals are also skillful at identifying portrayals that are unrealistic or have been enhanced by special effects. Overall, media-literate individuals tend to evaluate messages in terms of fairness and appropriateness, weighing ideas for themselves.

Media literacy instruction usually involves an informative, an analytic, and an experiential stage.

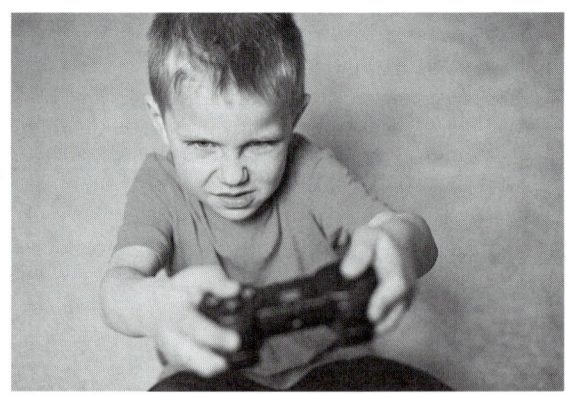

In one study, boys who played video games with highly muscular avatars were more likely to be dissatisfied with their own bodies afterward than boys whose avatars were normally proportioned (Sylvia, King, & Morse, 2014). Media literacy programs can help tykes realize how unrealistic media images can be.

Arli Quesada and Sue Summers (1998) described these stages well, and the discussion here is based on their work.

In the **informative stage**, participants in media literacy programs learn to identify different types of messages (persuasive, informative, and entertaining) and different types of media (television, radio, newspapers, and so on). They learn about the strengths and limitations of various media. For example, internet resources are vast and accessible, but some sources are not trustworthy. Participants also learn about production techniques and special effects.

In the **analytic stage**, participants discuss their perceptions of media in general and of specific media messages. In this stage they typically deconstruct messages with guidance from a trained leader. **Deconstructing** a message means breaking it down into specific components, such as key points, purpose, implied messages, production techniques, and goals. For example, beer commercials often present a social reality in which drinking is fun and sexy. In deconstructing a beer commercial (or any other media message), participants try to identify the message's purpose, what information is missing from it, and how it compares to their own social reality. They might conclude that beer companies make drinking look fun to sell their products, but the reality is different from what the commercials show.

Finally, in the **experiential stage**, media literacy programs challenge participants to write their own news stories, design ads, perform skits, and participate in other creative efforts to help them understand the process and demystify the way media messages are created. Adolescents who have taken part in tobacco-related media literacy programs are more likely than others to think carefully about tobacco commercials and to decide not to smoke (Pinkleton, Austin, Cohen, Miller, & Fitzgerald, 2007). A particularly useful technique is to have participants create their own anti-smoking messages (Banerjee & Greene, 2006).

Media literacy programs often yield promising results. Adolescent boys who took part in one program were subsequently less likely than their peers to consider advertisements for alcohol to be realistic (Chen, 2013). In another program, teenagers who studied the techniques that advertisers use to change models' appearance in photos were generally more satisfied with their bodies and less likely than their peers to have disordered eating, even more than two years later (Espinoza, Penelo, & Raich, 2013).

Media literacy can be taught at home when parents help children understand aspects of the media messages they encounter. This is known as **parental mediation**. Adults are often able to make children aware of inaccuracies and discrepancies in media messages. For example, "Why does this program show thin people eating fattening foods?" (Austin, 1995) or "Is the violence shown in this program realistic?" (Nathanson & Yang, 2003). Research suggests that children get maximum benefits from media (while minimizing unfavorable influences) when their parents (1) limit media exposure; (2) choose programs with care; (3) watch, listen, or read alongside them; and (4) discuss program content with them (Austin, 1993; Austin, Roberts, & Nass, 1990; Lee, 2013; Singer & Singer, 1998).

Summary

Health Images in the Media

- Excessive media use is associated with numerous social and health risks.
- Many media images are not what they appear to be. Images are often manipulated and "airbrushed to perfection" (Conlin & Bissell, 2014, p. 2). Unrealistic depictions have an influence on health when they affect people's self-esteem, their eating patterns, and more.
- Although media content can have harmful effects on health, it is also a means of sharing information that can help people better understand their health and health-related behaviors.

Theoretical Foundations

- Most people believe they are not personally susceptible to persuasive messages in the media but think that other people are. This is called third-person effect.
- Based on cultivation theory, children and adolescents may be especially susceptible to advertising messages because their frame of reference is limited.
- Social learning theory posits that people learn social behaviors by imitating others.
- Social comparison theory suggests that people strive to measure up to "idealized" characters in the media, even when the ideals are far from attainable.

Advertising

- It is difficult to say to what degree people's actions are affected by advertising, but significant influence is suggested by the number of people who eat the unhealthy food advertisers promote, drink the beverages they sell, and strive to emulate supermodels.
- Although advertising offers many advantages, it can be harmful if it encourages poor nutrition, drug and alcohol abuse, or an unhealthy reliance on cosmetics and fad diets.
- Sometimes advertisers make natural conditions seem bad or unnatural (pathological) so that people will pay money to change them.

Pharmaceutical Advertising

- Direct-to-consumer advertisements for pharmaceutical drugs increase consumers' awareness, but also present a number of challenges and ethical dilemmas related to social justice, research objectivity, full disclosure, and market agendas versus altruism.

News Coverage

- News coverage of health issues is important for sharing valuable knowledge. However, news audiences should remember that scientific findings are usually tentative, news stories tend to focus on unusual concerns, and coverage may be influenced by the desire to please advertisers or attract new audiences.

Media and Body Image

- Media messages often encourage an obsessive concern with physical appearance, sometimes to the detriment of people's health and self-esteem.
- Media consumers are consistently urged to believe that their skin, weight, hair, breath, clothing, and teeth are "problem areas." Theorists call this pathologizing the human body, making natural functions seem weird and unnatural (Wood, 1999). Teens are particularly susceptible to these kinds of messages.

Entertainment

- Entertainment portrayals may influence what people believe about medical care, risky behavior, and persons with disabilities.
- Sex and violence are shown mostly for entertainment value, not as serious subjects with health consequences. In reality, medical miracles are less common than depicted on television, and people are more diverse.
- Do not be surprised if the food, drinks, cigarettes, vehicles, and props in your favorite programs and movies were put in purposefully to please advertisers. Although product placements may not look like commercials, advertisers go to great expense hoping they will function like commercials.
- Health advocates sometimes use the same logic in inserting pro-health messages into entertainment programs, a practice known as education-entertainment programming.

Media Literacy

- Media literacy allows people some control over how media messages affect them. Wise consumers learn to distinguish between reliable and unreliable information by critiquing media messages to determine their purposes, strengths, and limitations.

Glossary

analytic stage In this stage, participants discuss their perception of media in general and of specific media messages. *See page 265.*

cultivation theory Proposes that people develop beliefs about the world based on a complex array of influences, media among them. *See page 240.*

deconstructing Breaking down a message into specific components such as key points, purpose, implied messages, production technique, and goals. *See page 265.*

direct-to-consumer (DTC) advertising Marketing that is aimed toward consumers when access to a product, such as prescription medication, requires an intermediary. *See page 247.*

entertainment-education programming Using media for entertaining and educating audiences. *See page 262.*

entertainomercials Sales pitches that resemble entertainment programming. *See page 261.*

experiential stage In this stage, media literacy programs challenge participants to write their own news stories, design their own ads, perform skits, and participate in other creative efforts to help them understand the process and demystify the way media messages are created. *See page 265.*

informative stage In this stage, participants in media literacy programs learn to identify different types of messages (persuasive, informative, entertaining) and different types of media. *See page 265.*

mass communication The dissemination of messages from one person or group to large numbers of people via media including television, radio, computers, newspapers, magazines, billboards, video games, and other means. *See page 239.*

media literacy Awareness and skills that allow a person to evaluate media content in terms of what is realistic and useful. *See page 264.*

parental mediation Media literacy that is taught at home when parents help children understand the aspects of media messages they encounter. *See page 265.*

pathologizing the human body Making natural functions seem weird and unnatural. *See page 253.*

product placement Paid inclusion of products or brand names in movies, television programs, video games, or other forms of entertainment. *See page 261.*

rape culture A society whose prevailing social attitudes have the effect of normalizing or trivializing sexual assault and abuse. *See page 259.*

sexual objectification The act of treating a person as a mere object of sexual desire. *See page 259.*

social comparison theory Proposes that people judge themselves largely in comparison to others. *See page 241.*

social learning theory Proposes that people learn how to behave by watching others, as well as media depictions of others, and by watching and attending to the consequences of others' behavioral choices. *See page 240.*

third-person effect Hypothesis that people believe mass media messages have a greater effect on others than on themselves. *See page 240.*

Discussion Questions

1. Consider the mediated images and messages that an elementary school student is likely to encounter in a typical day via television, billboards, the news, the internet, video games, and so on. Based on cultivation theory and social comparison theory, what is the child likely to believe about themselves and the larger world based on these messages?

2. Identify several DTC ads for pharmaceutical drugs. In your opinion, are the depictions in the ads realistic? Fair? Culturally inclusive? What are the advantages and disadvantages of these ads, as you see them? In your opinion, do the advantages outweigh the disadvantages or not? Why?

3. In what ways, if any, do media messages affect your food choices? Your body image? Your decision to drink or smoke, or not? Your preference for particular brands? Why do you feel you are or have been influenced, or why do you think media images have not influenced you?

4. You read about evidence that alcoholic beverage makers target underage youth? Have you seen evidence of this yourself? If so, how? Do you think it has an effect?

5. In what ways do some advertisers pathologize the human body? In what ways do some music videos dehumanize women? What are the health implications of these?

6. Identify several health items in the news. Does the information reflect ongoing health concerns (e.g., heart disease, cancer, asthma) or rarer conditions? Is the information helpful in terms of treating or preventing health concerns? What do you like best about the stories you have identified? What would you improve about them?

7. Do you ever struggle with the type of insecurities Rachel Hills describes, in terms of being attractive to others? In what situations, if any, do you feel sexually objectified? What evidence of objectification can you identity in the photos that appear in this chapter and in what you witness in the media?

8. What did Gerbner mean by the term *happy violence*? Can you give some examples from your own media experiences?

9. Analyze several media messages (an advertisement, a news story, a video game, or so on) following the steps in a media literacy program. What conclusions do you reach about the creators' agenda? The explicit and implied messages? The realistic nature of the images and messages?

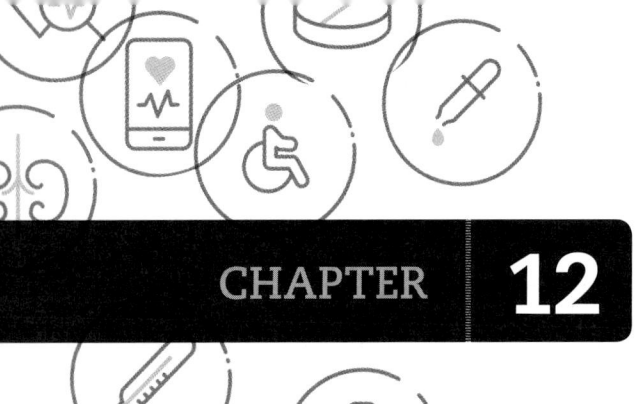
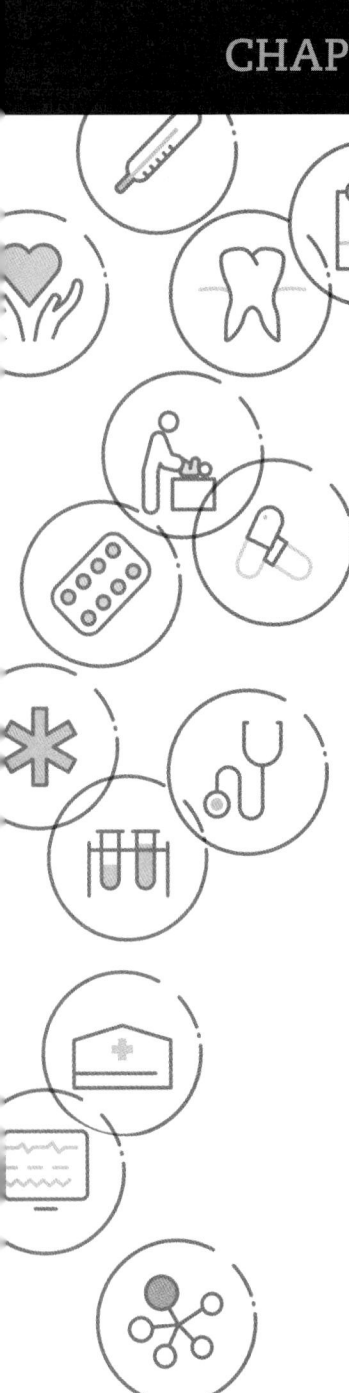

CHAPTER 12

Public Health and Crisis Communication

We began this book reflecting on one of the largest pandemics of all time. As of spring 2020, people in more than 200 countries had been infected with Coronavirus (COVID-19), and the numbers were rising. Communication challenges surround a health threat that has never been encountered before, especially when it escalates rapidly and crosses national borders. As this book goes to press, it's unclear whether world response to COVID-19 will ultimately be considered successful or not. What is clear is that we must continually learn from our mistakes and failures. This chapter is an attempt to do that.

This chapter explores the role of communication in promoting public health and managing health risks and crises. In contrast to chronic health conditions (covered in Chapters 13 and 14) that are often difficult to keep in the limelight, here we focus on the challenge of emergent threats that present health communication specialists with a different challenge—to make sense of rapidly emerging details and keep the public vigilant but not terrified. We explore real-life case studies about health crises to identify the best ways to prepare for and manage developing threats to public health. As you will see, an assortment of "lessons learned" appear in italics throughout this chapter and are summarized in Box 12.6 at the end of the chapter. We begin our discussion with an overview of public health.

What Is Public Health?

"The success or failure of any government in the final analysis must be measured by the well-being of its citizens. Nothing can be more important to a state than its public health; the state's paramount concern should be the health of its people." — Franklin Delano Roosevelt

Public health centers on the well-being of entire communities and involves thousands of agencies operating at local, national, and international levels.

You are already familiar with several such agencies. For example, in this book, you have read about the World Health Organization (WHO) and the Centers for Disease Control and Prevention (CDC). WHO coordinates international public health within the United Nations system and operates in 194 countries, while the CDC is the preeminent public health agency in the United States. Across the U.S., there are more than 2,800 local health departments (National Association of City & County, 2015), which employ more than 400,000 public health workers (Jones, Banks, Plotkin, Chanthavongsa, & Walker, 2015). (See Box 12.1 for more on career opportunities in public health.)

Apart from ensuring the well-being of communities, you may wonder what else public health encompasses and what public health workers do. Mary-Jane Schneider (2006) describes it this way:

> Just as a doctor monitors the health of a patient by taking vital signs—blood pressure, heart rate, and so forth—public health workers monitor the health of a community by collecting and analyzing health data. (p. 121)

But public health does not stop there. In the same way that physicians and other caregivers are devoted to keeping people well, public health professionals are concerned with maintaining the good health of the entire population (Schneider, 2006). They seek to accomplish this through education, community partnerships, health campaigns, and immunizations, and by maintaining healthy standards in restaurants, day care centers, schools, and other public spaces.

In the classic definition presented by Charles-Edward A. Winslow (1923), **public health** is

> the science and art of preventing disease, prolonging life, and promoting physical health and efficiency through organized community efforts for the sanitation of the environment, the control of community infections, the education of the individual in principles of personal hygiene, the organization of medical and nursing service for the early diagnosis and preventive treatment of disease, and the development of the social machinery which will ensure to every individual in the community a standard of living adequate for the maintenance of health. (Originally published in Winslow's The Evolution and Significance of the Modern Public Health Campaign, 1923, reprinted in the "History of Public Health," 2002, n.p.)

This definition prescribes that public health professionals be both proactive—seeking to avoid unhealthy conditions, illnesses, and injuries—and diligent about monitoring and responding to health needs that arise.

BOX 12.1 Career Opportunities

Public Health

Business or billing manager
Communication specialist
Emergency management director
Environmentalist
Epidemiologist
Fundraiser
Health campaign designer
Health department administrator
Health educator
Health inspector
Health researcher
Media relations professional
Nonprofit organization director
Nurse
Nutritionist/dietician
Patient advocate or navigator
Physician
Professor/educator
Public policy advisor
Risk/crisis communication specialist
Social worker

Career Resources and Job Listings

- American Public Health Association: apha.org/about-apha
- Partners in Information Access for the Public Health Workforce: phpartners.org/jobs.html
- U.S. Department of Health & Human Services Careers: hhs.gov/careers/
- Association of Schools & Programs in Public Health: https://www.aspph.org/
- World Health Organization: who.int/employment/vacancies/en

Also check the websites of your local hospitals and health departments.

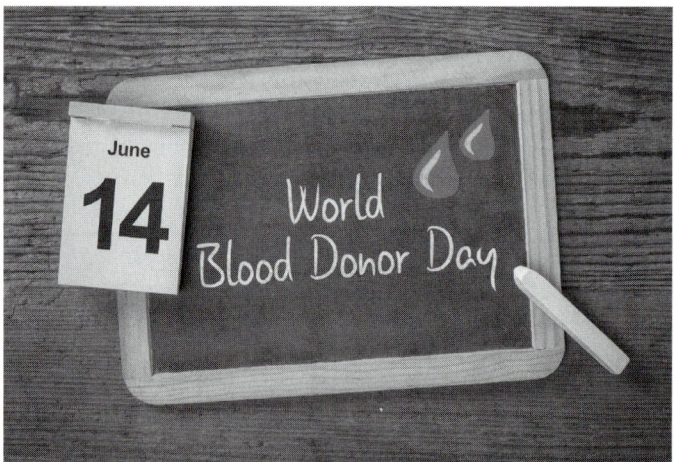

Think of an effort to mobilize the public. It might be a blood donation campaign, a stop-smoking PSA, a political campaign, or the like. Did it influence you? Did you take part? Why or why not?

Public health involves an array of health concerns. Traditionally, ongoing concerns like diabetes, cancer, and heart disease fall within the rubric of *health promotion* (Chapters 13 and 14). Typically, health promotion campaigns are designed with **social mobilization** in mind—large-scale efforts in which community members and professionals work interactively to define goals, raise awareness, and create hospitable environments for healthy behaviors. Social mobilization relies on teamwork, diversity, shared leadership, and active involvement (Patel, 2005).

Sometimes, public health agencies deal with other concerns, such as health emergencies—situations that occur in a particular time and place, including outbreaks of foodborne illnesses, epidemics, exposure to harmful substances, workplace dangers, natural disasters, and so on. During emergencies, public health agencies coordinate risk and crisis communication for affected communities. Risk and crisis messages differ from health promotion messages in a number of important ways. For one, risk and crisis communication traditionally has been largely one-way instead of collaborative. Social media, as we will see later in this chapter, is changing that. But first, let's explore what sets risk communication and crisis communication apart.

Risk and Crisis Communication

Risk communication is an ongoing process that involves disseminating information and engaging in interactive discussions about how people perceive risks and how they feel about risk messages (National Research Council, 1989, p. 21). Part of the challenge involves when and how to alert the public about health risks.

When people began falling ill after eating beef from cattle raised in Great Britain in the 1980s and 1990s, officials largely chose to downplay the risk and reassure people that British beef was safe to eat. The public gradually became skeptical, and even angry, about this claim. Six years before officials went public about what came to be known as "mad cow disease," the British journal *Nature* chided authorities for keeping people in the dark:

Never say that there is not danger (risk). Instead, say that there is always a danger (risk), and that the problem is to calculate what it is. And never say that the risk is negligible unless you are sure that your listeners share your own philosophy of life. ("Mad Cows and the Minister," 1990, p. 278)

The author of the article stressed that the minister of agriculture "should be obliged to tell it like it is" (p. 278) and admonished that the cost of officials' false reassurances was fear, distrust, and economic instability.

Downplaying risks may ultimately create a sense of distrust that discourages people from believing anything health officials say. Although risk communication professionals are sometimes in the business of soothing fears, in the mad cow disease scenario, they violated an important tenet of risk and crisis communication: *Be open about what you know, even if you do not have all the answers*. False reassurance—what Peter Sandman (2006a) calls "optimism masquerading as information" (para. 9)—can actually heighten fears and mistrust. This is supported by another lesson that belies conventional wisdom: *Citizens rarely panic when they are well informed*.

Reporting on 50 years of research about people's behavior during disasters, Lee Clarke (2002) observes that, despite the "panic myth," people rarely act irrationally or selfishly in crisis situations. Instead, emergencies usually bring out the best in people. "When danger arises, the rule—as in normal situations—is for people to help those next to them before they help themselves" (Clarke, 2002, p. 24). A notable example is the Cajun Navy, ad hoc groups of fishing boat owners who volunteer their vessels and expertise to aid in rescue efforts during major flood cancer diagnoses (Durkin, 2018). After a devastating earthquake in Nepal, so many untrained volunteers rushed to the country that they created a "second disaster"—escalating food shortages, clogging transportation routes, and adding to the chaos (Bennett, 2015). In such instances, risk communication is important because public health agencies must adequately convey potential dangers to both volunteers and victims.

Risk communication messages are usually tailored for specific audiences. Sandman (2006b) describes three "risk communication traditions": (1) helping people who are *insufficiently concerned* appreciate that a serious risk exists; (2) reassuring and calming people who are *excessively concerned*; and (3) working with people who are *appropriately concerned* (those who are "genuinely endangered and rightly upset") to help them cope and function effectively (p. 257). Let's shift gears for a moment and look at crisis communication.

In its broadest sense, crisis communication can involve any number of events—a natural disaster, a scandal that rocks a political campaign, an epidemic, a chemical spill, and so on. In this chapter, we focus on communication about crises that involve public health. The CDC (2008) defines health-related **crisis communication** as

> *an approach used by scientists and public health professionals to provide information that allows an individual, stakeholders, or an entire community to make the best possible decisions about their well-being, under nearly impossible time constraints, while accepting the imperfect nature of their choices.* (para. 2)

The definition is telling in that it acknowledges "the nearly impossible" demands and the inherently "imperfect" nature of crisis management. Public health expert Deborah Glik (2007) observes that a crisis involves "unexpectedness, high levels of threat, an aroused and stressed population, and media looking for breaking news stories" (p. 35). Practitioners work hard to lay solid groundwork and learn everything they can, but overwhelming demands and emotions can challenge even the most experienced public health professionals.

Managing Perceptions

In her review of risk communication research, Katherine McComas (2006) observes that people tend to perceive some risks, such as being attacked by

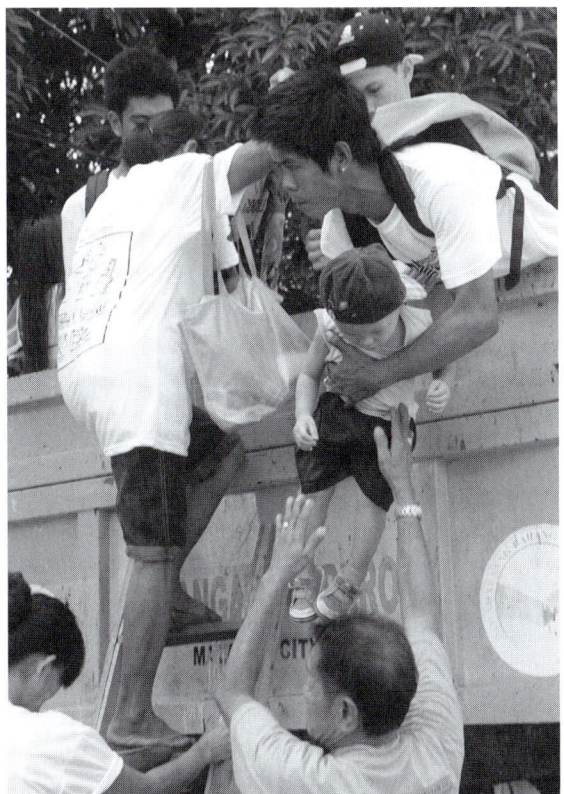

The "panic myth" says people act irrationally or selfishly in crisis situations. Research suggests the opposite: that emergencies usually bring out the best in people. However, timing is crucial. Rushing to the scene of a disaster can make things worse, particularly if you are not trained to offer assistance.

events (Wax-Thibodeaux, 2017). The Louisiana-based Cajun Navy emerged in the wake of Hurricane Katrina and reassembles as needed, as it did during the 2016 Baton Rouge floods and in Texas and North Carolina after Hurricanes Michael and Florence. There are now dozens of groups operating under the name "Cajun Navy," including Cajun Navy Relief, a federally recognized charitable organization that partners with regional and state disaster relief agencies and the Office of Homeland Security and Emergency Preparedness (Cajun Navy Relief, 2019).

But sometimes people with good intentions who rush to the scene of a disaster put themselves at risk and may hinder relief efforts. Consider these examples. Volunteers (as well as victims) in the immediate aftermath of the 9/11 terrorist attacks in New York City were exposed to toxic fumes and dust. Exposure to toxic substances released in the 9/11 attacks has been linked to more than 43,000 illnesses and 10,000

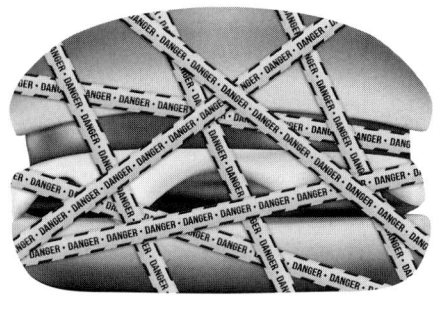

Exposed to too many "fear appeals," people become overwhelmed or indifferent; too few and they do not take risks seriously.

a shark while swimming at the beach, to be greater than they actually are, whereas people tend to have "optimistic biases" or "illusions of invulnerability" about other, statistically more threatening risks, such as smoking and sun exposure (p. 78). This is particularly true when the risky behavior has pleasant or socially rewarding implications. For example, despite warning messages that we have heard, we may tell ourselves that we are too young to get skin cancer, that we will put on sunscreen later, or that having a suntan is worth the risk.

Ratzan and Meltzer (2005) point out that people are not wrong when they see things differently from experts; they just have a different vantage point. "These two audiences receive different information, process it in unique ways, and respond to conclusions based on their own set of circumstances and concerns" (Ratzan & Meltzer, 2005, p. 324). It's complicated, of course, because members of the public are not uniform in their perceptions. For example, you may feel your anxiety rise while reading about Ebola, perhaps because you have been to western Africa, you have seen horrifying footage from the region, or your brother is a nurse who may have been exposed to Ebola. Meanwhile, some readers may feel insulated from the issue and wonder what all the fuss is about. There is no right way to feel. Instead, we must remember as health communication practitioners that belittling or ignoring diverse perspectives is typically ineffective and even unethical. (For more about diverse perceptions, see Box 12.2 about the controversy surrounding vaccines.)

BOX 12.2

Parents Grapple with Vaccine Information

By Patricia Barlow

More than 100 children brought home something more than memories when they visited southern California theme parks in 2015. They left with measles. "Disease detectives for months raced to contain the highly contagious disease, which surfaced at Disney theme parks and spread to a half-dozen U.S. states, Mexico and Canada," reported NBC News ("Measles Outbreak," 2015). In the end, 147 people were sickened in the outbreak, most of them children who had not been immunized as recommended or who were too young to be immunized.

Measles is caused by a virus that primarily affects the skin, nose, and throat. About 1 in 4 children with measles will require hospitalization, and 1 in 1,000 will experience swelling of the brain, which may cause brain damage and even death. When pregnant women get the virus, their babies may be born prematurely or of low birth weight (CDC, 2015a).

By 1998, measles had become so rare that experts at the CDC announced that it was "no longer an indigenous disease in the United States" ("Epidemiology of Measles," 1999, para. 1). It had become all but obsolete based on what scientists call herd immunity—people had been immunized with such consistency that the virus could no longer find a stronghold. However, that was about to change.

A 1998 article in the British medical journal *The Lancet* proposed a link between autism and a preservative (thimerosal) in the measles–mumps–rubella (MMR) vaccine (Wakefield et al., 1998). The study was later found to be faulty. It was based on only 12 children, and by the researchers' own admission, they misinterpreted the data (Willingham & Helft, 2014). Six years after the article was published, 10 of the 13

continued

continued

authors publicly disavowed its conclusions, and 12 years after publication, *The Lancet* retracted the story.

Extensive studies by other researchers have failed to indicate a link between autism and thimerosal. However, as a precaution, U.S. authorities ordered that it be removed from childhood vaccines beginning in 2001. Even so, the original article's impact on public sentiment has been profound.

Some parents (sometimes called anti-vaxxers) remain firm in their belief that vaccines cause autism. Consequently, about 1 in 12 children in the United States has not received the recommended MMR vaccination (Elam-Evans, Yankey, Singleton, & Kolasa, 2014). By 2014, some 16 years after the disease was deemed nearly nonexistent, the United States experienced a record-breaking number of measles cases (668 in all). In Europe, where measles had nearly died out as well, about 3,840 new cases a year are emerging (Fox & Connor, 2015).

Dialogue on the risks and benefits of vaccines has played out in the media with strong feelings on both sides. Actor/comedian Jenny McCarthy has been an outspoken opponent of vaccines. Other stars, such as Kristen Bell, have proclaimed, "No vaccines? You can't hold my children" (Cruz, 2015, headline). Health care providers are divided about whether to see patients who are not vaccinated, some of them fearful that contagious diseases will be spread to other children in their care (Bellafante, 2014). Government entities argue over strengthening mandates, eliminating exceptions, and imposing consequences on anti-vaxxers (Bernstein, 2015). For their part, anti-vaxxers worry that pharmaceutical companies are covering up evidence about vaccines so that people will continue to use their products.

Much of the conversation swirling within the vaccination controversy involves identifying the most effective strategies for communicating with parents who are concerned about the safety of vaccinations (Hendrix, 2015). Communication from public health professionals has emphasized empirical research about the benefits and safety of vaccines. However, this approach has not been highly successful with vaccination-averse parents (Nyhan, Reifler, Richey, & Freed, 2014), perhaps because they distrust government agencies and pharmaceutical companies. Some evidence suggests that the most effective messages emphasize the benefits of vaccinations (Friedersdorf, 2015; Hendrix, 2015), while other research indicates that it is more effective to describe the risks of diseases, especially if the news comes directly from trusted doctors (Nyhan et al., 2014).

What Do You Think?

1. What type of information do you consider most important on the topic of vaccines: news stories, scientific studies, physicians, parents, celebrities, or another source? Why?
2. If information is inconsistent, which sources are you most likely to trust? Why?
3. Are you more concerned about the safety of vaccines, or the ill effects of disease they are meant to prevent? Why?

How Scared Is Scared Enough?

While interacting with the public about health risks and crises, it's sometimes difficult to judge how much fear is productive and how much is disabling. It sometimes seems that public health advocates want people to be afraid of something nearly all of the time. As Dawn Hillier (2006) puts it, well-meaning health promoters sometimes feed the public "a steady diet of fearful programmes about impending calamities" (p. 30). After a while, people may be either too fearful to make effective choices or so weary of "fear appeals" that they discount them altogether. However, a *rational* fear of horrible outcomes is healthy and motivational. It's a fine line to walk. Sandman (2006b) captured the dilemma well when he wrote:

> *The Holy Grail of crisis communicators is to get people to take precautions without frightening them. This is like trying to write a novel without using the letter "e"; it may be possible, but it's certainly a handicap.* (p. 258)

By way of example, Sandman quotes a *New York Times* headline that read "Fear Is Spreading Faster Than SARS." He retorts, "As if it weren't supposed to. . . . If the purpose of fear is to motivate precautions, after all, then the fear must come before the

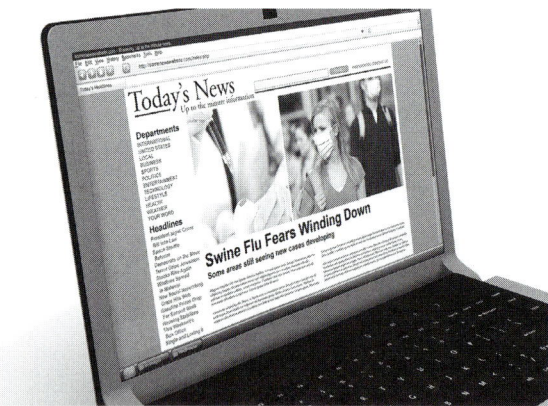

When the news is filled with frightening health information, how do you respond?

precautions are needed" (p. 259). We talk more about fear appeals in Chapter 14.

In the Heat of the Moment

Crisis communication looks easier on paper than it feels in reality. Vicki Freimuth (2006), former director of communication at the CDC, reflects on crises this way:

> Health communicators have a particularly difficult time with speed, as they are accustomed to conducting formative research, carefully segmenting audiences, planning messages, and pretesting before releasing them. [In a crisis] all of these activities have to occur in hours, not days, weeks, or months. Theory and research are still critical, but must be internalized by the communicators so they are available to use on the spot. (p. 144)

And a cool-headed commitment to safety can be even more difficult at the actual site of an emergency. Dave Johnson (2006) recalls the chaos at the World Trade Center in New York when it was attacked in 2001:

> A violent explosion rips through your office complex. Multiple fires are burning. An ominous plume of heat, fire, dust, debris and an unknowable mixture of perhaps asbestos, silica, lead and other metals floats into the atmosphere.... Firefighters and police and EMTs, over which you have no authority, arrive on the scene. The fire chief says "Get out of our way." His guys, and the police, don't wear proper protection.... Your own workforce is shocked. Some rush past the fires and debris, into the plume, searching for comrades.... It's chaotic. You're operating in a fog of disaster. (p. 58)

Johnson, who is editor of *Industrial Safety & Hygiene News*, presents some of the lessons learned about risk communication at Ground Zero.

- "*Beware of overly optimistic risk assessments*," as when an EPA administrator prematurely announced one week after the disaster that the air in New York City was "safe to breathe" (p. 58). False reassurance can undermine experts' credibility and put people in danger.
- *Understand the different information needs of various stakeholders*. After workers heard officials reassure the public that Ground Zero was safe, supervisors had a hard time convincing workers to exercise caution and use proper safety gear.
- "*Understand the emotions and fears you are dealing with*" (p. 60). People who are worried, anxious, angry, or grief-stricken are likely to brush aside safety concerns and then be sorry later.
- "*Expect resistance to your message*" *and don't give up* (p. 60). Use a range of methods if necessary. For example, when New York City mayor Rudy Giuliani balked at wearing a hardhat, the Ground Zero team presented him with one that said "VIP—Mayor" on the front. "It worked," said Stewart Burkhammer, an environmental safety and health consultant working at Ground Zero. At other times, Burkhammer said, bluntness worked better than subtlety. He once told the crew at a morning safety meeting, "I'm not going to be the one to tell the mayor we just killed somebody, so clean up your act" (quoted by Johnson, 2006, p. 62).
- *Foster relationships and open communication with partners* (media, emergency personnel, and so on) before, during, and after a crisis.
- *Be proactive rather than reactive.* "Communicate and instruct as much as possible in advance of an emergency," recommends Burkhammer. "We spent a lot of time being great reactors.... A lot of things were done by feel and guess. I think we were very poor proactors" (p. 62).

Box 12.3 presents a framework to help guide your efforts as you prepare for and manage health crises. Additional crisis communication models are described in the next section.

BOX 12.3

Risk Management/Communication Framework

Imagine that, after eating lunch in their school cafeteria, 125 local children have become ill, some of them requiring hospitalization. As the health education supervisor at the health department, you are expected to help manage the crisis. Your staff has received 25 calls from worried parents and 15 calls from media professionals, and the issue has not even hit the news yet. What do you do first? Following is a synthesis of advice from the models described in the chapter. After reviewing it, consider how you would handle the crisis.

Establishing the Foundations

If you are wise, the first step in managing the crisis actually began long before it occurred. Experts recommend developing interactive and trusting relationships with stakeholders when things are calm. They also recommend creating teams and crisis management plans and practicing what to do when a crisis occurs. This includes developing a following on social media and experience sharing information that way. Another precaution is to collect information in advance that will be helpful, quick at hand, and tailored to different audiences. There is not always time in a crisis to construct and pretest new messages carefully (Ratzan & Meltzer, 2005; WHO, 2018a). In your case, having ready access to good information about foodborne illnesses will make your job a great deal easier.

Partnering With Stakeholders

Stakeholders are important before, during, and after a crisis. Ratzan and Meltzer (2005) embrace a broad definition of *stakeholders* as "anyone and everyone touched by the event" (p. 325). In your case, this might mean parents, children, school employees, reporters, public officials, health professionals, food distribution and preparation personnel, state agencies, and more. Ratzan and Meltzer observe that there are several benefits of engaging stakeholders: (1) They can give you valuable, diverse input; (2) they can be (and should be) active partners in achieving shared goals; and (3) if you trust each other, you can engage in two-way communication that is honest and open.

In the current crisis, you might not know all of the stakeholders personally, but if you have made it a point to interact with at least a few key people in each group, you will be more effective in this crisis. In addition, you can activate your network to extend outreach to stakeholder groups. For example, if the health department supplies local schools with nurses, you might enlist the nurses' help in communicating with stakeholders. In the same way, you might call on health inspectors, media relations staff, PTA presidents, and others. If you have laid good groundwork and are open and trustworthy with stakeholders, a crisis can renew and strengthen relationships rather than damage them (Ratzan & Meltzer, 2005; Ulmer, Seeger, & Sellnow, 2007).

Communicating With the Public

You will also want to pass along information via mass and social media. Understanding media professionals' goals will help you work as partners rather than as adversaries. Be mindful that reporters have a stake in presenting immediate, accurate, and interesting information to the public. They look as foolish as you do if they pass along inaccurate information. But this doesn't mean you should keep them waiting until you know everything. "Today's media have a need for constant information updates to fill 24-hour broadcasts," Ratzan and Meltzer (2005) advise, adding, "Crisis communicators need to be aware that if they do not supply information, the media will report what they have" (p. 328). When using social media, keep in mind that posts should be updated regularly to reflect the latest information. Also, social media is a two-way communication channel—agencies should use social media to respond to the public's questions and comments.

In communicating with the public (either in person or through media channels), Ratzan and Meltzer (2005) recommend being "clear, honest and compassionate" (p. 330). Being clear requires that you consider the different needs and literacy levels of stakeholders. Information that might make sense to researchers and clinicians can bewilder and frighten members of the public. Your words and demeanor convey to the public how they should think and feel about the crisis. Always "think before you speak," urge Ratzan and Meltzer (p. 331).

continued

Internal Communication Strategies

In the general rush to meet public and media demands, it is easy to neglect teamwork in a crisis. But this oversight can lead to devastating mistakes. Ratzan and Meltzer (2005) underscore the importance of communicating regularly with members of your team. Depending on the duration of the crisis, you might call daily or twice-a-day briefings at which everyone can compare notes and impressions.

What Do You Think?

With regard to the "sick schoolchildren" crisis described at the opening of this box:

1. Where would you begin? What would you do first?
2. What stakeholders might you involve, and why? What questions would you ask each stakeholder group?
3. How would you enlist the stakeholders as active partners in the process?
4. How will you get (and convey) answers to reporters' questions such as the following: How sick are the children? Could this be deadly? Can you arrange interviews with some of the children or parents? How likely is it that other children will come down sick? Have you definitively linked the illness to food served at school? If so, what food was it? Who is responsible for food at school? Is there a chance that the tainted food was distributed to other schools as well? To restaurants? To grocery stores?
5. What will you do when your staff cannot keep up with all the phone calls, much less research the issue and contact stakeholders?
6. When the crisis has passed, how will you evaluate the success or failure of your efforts?
7. What might you do to prepare for future risks and crises?

Crisis Communication Models and Guidelines

Several theories and models help shape how crisis communication plans are developed and executed. The health belief model, for instance, informs many crisis communication strategies. The **health belief model** (Rosenstock, 1960; Stretcher & Rosenstock, 1997) proposes that people make behavioral choices based on six factors: (a) how susceptible they believe they are with respect to a particular risk, such as catching the flu or contracting measles; (b) the severity of the risk; (c) perceived advantages of the recommended behavior, like reducing the chances of becoming infected with the flu or measles by getting vaccinated; (d) perceived obstacles to carrying out the recommended behavior, such as the cost of getting vaccinated; (e) how confident they are in their ability to perform the recommended behavior (i.e., self-efficacy); and (f) cues to action or messages that suggest a specific behavior, like "Get Vaccinated." We'll talk more about the health belief model in Chapter 14, but this basic understanding will prove useful as we explore the following crisis communication models and guidelines.

In this section, we focus on three models: the *WHO Guideline on Communicating Risk*, which recommends how to prepare for and manage a crisis; the *IDEA Model*, which describes crisis messages and means of distributing them; and the CDC's *Crisis and Risk Communication Model*, which considers which messages are most needed at particular stages of a crisis. As you will see, there is some overlap between the models. All of them stress the importance of prior planning, relationship building, and careful message design and dissemination. Beyond that, each model presents unique nuances to enhance the value of crisis-related communication.

World Health Organization's Guidelines on Communicating Risk

In 2016, WHO commissioned dozens of scholars to assess hundreds of studies and reports on crisis communication to create the Guideline on Communicating Risk (Toppenberg-Pejcic et al., 2019, p. 437). The guidelines continually evolve based on new and emerging evidence, but the WHO (2018a) has issued several recommendations to date, which include:

- *Plan in advance.* Emergency communication infrastructures and strategies should be in place before crises occur. This requires adequate funding, trained personnel, interagency relationships, and multiple channels for communicating emergency messages.

- *Build trust.* Effective crisis communication is timely, transparent, easy-to-understand, addresses uncertainty, and promotes self-efficacy. Deborah Toppenberg-Pejcic and colleagues (2019), whose research helped shape the guidelines, stress that building trust boils down to two words: "Go local" (p. 440). The most effective campaigns are led and/or informed by community members.
- *Engage communities.* Identify and partner with local stakeholders. Involve them in decision making to ensure that messages are culturally and contextually appropriate. Some of the most important people to involve include religious leaders, community leaders, and women or women's groups (Toppenberg-Pejcic et al., 2019). Several studies find that targeting women during epidemics has been particularly effective. One report compared Ebola to fire and women to water—"water puts out the fire" (Toppenberg-Pejcic et al., 2019, p. 440).
- *Use multiple channels, including social media.* Newspapers, radio, and television have long been essential for disseminating information to the public in emergencies. These days, social media is increasingly seen as an important—if not vital—information channel that should be utilized in conjunction with traditional media during crises. Social media facilitates peer-to-peer communication and allows officials to monitor and respond to rumors. It also helps coordinate local-level response.
- *Monitor, evaluate, and adjust.* Use feedback from stakeholders to improve messaging and address concerns.

The IDEA Model

Several models focus on the impact of crisis-related messages and how they are shared. The **IDEA model** for instructional risk communication, as explained by Deborah Sellnow and Timothy Sellnow (2014), has four main components:

- **Internalization** refers to the process whereby people process risk messages based on personal relevance, proximity to the risk, potential impact, and timeliness (e.g., the time available to make preparations or respond to a crisis).
- **Distribution** refers to channels for sharing information, such as television, radio, newspapers, the internet, and social media.
- **Explanation** reflects the quality of a message, its accuracy, the credibility of its source, and how easily it is understood by the public.
- **Action** involves the specific steps people might take in an emergency.

Evidence shows that IDEA-shaped crisis messages can be more effective at promoting understanding and behavioral intentions than the messages typically conveyed by news media (Sellnow, Lane, Sellnow, & Littlefield, 2017).

Some scholars and crisis communicators pair the IDEA model with exemplification theory (Zillmann, 1999), which proposes that easy-to-understand examples can be used to convey complicated ideas in memorable ways that require little analytic thought. As explained by Deborah Sellnow-Richmond and colleagues, examples can have positive or negative connotations. For example, "superfoods" are typically considered healthy and "Frankenfoods" unhealthy (Sellnow-Richmond, George, & Sellnow, 2018, p. 141). Studies show that examples work best and are most memorable when they combine vivid images and emotional appeals (Sellnow-Richmond et al., 2018).

Even if they are widely distributed, messages missing one or more elements (internalization, explanation, action, exemplification) "often fail," observe Sellnow-Richmond and colleagues (2018). For instance, risk messages about the 2014 Ebola crisis in the United States were explanation-heavy and seldom used examples, which seemed to escalate public fear and uncertainty (Sellnow-Richmond et al., 2018, p. 153).

Sellnow-Richmond and colleagues (2018) offer the following recommendations when devising crisis messages:

- *Get attention and boost retention.* Provide information that will help people assess relevance (e.g., if they or their loved ones are likely to be impacted by the crisis). Describe where the crisis is happening and how much time people have to prepare and/or respond. Consider using examples to grab recipients' attention and make messages memorable.
- *Explain what is happening.* Give accurate information about the crisis and what is being done about it. Use and cite credible sources. Explain scientific terms and concepts in easy-to-understand language. If using examples, consider if or how they might lead to misunderstandings and revise accordingly.

- *Outline specific steps that message recipients should take.* Describe what people should do to prepare for and/or respond to the crisis.
- *Choose channels carefully.* Make certain the right channels are being used to reach the desired audience. Tailor messages for distribution over multiple channels.

The Crisis and Emergency Risk Communication (CERC) Model

The CDC developed the Crisis and Emergency Risk Communication (CERC) model to clarify the types of messages people need at various stages of a crisis. The model has been widely adopted for use in public health crises around the world (Lwin, Lu, Sheldenkar, & Schulz, 2018). The **CERC model outlines five crisis phases and accompanying** communication goals (CDC, 2014):

- *Pre-crisis*. Use communication to form partnerships with agencies, organizations, first responders, and the media. Develop recommendations in consultation with experts and first responders. Devise and test message strategies. Identify spokespersons and resources.
- *Initial event.* Inform and reassure the public, reduce uncertainty, and promote self-efficacy while acknowledging the event with empathy. Messages should explain risk in simple terms, recommend specific actions, and direct the public to sources for additional information. Timely updates should explain what is happening, how threats are being addressed, and the anticipated outcomes (e.g., health, social, and economic).
- *Maintenance*. Help the public more accurately understand the risk and what is being done. Explain response and recovery plans. Reiterate self-efficacy and restate recommended actions. Listen to feedback and correct misinformation.
- *Resolution.* Describe ongoing recovery efforts to the public. Encourage discussion about causes, blame, responsibility, and effectiveness of response efforts. Identify problems and mishaps.
- *Evaluation*. Evaluate response and communication effectiveness and identify specific actions for improving. Document and share lessons learned.

CERC materials (manuals, checklists, and worksheets) are regularly updated and are available for download at www.emergency.cdc.gov/cerc/resources.

Research shows that the CERC model is effective at helping people understand and follow officials' recommendations (Ophir, 2019), but news stories about public health crises often lack details about how individuals should respond to a crisis (Ophir, 2018). After studying the issue, Ophir (2019) recommended that journalists balance risk information with efficacy messages and refer the public to nonmediated sources of information such as health professionals or the CDC's website for additional details.

Many public health agencies, including the CDC and WHO, strongly encourage the use of social media in crisis situations to facilitate timely distribution of important information. Social media can also give agencies control over the content of risk messages—avoiding the risk that information will be sensationalized, shortened to fit available time/space, or otherwise altered by media outlets (Ophir, 2019). Let's focus our attention on some of the ways social media is being used in health crises and a few of the lessons learned to date.

Social Media and Crisis Communication

Most health agencies leverage social media to relay crisis messages to the public. Social media is a game changer when it comes to crisis communication for three main reasons—reach, speed, and interactivity.

- *Reach.* Facebook alone allows agencies to reach 2.4 billion users worldwide (Hutchinson, 2019).
- *Speed.* A Facebook post or a tweet can reach more people much more quickly than can a traditional television or radio news broadcast.
- *Interactivity.* Unlike traditional media, social media allows for back-and-forth, two-way communication. This means people "on the ground" can give minute-by-minute accounts as disasters unfold, summon assistance, coordinate local response (e.g., the Cajun Navy, described earlier), and correct misinformation.

Of course, social media can also be the source of misinformation. Health agencies that monitor messages others post may be able to spot rumors and respond accordingly.

Several examples illustrate the role of social media in sharing information and expediting two-way communication between affected publics and health officials (see, e.g., Eckert et al., 2018; Lwin et al., 2018;

Toppenberg-Pejcic et al., 2019). Health officials used the WhatsApp app to communicate with tens of thousands of subscribers during the 2014 Ebola epidemic in West Africa and in the aftermath of Hurricane Dorian in the Bahamas (McCarthy, 2019; Rubyan-Ling, 2015; Sugg, 2016), and Singapore effectively used Facebook during a Zika outbreak in 2016 to teach people how to prevent the spread of the virus; address the public's comments, concerns, and requests for information; and express gratitude for the public's cooperation (Lwin et al., 2018).

Despite these successes, social media tools "have not become routine practices in many government agencies" (Eckert et al., 2018, p. 1399) partly because there are not yet clear guidelines for using social media to promote health in general and respond to specific crises (see, e.g., Guidry et al., 2019). However, there are some valuable social media lessons that scholars have identified thus far:

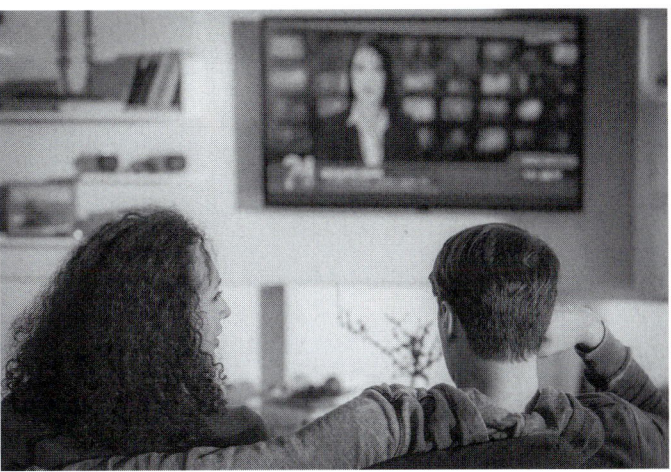

Do you trust information you see in the news about a health crisis? Why or why not? Are you likely to tune in to hear a public official update the public about a crisis? Why or why not?

- *Engage on social media daily.* For example, health promoters who engage on Twitter and Facebook every day will be familiar with them before a crisis happens. Additionally, agencies should make online "friends" to help establish trust and credibility ahead of crises (Eckert et al., 2018; Eriksson, 2018).
- *Use multiple channels and platforms.* Social media should not be used alone. Also involve traditional media to ensure maximum reach during a crisis. Social media has many advantages (e.g., quick dissemination, reach, ability to monitor the publics' reactions, etc.), but many people trust traditional media more (Eriksson, 2018).
- *Engage in two-way communication.* Use social media to respond to questions and comments (Eckert et al., 2018; Eriksson, 2018). Agencies should demonstrate that they are listening to the public's concerns.
- *Choose spokespeople carefully.* A trusted and identifiable spokesperson is usually more effective at getting a message across than are "anonymous" social media posts by health agencies (Eriksson, 2018).
- *Focus on message quality.* Social media posts are most likely to be read and shared if the information is up to date (Eriksson, 2018) and includes specific cues to action, confidence-inspiring advice, and clear benefits (Guidry et al., 2019).
- *Monitor how messages are received.* Health promoters can learn which messages are most valued by considering how often they are "liked" or shared (Lwin et al., 2018). For example, studies show that tweets with imagery, simple language, and infographics are liked and retweeted most often (Guidry et al., 2019).

Heeding these lessons when incorporating social media into a crisis communication plan is likely to prove beneficial.

Case Studies: A Global Perspective

In the past, it was largely feasible to contain contagious illnesses such as smallpox and yellow fever to geographic sectors. Now, because more than 2 billion people a day fly to locations that it would have taken days, weeks, or months to reach in the past, "an outbreak or epidemic in any one part of the world is only a few hours away from becoming an imminent threat somewhere else" ("World Health Report," 2007, p. x). Case in point: Thomas Duncan traveled from West Africa to the United States at the height of the Ebola epidemic in September 2014. He fell sick shortly after arriving in Dallas and though he did not know it, he was infected with Ebola. He sought help in an emergency room, where he spread the virus to two nurses and exposed dozens more before he died a week later. (See Box 12.4 for a profile of famous disease carriers

BOX 12.4

Typhoid Mary and TB Andy

Andrew Speaker, an Atlanta resident with drug-resistant tuberculosis (TB), traveled by plane to Europe and back in 2007, even though doctors say they told him not to fly because of the risk to others. Tuberculosis is dangerous and highly contagious, particularly in the recirculated air of an airplane cabin. Nearly 2 million people a year die from TB, mostly in developing countries (WHO, 2008). The disease has made a deadly comeback in recent years because new strains have emerged that do not respond to drug therapy, and people with immune deficiencies such as HIV and AIDS are particularly susceptible to TB whether they have been immunized or not.

In Speaker's case, authorities in Italy were alerted to his health status and refused to allow him to board a flight back to the United States. So Speaker and his wife (they were on their honeymoon) flew to Canada instead, where his status went unnoticed, and they were able to fly back to Atlanta. Many fellow airline passengers, angry that Speaker knowingly exposed them to a dangerous disease, later filed charges against him ("Plane Passengers Sue," 2007).

Some journalists nicknamed Speaker "TB Andy," referencing another famous figure in history, Typhoid Mary. In the years preceding 1906, Mary Mallon was a cook for wealthy families in New York. Authorities began to notice that, in the homes where she worked, an extraordinary number of people contracted typhoid fever. At the time, about 10% of people who got typhoid died from it. Mallon resisted being tested or being taken into custody. Indeed, she "brandished a meat fork and threats" so vociferously that it took five police officers to bring her in (*The Most Dangerous Woman*, 2004, para. 6).

Tests showed that Mallon was a typhoid carrier, although she manifested no symptoms herself. She was forcibly quarantined in a hospital on an island in New York City's East River. Her distraught letters from the time relate that she felt like a kidnap victim and a "peep show" ("In Her Own Words," 2004, last paragraph). Mallon was released after about six years. But when she disobeyed orders and returned to cooking professionally, she was taken into custody for the rest of her life. Historians have mixed feelings about whether Mallon was treated fairly or not.

What Do You Think?

1. Should the state take people into custody if they refuse to take actions (such as wearing gloves or face masks, agreeing not to fly, and so on) that would help protect others from catching their illnesses? Does it matter what illness it is? Do colds and flu count? What about illnesses that are somewhat, but not highly, contagious?

2. Should airlines beef up their "no fly" lists so that people with highly contagious diseases are not permitted aboard? Why or why not?

3. If a person knowingly exposes others to a contagious disease, should the people who are exposed have the right to sue? Would you? Why or why not?

4. Historians have noted that Mary Mallon had little means of earning a living besides being a cook. If protecting others means changing careers, should the government help pay for new vocational training or education?

5. Babies and people whose immune systems are compromised by illness, chemotherapy, or other conditions are particularly susceptible to diseases that would not endanger others. Should we exercise greater-than-usual precautions knowing that such people are in our communities? Why or why not? What precautions would you consider reasonable?

6. In some countries, people who have colds wear disposable face masks (like surgical masks) in public to protect others. Do you think people in other countries should adopt this practice as well? Why or why not? Would you wear a mask when you had a cold? Why or why not?

7. Many illnesses could be prevented if people washed their hands before eating. In Japan, even fast-food restaurants provide moist towelettes with every meal. Do you think other countries should adopt this practice? Why or why not?

8. A common means of transmitting illness is shaking hands with others and then touching food. Some people suggest that we would be healthier (and perhaps avert epidemics) if we bowed or waved in greeting instead of shaking hands. What do you think?

For an excellent video about Mary Mallon as well as discussion guides and ethical analyses, see www.pbs.org/wgbh/nova/typhoid.

and some tough considerations about personal liberties and public welfare.)

Another problem is that diseases—and their resistance to known drugs—are multiplying. Since 1970, about one new disease has surfaced every year, contributing to thousands of epidemics around the world ("World Health Report," 2007). Contact with other people, especially a *lot* of other people, can be hazardous to your health.

The good news is that globalization has also improved worldwide awareness of public health. After a devastating earthquake struck Nepal in 2015, people around the world contributed more than $69 million in the first three days alone (Petroff & Rooney, 2015). Just one day after Hurricane Dorian made landfall in the Bahamas in 2019, an international response team arrived and within a week more than 100,000 pounds of relief supplies were delivered to the hardest hit areas (see, e.g., Ali, 2019; Margesson & Sullivan, 2019; McCarthy, 2019; U.S. Agency for International Development, 2019).

We could fill volumes with descriptions of public health issues around the world. Instead, let's look at a few case studies that illustrate some key principles, challenges, and lessons.

Ebola

Ebola was first detected in humans in 1976, when two people in different regions of Africa were diagnosed with it. One of them lived near the Ebola River of Central Africa, which gave rise to the name. The Ebola virus resurfaced at various times over the next 38 years, killing about 1,000 people, mostly in remote regions of Africa (CDC, 2015b). However, nothing compared to the 2014 epidemic, in which more than 11,000 people died from the disease (WHO, 2015a) and more than 28,000 were infected (Turner, 2019). That crisis, which was daunting by medical standards, was further exacerbated by mistrust and poor communication. Communication challenges also hampered relief efforts during a 2019 Ebola outbreak in the Democratic Republic of the Congo (Turner, 2019).

Part of the fear surrounding Ebola stems from the dreadful nature of the disease. In early stages, the symptoms are much like the flu, making it difficult to diagnose accurately. There are few treatment options and most Ebola sufferers are likely to suffer internal and external bleeding and catastrophic organ failure (WHO, 2015b). At least half the people who contract the virus die. Health officials believe that people originally caught Ebola during contact with wild animals and then the virus mutated to spread between people. At the time of the 2014 outbreak, no vaccine was available to protect people from the contagion. Merck Pharmaceuticals began clinical trials on a vaccine in 2014, but it was not approved for provisional use until 2019, when health care workers in the Congo were allowed to take it because (although not fully approved) it was the only option available (Turner, 2019).

COMMUNICATION WITH THE WORRIED WELL

With limited information available during the 2014 epidemic, health authorities around the world scrambled to make people aware of the risks without unduly frightening them. After Thomas Duncan unknowingly brought Ebola into the United States, a variety of authorities, from the CDC to the president, sought to reassure an uneasy public. But their efforts often seemed disjointed and the information unclear and speculative. Public hysteria was fueled by the news media's "wall-to-wall coverage of the virus" and "was exacerbated by the conflicting and contradictory messages" from health officials (Sellnow-Richmond et al., 2018, p. 137). This led analysts/researchers Scott Ratzan and Kenneth Moritsugu (2014) to identify some of the first communication lessons from the crisis:

- *Provide the public with answers to three key questions.* "What do I need to know? What do I need to do or not do today to protect my health and that of my family? Where do I find information that I can trust and understand?" (p. 1214).
- *Designate a single spokesperson to provide* trustworthy, current information that is based on science and evidence.
- *Coordinate with local health officials so that advice and information is consistent at every level.*

At the height of the crisis, President Barack Obama urged, "We can't give in to hysteria or fear—because that only makes it harder to get people the accurate information they need" (Frizell, 2014). At the same time, however, people hungry for information watched the news and saw images of dead bodies in the streets of western Africa and heard predictions that Ebola would soon spread and claim more than a million lives (Ratzan & Moritsugu, 2014).

Observing disparate efforts such as these, Gaya Damhewage (2014), coordinator of the WHO Department of Communication in Geneva, urged people to conceive of public health communication as a "four-legged stool." In her model, the stool's legs represent:

- *specialists* in public health, social science, and communication who engage in ongoing, two-way communication with the public;
- *media professionals* with expertise in mass media, media relations, social media, and other means of reaching mass audiences;
- *policy-makers* engaged in leadership and resource management; and
- *scientists* and others who can provide data-based information and technical guidance.

From a communication perspective, this balance involves specialists in interpersonal, small-group, organizational, and mass communication, as well as leaders and coordinators to help diverse constituents communicate effectively with each other. The overall lesson is: *Engage in coordinated communication at every level—with individuals, community groups, policy-makers, health professionals, and scientists—utilizing media best suited for each type of interaction.*

As it turned out, nowhere did Damhewage's (2014) words ring truer than at the epicenter of the crisis, in western Africa.

COMMUNICATION IN THE MIDST OF TRAUMA

Since Ebola is transmitted via body fluids such as blood, patients in advanced stages of the disease are highly contagious, as are those who have recently died. Authorities believe that many people in Sierra Leone, Guinea, and Liberia contracted the disease while caring for infected loved ones and handling their bodies after death.

"Anyone who touches a droplet of sweat, blood, or saliva from someone about to die or just deceased is at high risk of contracting the disease," explains Amy Maxmen (2015, para. 12). Considering that, it is understandable from a scientific perspective why health authorities were eager to remove ill individuals and corpses from their homes. However, they initially failed to consider other factors that were equally as important to the people involved.

"The problem," says anthropologist Julienne Anoko, "was that the people handling the intervention only looked at this as a health issue; they did not try to understand the cultural aspects of the epidemic" (quoted by Maxmen, 2015, para. 10). In communication terms, they acted on the facts as they saw them, but they frequently overlooked issues of culture and history that made their claims unbelievable to the people they sought to influence.

During the crisis, people in western Africa often refused to believe that Ebola was real. Instead, they suspected that officials were kidnapping and killing their loved ones. As a consequence, citizens often hid their ill and dead family members and unwittingly infected themselves and others (Maxmen, 2015). The citizens' response may seem irrational on the surface. However, it becomes clearer considering their past experiences.

In the areas of Africa hardest hit by Ebola, a history of poverty, corruption, killings, and civil war has made citizens skeptical that local authorities have the public's best interests at heart. People there also tend to be distrustful of foreigners, whom they may associate with violent "blood diamond" warlords of the past who killed and enslaved millions in wars over the region's diamond mines (Thompson, 2014).

As you might imagine, citizens' fears escalated when health officials—many of them from other countries and all of them dressed in what looked like protective spacesuits—began forcibly removing the ill and recently deceased from their homes. With inadequate resources, health professionals frequently forwarded ill patients to larger hospitals, where patients were sometimes transferred to other facilities. And to stem the contagion, health officials

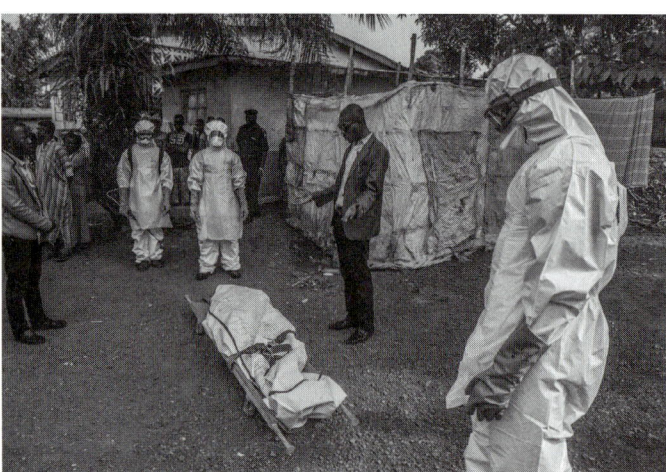

Empathic communication led relief workers in Sierra Leone to rethink the way they intervened when community members died from Ebola. Here, health workers in protective "spacesuits" pause before removing a body to allow loved ones to pray over it from a safe distance.

quickly buried the dead, often without clearly recording their identities, if they even knew them in the first place. Consequently, once their loved ones had been removed, families were often unable to locate them or even determine if they were alive. They knew only that they had "disappeared" at the hands of people they did not know or trust.

"These disappearances stoked conspiracy theories that Ebola was a hoax," explains Maxmen (2015, para. 21). "In one, doctors were said to be killing patients to steal their organs. The less people believed that Ebola was real, the less likely they were to bring deathly ill relatives to clinics and to stop honoring their dead relatives in the traditional way."

One turning point involved listening and empathic communication. At some point, officials appealed to community chiefs, religious leaders, and healers for insight and help. These leaders, who were trusted within their communities, educated health professionals about local customs and began to reassure their fellow citizens that it was okay to forgo the traditional (and highly dangerous) burial rituals (Maxmen, 2015). Officials in charge of confiscating bodies for burial recruited trusted community members to help them communicate with families throughout the process. Together, these teams began explaining their reasons to family members, assuring them that their loved ones' burials would be "safe and dignified." They also began to pause once they had wrapped an infected body in protective plastic, to allow loved ones to gather around it at a safe distance for prayer and goodbyes. Whenever possible, the officials agreed to dress the deceased loved ones in garments chosen by the family and bury them with family keepsakes.

Once these changes were made, families began to cooperate more willingly with authorities, which was a vital step in controlling the epidemic. By early 2015, cases had dwindled. Midway through 2015, new cases were as few as nine a week (WHO, 2015a). The lesson was clear: *However well intentioned, communication that is not built on trust and mutual understanding is unlikely to be effective.*

AIDS

AIDS has been called the greatest public health challenge of the last half-century. About 38 million people are now living with HIV or AIDS. The crisis is particularly bad in Africa, where nearly 1 in every 25 adults has HIV, accounting for "more than two-thirds of the people living with HIV worldwide" (WHO, 2018b, para. 1). One challenge of AIDS is that related behaviors are sometimes considered taboo, immoral, or too personal to be discussed. Cultural rules about these behaviors vary widely from culture to culture. For example, although members of Western cultures mean well, their Judeo-Christian worldview can be baffling to others. Americans missed the mark when they designed public health messages urging people in Namibia, Africa, to prevent HIV by abstaining from premarital sex and by being faithful to their spouses. These concepts are not meaningful to most Namibian citizens, who are accustomed to polygamy and who tend to define marriage very loosely (Hillier, 2006). Hillier concludes, "Prevention campaigns have been silent about polygamous sexual cultures. . . . [They have] elevated the Christian monogamous marriage to the most desirable norm but it is not the only or most common form of sexual union" (p. 18). As a result, many foreign efforts are culturally unacceptable and are therefore ineffective when it comes to changing people's behavior.

There are medications that can help prevent HIV infection, but they are not widely used for a variety of reasons. One combination of drugs (marketed as PrEP) can reduce the risk of HIV infection by 99% in some instances, but treatment is generally only recommended for those who are at very high risk of infection—persons who have unprotected sex with multiple partners or with HIV-positive partners and/or persons who inject drugs (CDC, 2019). The problem is that PrEP is expensive and, consequently, many people who would benefit from taking it cannot afford it. To be effective, a PrEP pill must be taken every day, but a 30-day supply costs around $2,000 in the United States (Citroner, 2018). In the first two years after its U.S. release (from 2012 to 2014), only

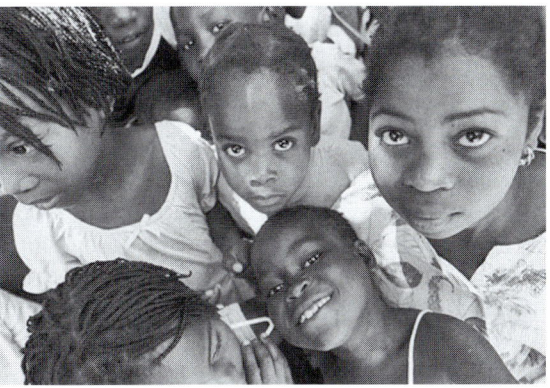

Children in sub-Saharan Africa can only hope for a brighter future than current conditions predict. That region now has the highest concentration of HIV infection in the world.

3,200 prescriptions for PrEP were filled, amid about 80,000 new HIV infections in the same period. Since then, the price for PrEP has gone up more than 45% (Citroner, 2018).

In Africa, where PrEP adoption could turn the tide in the global battle against HIV, cost is just one barrier preventing widespread PrEP adoption. Nelly Mugo and colleagues (2016) identified several obstacles, including lack of knowledge about PrEP (even among some health care workers, PrEP's potential is not fully understood); low availability; and the stigma surrounding HIV, especially for sex workers and for men who have sex with other men (Mugo, Ngure, Kiragu, Irungu, & Kilonzo, 2016). Risk and crisis communicators are tasked with educating local health care workers, policy-makers, and the public about PrEP while dispelling misconceptions, addressing stigmas, and respecting local beliefs.

Mugo and colleagues (2016) recommend that public health workers partner with community members to devise strategies for promoting PrEP, citing the adage, "Nothing for us without us" (p. 83). And, as the Ebola epidemic taught us, the best communication and behavioral change strategies can "be summarized in two words: Go local" (Toppenberg-Pejcic et al., 2019, p. 440). Communication strategies, however, must address a number of concerns. For instance, some worry that PrEP will be seen as a "promiscuity pill" in certain communities, which may deter people from asking about it. In Kenya, PrEP pills look like a commonly abused mood-altering drug (i.e., both pills are blue), which may discourage potential users from asking about or taking PrEP. And there are fears that PrEP will reduce condom use, thereby causing other sexually transmitted infections to run rampant (Mugo et al., 2016).

Until the factors preventing PrEP's widespread adoption are addressed, the most feasible way to prevent HIV transmission is by changing people's behavior (Schneider, 2006), but that is a tremendous challenge. Some health communication specialists have concluded that it is naive to assume that most people *will not* have sex. The trick, they feel, is to make safer sex sexier. The Pleasure Project, based in Oxford, England, is a cooperative effort to emphasize the erotic appeal of safer sex. The project's website explains:

> While most safer sex and HIV prevention programmes are negative and disease-focused, The Pleasure Project is different: we take a positive, liberating and sexy approach to safer sex. Think of it is as sex education . . . with the emphasis on "sex." ("About Us," 2013)

Project coordinators present condoms and alternatives to sexual intercourse as exciting and erotically stimulating. The website includes a racy directory of related organizations and programs, erotic tips for safer sex, and links to organizations that sell condoms and sex toys and donate the proceeds to the safer sex campaign.

The "safer sex is better sex" effort has been applauded by a range of public health experts. After reviewing relevant research, the authors of a "Viewpoint" article in *The Lancet* concur:

> Since pursuit of pleasure is one of the main reasons that people have sex, this factor must be addressed when motivating people to use condoms and participate in safer sexual behaviour. (Philpott, Knerr, & Maher, 2006, p. 3)

These are just a few of the many approaches to preventing HIV and AIDS. The good news is that the number of AIDS deaths worldwide has fallen by more than half since peaking in 2004 (from 1.4 million to 770,000 in 2018), but "the pace of progress" is slowing down, according to analysts (HIV.gov, 2019, para. 12). As the fight against HIV/AIDS continues, the following lessons may help ongoing crisis and risk communication efforts.

- *Listen and learn.* Knowing what the public believes and is willing to do is just as important, sometimes more important, than knowing what experts think people *should* do (Covello, 2003).

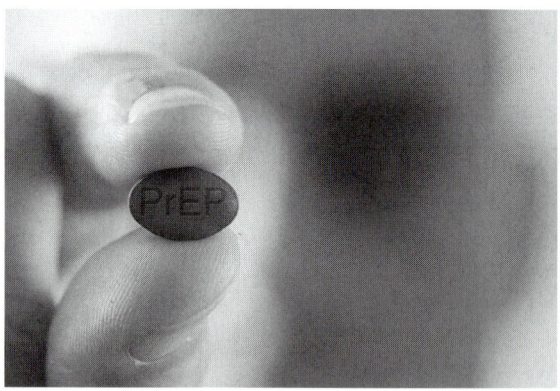

How would you go about designing messages that address PrEP's perceived risks while highlighting its potential advantages? Of the communication theories or models that we have discussed, which would you consider using? Why? Would you include social media in your message strategy? If so, how?

- *Vary your approach*. Fear appeals can be highly motivational, but particularly for frightening and long-term crises such as AIDS, people may tune out fear messages because they are overwhelming or overly familiar. Innovative, culturally sensitive appeals may regain people's attention.

SARS

One of the great success stories in managing a public health crisis arose from worldwide efforts to contain severe acute respiratory syndrome (SARS). The issue first drew attention in February 2003, when a man in Vietnam was admitted to a hospital with a respiratory disorder. His condition deteriorated, and, although he was transferred to a Hong Kong medical center, he died within four days. Soon, seven caregivers who had been involved with the patient became sick as well. The disorder spread so quickly that, in slightly more a month, there were 150 cases of SARS in eight countries (WHO, 2003b).

By May 2003, SARS had become a pandemic. New cases were emerging at the rate of 200 a day. The disease had spread to almost every continent. A total of 8,000 people in 28 countries were infected (WHO, 2003a). SARS was especially hard to contain because it was easily spread from person to person, it was infectious for more than a week before symptoms appeared, and it was hard to diagnose because the initial symptoms were similar to those of many other illnesses. Worst of all, SARS was deadly. About 10% of people who were infected (many of them hospital personnel) died.

The authors of the World Health Report (2007) recall:

> SARS incited a degree of public anxiety that virtually halted travel to affected areas and drained billions of dollars from economies across entire regions.... It showed that the danger arising from emerging diseases is universal. No country, rich or poor, is adequately protected from either the arrival of a new disease on its territory or the subsequent disruption this can cause. (p. xix)

However, it could have been worse. Remarkably, just 100 days into the crisis (in June, 2003), spokespersons for WHO announced that the pandemic was under control and that new cases had dwindled to a handful a day. The crisis that began in February was largely over by July. How was that possible? The turnaround resulted partly from effective quarantines. Much of the success also involved communication. Lessons from the experience illustrate the role communication played:

- *Develop strong teams*. WHO credits "monumental efforts" by governments, health professionals, and public health agencies. Because officials around the world reported cases promptly, WHO and other agencies were able to monitor and contain new outbreaks as much as possible. WHO dubbed it "solidarity" and "interdependence" on a global scale never seen before (WHO, 2003a, para. 8).
- *Make the most of communication technology*. Communication technology allowed researchers and health experts to share data and new developments quickly and accurately. Because of this, they figured out how SARS was transmitted "in record time" (WHO, 2003a, para. 11).
- *Keep everyone informed*. Although experts did a good job communicating with each other, members of some affected populations were out of the loop. In China, because of tight government controls on media content, many people were frustrated by the lack of SARS news

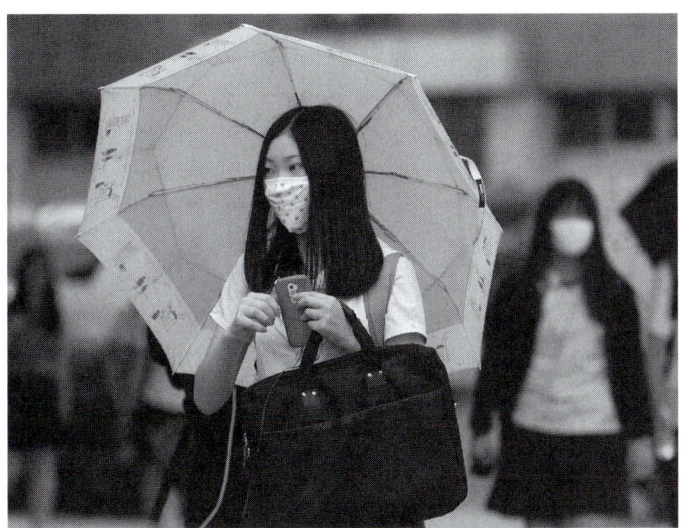

A high school student in South Korea wears a mask as protection from Middle East respiratory syndrome (MERS). The challenge for public health communicators is to gauge when it is helpful to recommend such precautions and when they might frighten the public unnecessarily.

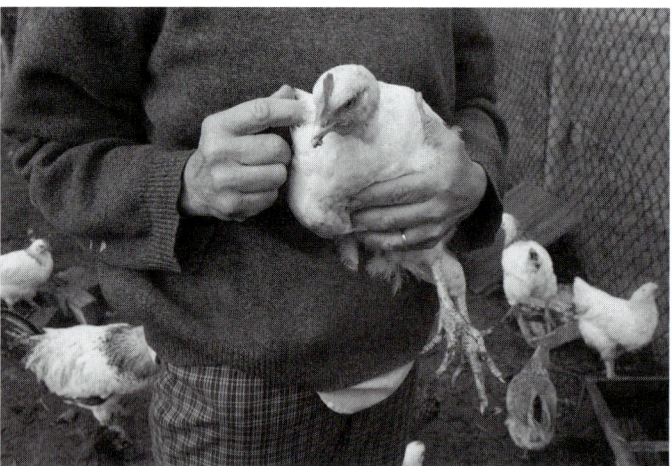

When tens of millions of poultry in the United States were found to have bird flu, part of public health officials' job was to educate farmers about precautions they could take to minimize the chance of human infection.

coverage. Some of them there used the internet to seek and share information about SARS that they could not get otherwise (Tai & Sun, 2007).

- *Educate the people involved.* Once officials knew that SARS was transmitted via droplets spread through coughing and sneezing, they were able to tell health care workers how to minimize the risk of infection.

In just a few months, SARS took a heavy toll. By the time it was contained, 8,098 people had been infected and 774 of those had died (CDC, 2005). However, containing the disease so quickly saved millions of lives. The SARS case is regarded as a model response to a nearly unthinkable public health threat.

Avian Flu

One of the threats keeping public health professionals on high alert is avian flu, also called bird flu. As the name suggests, the virus originated in poultry. There are several strains of avian flu that can infect humans, but the deadliest to date is H5N1. About half of the people diagnosed with the H5N1 strain of avian flu have died from it (WHO, 2019). In serious cases, there is nothing doctors can do. Within days, lung tissue dies, and so does the patient. As in the case studies we have reviewed already, communication plays a pivotal role in managing this ongoing threat.

The first documented case of the H5N1 strain of avian flu occurred in Hong Kong in 1997. After that, the government oversaw the killing of every chicken in Hong Kong (about 1.5 million birds; Appenzeller, 2005). The disease seemed to go away, but it resurfaced and it spread. By May 2015, the media reported that turkeys and chickens in 220 poultry farms in 20 states of the United States were infected ("Secretary of Agriculture," 2015, para. 1). As of this writing, 455 people worldwide have died from H5N1 since 2014, which represents about half of the people who have contracted the virus (WHO, 2019), and avian flu remains an ongoing public health crisis.

The virus often kills birds in a matter of hours by destroying their lungs, brains, muscles, and intestines (Appenzeller, 2005). So far, people with H5N1 seem to have caught it from direct contact with affected animals. Although scientists are not certain how the disease jumps to humans, they caution people to cook poultry fully, to use gloves and masks when handling live or dead birds, and not to use bird-dropping fertilizer.

But the danger that most worries public health officials is that this virus will mutate so that it can spread among humans. Past flu viruses have been remarkably adept at doing that. "It's bound to happen," predicts Jeremy Farrar, an Oxford University physician who specializes in avian flu, "and when it does, the world is going to face a truly horrible pandemic" (quoted by Appenzeller, 2005, para. 11).

If H5N1 becomes a pandemic, millions of people could die. It has happened before. During World War I, some 50 million people died from Spanish flu—more than three times the number of soldiers who died in the war (Appenzeller, 2005). Like avian flu, Spanish flu probably jumped from animals to people. That type of mutation is extremely dangerous because humans have few antibodies to protect them from the novel virus.

So, you may wonder, why not get a flu shot to guard against infection? For one, "regular" influenza vaccines do not prevent avian flu. And two, although an H5N1 vaccine has been available in the United States since 2007, the federal government has purchased all available dosages to vaccinate "priority recipients" (e.g., first responders and people in high-risk zones) in case of an epidemic (FDA, 2018, para.1). (See Box 12.5 for more about ethical dilemmas concerning who should receive the limited number of H5N1 vaccines available.)

And if you are thinking that you rarely get the flu or that you get over it quickly when you do, beware.

BOX 12.5 Ethical Considerations

Who Should Be Protected?

The good news is that the vaccine for H5N1 reduces the risk of infection in 45% of the people who receive it (FDA, 2018). It's not perfect because researchers don't know exactly how the virus will mutate. Also, they must ensure there are no harmful side effects. But "the production capacity in the United States currently is not sufficient to make vaccine rapidly available for the entire population" (FDA, 2018, para. 21). So public health experts face a dilemma. After reading about bird flu in this chapter, consider what you would do in their shoes.

1. If you had to choose, which of the following populations would you vaccinate and why? (a) people who are most likely to die from the disease if they get it; (b) service providers such as health care professionals, firefighters, and police officers; or (c) another population of your choosing.
2. Would you first vaccinate people in communities in which avian flu cases have already been diagnosed? Why or why not? If those citizens or their governments are unable to afford the vaccine, do you believe people in other countries should help pay for it? Why or why not?
3. Viruses such as the flu often spread quickly among children. Would you vaccinate them early on? Why or why not?
4. Are you in favor of *requiring* people at high risk for avian flu (such as those who regularly handle birds) to get vaccinated? Why or why not?
5. Depending on how the virus mutates, the vaccine might not be especially effective. Do you think governments should invest in it anyway? Why or why not?
6. Given the opportunity, would you choose to be vaccinated? Why or why not?

This version of the flu is especially dangerous for people who have well-functioning immune systems. In serious cases, avian flu so overstimulates the body's immune system that the lungs become grossly inflamed with white blood cells, and life-sustaining tissues die (Appenzeller, 2005).

It is difficult to imagine overplanning for a crisis such as avian flu. As Barbara Reynolds (2006) points out, in any health crisis, "the devil is most certainly in the details" (p. 249). WHO (2007) has released rapid-response guidelines for containing a deadly flu pandemic. Public health personnel in your community are probably already working on the local plan. WHO guidelines include the following:

- Create a geographic "containment zone" when the first cases surface in order to separate people who have the disease, as well as those who have been exposed to it, from other people;
- Create a "buffer zone" around the containment zone to reduce further the risk of contagion; and
- Communicate effectively with the public to maintain barriers, keep people informed, ensure that people within the containment zone have adequate care and supplies, and minimize stigmatization of people with the disease.

How will this work exactly? It sounds a bit frightening, but it's not as scary as the alternative. Imagine your community partitioned with roadblocks, warning signs, and guarded screening stations. No one except essential personnel will go in or out of containment zones for at least 20 days. It sounds like something from a movie, but it's no exaggeration. Health officials realize that the only way to save lives is to limit the spread of the virus. Inside the containment

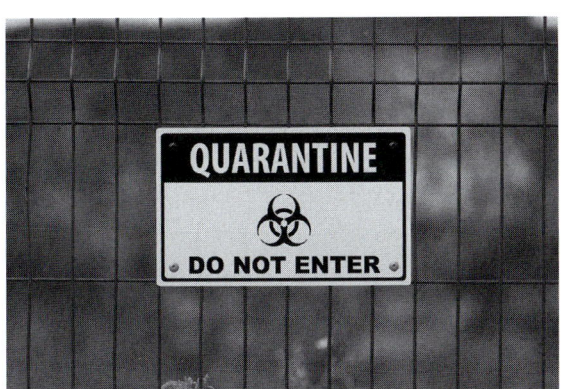

Would you be frightened if a containment zone were declared in your area? Why or why not? Do you feel adequately informed about, and prepared for, such a crisis?

zone—which could be your neighborhood or a portion of your hometown—health officials will monitor people's health, care for and quarantine (in a hospital or at home) people who are infected, watch for new outbreaks, and help distribute antiviral medication to those who are still healthy.

This means that, if a person in your household becomes ill, you may all be confined to your home until officials can be sure you are not contagious. And even if everyone in your household is healthy, if an outbreak occurs in your area, it would be advisable to remain in your home. Public health experts recommend that everyone maintain a two-week supply of food, water, and needed medications just in case. They also recommend that people wash their hands frequently and cover their mouths when sneezing or coughing.

As we reflect on world response to the Coronavirus pandemic of 2020, it will be interesting to see whether communication lessons learned in the SARS case were implemented, and if so, if they were useful. It's likely that new lessons will emerge as well.

A visit to the WHO, CDC, or PandemicFlu.gov website reveals an extensive collection of materials, including health-tracking software, government agency contact lists, brochures, and checklists for a wide range of stakeholder groups.

As with many other components of public health and risk/crisis management, success depends largely on effective communication (Seeger, 2006). It's no longer defensible to think of avian flu as an Asian crisis or a future scenario. Sandman (2006b) advises crisis communicators to imagine "that the crisis has just begun and to make a list of things they wish the public had already learned or already done" (p. 259). The Coronavirus outbreak forced people to consider answers to questions such as: *Are we aware and prepared for a deadly flu pandemic? If containment zones were created in our community, would we understand what was happening? Are we (and our neighbors) prepared to stay in our homes for weeks at a time?* Ideally, the public should answer yes to these questions well in advance of a crisis.

Zika

Zika dominated headlines as it spread from Brazil throughout South and Central America, and eventually to the United States in 2016. One reason Zika was so heavily covered was that athletes from around the world were scheduled to visit Brazil in 2016 for the summer Olympic Games (Ophir & Jamieson, 2018, p. 2). Another reason was that the mosquito-borne virus can cause severe birth defects in infants, most notably, microcephaly (brain damage and small head size). Some members of the media sensationalized the threat of microcephaly, owing to the condition's disturbing appearance (see Chapter 11). But, as with most headline-making stories, media coverage of the Zika epidemic eventually waned (coverage declined sharply after the Olympics ended) and journalists moved on to other stories. This may have given people, especially those who live in the United States, the impression that Zika is no longer a threat. In fact, the virus is still a threat worldwide (Broussard et al., 2018). Although there is much we still don't know about Zika and its long-term effects, scientists agree that "most people in the world . . . are susceptible to infection" (McDonald & Holden, 2018, p. 139).

Zika is spread in a few ways. Several mosquito species transmit Zika, two of which are present in the United States. Perhaps more alarming, Zika is the first virus transmitted by insects that can also be spread from person to person during sex (McDonald & Holden, 2018). There is no vaccine against Zika, so prevention efforts center on avoiding mosquito bites and taking precautions during sex. Unfortunately, some studies find that many people believe their perceived risk is relatively low and think Zika is mainly a concern for pregnant women. Consequently, many people neglect to engage in protective measures such as wearing insect repellant and/or using condoms (McDonald & Holden, 2018). Risk and crisis communication also play an important role.

As described earlier in this chapter, Singapore has been lauded for its communication strategy—especially its use of Facebook—during a Zika outbreak there. News media in the United States took a different approach. The CDC stressed that the public needed to know three important things: (a) Zika was transmitted through mosquitoes and sex (therefore prevention hinged on avoiding mosquito bites and refraining from unprotected sex), (b) its consequences included birth defects, and (c) it was largely asymptomatic in adults (Anderson, Thomas, & Endy, 2016). However, media coverage did not uniformly follow the CDC's guidelines.

For example, one study found that the news media's coverage of Zika focused on mosquitoes as a vector much more than on transmission through sex, and microcephaly was mentioned far more often than was the lack of symptoms in adults (Ophir & Jamieson, 2018). The authors of another study found that 80% of newspaper stories about Zika mentioned the worst possible outcomes—microcephaly and Guillain-Barré syndrome—but provided scant information about how readers could protect themselves (Jerit, Zhao, Tan, & Wheeler, 2018).

The models and guidelines for effective crisis communication we have reviewed in this chapter stress the importance of self-efficacy messages—helping people understand how they can protect themselves. In this respect, many media outlets failed to effectively communicate the full scope of the Zika crisis to the American public.

One option is for health agencies to "compensate for the gaps in media coverage" by communicating with the public directly through channels such as social media (Ophir, 2019, p. 553). The CDC did use Twitter to inform the public about Zika, but when Shi Chen and colleagues (2018) analyzed the CDC's Zika-related tweets from 2016, they found that almost 85% of them were sent in the first four months of the year, *before* Zika cases began appearing in the United States. Public engagement was high during the CDC's information campaign, as determined by the number of retweets. But as the number of Zika cases climbed, the CDC's Twitter activity decreased significantly, as did public engagement. The study's authors don't speculate on the CDC's reasons for scaling back Twitter activity, but that decision stood in stark contrast to Singapore's highly successful approach of maintaining a social media presence throughout every phase of the Zika outbreak there in 2016 (Lwin et al., 2018). How Zika was handled (or mishandled) in the United States thus offers some important lessons:

- *Health crises often persist after the news media have stopped reporting on them*. Zika remains a serious health concern, even though it may receive little attention in the media. Public health agencies are challenged with finding ways to keep the public informed about ongoing risks.
- *News media often fail to report health crises in accordance with guidelines and best practices*. Health officials often believe that the information they provide the news media will be reported in its entirety because it is important (Parmer et al., 2016). However, news stories average about two out of seven "best practices" based on the CERC model described earlier in this chapter (Parmer et al., 2016). Because public health officials and journalists have different professional objectives, it's important that they work together so the public is sufficiently informed during crises.
- *Maintain a consistent social media presence throughout public health crises*. The CDC's Twitter activity slowed down as the Zika crisis ramped up. While the CDC continued pushing messages to the public through media releases and its website, research tells us that such a strategy does not guarantee the public will be, or will remain, sufficiently informed about health risks. To make matters worse, the CDC's website is underutilized as an information source. During the Zika outbreak, only 16% of people surveyed reported that they went to the CDC's website to learn about the virus. About 85% got their information from television or radio and 39% relied on social media (McDonald & Holden, 2018). The implication is that many people rely on multiple sources, but social media had a greater reach than the CDC website.

Next, let's turn our attention to ways medical and public health professionals have addressed addiction.

The Opioid Epidemic

The opioid "situation" in the United States has been described as a *crisis*, an *emergency*, and an *epidemic* (respectively, National Institute on Drug Abuse [NIDA], 2019; U.S. Department of Health and Human Services [HHS], 2017; CDC, 2018). So, what's the difference between a crisis, an emergency, and an epidemic? Moreover, does it matter? Some say how we talk about health—and how we describe addiction—matter a great deal. For instance, in a study described by Lily Frank and Saskia Nagel (2017), when physicians were queried about hypothetical patients labeled as either "substance abusers" or persons "with a substance abuse disorder," physicians were more likely to conclude that "substance abusers" were more responsible for their own problems and deserving of punishment. We may reasonably conclude, based on this example, that persons with "substance abuse disorders" likely receive more compassionate care from their physicians than do persons labeled "substance abusers." In sum, labels matter.

Labeling an event "a crisis," "an emergency," or "an epidemic" denotes the degree of seriousness bestowed

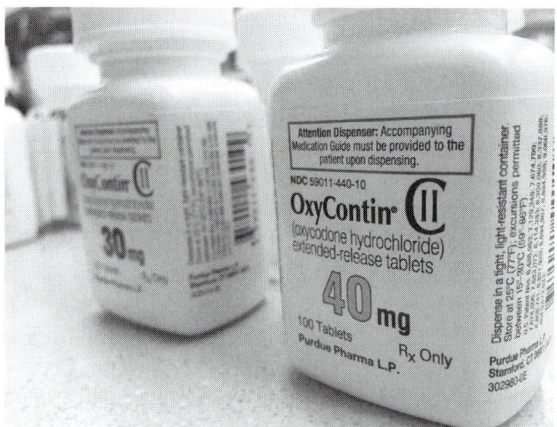

About 130 Americans die from opioid overdoses every day (NIDA, 2019). Some people view addiction as a matter of choice, whereas others see it as a disease. What do you think? Do the labels we assign to certain conditions affect our health? If so, how? Does calling a condition such as addiction or obesity a "choice" affect public health policy? Explain.

upon the event by the persons or agencies doing the labeling. A *crisis* suggests a time of intense difficulty or trouble. An *emergency* connotes a serious, unexpected, and often dangerous situation requiring immediate action. And an *epidemic* refers to a disease widely occurring in a community at a particular time.

Arguably, an epidemic is more serious than a crisis. But the real distinction here hinges on the word "disease." There is a long-standing debate as to whether addiction is a disease or a choice. Diseases are treated by medical professionals, whereas choices—especially choices that harm health—are moralized, leading to shame, blame, and stigma. Consequently, many people, including some health professionals, think addiction reflects a person's poor character (see, e.g., Kean, 2013; Frank & Nagel, 2017). The American Medical Association classified drug addiction as a disease in 1989, but "public attitudes have yet to catch up with science," says Janina Kean, citing a 2005 survey that revealed 63% of the general public and 43% of physicians viewed addiction as a moral or personal weakness (Kean, 2013, para. 10). While there is credible evidence that addiction is a brain disease, persistent moralization harms addicted persons, the public health, and society at large (Frank & Nagel, 2017, p. 138). Opioid addiction, which may rightly be called an epidemic, is proof.

Let's consider some of the ways the opioid epidemic has harmed people, public health, and society. Between 1999 and 2017, opioid overdoses killed about 400,000 people (CDC, 2018). Today, on average, 130 Americans die from opioid overdoses every day (NIDA, 2019). According to NIDA (2019), the problem has intensified in recent years. Here are a few facts from NIDA's website proving as much:

- Between July 2016 and September 2017, opioid overdoses increased 30% in 45 states.
- During that same period, overdoses in the Midwest increased by 70% and big cities in 16 states saw a 54% increase in opioid overdoses.
- 47,000 people died as a result of opioid misuse in 2017.
- About 1.7 million people have substance abuse disorders tied to prescription opioids.

With respect to public health, opioids are problematic for a number of reasons. In addition to killing hundreds of thousands of people, injecting opioids spreads infectious diseases like hepatitis C and HIV, and opioid abuse during pregnancy has led to an increase in neonatal abstinence syndrome, a collection of health issues experienced by newborns exposed to drugs before birth (NIDA, 2019). Addiction is more common than heart disease, diabetes, and cancer—and according to substance-abuse expert Janina Kean (2013), that makes addiction the biggest and most costly public health problem in the United States.

Regarding society at large, lost productivity, lost wages, and overburdened health care systems are just a few of the problems tied to the opioid epidemic. Consider that opioid overdoses account for 750,000 emergency room visits each year (Skolnick, 2018), which means already overcrowded, understaffed emergency rooms are further taxed. So too are legal and criminal justice systems dealing with increasing numbers of opioid-related cases, partly owing to an uptick in heroin and synthetic opioid abuse (CDC, 2018; Skolnick, 2018). A sizeable majority of heroin users start off abusing prescription opioids but switch to heroin because it is "less expensive and often more accessible" (Skolnick, 2018, p. 144).

How did all of this happen? It started in the 1990s when the American Pain Society (APS) advocated that pain be classified as "the fifth vital sign," arguing the move was necessary because physicians undertreated pain (Lyapustina & Alexander, 2015). Coinciding with APS's fifth vital sign campaign, "Purdue Pharma

BOX 12.6

Lessons for Public Health and Crisis Communication

Following is a summary of the tips provided in this chapter.

Have a Plan

- Create a well-developed crisis management plan.
- Designate who will speak on behalf of the issue or organization.
- Practice what to do when a crisis occurs.

Cultivate Ongoing Relationships

- Nurture interactive and trusting relationships with stakeholders (community members, leaders, media, emergency personnel, and so on).
- Listen well. Focus on stakeholders' beliefs, expectations, and information needs.

Build an Information Library

- Collect information in advance that will be helpful, quick at hand, and tailored to different audiences.

Emphasize Teamwork

- Develop strong teams within and between organizations.
- Even if you do not specialize in crisis management, learn as much as you can about it and be prepared to take part.
- Even in the midst of a crisis, do not be afraid to restructure the system if it helps you respond to stakeholders more effectively.

Be Honest and Consistent

- Present trustworthy, current information that is based on science and evidence.
- Provide the public with answers to three key questions: "What do I need to know? What do I need to do or not do today to protect my health and that of my family? Where do I find information that I can trust and understand?" (Ratzan & Moritsugu, 2014, p. 1214).
- Coordinate with local health officials so that advice and information is consistent at every level whenever possible.
- When information is unavoidably inconsistent, acknowledge that and explain why.
- Be proactive rather than simply reacting to developments as they occur.
- Do not downplay legitimate risks and dangers.
- Vary your approach.
- Use multiple channels, including social media.
- Make the most of communication technology.

Recognize Diversity

- Remember that crisis is a matter of perception. People may assume that issues are more or less threatening than they seem to you.
- Don't overlook "forgotten publics."

Keep Communicating

- Expect resistance to your message and do not give up.
- Keep everyone involved (internally and externally) well informed and educated about risks and precautions.
- Communicate regularly with the public, members of the team, and with external agencies.

---

marketed and promoted OxyContin aggressively" (Skolnick, 2018, p. 145). Purdue's marketing, however, downplayed the fact that OxyContin could be addictive (Lyapustina & Alexander, 2015). By 2004, OxyContin was making billions of dollars for Purdue Pharma and was the most abused opioid pain reliever on the market. (Purdue Pharma sought bankruptcy protection in 2019, citing financial burdens stemming from 2,900 OxyContin-related lawsuits; Johnson & Mulvihill, 2019.)

Although it was clear in the early 2000s that prescription opioid abuse was a problem, HHS did not declare "a nationwide public health emergency" until 2017. Because the disease of addiction was (and remains) moralized and addicted persons stigmatized, opioid abuse was not held up as a public health problem—but instead as a personal problem. Some people believe that race also was a factor that shaped the public's response. Researchers have found evidence that addictions are moralized and stigmatized along racial lines (Frank & Nagel, 2017). In a piece written for *The Guardian*, Brian Broome (2018) observed that Whites are seen as "victims" in the opioid epidemic whereas African Americans are labeled "addicts." In recent years, the news media have given considerable attention to White, middle-class opioid abusers who are dying at twice the rate of African Americans (Nolan, 2016). Widespread media attention focused on White victims may have helped turned a "problem" into an "epidemic."

Although the situation is unfolding (as of the writing of this book) and we still have a lot to learn about communicating the risks associated with opioid abuse, there are a few lessons that stand out:

- *Language matters.* Be attentive to the ways words and phrases might negatively moralize health behaviors such as smoking, eating fatty foods, becoming obese, and not getting a flu shot (Frank & Nagel, 2017). By shifting blame to individuals, we might overlook social and/or economic factors that affect health. Consider persons living in food deserts who may not have access to fresh fruits and vegetables. If their only available food sources are convenience stores and fast food restaurants, can they be entirely to blame if they become overweight or obese? Societal forces that perpetuate income inequality and health disparities are partly to blame and should not be overlooked.
- *Don't overlook "forgotten publics."* News coverage of the opioid epidemic has, to date, focused on White, middle-class "victims" while underreporting—and sometimes misreporting—African Americans' experiences. We know from Chapter 11 that media images influence our thinking, so it's conceivable that news stories about "White victims" and "Black addicts" have skewed our understanding of this epidemic. While we are not accountable for most of what appears in the news, it's important that we be sensitive to and (if necessary) correct messages that imply that the health and safety of some people are more important than those of other people.

As we wrap up coverage of international health crises, it helps to remember that challenges are happening all the time, but so are victories. In his article "Still a Privilege to Be a Doctor," pediatrician Lawrence Rifkin (2008) pauses to reflect on the small miracles that health advocates accomplish every day:

> Ashley's in Room 3, with a positive rapid strep. It doesn't get more commonplace than that. Then, with a sense of wonder, I remember: A century ago, rheumatic fever complications from strep were the No. 1 cause of death in school-age children. Now, we hardly see rheumatic fever in this country; a few generations ago, Ashley may have been one of the victims. As I write out yet another prescription for amoxicillin, I think maybe I just saved a life. (p. 28)

Summary

What Is Public Health?

- Public health centers on the well-being of entire communities and involves agencies operating at local, national, and international levels.
- Public health agencies often deal with health emergencies—situations that occur in a particular time and place, including outbreaks of food-borne illnesses, epidemics, and natural disasters.
- During emergencies, public health agencies coordinate risk and crisis communication for affected communities.

Risk and Crisis Communication

- Risk communication is an ongoing process that involves disseminating information and engaging in interactive discussions about how people perceive risks and how they feel about risk messages.
- Crisis communication is an attempt by public health professionals to provide information that allows individuals, stakeholders, and entire communities to make the best possible decisions for their well-being during a crisis or emergency.
- Even when scientists cannot provide definitive answers, it is dangerous and unethical to keep the public in the dark about a potential health threat.
- Although public officials naturally worry about creating panic, the majority of evidence suggests the opposite: People typically want to assist others in emergency situations. This can make it difficult to convince citizens and rescue workers to use safety precautions, as we saw following the 9/11 terrorist attacks.

- Public health experts are advised to use fear appeals with sensitivity. Overloading the public with frightening messages can cause undue worry. Conversely, offering false reassurance can mislead people and damage their trust in public officials.

Crisis Communication Models and Guidelines

- Several crisis communication models and guidelines are based on the health belief model, which posits that people make behavioral choices based on six factors: perceived risk, severity of the risk, recommended actions, advantages of complying with recommendations, their belief in their ability to carry out recommendations, and specific cues to action. Successful crisis communication takes these factors into account.
- The models and guidelines explored in this chapter remind us that the best crisis communicators lay solid groundwork before a crisis emerges so they have information at hand, trusting and open relationships with stakeholders, and well-developed and well-rehearsed plans in place.
- The WHO Guideline on Communicating Risk recommends how to prepare for and manage a crisis.
- The IDEA Model describes crisis messages and means of distributing them.
- The CDC's Crisis and Risk Communication Model considers which messages are most needed at particular stages of a crisis.

Case Studies: A Global Perspective

- The Ebola experience reminds us that it is critical for health officials to understand the fears, customs, and expectations of people involved and to communicate with them in respectful and consistent ways.
- A different challenge is keeping an ongoing health crisis such as AIDS on the public agenda. Prevention efforts are complicated by the sensitive nature of transmission-related behaviors and the wide diversity of cultures affected. The AIDS example underscores how important it is to listen to, respect, and understand the people we are trying to help.
- The global nature of commerce and travel makes it imperative that health advocates around the world work together to monitor emerging concerns, track their incidence, and stop the spread of contagious illnesses as quickly as possible. The SARS example represents a successful effort to do just that. Efforts are under way to respond to an avian flu pandemic if it occurs.
- How Zika was covered by the U.S. news media reminds us that health agencies cannot rely on news media alone to distribute accurate and complete crisis messages to the public. Social media, if used consistently, can help fill gaps in media coverage.
- The opioid epidemic teaches us that the words we use to describe conditions like addiction can lead to moralizing, blaming, and stigmatizing.
- Although these lessons look easy on paper, the stress and demands of an actual crisis make them difficult to follow.

Glossary

crisis and emergency risk model (CERC) Developed by the CDC, the CERC model outlines five crisis phases and accompanying communication goals. In the pre-crisis phase, partnerships with agencies, organizations, first responders, and the media are formed. During the initial event, aims include informing and reassuring the public, reducing uncertainty, and promoting self-efficacy. The maintenance phase involves helping the public more accurately understand the risk and what is being done. During the resolution phase, ongoing recovery efforts are shared. The evaluation phase includes evaluating response and communication effectiveness and identifying specific actions for improving. *See page 278.*

crisis communication An approach used by scientists and public health professionals to provide information that allows individuals, stakeholders, or an entire community to make the best possible decisions about their well-being, under nearly impossible time constraints, while accepting the imperfect nature of their choices. *See page 271.*

health belief model Model positing that people make behavioral choices based on six factors: perceived risk, severity of the risk, recommended actions, advantages of complying with recommendations, their belief in their ability to carry out recommendations, and specific cues to actions. *See page 276.*

IDEA model The IDEA model has four main components. Internalization refers to the process whereby people process risk messages based on personal relevance, proximity to the risk, potential impact, and timeliness (e.g., the time available to make preparations or respond to a crisis). Distribution refers to channels for sharing information, such as television, radio, newspapers, the internet, and social media. Explanation reflects the quality of a message, its accuracy, the credibility of its source, and how easily it is understood by the public. Action involves the specific steps people might take in an emergency. *See page 277.*

public health The science and art of preventing disease, prolonging life, and providing physical health and efficiency to organize community efforts for the sanitation of the environment, the control of community infections, the teaching of the individual and principles of personal hygiene, the organization of medical and nursing service for the early diagnosis and preventive treatment of disease, and the development of the social machinery that will ensure standards of living adequate to maintain health. *See page 269.*

risk communication An ongoing process that involves, not just one message, but many diverse messages about risk factors as well as interactive discussions about how people perceive these factors, how they judge the risks, and how they feel about the risk messages themselves. *See page 270.*

social mobilization Large-scale efforts in which community members and professionals collaborate to define goals, raise awareness, and create hospitable environments for healthy behaviors. *See page 270.*

World Health Organization's guidelines on communicating risk The WHO's guidelines recommend specific steps to prepare for and manage a crisis. The steps include planning in advance, which means having communication infrastructures and strategies in place before crises occur; building trust with the public; engaging stakeholders; using multiple channels, including social media; and monitoring, evaluating, and adjusting crisis communication using feedback from stakeholders. *See page 276.*

Discussion Questions

1. How would you feel if health officials in hazardous-material suits showed up at your home and the homes of your neighbors, demanding that you turn ill family members over to them? What if you heard that many families who turned their loved ones over to authorities never knew what happened to them afterward?

2. What advice do you have for health crisis communicators who are worried about creating panic? For those who are worried that too many warnings will make people indifferent when true emergencies arise?

3. Of the three risk communication traditions presented by Peter Sandman, which is most descriptive of risk communication? Of crisis communication?

4. Describe the risk management/communication framework that Scott Ratzan and Wendy Meltzer present.

5. Compare the WHO's guidelines on communicating risk, the IDEA model, the CERC model, and the adapted CERC model. How are the recommendations alike and where do they diverge?

6. Discuss the ethical implications raised by the Andrew Speaker (TB Andy) and Mary Mallon (Typhoid Mary) cases. Why might such public health risks be even more salient today than in Mallon's time? What do you think we should do to protect individual liberties while preserving the public's health interest?

7. Describe how the CDC and news media handled the Zika crisis and what we can learn from the experience.

8. Discuss the implications of moralizing health behaviors. Describe examples in which behaviors are moralized positively and examples showing negative moralizations. Do you think moralization can be justified in some situations? If so, explain.

9. Trace the development of the avian flu so far. Would you be frightened if a containment zone were declared in your area? Why or why not? Do you feel adequately informed about and prepared for such a crisis? Why or why not?

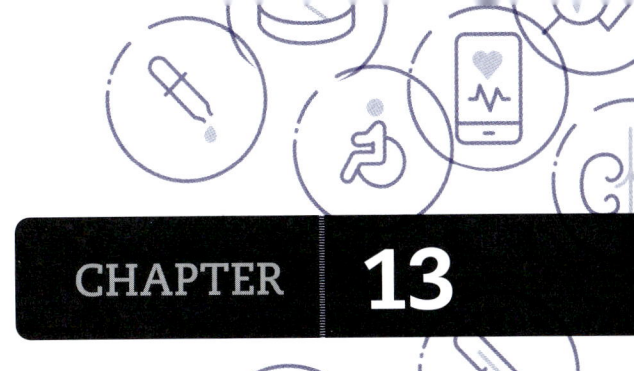

CHAPTER 13

Planning Health Promotion Campaigns

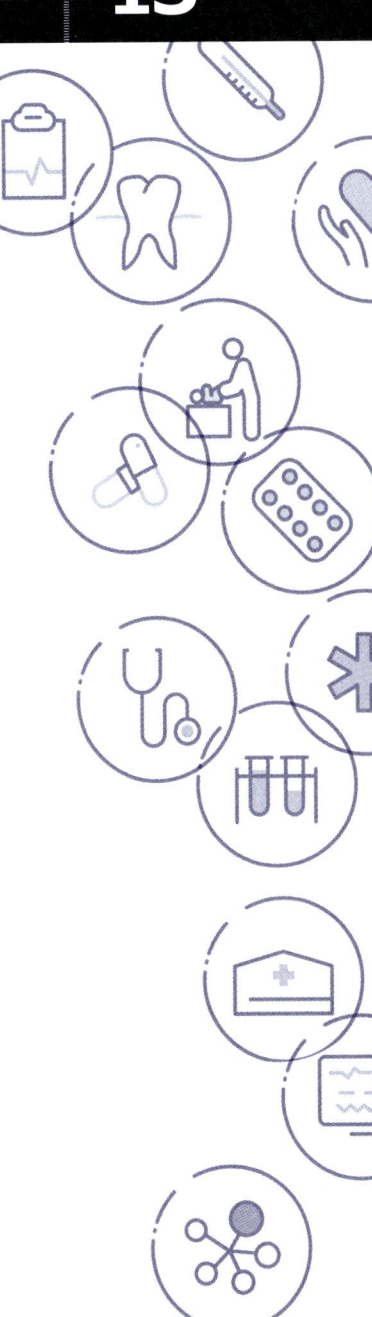

The truth is all around you—the truth® campaign, that is. You might remember images of public spaces filled with life-sized mannequins, each one representing a person who died as a result of smoking. Or you might have seen the "Catmageddon" videos, compilations of the some of the Web's best viral cat videos set to music and featuring graphics warning viewers that cats are twice as likely as their owners to die from smoking-related cancer. "The Internet is fueled by cat videos, and because cigarettes can kill cats, too, we're freaking out, and you should, too" says a truth® campaign message. "#CATmageddon is truth®'s most successful campaign ever in terms of cultural impact and changing teen attitudes towards smoking," according to truth® representatives who described the campaign to the Shorty Awards (the internet's version of the Oscars). The campaign generated more than 100,000 mentions and even more views online (Shorty Awards, 2017).

Many truth® campaigns, like #CATmageddon, are irreverent and entertaining, but they mean business. truth® is the nation's longest running and most successful youth smoking-prevention campaign series designed for a highly specific target market—youth ages 12 to 17. As truth®'s creators explain:

> truth speaks to youth and young adults on their terms, through the channels they understand and trust. truth delivers the facts about the health effects and social consequences of tobacco and the marketing tactics of the tobacco industry so that youth and young adults can make informed decisions and influence others to do the same.

The campaigns get results. When truth® launched in 2000, teens' awareness of antitobacco messages almost immediately doubled (Farrelly, Healton, Davis, Messeri, & Haviland, 2002). Since then, the percentage of teen smokers in the

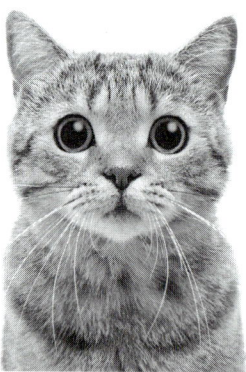

truth®'s #CATmageddon campaign taught viewers that cats exposed to second-hand smoke are twice as likely as their owners to die from smoking-related cancer. To date, #CATmageddon is truth®'s most successful campaign.

Why do you think the #CATmageddon campaign was so successful?

United States has dropped to its lowest level in more than 20 years (Johnston, O'Malley, Miech, Bachman, & Schulenberg, 2014). According to truth®:

> Youth and young adults exposed to truth ads are almost 2.5x more likely to agree with anti-tobacco attitudes and 70% less likely to intend to smoke cigarettes in the next year. We saw a 21% increase in agreement with "Tobacco companies make me angry" among those aware of #CATmageddon and a significant increase in knowledge and change in attitudes about secondhand smoke. (Shorty Awards, 2017, para. 3)

The truth® campaigns are not solely responsible for reducing teen smoking, but analysts give truth® kudos for having a huge impact. *Advertising Age* named truth® one of the Top 15 Ad Campaigns of the 21st Century ("truth® Named," 2015).

Just as teen smoking rates reached a record low, vaping threatened to undo decades of public health work. In response, truth® started a #DITCHJUUL campaign in 2019. JUUL is the most popular brand of e-cigarette among teens and its "nicotine content is one of the highest among e-cigarettes on the market" (Truth Initiative, 2019, para. 12). Nicotine is a *big* problem—it "can harm brain development, alter nerve cell functioning and change brain chemistry in ways that make adolescent brains more susceptible to other addictive drugs" (Truth Initiative, 2019, para. 13).

truth® campaigns are sponsored by Truth Initiative, a national public health organization dedicated to achieving a culture in which all youth and young adults reject tobacco. It is funded by a settlement reached between the tobacco industry and 46 states and five U.S. territories in 1998. In the early years, truth® messages were mostly about the health threats of tobacco use (Lavoie & Quick, 2013). Campaign advocates published the ingredients of cigarettes (including chemicals also found in "cat pee" and "dog poop") and presented the "hard facts" about tobacco companies' deceptions and unfair practices. Today, truth® continues its assault on big tobacco, while also tackling vaping and the opioid epidemic.

In this chapter we walk through the first steps in creating an effective health-promotion campaign. In Chapter 12, we discussed the overlap between public health and crisis communication. Here we turn our attention to another side of the same coin—efforts to help people protect themselves from more chronic health threats such as cancer, obesity, diabetes, and accidents. Keeping health issues on the public agenda and working with people to change their everyday behaviors can be as challenging as managing a crisis.

Health-promoting behaviors are those that "enhance health and well-being, reduce health risks, and prevent disease" (Brennan & Fink, 1997, p. 157). These behaviors include lifestyle choices, medical care, prevention efforts, and activities that foster an overall sense of well-being.

Health promotion campaigns are systematic efforts to influence people to engage in health-enhancing behaviors (Backer & Rogers, 1993). These efforts may involve the use of many communication channels, from face-to-face communication to mass media. The term *health promoter* includes anyone involved in the process of creating and distributing health promotion messages. This includes volunteers in the community, employees of nonprofit health agencies, public relations and community relations professionals, production artists, media decision makers, and more. As this list suggests, health promotion offers diverse career opportunities for communication specialists. (See Box 13.1.)

We will consider the challenges of promoting health behaviors among diverse members of the population, beginning with a brief overview of some notable

> **BOX 13.1 Career Opportunities**
>
> ## Health Promotion and Education
>
> Community health educator
> Corporate wellness director
> Director of nonprofit organization
> Fitness instructor
> Health information publication designer
> Hospital-based health educator
> Patient advocate or patient navigator
> Professor/educator
> School-based health educator
>
> **Career Resources and Job Listings**
>
> - Society for Public Health Education: sophe.org
> - Area Health Education Centers: nationalahec.org
> - National Commission for Health Education Credentialing (NCHEC): nchec.org
> - U.S. Bureau of Labor Statistics Occupational Outlook Handbook: bls.gov/ooh
> - *Chronicle of Higher Education* Job Search: chronicle.com/jobs
> - Centers for Disease Control and Prevention Division of Health Communication: cdc.gov/healthcommunication
> - National Institutes of Health: nih.gov
> - World Health Organization: who.int/employment/vacancies/en

health campaigns. Then we walk through the first four stages of designing a health promotion campaign:

Step 1: Defining the situation and potential benefits
Step 2: Analyzing and segmenting the audience
Step 3: Establishing campaign goals and objectives
Step 4: Selecting channels of communication

Steps 5 through 7, on designing and implementing a campaign, are covered in the next chapter. Keep in mind that it's important to know all the steps before you actually begin. Although evaluating and refining the campaign is the final step, you must consider from the beginning how you will accomplish those goals later on.

Background on Health Campaigns

Live long and prosper.

The Vulcan salutation made famous by *Star Trek's* Mr. Spock seems to say it all. A long and healthy existence—isn't that what life is all about? You might think so. But it turns out that Vulcan logic cannot always explain human behavior, as Mr. Spock discovered.

Early health campaigns were designed with the confidence that, as humans, we want nothing so much as our own health and longevity. From that viewpoint it follows that if we know a behavior is unhealthy, we will not engage in it. In fact, we should go to great lengths to pursue health-enhancing outcomes. Seen this way, persuasion is not an issue. People only need reliable information. The motivation to comply with it is presumably already there, as innate as the animal instinct for survival.

Motivating Factors

It turns out that influencing human behavior is not that simple. We are motivated by a number of factors that make us more or less receptive to health information and more or less motivated to change our behavior. Sometimes we do things we know to be unhealthy because the behavior is inexpensive, convenient, socially rewarding, or fun. For instance, research indicates that people may drink alcoholic beverages even though they believe alcohol to be unhealthy because people are reluctant to give up the social ritual of drinking with friends. Conversely, we sometimes change our behavior without thinking or knowing much about the change or our reasons for it. We may try a new behavior (like taking vitamins) simply because someone tells us to or because the change seems easy, fashionable, or so on. In these instances, knowledge may *follow* behavior change.

When it comes to health campaigns' ability to change our behaviors, research has not always been encouraging. Campaigns have been criticized for naively seeking to change people's behavior without changing or acknowledging their circumstances and for assuming that knowledge reaches and affects all people equally.

In reality, campaigns may raise awareness, but they are not likely to change behavior unless the recommended behaviors are compatible with people's beliefs and are supported within their social networks. Health promoters have discovered that we cannot simply educate people about health and presume they will adjust their lifestyles accordingly. We must take a range of factors into account. It is crucial to know a campaign's intended audience and to consider not just how they might benefit from certain behaviors, but whether they are willing to change their behaviors, how difficult the changes might be to implement, and what obstacles they may face.

Exemplary Campaigns

This section describes a few exemplary health promotion campaigns. Each provides an inspiring lesson for promoters. Together, these examples illustrate that, as health promoters, we must often do more than simply disseminate information if we are to succeed. Sensitivity to audience needs, problem-solving skills, assessment, community involvement, and careful planning and follow-through are required as well.

GET TO KNOW THE AUDIENCE

One quality of effective health promoters is that *they know their audiences well and design campaigns to suit those audiences*. Analysts say truth® has been successful largely because its creators take time to understand and engage with the target audience. Whereas health promoters have long been frustrated by teens' tendency to do the opposite of what they are told, the truth® campaign honors their rebellious nature (Farrelly et al., 2002). The campaign "never preaches and never talks down to teenagers," explain truth® sponsors ("truth® Overview," n.d.). Instead, it honors adolescents' sense of independence and personal choice. As the truth® website puts it:

> WE DON'T HATE. **WE INSTIGATE.**
> We're not here to criticize your choices, or tell you not to smoke. We're here to arm everyone—smokers and non-smokers—with the tools to make change.

> EXPOSING **BIG TOBACCO**
> We've always been about exposing Big Tobacco's lies and manipulation. And while they keep adapting their tactics, we keep it real. (thetruth, 2015, "About Us")

The people behind truth® wager that when teens are exposed to the deceit and manipulation behind tobacco companies' efforts, they will rebel against corporate greed by *not* smoking.

If you do not know your intended audience well, then get to know them! For example, researchers in Singapore wanted to convince men to wear condoms when hooking up with women in entertainment establishments (e.g., bars, karaoke lounges, dance clubs, etc.), so they asked men who frequented those types of places for advice. Raymond Boon Tar Lim and colleagues (2019) spent more than a year surveying and interviewing heterosexual men about their sexual practices, their thoughts on using condoms, and their knowledge about HIV. They also asked men about the types of messages they would pay attention to and their opinions on possible campaign strategies. The men who were interviewed suggested staging entertaining interventions in popular hangouts, such as talk- or quiz-show–style interactive performances. The men even came up with a name for the campaign—THINK. The name "carried a subtle yet non-stigmatizing meaning, as it would prompt them to think twice before engaging in unprotected sex" (Lim, Tham, Cheung, & Adaikan, 2019, p. 50). By taking the time to really get to know (and listen to) their audience, Lim and colleagues (2019) ended up designing a fun and effective intervention that worked.

INVEST IN COMMUNICATION INFRASTRUCTURES

A community health initiative involving Matthew Matsaganis and colleagues illustrates another best practice in health promotion: *Create enduring infrastructures that support relationship development and collaborative problem solving*. The research team helped to increase reproductive health care received by low-income African American women in one community by helping underserved community members and service providers get to know each other better (Matsaganis, Golden, & Scott, 2014). The program was based on four main premises. One was that storytelling can be a powerful means of bridging social gaps. Another was that outreach efforts should be initiated within the places and circumstances of people's everyday lives. A third was that underserved individuals are capable of and deserving of collaborating with care providers to structure how services are provided. A fourth premise was that long-term success relies on the creation of an enduring communication infrastructure. For more about this remarkable project, see Box 13.2.

BOX 13.2

Storytelling Connects Underserved Women and Care Providers

It was a common dilemma. A publicly funded health care center was available to the residents of a small, rural community. However, many of the people most in need of its services were not receiving them. Here is what happened when a team of three health communication scholars took on the challenge.

Aware that low-income African American women were underutilizing a reproductive health care center in their community, scholars Matthew Matsaganis, Annis Golden, and Muriel Scott (2014) focused on the reasons why. They soon realized that there was a general disconnect between the women and local services organizations. Although organizational members wished women would make greater use of their services, most of them felt unsure how to bridge the gap that separated them from the women. For their part, the would-be clients were often unsure what was available to them, unable to find reliable transportation, and skeptical that they could trust care providers.

Over the course of four years, principal investigators Matsaganis and Golden served not only as researchers, but as interstitial actors in the effort to help. That is, they were intermediaries who helped to bridge the gaps between people, organizations, and larger public entities. They reached out to underserved women in gathering places (communication hotspots) the women frequented in everyday life. In this way, they sidestepped some of the barriers—such as transportation difficulties and distrust—that might have prevented the women's participation (Matsaganis, Golden, & Scott, 2014).

The objective was to listen to and partner with African American women, not to engage in one-way communication or to privilege organizational agendas. As the women interacted with each other and with organizational representatives, storytelling emerged as a natural means of getting to know each other.

Significantly, Matsaganis and colleagues (2014) helped to create enduring communication infrastructures. They founded a community advisory board, recruited and trained peer health advocates, and spearheaded the creation of a field office at a local public housing complex, which they staffed with an African American community outreach associate who was familiar in the community and knowledgeable about health resources.

The field office was critical to the project's success, reflects Matsaganis. It became a "comfort zone" within the community, "a great place to connect with residents and foster the development of trust between the research team and residents" (Matsaganis, personal correspondence). Based on the relationships that emerged in the field office, women in the community were more comfortable taking part in other activities sponsored by the team, such as health fairs and entertainment events, and ultimately, in seeking reproductive health care and other services (Matsaganis et al., 2014).

With a clearer understanding of underserved women's needs, staff members at the field office and other locations initiated new support services. For example, they began to assist women in making health appointments, and they provided taxi vouchers so they could reach the health center.

As with any program of this magnitude, participants faced hurdles in terms of limited resources and resilient distrust. However, with the benefit of a communication infrastructure that invited their involvement, local residents and members of the health community gradually developed more trusting partnerships. Utilization of reproductive health services increased 25% (Matsaganis et al., 2014).

MAKE HEALTHY OPTIONS ACCESSIBLE

Another lesson is that health promotion comes in many forms, and *sometimes actions are more empowering than words alone*. For example, realizing that healthy eating is not an affordable option for everyone, programs such as Feeding America offer nutritious take-home food for school children in need.

Another example involves **nudging, the practice of making healthy options readily apparent**, appealing, and available. Some nudging efforts are nonverbal, such as displaying healthy food in a prominent location of the grocery store. Others are more explicit, as when health promoters provide discount coupons for child safety seats. Astrid Junghans and colleagues (2015) surveyed consumers in the United Kingdom to see whether they mostly considered nudges in the supermarket to be manipulative or empowering. Most of them felt that nudges were helpful if they were not overpowering and if they were motivated by a desire to help people rather than to make a profit (Junghans, Cheung, & De Ridder, 2015). However, some people felt that nudges have a paternalistic downside in that they seek to influence people's behavior at a subconscious level rather than presenting a persuasive message outright.

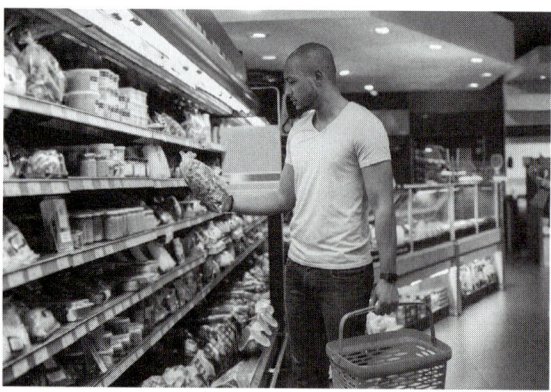

Do you feel it is ethical to locate the supermarket bakery near the front of the store so that shoppers will immediately smell the scent of bread and sweets? Why or why not? Do you feel it is ethical for supermarket personnel to display fresh produce in highly visible places throughout the store? Why or why not? What might supermarket personnel do to make healthy choices accessible without being unfairly manipulative or paternalistic?

TAKE A MULTIMEDIA APPROACH

A *multimedia approach may be more beneficial than using only one channel*. To test this idea, Grace Ahn (2015) invited a group of university students to don headsets and experience a virtual world in which they observed time-lapse images of a person drinking sugary soft drinks over a two-year span and gaining 20 pounds. The experiment was immersive in that the students could "look around the virtual world as they would in the physical world" and hear the sound of "fat splattering onto a digital scale" as the person gained weight (Ahn, p. 548). Ahn asked other students to review only a printed pamphlet that described the same process. Still a third group both reviewed the pamphlet *and* took part in the virtual experience. One week later, participants in the third group were the most likely of all to say that they would not have sugary drinks, which suggests that the combined impact of multiple experiences may be a particularly powerful means of conveying health information.

SET CLEAR GOALS AND MEASURE YOUR SUCCESS

Another best practice is to *establish clear goals and measure your success*. Take the "designated driver" campaign. The campaign was launched in 1988 by members of the Harvard School of Public Health's Center for Health Communication, who were inspired by a similar concept in Scandinavia. It is estimated that the program and related spin-offs have saved the lives of at least 50,000 people ("Designated Driving Statistics," 2020). Public health expert Jay Winsten (2010) proposes that the campaign was successful largely because the goal (to reduce drunk-driving accidents) was clear and measurable and it involved a modest change in behavior (agreeing to be a sober driver for one's friends). Plus, the entertainment industry embraced the idea and wove it into prime-time storylines—as many as 160 of them.

Another example is Lim and colleagues' (2019) condom project. Their goal was to see a 50% increase in condom use among casual sexual partners in 6 months' time. Participants in the study went from using condoms 52% of the time to using them 80% of the time. Another valuable lesson we can take from this campaign: *Don't forget to get a baseline measurement before you launch a health campaign (you will need it for comparison later)*.

Next let's consider how we would create our own health campaign.

Step 1: Defining the Situation and Potential Benefits

To illustrate the steps in planning a health campaign, imagine that staff members of a university sports recreation department have asked us to help recruit new participants. Specifically, they would like to increase the number of people who go to the campus fitness center in their free time. The recreation department will not benefit financially from the added enrollment, but the staff wishes to increase participation because physical activity improves people's health. The rest of the chapter guides us through the initial steps of creating a campaign. The hypothetical sports recreation campaign is admittedly a small-scale effort, but many influential campaigns are aimed at limited audiences, and improving health habits among even a small group is a momentous goal. Furthermore, the steps given apply well to large and small campaigns.

If you are like many people, your first instinct is to hang fliers or post promotional messages on Facebook or Instagram. Those may be effective steps, but before we begin, let's take the advice of professional campaign planners and do some preliminary research.

Benefits

At this stage, we should be interested in learning what benefits (if any) our efforts might yield. Following are some questions we might research.

- Would exercising at the fitness center actually improve people's health?
- Would everybody benefit?
- Are there some people who would not benefit?
- Are there alternative ways to get the same benefits?

Answers to these questions can be obtained by reading published literature and talking with experts in the field. This kind of preliminary research may help us decide if the project is worthwhile.

Current Situation

Assuming that we find reasonable evidence to believe that people might benefit from exercising at the gym, the next step is to assess the current situation. Following are some questions to guide our

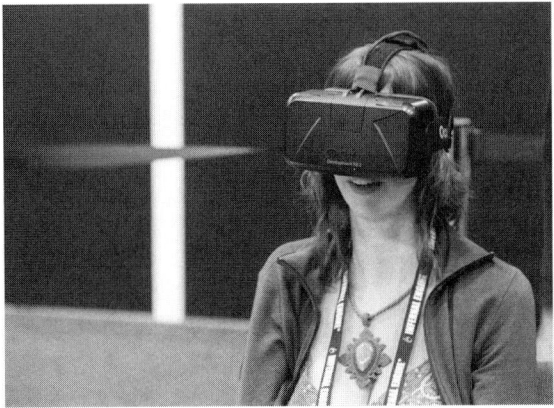

Virtual reality headsets such as this one are a means of making health-related images vivid, immersive, and tailored to individuals. In one study, participants were more likely to swear off sugary soft drinks after they read a pamphlet about their ill effects and watched a virtual-reality time-lapse presentation of a soft drink consumer gaining weight (Ahn, 2015).

preliminary research. The same questions will be useful later in guiding audience analysis. Remember that experts, program leaders, current participants, and nonparticipants are all valuable sources of information. In addition to these general questions, we may want to add some specific questions relevant to the campaign.

- How many people currently participate in the recommended behavior?
- What types of people participate and for what reasons? (Of interest is demographic information, such as age, sex, and income, as well as cultural, personal, social, or personality variables that might be relevant.)
- What are the strengths and weaknesses of the program (from the perspective of participants and nonparticipants)?
- What types of people do not participate?
- What are their reasons for not participating?
- What factors are most important to participants and nonparticipants (e.g., cost, convenience, social interaction)?
- Do people consider the potential benefits of this behavior important? Why or why not?
- Are there any conditions under which nonparticipants might participate?
- How do the people in the audience usually receive information (i.e., fliers, radio, email, social media, etc.)?

- Through what channels do they prefer to get information?
- What information sources do they trust?

Preliminary answers to our questions may be surprising. We may find, for instance, that current sports recreation participants are not primarily concerned about health benefits. They go to the fitness center because their friends are there and they enjoy the social interaction. Or we might find that some people will not participate no matter how healthy physical activity is because they are afraid of looking foolish on the basketball court or out of shape in group fitness classes. Perhaps recreational programs are scheduled when many people cannot attend them. Simply educating people about the health benefits of exercise may not do much good.

Diverse Motivations

Keep in mind that health concerns are not people's only motivation. We are all most receptive to options that satisfy us on many levels (intellectual, emotional, personal, social, and so on). In assessing the situation, it's important not to assume that everyone is motivated in the same way we are. Consider (and ask about) the diversity among people who might participate in the sports recreation program. Our audience is probably not just traditional college students (a diverse group in itself), but international students, people with disabilities, middle-aged and older adults, experienced students and newcomers, university faculty and staff members, and maybe even community members and children.

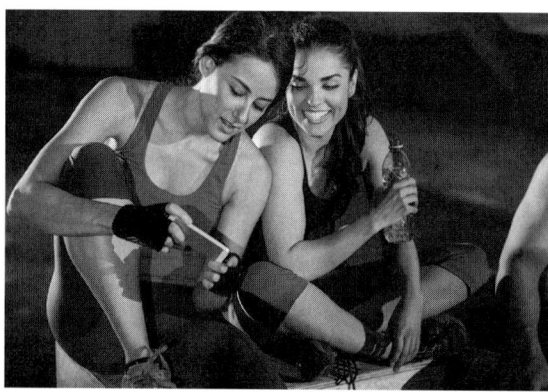

People have diverse motivations for taking part in health-related behaviors. Some may enjoy the social aspect of going to the gym, whereas others are motivated primarily by the desire to have quiet time, lose weight, or reach other goals.

In Step 2, we will attempt to learn about our audience and choose a portion of it to target. Being sensitive to diverse beliefs and motivations can help us understand why people behave as they do and what is important to them. This understanding is crucial to our success as we partner with them.

Step 2: Analyzing and Segmenting the Audience

After assessing the health benefits and the current situation at the sports recreation department, we are ready to analyze potential audiences for our campaign. This will involve asking a larger number of people many of the same questions we asked in preliminary research.

Audience research may seem like an unnecessary or even repetitive step, but experienced campaign planners know better. Audience analysis allows us to collect important data about people's behaviors and preferences. It pays to know, in advance, what information sources our target audience members use and trust, how they view their overall health, what their main concerns are, and more (Ledlow, Johnson, & Hakoyama, 2008). Edward Maibach and Roxanne Parrott (1995) applaud promoters for considering the audience's needs before they determine campaign goals. As they put it, audience-centered analysis "means that health messages are designed primarily to respond to the needs and situation of the target audience, rather than to the needs and situation of the message designers or sponsoring organizations" (p. 167).

Data Collection

There are several ways to learn about potential audience members. Preexisting databases are a good place to start. For example, we might request demographics about the people who do go to the gym from the campus recreation department. We might also request information from the campus registrar about the student body (e.g., how many from each class, their majors, ages, genders, etc.). We should also try to get more specific information about the target audience's beliefs, values, and habits. We probably won't find this information in an existing database, so we will have to collect it ourselves.

This section describes how to get started, including how and when to get ethics-board approval for our research. We will also look at the comparative advantages of using interviews, questionnaires, and focus groups to learn about the people we hope to help.

ETHICAL COMMITMENTS

Before we discuss the research phase, keep in mind that to uphold the highest standards of ethics, we must get an official go-ahead from the university to carry out the research procedures we design. Usually, this means submitting the research plan (e.g., questionnaires and/or interview questions) to an **institutional review board** (**IRB**), an ethics panel that reviews and monitors research efforts to ensure that participants are treated fairly. Universities have IRBs, as do many organizations, especially in health care. If our research involves people from more than one organization, it may be necessary to get IRB approval from each of them.

The IRB will be interested to know how we will secure informed consent from participants (see Chapter 4), maintain their anonymity or keep their identities confidential, and avoid causing them unnecessary distress. We will need to make special efforts to protect the needs and rights of vulnerable populations if they are involved in our study, including children, people with cognitive disabilities, people recovering from abuse, seriously ill people, and so on. It is advisable to check IRB guidelines and timelines early on so that ethics will be first on our minds and we can avoid unexpected delays.

DATA-GATHERING OPTIONS

There are a number of ways we might learn more about the audiences our campaign may target. Approach data gathering with avid curiosity and a respect for multiple viewpoints. Here is a quick overview of some information-gathering methods we might consider.

INTERVIEWS. You might be surprised by what you can learn from asking and listening. Here are different interview strategies and the advantages and limitations of each (based on Frey, Botan, Friedman, & Kreps, 1999).

- **Highly scheduled interviews**. Interviewers are given specific questions to ask and are not allowed to make comments or ask additional questions. This helps minimize the interviewers' influence on respondents' answers, but it doesn't allow for follow-up questions or clarifications. Answers are typically brief but easy to tally and compare.

- **Moderately scheduled interviews**. Interviewers are given a set of questions but are allowed to ask for clarification and additional information as they see fit. These interviews are more relaxed and conversational, but less precise, than highly scheduled interviews.

- **Unscheduled interviews**. Interviewers are given a list of topics but are encouraged to phrase questions as they wish and to probe for more information when it seems useful and appropriate. These interviews are useful for collecting information about respondents' feelings, but they do not yield answers that can easily be compared or tallied.

QUESTIONNAIRES. Because they can be administered to large numbers of people in less time than it would take to conduct interviews, questionnaires are a popular way to collect audience information. A **questionnaire** asks respondents to indicate their answers to a list of questions. In general, written responses are more limited in scope than interview responses, but the upshot is that people may be more willing to answer sensitive questions in writing or online, especially if surveys are conducted anonymously.

Here are some guidelines for designing an effective questionnaire:

- *Keep it brief.* People are unlikely to complete surveys that take more than 10 minutes.
- *Seek immediate response.* If people take time to complete the survey right away, the response rate will be higher.
- *Collect demographic information.* This may include factors such as age, sex, income, college major, occupation, and the like, if they are relevant to the campaign. **Fixed-alternative questions** ask respondents to select the appropriate response(s) from a list of all possibilities (e.g., African American, Asian, Hispanic, or White, etc.). These types of questions make it easy to count and compare answers, but it's important to include an "other" option when the list is not comprehensive.
- *Ask about knowledge and behaviors.* A mixture of open and closed questions will yield the most useful information. **Open-ended questions** allow respondents to express ideas in their own words (e.g., *How do you feel about basketball and aerobics?*). **Close-ended questions** require very brief answers (e.g., *Do you prefer to work out with free weights or weight machines?*).

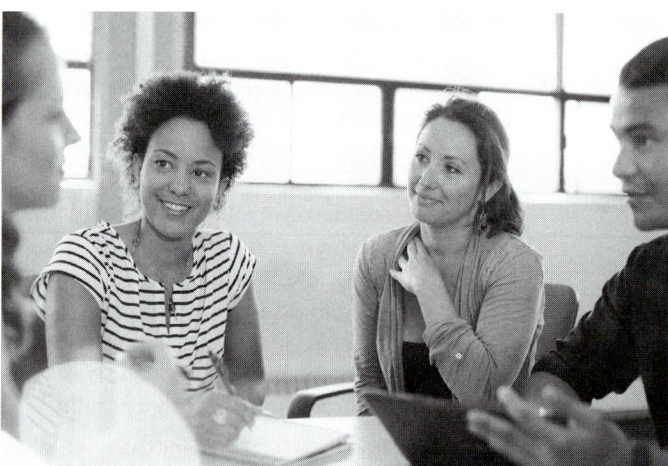

Conducting interviews, administering questionnaires, and holding focus groups are good ways to learn about a health campaign's intended audience.

- *Pilot (pretest) the questionnaire.* We will test the questionnaire on a few representative people before administering it to everyone in our sample, and we will ask the respondents to indicate if any questions are confusing or leading, if fixed-alternative questions include all possible answers, and if they can think of other questions we should add.
- *Allow for anonymity.* Whether the questionnaire is on paper or online, it is ideal if people can respond anonymously.

FOCUS GROUPS. A third option for collecting information is the use of focus groups. A **focus group** involves a small number of people who respond to questions posed by a moderator. The moderator encourages the group members to speak openly on topics relevant to the campaign. Members' comments are usually recorded so that they can be studied later. Focus groups are useful for learning the target audience's feelings about an issue. For example, a research team led by Rose Clark-Hitt conducted focus groups with military members to see how they reacted to campaign materials that encouraged them to "help a buddy take a knee"; that is, to support their comrades in seeking mental health counseling without shame (Clark-Hitt, Smith, & Broderick, 2012).

Whether we use surveys, questionnaires, or focus groups, it's important to think carefully about whom to include. Choosing people to include is called **sampling** the population. Interviews and surveys allow us to collect information from people who reflect the diversity in the population we are considering. In contrast, focus group participants are members of a target group such as nontraditional students or freshmen. Too much diversity within one group of respondents can make it hard to develop a focused discussion. For example, when Mary Frances Casper and colleagues (2006) conducted focus groups about college students' drinking patterns, they had student participants fill out questionnaires in advance. Then they assigned students to one of three focus groups. The students didn't know it, but the groups reflected their typical drinking levels—nondrinkers, moderate, and more-than-average drinkers (Casper, Child, Gilmour, McIntyre, & Pearson, 2006). The researchers knew that participants were more likely to engage in open discussion if it emerged that other people in the room had similar feelings.

Although we should keep membership in any one focus group fairly homogenous, it is important to hold focus groups that, together, represent a wide array of perspectives. Depending on the campaign, consider how you might include diversity in terms of culture, race and ethnicity, gender identity, age, ability, and other factors.

In our case, we might conduct separate focus groups with people who use the workout facilities and those who do not. Throughout the process, we must be careful not to assume that one group speaks for the others or for the population overall.

Following are some tips for conducting effective focus groups:

- *Determine what type of information you most want to collect.* For example, concerning our fitness campaign, consider whether you are more interested in the opinions of people who already use the fitness center or people who are not yet involved.
- *Design a list of open-ended questions to get the information you most want.*
- *Appoint (or hire) a facilitator to lead the focus group discussion.* A good facilitator helps people feel comfortable expressing their opinions, allows everyone to contribute to the discussion, and does not influence members' responses. Many experts recommend using a facilitator not associated

with the promotion effort because focus group members may feel more comfortable voicing criticisms and because the facilitator may be more objective.

- Choose 7 to 10 people from the target audience to make up each focus group.
- Arrange to conduct the focus group in a conference room or other comfortable area. (It is customary to provide refreshments for focus group participants.)
- Arrange to audio- and video-record the session unobtrusively (with participants' permission).
- Review the information collected.
- Consider conducting multiple focus groups with different members of the target audience.

Choosing a Target Audience

It's part of our ethical responsibility as health promoters to identify the group that we most want to reach and to make every effort to understand that audience. In this section we talk about the vulnerabilities and needs of various groups we might target. We start by examining the irony that the people who are easiest to reach and who are most receptive are probably already aware of what we would like to tell them. Often, a more worthwhile challenge is to connect with people who are not already information rich.

THEORETICAL FOUNDATIONS

The **knowledge gap hypothesis** proposes that people with plentiful information resources (such as televisions, computers, and well-informed friends and advisors) are likely to know more and to continue learning more than people with fewer information resources (Tichenor, Donohue, & Olien, 1970). Income and education are highly linked to resource availability and media habits. Consequently, people of high socioeconomic status tend to be knowledge rich, and people of low status tend to be knowledge poor. New information often increases the knowledge gap rather than diminishing it. In other words, the people who already know a lot learn more, and the others fall farther behind.

Unfortunately, people who are information poor are often most in need of health information. Here are a few examples:

- Three years after a state medical assistance program for the uninsured was implemented in their community, 50% of low-income families were still unaware of it (Rucinski, 2004).
- Mexican American women in rural areas more frequently die from breast cancer than other women, but they often know little about breast self-exams and the severity of the disease (Hubbell, 2006).
- Girls who have sex before age 16 are at highest risk for sexually transmitted infections, but they are the least likely to know about or to be offered preventive care such as the human papillomavirus (HPV) vaccine (Sacks, Copas, Wilkinson, & Robinson, 2014).

There are several reasons that underprivileged persons are hard to reach with health messages. One barrier involves trust. Underprivileged audiences tend disproportionately to be people from minority cultures. They may be skeptical about mainstream messages, either because they seem irrelevant (aimed at Whites rather than Blacks, for example) or because they mistrust the sources (Holland, 2014).

Second, underprivileged individuals are more likely than others to rely on television for information than on more detailed sources, such as health information websites. A so-called **digital divide** separates the information rich, who have easy access to the internet (predominantly young, well-educated city dwellers), and the information poor, who are often rural residents with limited or no online access (Rains, 2008b). As you might expect, people with quick, convenient access to online sources are more likely to use them to access health information (Rains, 2008b).

Third, although they may watch television, members of ethnic co-cultures are more likely to believe interpersonal sources (such as friends and health professionals) than the mainstream media (Cheong, 2007). That's fine if they have ready access to health experts, but many do not. Female African American and Latina adolescents in one study were familiar with breast and lung cancer because they knew of people with those diseases. However, most of the girls had never heard of cervical cancer, even though it was receiving abundant media attention in connection with a new HPV vaccine (Mosavel & El-Shaarawi, 2007). Their lack of knowledge is especially unfortunate because the vaccine is designed primarily for girls their age (Mosavel & El-Shaarawi, 2007).

Fourth, people may filter out new information because it doesn't mesh with what they know or believe. For example, Mexican American women over age 65 often feel that they are expected to spend their time cooking, cleaning, caring for children, and going to church rather than engaging in physical activity for the purpose of staying fit (Balbale, Schwingel, Wojtek, & Huhman, 2014). This proposes a dilemma, as Dutta-Bergman (2005) explains:

> Campaign materials that propose to alter the belief structure of the receiver of the message are not likely to be adhered to. Instead, those individuals who are already interested in the issue end up learning more from the message. (p. 112)

Finally, underprivileged audiences may have different priorities. People who are worried about violence and hunger may feel that long-term health issues are the least of their concerns.

REACHING UNDERINFORMED AUDIENCES

In their article "Lessons From the Field," three noted health promotion specialists urge campaign designers not to overlook marginalized members of society. They write:

> Conducting communication research within diverse ethnic/racial/underserved communities will be especially important in the future. Attention to these audiences is a necessity, not a nicety.... Working with an audience for the first time inevitably brings frustrations as one discovers that principles applied successfully in the past with other populations do not necessarily fit in other contexts. Our experience has been that the potential payoff is worth the initial frustration. (Edgar, Freimuth, & Hammond, 2003, p. 627)

It is not enough to encourage people to engage more with media. We must think, as well, about the subtext, values, and trust issues involved. The term **social capital** encompasses the benefits possible when members of a community build positive social connections and a mutual sense of trust. In terms of social capital, Christopher Beaudoin and Esther Thorson (2006) found that watching television news benefits European Americans significantly more than African Americans. This is mostly because African Americans are so often portrayed negatively in news and entertainment that media images may strengthen prejudice and feelings of powerlessness rather than provide information that African American audiences feel they can trust and use. This may be true even when the messages are well intentioned. For example, highlighting the high incidence of HIV among African Americans and among gay men may get their attention, but it may also strengthen others' prejudice against them.

The challenge for health promoters is to earn trust, respond to community needs, and inform and enable people, at the same time being careful to avoid stigmatizing communities at risk (Smith, 2007). Here are a few suggestions:

- *Focus on social capital*. Recognize that health is not merely a matter of individual control. Prejudice, trust, community resources, social networks, and confidence have profound effects as well. (We cover this idea more thoroughly in Chapter 14.)
- *Tailor materials to audiences' literacy levels*. For example, clinics might educate people with low reading skills by showing instructional health videos in medical waiting rooms. (We'll talk more about tailoring later in this chapter.)
- *Help build online skills and confidence*. For some people, access to health information is limited because they lack a computer or online capability. Even for those with access, a sense of self-efficacy is often missing (Rains, 2008a). Evidence suggests that members of underinformed audiences benefit when they are coached to use the Web knowledgeably and confidently. The National Cancer Institute has helped fund a number of projects to narrow the digital divide by designing websites tailored to the needs of underserved populations and offering community workshops to teach people how to use them (Kreps, 2005).

With these issues in mind, let's turn to the important task of determining exactly whom to target with our campaign.

Segmenting the Audience

As we consider who should receive information about the sports recreation program, it may be tempting to target everyone possible. However, research suggests that appealing to an entire population at one time usually doesn't pay off. Because people tend to evaluate information based on its relevance to them, a broad message may seem too general for anyone to take personally. On the other hand, people tend to take messages more seriously when they identify with the people in them (Moran & Sussman, 2014).

The odds are that, even on small campuses, the population is varied enough to make audience segmentation preferable.

Segmenting an audience means identifying specific groups who are alike in important ways and whose involvement is important to the purpose of the campaign. As we attempt to segment the audience, we must avoid grouping people based on superficial attributes. Characteristics such as race and income are not reliable indicators of how people think and behave. People within those categories may have very divergent viewpoints. Identifying groups on the basis of similar goals and experiences is harder to do but is usually more productive. Following are some questions to consider:

- Who is currently involved (and not involved) in the recommended activity?
- What are people's reasons for participating (or not)?
- Who stands to benefit from the recommended behaviors?
- Who is in most need of these benefits?
- Who might reasonably be expected to adopt these behaviors?
- Is there anyone who should *not* be encouraged to participate?

Remember that some campaigns do more harm than good by recommending behaviors inappropriate for the audience. For example, vigorous exercise is not right for everybody.

Also be open to unexpected combinations. For instance, freshmen and university staff members may be alike in feeling out of place at the campus gym. Where our campaign is concerned, this similarity may be more important than the differences between these groups. Based on these similarities, we might decide that both freshmen and staff members would respond more enthusiastically to personal invitations than to bulletin board notices or Facebook posts.

It's sometimes difficult to decide where to draw the line in segmenting an audience. The choice may be to target a small audience of high-need individuals or a large audience whose needs are less severe. Sometimes campaign designers overlook great opportunities to help small audiences. For example, tobacco harvesters are a relatively isolated and overlooked community within the overall population, but they have serious health concerns. For one, they often suffer from nausea, dizziness, and heart rate disruptions caused by exposure to green tobacco leaves (Parrott & Polonec, 2008). They can minimize their risk by wearing thicker clothing and changing into dry clothes when moisture from the plants soaks them, but little effort has been devoted to educating farmers about this (Parrott & Polonec, 2008). This health concern might not be as widespread as some others, but it is a serious issue for the people involved, and results are reasonably attainable. All in all, there is no definitive rule for choosing between highly focused and more generalized approaches, but health promoters who are sensitive to audience needs and health benefits are most likely to make reasonable judgments.

Based on our audience analysis, we might decide to target our sports recreation campaign toward people new on campus (students, staff, or both), to community members, or to nontraditional students. We might find that current participants do not reflect the racial and ethnic diversity on campus, or that the current membership is mostly men or women, or that people with disabilities are not as involved as they could be. Consequently, we might direct the campaign toward groups that are currently underutilizing the sports recreation program or those people who most need the benefits it offers. And don't forget the current participants. Maybe their involvement can be improved. The possibilities are numerous, making it especially important to know the audience well before choosing a segment of it to target.

Audience as a Person

Once a target focus community has been identified, imagine that audience as a single person, complete "with name, gender, occupation, and lifestyle" (R. Lefebvre et al., 1995, p. 221). With this "person" in mind, Lefebvre and colleagues (1995) pose the following questions for consideration:

- What is important to this person?
- What are the person's feelings, attitudes, and beliefs about the behavior change (including perceived benefits and barriers)?
- What are their media habits?

Imagining the audience as a person is useful in focusing the campaign and in creating messages that seem personal and immediate.

Every audience and every audience member is unique, but some overall characteristics may help guide our efforts. Here is some information that may be useful to us as we attempt to understand our focus community.

Young Audiences

Age may have some effect on how members perceive health messages. Although it's difficult to make generalizations about adult audiences, the developmental stages of youth often have relatively predictable effects.

Children are an important audience. As Erica Weintraub Austin (1995) points out, it's easier to prevent bad habits than to break them. Sending consistent messages to children early on may prevent them from developing unhealthy behaviors later. Evidence supports that children are strongly influenced by adults. On the bright side, young people tend to follow their parents' advice (Moran & Sussman, 2014). However, children often seek to emulate adult behaviors—even the unhealthy ones. Portraying behaviors such as smoking as "adult-only" may actually make them seem more appealing to youngsters.

Adolescents often believe they are unlike other people and that others don't understand them (this is called **personal fable**). Consequently, they are likely to assume that health warnings don't apply to them (Effertz, Franke, & Teichert, 2014). Teenagers also tend to be extremely self-conscious and to feel that people are scrutinizing their appearance and behavior (this is called **imaginary audience**). This makes them sensitive to peer pressure and social approval, which can work for or against health promotion efforts (Helms et al., 2014). A third factor, called **psychological reactance**, characterizes adolescents' desire to assert their independence and sense of personal control (Brehm, 1966). They often resent it when they feel that other people are telling them what to do, and they may rebel just to avoid feeling controlled.

Despite the challenges, there is some promising research about reaching adolescents.

- *Focus on immediate concerns*. Austin (1995) reminds health promoters that teens' immediate social concerns may outweigh their long-term health considerations. In Austin's words, adolescents may "care more that smoking will make their breath smell bad than that they could develop cancer" (p. 115).
- *Emphasize personal choice*. Adolescents tend to react negatively to messages that restrict their freedom of choice (Rains & Turner, 2007; Lee, 2010). Message resistance might be reduced with a passage like this: "You might feel that your freedom to choose how you will consume alcohol is being threatened. However, the facts about binge drinking . . . are pretty powerful when you think about them" (Richards & Banas, 2015, p. 455). It may also be useful to conclude messages with "restoration of freedom" passages such as, "We all make our own decisions and act as we choose to act. Obviously, you make your own decisions too. The choice is yours. You're free to decide for yourself" (Miller, Lane, Deatrick, Young, & Potts, 2007, p. 240).
- *Remember that there are many stages of youth*. A few years can make a big difference in how young audiences respond. Hye-Jin Paek's (2008) data indicate that younger children respond well to school-based programs, whereas older teens benefit more from high-sensation appeals and fact-based information, such as the truth® campaign's presentation of tobacco-related statistics and tobacco-industry memos.

Sensation-Seekers

The **activation model for information exposure** supports two premises: first, that persuasive messages are most effective when they stimulate an optimal amount of arousal in the reader/viewer; and second, that what is "optimal" for one person may be boring or too intense for another (Donohew, Palmgreen, & Duncan, 1980). For example, reactions were mixed when a police

The danger with high sensation-seekers is that risky behaviors appeal to them. Not only are they less likely than others to take recommended precautions, they are more likely to be in dangerous situations in the first place.

department in Wales released don't-text-while-driving PSAs that showed bloody images from automobile accidents. American broadcasters declined to air the PSAs, but the campaign's creators argued that people should know how horrific the outcomes of distracted driving can be (Inbar, 2009). Graphic images on cigarette packages (see photo below) are another example. Some countries now require that tobacco companies dispense with attractive colors and instead package their products with realistic images of tobacco and nicotine's effects on the body. The argument is the same—that, while some people may be offended, the shock value is necessary to impact audiences who tend to ignore health threats otherwise. The Meth Project is yet another example, which we will address later in this chapter.

The activation model can apply to audiences of any age or description. So far, researchers and campaign designers have used it most extensively for adolescent and young-adult audiences, who are more likely than others to be high sensation-seekers, meaning that they enjoy new and intense experiences (Everett & Palmgreen, 1995; Zuckerman, 1994). The danger with high sensation-seekers is that risky behaviors appeal to them. Not only are they less likely than others to take precautions, they are more apt to be in dangerous situations in the first place. For instance, compared to their peers, high sensation-seekers are more likely to think smoking is appealing (Paek, 2008). They are typically more impulsive about having sex, yet less willing than others to use condoms (Noar, Zimmerman, Palmgreen, Lustria, & Horosewski, 2006). And they tend to associate with other high sensation-seekers, which can make their behaviors seem normal rather than dangerous or extreme (Wang et al., 2014). These factors may be challenging for health promoters. But also keep in mind that because high sensation-seekers are receptive to novel situations, they typically welcome diversity and intercultural communication (Arasaratnam & Banerjee, 2011). Thus, they may be less ethnocentric and more open minded than other people are, which may make them receptive to a range of health-related messages and spokespeople.

Here are a few promising lines of research about appealing to high sensation-seekers:

- *Make messages varied and intense.* Messages that have quick and vivid visual edits and loud and fast music typically have the most impact on high sensation-seekers, teens, and tweens (9- to 12-year-olds) (Lang, Schwartz, Lee, & Angelini, 2007; Niederdeppe, Davis, Farrelly, & Yarsevich, 2007).
- *Make the most of low-distraction environments.* Both intense- and mild-content antismoking PSAs had an impact on high sensation-seekers when they were exposed to the messages in a controlled classroom environment (Helme, Donohew, Baier, & Zittleman, 2007).
- *Run PSAs during popular programs.* High sensation-seekers who watch a lot of television don't necessarily remember a lot about the PSAs they see. But they do typically remember the PSAs that appear during their favorite programs (often sports, comedies, and cartoons for 16- to 25-year-olds) (D'Silva & Palmgreen, 2007).

Part of the dilemma, of course, is that the intense messages that sensation-seekers enjoy may be too much for most audiences, making it difficult to target high-risk individuals without offending others. (For other ethical considerations about health promotion, see Box 13.3.)

As we complete Step 2 in creating a health campaign, it may seem that, although we have already done a lot of work, we still don't know what the

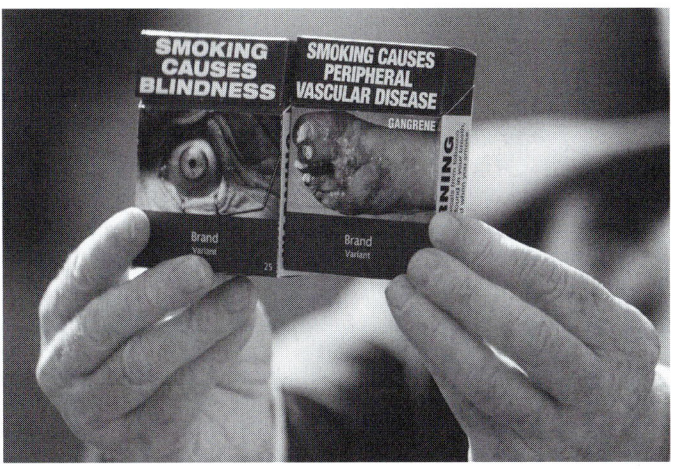

In 2015, regulators in Ireland followed Australia's example by ruling that cigarette packages depict graphic warning images such as those above rather than splashy brand-name packaging. There is some evidence that graphic images discourage teens from smoking, particularly if they are not already heavy smokers (Andrews, Netemeyer, Kees, & Burton, 2014).

BOX 13.3 Ethical Considerations

The Politics of Prevention—Who Should Pay?

Health promotion may seem like a win–win situation. If people can be encouraged to prevent disease and injuries, they will enjoy better health and the nation's health costs will be minimized. How far should we carry this line of reasoning? Should people who work hard to be healthy get discount prices on health care and insurance? Should they be given advantages when competing for jobs? If people knowingly engage in unhealthy behaviors, should society help pay for their medical bills?

Some 86% of America's health care dollar pays for care of people with chronic health conditions, many of which could have been avoided with healthier diets, more exercise, and abstention from alcohol and tobacco (CDC, 2015). The added expense eats up tax money and leads to hikes in health insurance rates. As Daniel Wikler (1987) puts it, "The person who takes risks with his [or her] own health gambles with resources which belong to others" (p. 14). Some theorists argue that people who continue risky behavior (such as smoking, overeating, or driving without seatbelts) when they know it is bad for them should pay from their own pockets when their behavior leads to medical expenses.

In a related issue, some feel that companies that profit from selling unhealthy products should pay part of the health bill. State governments have successfully sued tobacco companies for damages, charging that it's unfair for them to make huge profits while others foot the enormous bill of treating tobacco-related illnesses. Experts estimate that smoking costs Americans $193 billion a year in medical expenses and lost productivity (CDC, 2011). Around the world, more than 5 million people a year die from tobacco-related illnesses, including 600,000 who are killed by the effects of secondhand smoke (WHO, 2012).

Some companies now refuse to hire smokers or people who are extremely overweight because they are at greater health risk, and thus are likely to cost the company more money than others in terms of health benefits and sick leave. Similarly, some insurance companies offer a discount to people who do not smoke and those who remain accident free or who complete informational programs such as defensive-driving courses.

On the other side of the issue, some worry that governments and employers are becoming too involved in people's lifestyle decisions. Some charge that groups like Mothers Against Drunk Driving (MADD) are taking a good thing too far by seeking to punish people for drinking even small amounts of alcohol. Some people say that increasing the "sin taxes" on alcohol and tobacco will hurt consumers, not companies, and they are afraid the taxes will be extended to cover snack foods and other not-so-healthy items. A third argument is that health concerns such as obesity are not always matters of individual control. Obesity has many causes, including social norms and heredity. People may gain weight because of medications or other health conditions. However, media coverage tends to sway the public toward considering obesity as either an individualistic or a societal issue (Kim & Willis, 2007). All in all, opponents of tighter health requirements say you cannot assume people are fully in control of their health, and you cannot control the risks people take without also controlling their freedom of choice.

What Do You Think?

1. Should people who knowingly take health risks pay more than others for health insurance? Should they be denied insurance? Should they be denied health services?
2. Should people be required by law to engage in healthy practices such as being immunized and exercising regularly?
3. Should it be against the law to sell or advertise products known to have a high health risk? Does it matter if such products are addictive?
4. Do you agree with the rationale behind many states' seatbelt and motorcycle helmet laws—that people who neglect safety precautions not only endanger their own lives but also increase the trauma and expense for everybody?
5. How do you weigh the argument that some people are not well informed about health issues (perhaps because they cannot read or cannot afford a computer) and that it is unfair to expect them to follow health guidelines about which they know little?

continued

6. In your opinion, which of the following behaviors (if any) should be grounds for denying or limiting health benefits? On what criteria do you make your judgments?
   Smoking
   Engaging in unprotected sex
   Exceeding the speed limit
   Snow skiing
   Neglecting to exercise regularly
   Overeating
   Playing football
   Rescuing accident victims

7. If a person has a family history of a disease, should that person be required by society to take extra health precautions?

campaign will involve. Our efforts to this point will not go to waste. Research shows that health campaigns launched without a clear understanding of the audience, current situation, and potential benefits are often frustrating to create and ineffective at reaching their goals. With a focus community in mind, we are ready for Step 3.

Step 3: Establishing Campaign Goals and Objectives

By this point we should have a fairly clear impression of the sports recreation department, its potential benefits, and the people we most want to reach with our campaign. Collecting and analyzing data have prepared us to establish specific objectives for our campaign. **Objectives** state in clear, measurable terms exactly what we hope to achieve with the campaign. We might consider the following questions:

- What exactly do we want people to start/stop/continue doing?
- If we hope to encourage a particular behavior, when (and for how long) should it occur to be of benefit?
- How will we know if our campaign has been successful?

Relevant to the sports recreation campaign, we may decide that signing up 40 freshmen in three months would constitute success. Or perhaps we have decided to focus on students with disabilities or on newcomers. Our objective may be to get at least 20 current participants to bring an individual from one of those groups to an event.

We must make sure our objectives are oriented to the overall purpose of the campaign. For instance, if people participate in one climbing-wall session or one yoga class, will there be health benefits? Will our campaign have succeeded in reaching its goal(s)? If better health is the goal, then it may be important that campaign messages aim for ongoing attendance—perhaps participating in activities once a week for at least two months.

Let's think ahead about exactly how we will measure the effects of the campaign. This may involve follow-up surveys or sign-up sheets to keep track of participation. Setting measurable goals will allow us (and others) to determine if the campaign has been a success.

Health promoters are increasingly being held accountable for their efforts. **Accountability** means demonstrating how the results of a project compare to the money and/or time invested in it. Consider once again the condom promotion campaign mentioned earlier in this chapter. Lim and colleagues (2019) spent several years working on the project and, in the end, they successfully increased condom use among their target audience by a considerable amount. The project was funded by the Singapore Ministry of Health and—given the campaign's great success—ministry officials may continue funding it or similar campaigns, especially given the benefit to society when HIV risk is reduced.

Sometimes, however, campaign results are inconclusive or underwhelming. Even then, by analyzing and accounting for a campaign's results, researchers can learn valuable lessons about what works and what doesn't. For instance, when researchers replicated anti-vaping PSAs and showed them to smokers and persons who both smoked and vaped, the researchers discovered that the PSAs had the opposite effect than intended—they actually stimulated audience members' urge to vape (Sanders-Jackson, Clayton, Tan, & Yie, 2019)! It turns out that PSAs that show e-cigarettes being used along with visible vapor (i.e., the "smoke" that is exhaled while vaping) activate the brain's motivational system, stimulate positive emotion, increase memory formation, and trigger urges (Sanders-Jackson et al., 2019). PSAs without the vapor do not have the same effects, leading researchers to recommend that future anti-vaping campaigns omit vapor altogether (Sanders-Jackson et al., 2019). This lesson (if heeded) can help ensure that health promoters' time and campaign dollars are not squandered producing counterproductive messages.

When public funds finance health campaigns, it is especially important to show that the campaigns work. Otherwise, money that might be spent on other (proven) prevention campaigns and/or treatment programs is wasted. Consider the Meth Project. It started as a privately funded campaign in Montana in 2005, quickly becoming famous for its use of graphic images and shocking scenarios—decaying teeth, skin sores, skeletal bodies, teens trading sex with older men for meth, attempted suicides, overdoses, and more (you can view the ads at http://www.methproject.org/ads/tv/). Meth use in Montana declined after the campaign launched—by as much as 63% among teens, according to campaign directors ("Meth Project," 2010). The campaign won dozens of awards and was praised by the White House as "one of the country's most powerful and creative prevention programs, and a model for the nation" ("Meth Project," 2010, para. 8). The Meth Project was replicated in several other states, supported largely by millions of dollars in state and federal funds.

But when the original Montana campaign was examined by two researchers working independently, each concluded that there was no statistical evidence that the Meth Project worked and, surprisingly, the campaign was associated with lowered perceived health risks and increased meth use among some teens (Anderson, 2010; Erceg-Hurn, 2008). The campaign producers were faulted for not capturing a baseline for comparison and for not taking into account a preexisting downward trend in meth use, which was attributable to other factors (e.g., beefed-up law enforcement efforts). When D. Mark Anderson (2010) compared Montana's rate of meth use against 10 years' worth of state and national data, he found the campaign "had no discernable impact" (p. 732) and recommended against continued public funding. Although law enforcement and government officials believe the Meth Project works, the studies' authors question the appropriateness of allocating public

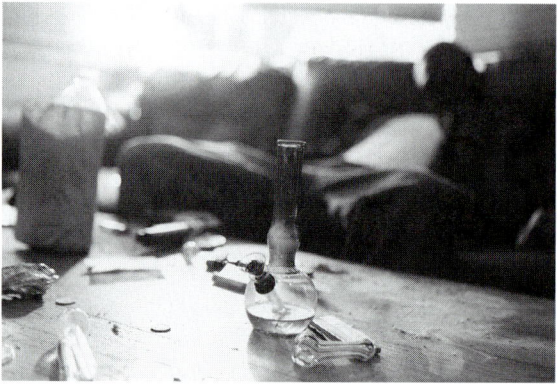

Have you seen Meth Project PSAs? Do you believe the ads are effective? Why or why not? Do you think public funds should be used to finance the campaign? How do you reconcile law enforcers' and legislators' insistence that the campaign works, despite statistical evidence suggesting it doesn't?

funds for the project and, as we will discuss in Chapter 14, the utility of fear appeals.

Step 4: Selecting Channels of Communication

A **channel** is a means of communicating information, either directly (in person) or indirectly (via technology). The term "channel" often has been used to refer to media channels, such as TV, radio, and newspapers. But "channel" can also describe health fairs, church meetings, community theater productions, game shows (e.g., the THINK campaign), and one-on-one interventions.

Sometimes channel selection is limited by time or money. Our sports recreation enrollment effort will probably not involve full-color magazine ads, billboards, or sophisticated television commercials. Nevertheless, as health promoters, we should be familiar with all types of channels. Moreover, let's not assume too quickly that a channel is out of our reach. For example, we may not produce television commercials, but we might book appearances on campus or community television talk shows.

Channel Characteristics

Let's consider the advantages and limitations of different channels. Experts suggest that channels for a health campaign be evaluated in terms of reach, specificity, and impact (Schooler, Chaffee, Flora, & Roser, 1998). **Reach** refers to the number of people who will be exposed to a message via a particular channel. **Specificity** refers to how accurately the message can be targeted to a specific group of people. **Impact** is how influential a message is likely to be.

Television and the internet usually have larger and more diverse audiences than other media. As such, they have immense reach. However, when audiences are large and diverse, it can be hard to tailor messages to particular people. Television, especially, has low specificity, although that has changed somewhat with the creation of special-interest cable and satellite, and streaming programs. The internet and social media can be more specific, if we put the effort into selecting people within the target audience and/or posting information with specific identifiers that will lead interested people to it.

Although it may be tempting to aim for the broadest reach possible, it's advisable to focus on our target audience. Exposure that is broader than necessary can waste resources and contribute to information overload, making it difficult for people to identify which messages are most important and relevant to them (Lang, 2006).

Message Impact

The channels we select influence the nature and impact of our messages. In the interest of selecting the most effective channels, we next consider two factors relevant to message impact: arousal and involvement.

AROUSAL

Arousal refers to how emotionally stimulating and exciting a message is (Schooler et al., 1998). When we view words and images about risky products—such as condoms, liquor, and cigarettes—we typically experience greater emotional and physical arousal than with more innocuous products such as water and vegetables (Lang, Chung, Lee, & Zhao, 2005). We tend to identify the risky products more quickly and remember them longer (Lang et al., 2005). This can make it difficult for healthy campaign messages (especially if they are sedate) to compete with advertisements for unhealthy products.

Interactive computer programs are a good example of high-arousal messages that can be used to promote healthy behaviors. Interactive, on-screen messages are often very engrossing, with colorful graphics, moving images, and sound. Roberto and colleagues (2007) report success using an interactive computer program to involve high school students in safer sex and pregnancy-prevention efforts. Compared to other students, those who took part in the online program were more knowledgeable about STIs, more aware of their personal risk, more reluctant to have sex, and more confident about their ability to use safer sex practices if they did have sex. The THINK campaign, in addition to putting on shows in entertainment establishments, directed men to a website that had videos and an interactive HIV risk calculator. As mentioned, the campaign succeeded in getting men to use condoms during casual sex and it contributed to their HIV-risk knowledge (Lim et al., 2019).

INVOLVEMENT

Involvement is the amount of mental effort required to understand a message. Interpersonal communication is high involvement. It requires a great deal of thought and action. Thus, health professionals, family members, and friends tend to have high impact. Reading is also high-involvement, because people must use their imaginations. Television is low involvement, because viewers more passively observe the sounds and sights displayed for them.

The **elaboration likelihood model** proposes that when we are highly involved with a message, we pay close attention to details and evaluate the message thoroughly. As a consequence, we tend to remember high-involvement messages longer than others and are more likely to act on them (Briñol & Petty, 2006; Petty & Cacioppo, 1981). In short, people usually pay closer attention when using high-involvement channels, such as reading and talking, and this affects how much they are influenced by the information. Surveys show that people who use high-involvement channels are usually better informed about health than people who rely on low-involvement channels such as television.

Evidence suggests that **tailored messages—those that are designed to be personally relevant to the recipients**—generally have greater impact on recipients' behaviors than messages that are more generic in nature (Lustria et al., 2013). The impact and degree of tailoring differs widely. At one level, images might be tailored to match the age group and general appearance of a media consumer (Ahn, 2015). At another level, messages may be tailored in multiple ways using

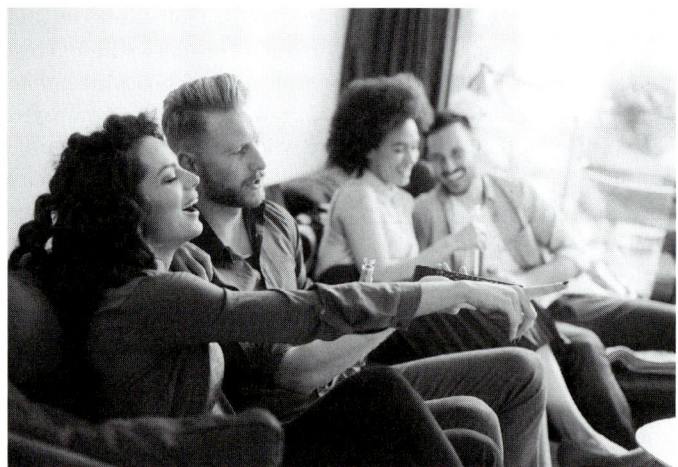

Audiences in positive moods, as when they are watching comedies, tend to be more receptive than others to detection messages (e.g., breast self-exam, cancer screening, and so on). Audiences in negative moods—when, say, they are watching dramas or news shows—are typically more receptive to prevention messages, such as using sunscreen (Anghelcev & Sar, 2011).

complex computer algorithms. For example, rather than sift through dozens of web pages for information that is useful to you, you might log onto an interactive site and answer a number of questions about your background, lifestyle, goals, frustrations, and so on. Based on your responses, the system will sift through information for you and present a collection of resources (information, videos, photos, community resources, live links, and so on) chosen specifically to suit your needs. Some programs paraphrase and reflect your input much like a real-life counselor would. For example, you might get an on-screen message that reads something like this:

> On the one hand you think it is not that important to become more physically active because you have a very busy life. On the other hand you do think it is important to become more active because physical activity helps you to relax. . . . This is a very common and very understandable situation. Many people find it convenient to deal with this situation by assessing what their current activity schedule is like on a typical day in their lives. As the next step, they decide whether they spend enough time doing things they really think are important. Maybe this could be an interesting idea for you, too? (Friederichs et al., 2014, p. 11)

Based on the tenets of the elaboration likelihood model, we are likely to pay close attention to messages such as these that feel relevant to us as individuals.

Valerie Pilling and Laura Brannon (2007) took a tailored approach in creating a responsible-drinking website for college students. Some students in the study viewed a website tailored to suit their personalities (either responsible, communicative, logical, or adventuresome), while others viewed more general messages about the dangers of binge drinking. Students who viewed the tailored messages were significantly more likely than the others to consider the website interesting, to predict that it would be effective, and to say that the materials affected their attitudes about drinking.

Messages can also be tailored based on culture, ethnicity, literacy, educational attainment, health status, and so on. Health promoters often use multiple strategies to tailor health messages. As described by Marisa Torres-Ruiz and colleagues (2018), five common strategies are:

- *Sociocultural:* Using cultural values, beliefs, attitudes, and behaviors to contextualize health messages for the target audience.
- *Constituent-Involving:* Soliciting input from members of the target community to aid/improve message tailoring (e.g., the THINK campaign).
- *Linguistic:* Translating messages into the targeted group's preferred language.
- *Evidential:* Using evidence to show how the issue/topic is relevant to members of the target audience and why they should pay attention.
- *Peripheral:* Designing campaign materials and messages to appeal to a specific group (e.g., using fast edits and loud music to appeal to young audiences).

Research suggests that relying on just one strategy to tailor your message might not be enough. Instead, use multiple strategies to ensure that the message resonates with your intended audience. For example, analyzing anti-meth PSAs led Joseph Scarpaci and Christine Burke (2016) to advise against "merely translating Anglo spots into Spanish" (p. 168).

Without attending to sociocultural concerns, translation alone "is an insufficient strategy to reach Hispanic youth because it targets rather than tailors its message" (p. 168).

Even if we cannot create tailored versions of our campus fitness campaign for individual users or groups of users, it's clear that directing our message to a clear target audience will likely enhance its impact.

Multichannel Campaigns

As you have seen, broadcasting and narrowcasting have advantages. Many times, the best chance of making a difference is to reach people through several channels. Multichannel efforts are important because people have different communication patterns and preferences. What reaches and appeals to some people may not reach and/or appeal to others. For these reasons, multichannel campaigns are the norm these days. For instance, consider the culture-centered community campaign overseen by Mohan J. Dutta and colleagues (2019). While addressing health disparities and information resources in African American communities, Dutta led a team of researchers and community members who devised a multichannel approach for educating audiences about cardiovascular disease. Community members created a powerful and effective campaign that relied on mass media (television, radio, and print ads), health fairs, church meetings, information cards passed out by community leaders, postcards distributed by providers in health clinics, face-to-face interventions, community events, community-based performances, websites, and Facebook (Dutta et al., 2019). Compared with a control group, community members who were exposed to the campaign "showed higher overall knowledge levels" (Dutta et al., 2019, p. 1081) about certain cardiovascular issues such as atrial fibrillation and treatments like heart medications.

Social media was an important channel in Dutta et al.'s (2019) study and, increasingly, health promoters are encouraged to use social media in health campaigns because it is cost-effective and has tremendous reach. While some researchers are divided over social media's impact, Liang Chen and Xiaodong Yang (2019) found that there was no difference between social media and traditional media when they studied messages that encouraged breast self-examinations. Women exposed to high-threat/high-efficacy fear appeals in printed brochures and on social media had near identical responses—increased intention to perform breast self-exams—when compared with women who viewed low threat and/or low efficacy messages. It was message content, not the channel, that influenced participants' behavior. Thus, social media can be just as effective as traditional media when it comes to changing people's health behaviors.

Mass-media, social media, and interpersonal channels are complementary, in that media messages often influence what people think and talk about; at the same time, people are influenced by discussions with neighbors and family members (i.e., interpersonal channels). **Diffusion of innovations** theory describes a multistep process in which new information is filtered and passed along throughout a community (Brosius & Weimann, 1996; Lazarsfeld, Burleson, & Gaudet, 1948; Rogers, 1983). Research shows that some community members are opinion leaders who have credibility by virtue of their expertise or social standing. They often pass along new ideas and information from the media to other people. In this way, mass media messages may influence people indirectly, whether they use the media or not.

In our campaign, we may find that in addition to using multiple channels, targeting opinion leaders on campus (e.g., popular professors, athletes, or student groups) will help spread our message. This tactic has proven successful in other health campaigns. For example, researchers found that there was a 22% reduction in the odds of becoming a smoker among students whose schools participated in an antismoking campaign that involved "peer supporters" sharing information with other students (Holliday, Audrey, Campbell, & Moore, 2016). "Peer supporters" were students who had large social networks (i.e., they knew and were known by many students). Additionally, researchers working in China found that people with a lot of social media connections and followers were uniquely positioned to spread messages encouraging organ donation because the messages they post are likely to be retweeted or reposted, thereby expanding the messages' reach (Shi & Salmon, 2018). The study's findings were so promising that the researchers strongly encouraged health promoters to target well-connected social media opinion leaders when devising health campaigns.

As you can see, a lot of planning goes into crafting an effective health campaign. The steps necessary for designing and implementing a campaign are covered in the next chapter.

Summary

Planning Health Promotion Campaigns

- Health promotion campaigns are systematic efforts to influence people to engage in health-enhancing behaviors.
- A health promoter is anyone involved in the process of creating and distributing health promotion messages.
- Successful health promotion recognizes that people do not necessarily change their behaviors because they have been presented with new health information.
- As campaign designers, we must take into account the concerns, habits, and preferences of the people we wish to influence.
- Campaigns with the best chance of succeeding talk to people where they are, whether it is the beauty salon, the athletic field, or the doctor's office.

Background on Health Campaigns

- Early health campaigns were designed with the view that people act to ensure their own health and longevity. From that viewpoint it follows that if people know a behavior is unhealthy, they will not engage in it. But influencing people's behavior is not that simple.
- People are motivated by a number of factors that make them more or less receptive to health information and more or less motivated to change their behavior.
- The best campaigns involve members of the focus population as active participants and recruit social support for healthy behaviors. Furthermore, they speak with many voices, including the concerned tones of loved ones, the calm assurance of experts, and the printed and recorded messages of mass media and social media.
- Good campaigns also make it practical for people to adopt healthy behaviors, even if it means changing public policy, offering free or easy-to-access options, and building communication infrastructures.
- Health campaign success stories show that it is important to know the audience well, take positive action, establish clear goals, measure success, and make behaviors socially rewarding.
- Whereas illness and disease prevention seem to benefit everyone, ethical dilemmas are involved, such as: Should people be rewarded or penalized based on their health-related behavior? How should we balance people's right to choose for themselves with society's interest in keeping costs down? Where do we draw the line between healthy and unhealthy behaviors?

Step 1: Defining the Situation and Potential Benefits

- The first step in creating a health campaign is to research potential benefits of the campaign. Find out who stands to gain, who is already behaving according to campaign recommendations, and what alternatives exist.
- In assessing the situation, it's important not to assume that everyone is motivated in the same way. People are most receptive to options that satisfy them on many levels (intellectual, emotional, personal, social, and so on).

Step 2: Analyzing and Segmenting the Audience

- The second step is to choose a target audience.
- Because people are inclined to pay more attention to messages that seem relevant to them, campaigns directed at "everyone" may not pique the interest of anyone.
- Interviews, questionnaires, and focus groups are useful ways to learn about potential audience members—what they like, what they know, how they typically behave, what they consider important, and more.
- We may wish to target people in great need or those who are most likely to respond to the campaign. At the same time, keep in mind audience characteristics such as self-consciousness, sensation hunger, confidence, need for independence, and psychological reactance.
- It is often challenging to reach audiences who are culturally different from the mainstream. However, considering the knowledge gap hypothesis, these audiences are often the most in need of health information and assistance.

Step 3: Establishing Campaign Goals and Objectives

- The third step in creating a health campaign is to establish clear and measurable objectives so we can accurately assess a campaign's effects.

Step 4: Selecting Channels of Communication

- Fourth, we select channels through which to communicate campaign messages.
- Channels typically differ in terms of reach, specificity, and impact.
- Often, the best campaigns make use of several channels.
- People usually pay closer attention when using high-involvement channels, such as reading and talking, and this affects how much they are influenced by the information. People who use high-involvement channels are usually better informed about health than people who rely on low-involvement channels such as television.
- Sometimes tailored messages are more effective than broadcast ones, in that tailored messages focus on information that is well suited to an individual's interests, abilities, and resources.
- All in all, the media play an important role in promoting health issues, but media impact is limited without interpersonal reinforcement.

Glossary

accountability Demonstrating how the results of a project compare to the money and/or time invested in it. *See page 311.*

activation model for information exposure An idea that encompasses two premises: first, that persuasive messages are most effective when they stimulate an optimal amount of arousal in the reader/viewer; and second, that what is "optimal" for one person may be boring or too intense for another. *See page 308.*

arousal How emotionally stimulating and exciting a message is. *See page 313.*

channel A means of communicating information, either directly (in person) or indirectly (via technology). *See page 312.*

close-ended questions Questions that can be answered with brief replies. *See page 303.*

diffusion of innovations Theory that describes the multistep process in which new information is filtered and passed along throughout a community. *See page 315.*

digital divide The gulf that separates the information rich, who have easy access to the internet (predominantly young, well-educated city dwellers), from the information poor, who are often rural residents with limited or no online access. *See page 305.*

elaboration likelihood model A model that proposes that when people are highly involved with a message, they pay close attention to details and evaluate the message thoroughly. *See page 313.*

fixed-alternative questions Questions that provide multiple-choice answers. *See page 303.*

focus group A small number of people who respond to questions posed by a moderator. *See page 304.*

health-promoting behaviors Actions that enhance health, reduce health risks, and prevent disease. *See page 296.*

health promotion campaigns Systematic efforts to influence people to engage in health-enhancing behaviors; may involve the use of many communication channels, from face-to-face communication to mass media. *See page 296.*

highly scheduled interviews A type of interaction in which interviewers are given specific questions to ask and are not allowed to make comments or ask additional questions. *See page 303.*

imaginary audience The belief among adolescents that people are scrutinizing their appearance and behavior. *See page 308.*

impact How influential a message is likely to be. *See page 313.*

institutional review board (IRB) An ethics panel that reviews and monitors research efforts to ensure that participants are treated fairly. *See page 303.*

involvement The amount of mental effort required to understand a message. *See page 313.*

knowledge gap hypothesis Belief that people with plentiful information resources (such as televisions, computers, and well-informed friends and advisors) are likely to know more and to continue learning more than people with fewer information resources. *See page 305.*

moderately scheduled interviews Interactions in which interviewers are given a set of questions but are allowed to ask for clarification and additional information as they see fit. *See page 303.*

nudging The practice of making healthy options readily apparent, appealing, and available. *See page 300.*

objectives Clear and measurable terms that state exactly what a campaign's designers hope to achieve. *See page 311.*

open-ended questions Questions that require more than a simple one-word answer and allow respondents to express ideas in their own words. *See page 303.*

personal fable An egocentric belief often held by adolescents that they are unlike other people and that others don't understand them. *See page 308.*

psychological reactance An unpleasant reaction to persons, rules, or regulations that threaten or eliminate behavioral freedoms. Reactance occurs when people feel that their choices are limited. *See page 308.*

questionnaire A set of printed or written questions with a choice of answers, devised for the purposes of a survey or statistical study. *See page 303.*

reach The number of people who will be exposed to a message via a particular channel. *See page 313.*

sampling Process of selecting people from a larger population for measurement. *See page 304.*

segmenting an audience Identifying specific groups who are alike in important ways and whose involvement is important to the purpose of the campaign. *See page 307.*

social capital Encompasses the benefits possible when members of a community build positive social connections and a mutual sense of trust. *See page 306.*

sensation-seekers People who enjoy new and intense experiences. *See page 309.*

specificity How accurately the message can be targeted to a specific group of people. *See page 313.*

tailored messages Messages that are designed to be personally relevant to the recipients. *See page 313.*

unscheduled interviews Interactions in which interviewers are given a list of topics but are encouraged to phrase questions as they wish and to probe for more information when it seems useful and appropriate. *See page 303.*

Discussion Questions

1. Describe the strategy and principles of the truth® campaign. How do they relate to the principles suggested throughout the chapter?

2. What are five qualities of good campaigns, as illustrated by the exemplary campaigns in this chapter? Find or think of other campaigns that embody one or more of these best practices.

3. Using your classmates as a target audience, conduct a quick focus group to identify an important health interest they have in common. Then develop a simple survey to find out more about their current practices, goals, barriers, and preferences regarding this health issue.

4. Using the knowledge gap hypothesis, explain why people of low socioeconomic status are often underinformed about health issues. How does the digital divide figure in? What are some tips for reaching underinformed audiences?

5. Explain the activation model for information exposure. Link it to the concept of sensation seeking.

6. Deliver campaign messages via a variety of channels. Compare them in terms of reach, specificity, impact, arousal, and involvement.

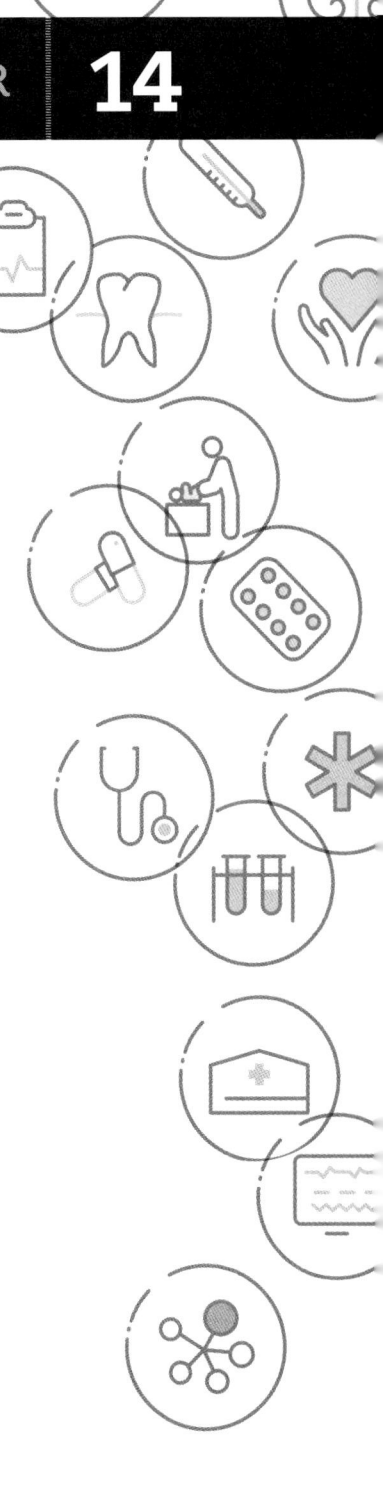

CHAPTER 14

Designing and Implementing Health Campaigns

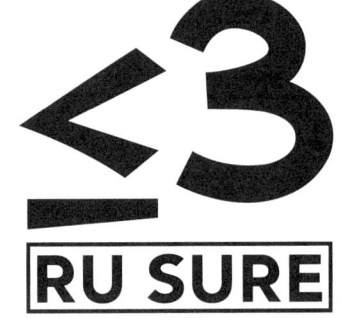

One of the most widely emulated health communication campaigns on college campuses is RU SURE, developed in the 1990s at Rutgers University to curb dangerous alcohol consumption. The campaign, which is still going strong today, challenges students to reconsider the notion that most young adults drink to excess. RU SURE materials make the point (as in the graphic to the right) that two-thirds of Rutgers students actually stop drinking after three or fewer drinks ("RU SURE," 2015). In fact, one in five students don't drink at all ("RU SURE," 2019). By providing students with accurate statistics, campaign sponsors hope to clarify that the norm is less extreme than many students may think; thus students need not drink excessively to fit in with their peers (Lederman & Stewart, 2005; Lederman et al., 2001; Menegatos, Lederman, & Hess, 2010).

The RU SURE campaign is famous for its high level of student involvement and its novel ways of integrating campaign messages into everyday campus life. The campaign is designed by students for students. "Communication majors are involved in all aspects of this campaign, from designing ways to deliver campaign messages to gathering evaluation data," says Lea Stewart, professor and director of the Rutgers Center for Communication and Health Issues. "Since no one works on the campaign without first learning about the scope and consequences of dangerous drinking among college students, we reach two audiences: our target audience of first-year students and a secondary audience of upper-level students."

Through the years, students in the campaign have designed and distributed free T-shirts featuring a "Top Ten Misperceptions" list about life at Rutgers, including three misperceptions about drinking as well as humorous myths such as, "You don't need shower shoes for the dorms." They have also engaged students in RU SURE Bingo games, developed curricula supplements for campus courses, and developed partnerships with community leaders and others. The campaign seems to be effective. Students' estimates of peer drinking at Rutgers dropped considerably once RU SURE began (Lederman, Stewart, & Russ, 2007; Stewart et al., 2002).

Like many health-promotion efforts, the RU SURE campaign is based on social norms, which we talk about later in this chapter (see Box 14.3), and on social marketing. **Social marketing is an approach wherein campaign designers** apply principles of commercial advertising to prosocial campaigns, such as health-promotion efforts (Lefebvre & Flora, 1988). The rationale is that many of the techniques used to sell goods and services also work well when promoting healthy lifestyles.

Social marketers are often guided by the classic 4Ps of marketing: price, product, promotion, and place (Borden, 1964). From a social marketing perspective,[1] health-related behaviors have a price tag of sorts—they cost something in terms of money, time, energy, or some other investment. The product may be tangible (such as healthy food, condoms, or cleaner drinking water) or intangible (better health, more opportunities, or greater control over one's circumstances). Promotion describes the process, design, and means of sharing information. Place refers to where messages are received (such as online, at a friend's house, or on television) and where the effects may be most felt (within the family, at school, or in the workplace, and so on.)

While the 4Ps may be a good place to start when planning a campaign, many theorists question their utility as a stand-alone model for social marketing. Some advocate adding additional Ps to the model that recognize the importance of people, public policy, physical evidence (used to weigh various options and to evaluate outcomes), purse strings (resources), and processes (conventional ways of doing things and potential alternatives) (Booms & Bitner, 1981; Goyal Wasan & Tripathi, 2014; Kotler & Zaltman, 1971). The two most fundamental challenges to the 4P model are that (a) it focuses on "sellers'" needs (i.e., the need to sell something and make a profit) more than it focuses on "buyers'" needs and (b) it is more oriented to one-time transactions than to ongoing efforts and relationship-building (Grönroos, 1994; Gordon, 2012). In contrast to commercial marketing efforts, social marketers sometimes function more as lobbyists, advocates, and facilitators than as salespeople. For example, they may "go upstream" to address the source of a health issue, as when they advocate for new legislation or stand up to factories that pollute the environment (Gordon, 2012).

Components of social marketing appear throughout the chapter as we continue our conversation about health campaign strategies. But first let's recap. Chapter 13 provided a guide to the first four stages of creating a health campaign:

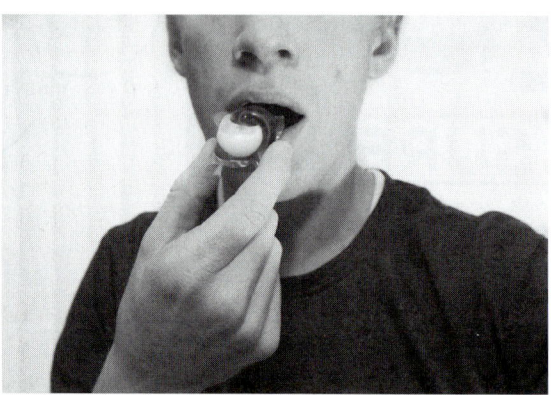

Social norms theory suggests that people base their behavior partly on what people around them do. The RU SURE campaign shows how social norms can be used to improve health. But social norms can also harm health. As proof, consider the popularity of social media challenges. The Tide Pod Challenge involves people recording themselves eating laundry detergent pods, which contain bleach and other dangerous chemicals, and then posting the videos online. One such video garnered over 2 million views!

Have you noticed other social media challenges? If so, what do you think of them? Have you participated in a social media challenge? Why or why not?

---

[1] Be careful not to confuse social marketing with social norms theory, which we talk about later in the chapter. Social marketing is a general approach, whereas social norms theory proposes that people base their behavior partly on what they consider to be normal among their peers.

Step 1: Defining the situation and potential benefits
Step 2: Analyzing and segmenting the audience
Step 3: Establishing campaign goals and objectives
Step 4: Selecting channels of communication

The process continues in this chapter with a description of key theories and techniques to create health-promotion campaigns. The hypothetical sports recreation campaign we began in Chapter 13 helps illustrate how a health-promotion effort comes together. We will continue it in this chapter. Keep in mind that the same steps apply to campaigns of various sizes on any number of health topics.

This chapter begins by introducing four influential models of behavior change: the health belief model, social cognitive theory, the theory of reasoned action, and the transtheoretical model. We then explore the critical-cultural approach and describe the three final stages in campaign development:

Step 5: Designing campaign messages
Step 6: Piloting and implementing the campaign
Step 7: Evaluating and maintaining the campaign

Along the way, we will touch on a number of message-design perspectives, including the role of affect, social norms theory, the theory of normative social behavior, and the extended parallel process model.

Theories of Behavior Change

The theories described here emphasize that people make lifestyle decisions based on a complex array of factors, including personal perceptions, skills, social pressure, convenience, and more. Understanding these factors—and the theories that describe them—can help us design better campaign messages. Moreover, "theory-driven interventions are more likely to be effective than atheoretical approaches to health promotion" (Gothe, 2018, p. 744).

Each of the theories discussed here has earned considerable respect among health communication scholars and health promoters. Space is not available to discuss each model in great detail, but this introduction should help orient you to the rich scholarship behind health campaign efforts and provide opportunities for further investigation. Applying these theories to health campaigns can have a positive effect—at least some of the time. Keep in mind that theories are only guiding principles, not magic formulas. No one theory works all of the time or with every audience.

Health Belief Model

The **health belief model** proposes that we base our behavior choices on five primary considerations (Rosenstock, 1960; Stretcher & Rosenstock, 1997). Namely, we are most motivated to change our behaviors if we believe that:

- we will be adversely affected if we do not change;
- the adverse effects will be considerable;
- behavior change will be effective in preventing the undesired outcome;
- the effort and cost of preventive behavior is worthwhile; and
- we are moved to action by a novel or eye-opening occurrence, such as a brush with danger, a compelling warning message, or an alluring incentive.

In short, motivation is based on an individual's perception of personal susceptibility, serious consequences, worthwhile benefits, barriers/costs, and cues to actions.

Critics have pointed out that the health belief model does not specify how the variables should be ordered, which variables are more important (or if they are equally important), or if the variables interact with one another (Jones et al., 2015). Consequently, one may wonder if a campaign message must have all five variables in order to be effective (i.e., susceptibility, consequences, benefits, barriers/costs, and action cues). Researchers have explored this issue and drawn some interesting conclusions. For example, Christina Jones and colleagues (2015) studied an influenza vaccination campaign and found that perceived barriers mediated the relationship between exposure to the campaign and audience behavior. In other words, "researchers and practitioners should focus their efforts on identifying and countering perceived barriers" (Jones et al., 2015, p. 573) before debuting messages that highlight other variables, such as benefits, consequences, or cues to action.

Understanding where audience members are, in terms of their thinking about a certain health issue, means that campaign planners can play up one or more of the model's variables at different stages in a campaign or modify messages for different audiences.

Kami Silk and colleagues (2006), for instance, used components of the health belief model to guide focus groups with female adolescents and adults prior to developing breast cancer prevention materials. They found that participants of all ages understood the severity of breast cancer, but they defined the consequences somewhat differently. The adolescents tended to focus on the appearance-altering effects of the disease, such as hair loss during chemotherapy. The adults were more likely to know a lot about the disease and to feel personally susceptible. Thus, in this case, understanding how teens and adults diverge when it comes to consequences and perceived susceptibility helps campaign planners craft unique, targeted messages for each group.

Of course, people will not get vaccinated against the flu or perform regular breast self-exams simply because someone tells them to do so. A campaign message may be a cue to action, but unless someone has reason to believe that the recommended behavior is useful and worthwhile, and that it will prevent an outcome that is otherwise likely to occur, the recommendation will probably not be motivation enough.

If we are trying to increase participation in our university's sports recreation program, we might consider how strongly members of our target audience believe the benefits we propose may actually help them. Let's say that audience analysis reveals a common sentiment such as this: "I know exercise is good for people. But I'm young and healthy. I don't have to worry about that yet." According to the health belief model, people who feel this way will not be motivated

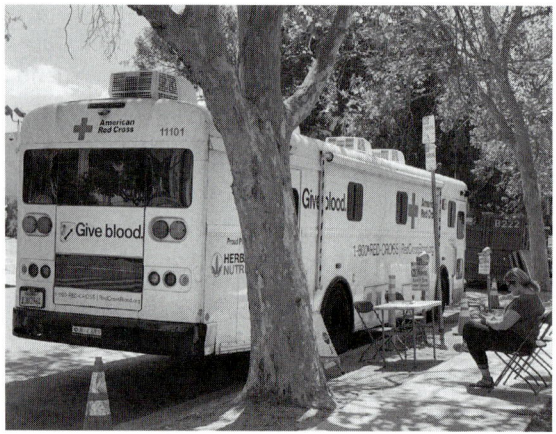

Can you think of a time when an event or message spurred you to action? If so, why do you think it had that effect?

to seek the benefits proposed because they do not believe they need them. Therefore, we might focus on other goals—such as looking good, meeting people, and winning awards—that are relevant to gym membership and more important to members of the target audience. Conversely, if people don't know about the benefits of exercise, the health belief model advocates educating them. Knowledge does not ensure behavior change, but it is an important foundation for it.

Social Cognitive Theory

Returning to the sports recreation campaign, imagine that everything seems to be in our favor. People are aware of the recreation program. They know about the benefits. They even feel they would benefit personally. Yet, they do not plan to participate. This may seem puzzling.

A promoter familiar with social cognitive theory would consider the environment. **Social cognitive theory** holds that we make decisions by considering the interplay of internal and environmental factors (Bandura, 1986, 1994). **Internal factors** include knowledge, skills, emotions, habits, and so on. **Environmental factors** include social approval, physical environment, institutional rules, and the like. According to the theory, we are most comfortable when internal and environmental factors are in sync. This may explain why changing people's minds does not necessarily change their behavior. Elements of the environment have a persuasive appeal of their own, which may run counter to experts' advice. For example, people may knowingly expose themselves to the risks of indoor tanning because they believe it will make them more attractive (Noar et al., 2015). And as Neha Gothe (2018) found, many older adults, and older African Americans in particular, rarely get the recommended amount of physical activity because they doubt they have the skills necessary to work out regularly and they don't believe the outcomes will be worth the effort. Even when presented with compelling evidence regarding exercise's health-boosting properties, some people still don't do it regularly. As health promoters, we have our work cut out for us!

Let's apply social cognitive theory to our sports recreation campaign. The theory suggests that, as health promoters, we must do more than simply make people aware of health risks. We already know that awareness is not enough to get people to change their behavior (see Gothe, 2018). We have to make healthy behaviors practical and socially acceptable. We may find that, although people believe it's healthy to work out, they are discouraged from doing so because they fear others will laugh at them, the gym's hours are not convenient, or they don't know anyone at the gym. If so, we may dedicate our efforts to improving the social atmosphere at the fitness center, suggesting different hours, or making other changes that build people's confidence and reduce the perceived risks of participating.

Theory of Reasoned Action

The **theory of reasoned action** (**TRA**) is based on the assumption that we are rational decision makers. We do not just *happen* to behave one way or another. Instead, we make decisions and deliberate choices based on two primary considerations: (1) how strongly we believe a behavior will lead to positive outcomes, and (2) the perceived social implications of performing that behavior (Ajzen & Fishbein, 1980).

TRA is similar to social cognitive theory in that both consider personal and social influences. However, TRA is more global in focus. Its predictive power lies in assessing the attitudes and behaviors of large numbers of people (Ajzen & Fishbein, 1980). For example, using TRA determinants, researchers have developed models that successfully predict how likely it is that patients with type 2 diabetes in rural communities will say that they plan to exercise. As it turns out, self-efficacy is the strongest predictor of their intention to exercise (Sarbazi, Moradi, Ghafari-Fam, Mirzaeian, & Babazadeh, 2019). Knowing this means health promoters can develop campaigns for patients with type 2 diabetes that, first and foremost, address patients' beliefs that they do not have the skills needed to stick with an exercise program. Then, campaigns can tackle other determinants, such as subjective norms or patients' attitudes.

Because TRA is designed to make generalizations, its founders don't consider it necessary (or even helpful) to focus on specifics such as personality, rules, and emotions. The effects of these variables tend to even out over large populations. By the same token, TRA does not assume that small changes will make much difference overall. As Ajzen and Fishbein put it, "Changing one or more beliefs may not be sufficient to bring about change in the overall attitude" (p. 81).

Icek Ajzen, one of the cofounders of TRA, extended the theory several years after its inception with the theory of planned behavior (Ajzen, 1985, 1991), which addresses circumstances in which the conditions set forth in TRA are met. For example, a person may believe strongly that a behavior would be useful and socially supported but still encounter circumstances in which it is difficult to follow through with the behavior. Maybe the person has said for months that they are going to start a new diet, but something always seems to prevent them from doing it. According to the **theory of planned behavior** (**TPB**), the difference between wanting to do something and actually doing it may lie partly in the strength of a person's intentions, which are shaped by three main factors: the person's attitudes about the issue and behaviors (*maybe they are not sure which diet to choose*), how socially rewarding and acceptable they consider it to be (*it might be easier if their friends were not always eating hamburgers and French fries*), and the extent to which they feel—all things considered—that they can carry out the behavior (*they may mean to make healthy dishes but it seems there is never time to buy and prepare healthy food*). The theory is empowering in that it sensitizes us to some of the factors that underlie our choices.

The theory also reminds us that our intentions often affect the people around us. When Kyle Andrews and collaborators studied the link between parental behavior and childhood obesity, they found that parents are least likely to proactively guide their children's eating and TV-watching habits if (1) they do not feel strongly that those behaviors are important; (2) they do not see other parents they admire doing so; and/or (3) they are not sure those behaviors make much difference anyway—maybe because they have been frustrated by attempts to manage their own

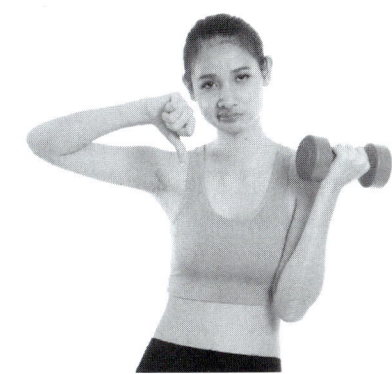

According to the theory of planned behavior, the difference between wanting to do something healthy and actually doing it lies partly in the strength of our intentions and partly in how confident we are that we can actually follow through with them.

weight (Andrews, Silk, & Eneli, 2010). More recently, researchers have found that active parental guidance is positively associated with all three of TPB's behavior predictors with respect to children's fruit and vegetable consumption. When parents talk about and teach the importance of healthy food (as opposed to simply governing what children can and cannot eat), there is often a positive impact on children's attitudes about eating healthy foods, their understanding of relevant social norms, and their perceived level of control over their diet (Yee, Lwin, & Lau, 2019). In turn, these factors—attitudes, norms, and perceived behavioral control—are associated with children eating more fruits and vegetables (Yee et al., 2019). These lines of research suggest that health promoters should keep in mind that knowledge is just one part of the equation—attitudes, role models, and confidence are also significant factors in achieving long-lasting change.

It may seem that the macro focus of TRA (and, by extension, TRB) is not very helpful in planning our sports recreation campaign. Indeed, our target audience may be too small to make broad generalizations very useful. But TRA is of interest theoretically because it suggests that people make behavior changes based on their *overall* beliefs and perceptions. Small changes may not have much effect if they are outweighed by larger concerns. For example, imagine that a new study suggests that the best sunscreen is a thick coat of zinc oxide ointment. Do you suppose you could get students at your school to cover their faces with white goop every day? Probably not. Their belief in the health benefits is probably outweighed by their desire to be socially acceptable. Luckily for us, physical exercise *is* widely accepted. What we propose is already in line with most people's overall intentions.

Transtheoretical Model

In analyzing the audience for our sports recreation campaign, imagine that we find some people *want* to exercise but that many of them are not doing so. We may even find that people *plan* to go to the gym but don't make it there. This is an important finding because it helps us understand our audience's state of mind. According to the **transtheoretical model** (**TTM**), we may not proceed directly from thinking about a problem to changing our behavior (Holtgrave, Tinsley, & Kay, 1995; Prochaska & DiClemente, 1983; Prochaska, DiClemente, & Norcross, 1992). Instead, we tend to change in stages. According to the model, change typically involves the following five stages:

- *Precontemplation:* Not aware of a problem
- *Contemplation:* Thinking about a problem
- *Preparation:* Deciding to take action
- *Action:* Making a change
- *Maintenance:* Sticking to the change for six months or more

The implication is that people react differently to health-promotion efforts depending on their current stage. Attention-getting information may be useful when they are unaware of a problem. But skills training and encouragement may be more useful if they are already prepared to make a change. Furthermore, if they have already adopted the recommended behavior, they may be encouraged to continue it.

Hyunyi Cho and Charles Salmon (2007) found support for this concept when they exposed students to a variety of messages about skin cancer. Participants in precontemplation stages who viewed highly threatening messages were highly motivated

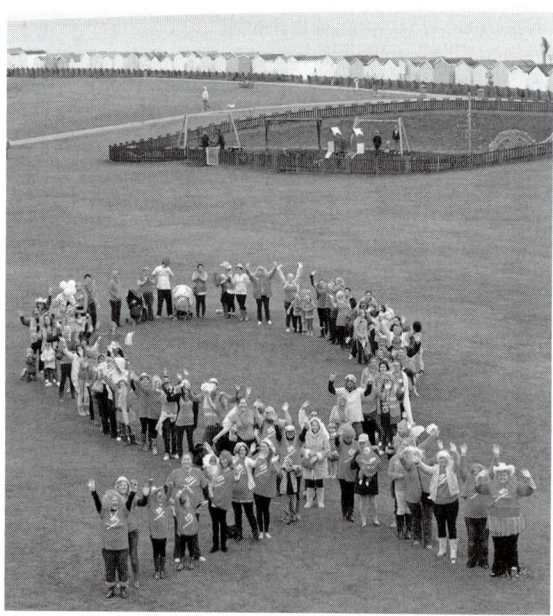

The Pink Ribbon campaign has raised awareness about breast cancer, but some critics charge that the rhetoric has not translated into effective support for cancer research (Jenkins, 2012), highlighting the lesson that publicity is not the only measure of a health campaign's success.

to protect themselves, but they also reported higher-than-average feelings of hopelessness and fatalism. The authors concluded that fear appeals can call attention to previously unattended issues, but they may be counterproductive unless accompanied by clear and useful guidance.

Of course, not everyone moves sequentially through the stages. Research suggests that people can skip stages, revert to previous stages, and/or cycle through stages more than once. As described by Ahmed Jerôme Romain and colleagues (2018), progression/regression through the stages is based on four theoretical constructs:

- *Decisional balance*: The perceived pros and/or cons of changing a behavior.
- *Temptation*: The urge to enact particular behaviors or habits, especially during difficult situations (e.g., eating ice cream when depressed or drinking alcohol when stressed out).
- *Self-efficacy*: How confident people are in their abilities to carry out new behaviors.
- *Processes of change*: Strategies people use when actively changing their behaviors. Examples include (a) substituting healthy behaviors for unhealthy ones, such as going for a walk instead of eating junk food, and (b) rewarding oneself for sticking with healthy behaviors, such as shopping for new shoes or clothes after meeting a weight-loss goal.

When analyzing 33 TTM-based studies about physical activity interventions, Romain et al. (2018) found that campaigns that factored in TTM's theoretical constructs were considerably more effective than those that didn't. For example, interventions that included at least three constructs were three times more likely to boost physical activity (Romain et al., 2018).

Two constructs—self-efficacy and processes of change (i.e., strategies)—are particularly important when it comes to increasing physical activity. By some estimates, campaigns that address these are twice as likely to increase physical activity as campaigns that don't (Romain et al., 2018). For instance, self-efficacy is positively associated with the likelihood that breast cancer survivors will advance from one stage to the next in terms of contemplating, preparing, and then actively participating in an exercise program (Scruggs et al., 2018). And, according to one study, strategies are the most important predictors of physical activity (Romain, Horwath, & Bernard, 2018). The take-away for health promoters is to remember TTM's stages *and* constructs—especially self-efficacy and processes of change—when devising campaign messages.

Considering change as a stage-based process reveals some key challenges and opportunities for health campaign managers. One challenge is that people don't simply overhaul their behavior as soon as they hear new information. Change agents must be sensitive to barriers and motivations as well. Second, TTM reveals why prevention efforts are particularly challenging. Inundating audience members with messages inappropriate to their stage of change may actually discourage them from proceeding. Rather than changing, people may avoid the issue entirely.

The TTM presents opportunities for important contributions as well. Without motivational health campaigns, members of at-risk populations may "remain stuck in the early stages" (Prochaska, Johnson, & Lee, 1998, p. 64). The model also suggests that changes, once initiated, must be supported. A team led by Elisia Cohen (2015) showed a video about the importance of HPV vaccines to women who had just had the first dose of the vaccine. Those women were subsequently 2.5 times more likely than others to return for the second and third doses of the vaccine than women who did not view the video. Cohen's team also found that, with slight modifications, the video was helpful for women in other stages of decision making as well. The project is a good reminder that effective campaigns are not simply one-shot affairs, but ongoing programs that support change and commitment.

Wrapping It Up

In closing our discussion of behavior change theories, it's important to point out that, as health promoters, we need not limit ourselves to any one model. The beauty of these theories is that they often overlap and call attention to different shades of meaning within the same process. Theories are like camera lenses, in that they help us achieve focus and clarity. This can be immensely helpful. But if we are not careful, a focus can be a limitation. In the next section we explore a different perspective.

Critical-Cultural Perspective

Return for a moment to the idea of a camera. When you look through the viewfinder you can zoom in on elements in the environment. But while you are focusing on one thing—even a very big thing like a sunset—there are other things you don't see. That's natural. This becomes a problem if you start to think that what you see in the viewfinder is all there is. No matter what our perspective, there is usually more there than meets the eye. In this spirit, critical theorists remind us that cognitive theories—despite the many contributions we have discussed—share a common focus: They treat health as primarily the product of choices people make as individuals (Dutta-Bergman, 2005). Granted, cognitive theories acknowledge that people's choices are influenced by a range of factors. But the nexus is still individual thought and decision making. What if we assume that this is only part of the story and look at health issues through a wider-angle lens?

Communication theorist Mohan J. Dutta has emerged as a leading advocate of the **critical-cultural approach**, which proposes that health is not merely the result of individual choices, but is intertwined with issues of culture, power, control, identity, and social consciousness. From this perspective, health-related behaviors are profoundly influenced by dynamics that are larger and more pervasive than any individual (Dutta-Bergman, 2005).

There is plentiful evidence to support the idea that health is, to a great extent, a socially enacted phenomenon. As you may remember from Chapter 6, health disparities typically reflect social boundaries. The overall health of some groups is worse or better than the health of others for a range of reasons such as resources, prejudice and discrimination, trust, cultural mores, information, stress, living and working conditions, and more. Assuming that people who are poor in information and resources have the same choices as other people requires that we overlook a host of factors that are very real to the people who experience them.

Moreover, it's not simply a question of having or not having. Cultural values and identities influence what is "good," "healthy," and "acceptable." The way a health expert views a particular behavior (such as smoking, drug use, driving fast, wearing a helmet, monogamy, and so on) may be very different from the way members of diverse cultures view it. Slater (2006) observes that health-related behaviors are often tied to issues of personal identity:

> *Risk-taking teens may believe that alcohol or marijuana experimentation is part of what defines them as adventurous, fun party people. Farmers may believe that accepting risk of injury [as in deciding not to have rollbars mounted on their tractors] in the interest of keeping costs low is part of what makes them farmers.* (p. 155)

And, as Helme et al. (2019) found, adhering to traditional conceptions of masculinity doubles the chances that rural teens will use smokeless tobacco products. Moreover, health-related behaviors may be attributed moral qualities such that they are considered bad, irresponsible, or evil. (This is especially true of issues such as sex and drug use, as discussed in Chapter 12.)

Considering these diverse viewpoints, a number of questions present themselves: *Whose view is right? Who should decide how people ought to behave? And how is one's quality of life improved or diminished by the behaviors in question?* These are difficult questions. The answers, say critical theorists, are not simple or

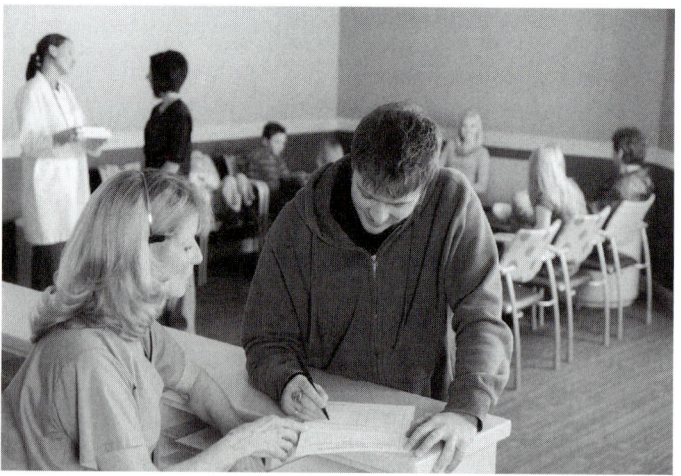

What factors influence your own health-related behaviors (e.g., how often you visit a doctor, whether you exercise every day, eat right, and so on)? How are these behaviors affected by larger issues such as resources, culture, and social support?

universal. Rather than privileging one perspective over another, they advocate open and respectful dialogue about the issues—involving the active participation of theorists, practitioners, and, most notably, members of the social group themselves (Dutta-Bergman, 2005).

Critical-cultural theorists observe that health promotion efforts that don't recognize the social contexts in which people live often fail to do much good. In fact, they often do harm—by reifying power differences, dominating the cultural landscape, and reinforcing the idea that people whose health is "poor" are not trying very hard or are like children who should be instructed by others. (See Box 14.1 for more on these ethical dilemmas.)

This is not to say that health promoters mindfully oppress the people they are trying to serve. It is more that their good intentions are often based on tacitly held assumptions about whose ideas are most valuable and who should be telling whom how to behave. You may say, "But they are only trying to teach people how to have better health." That's undoubtedly true. But let's unpack the baggage within that assertion. The idea of teaching implies that one person has knowledge or insight that they help others comprehend. That is relatively unproblematic if we assume that the information is straightforward and value-free. One thing we know about health: It is never impersonal or value-free. So, who defines what "better health" means? And

BOX 14.1 Ethical Considerations

Three Issues for Health Promoters to Keep in Mind

Health promoters are faced with a number of ethical considerations. Among them is deciding how to warn audiences without needlessly frightening them. They must also be careful not to blame people for ill health, while also encouraging them to prevent any illnesses and injuries they can. All the while, they must walk a fine line between making people concerned about illness and making them worried sick.

Timing

When early evidence of a health risk surfaces, is it better to warn the public right away or to wait for more conclusive evidence? This question poses a dilemma for health promoters. On the one hand, researchers suggest that people are wary of premature announcements that are later shown to be inaccurate. For example, people were long urged to increase their exposure to sunlight to ensure sufficient amounts of vitamin D. Now people are encouraged to avoid sunlight to lower their risk of skin cancer. Conflicting messages such as these may confuse people and cause them to ignore health advisories.

On the other hand, it may take months or years to compile conclusive evidence. During that time, people may be exposed to health risks they might have avoided. People are likely to be angry if health officials are aware of potential risks yet do not warn the public.

Scapegoating

It's difficult to know where the responsibility for personal health lies. For example, if children with the flu go to school and spread it to others, is it (1) the parents' fault for not keeping them home, (2) employers' fault for making it difficult for parents to stay home with sick children, or (3) health officials' fault for not educating parents about the need to keep children home? Although all of these factors probably contribute to the problem, part of a health promoter's job is to identify the conditions that most need improvement. In doing so, however, it is easy to scapegoat—to blame one person or group for the whole problem.

Scapegoating presents an ethical dilemma. It makes sense to focus attention on the condition or people with the greatest chance of making a difference. The typical health-promotion message cannot describe all the factors that contribute to a problem. However, focusing on one aspect or group of people may seem to place blame. For example, a campaign that admonishes parents to keep their sick children home may alienate parents who cannot

continued

continued

afford to miss a day of work. These parents may feel frustrated and criticized, and they may resent promoters' efforts. Second, people not held to blame may feel that the problem is no longer their responsibility. Ruth Faden (1987) asserts that government officials sometimes promote the idea that people are personally responsible for their health partly because this lets government off the hook. There is little imperative to make sweeping social changes or health care reform if it seems that health is solely the product of voluntary lifestyle changes.

Evidence fuels both sides of the debate, suggesting that personal choices and empowerment are important to health but that, at the same time, personal efforts are often constrained by environmental factors beyond individuals' control (such as money to afford medical care or sanitary living conditions). Health promoters may find themselves trying to identify key objectives without ignoring that every objective is intertwined with others.

Stigmatizing

Prevention is the process of avoiding undesirable outcomes. People wear helmets to avoid head injuries, they are immunized to avoid diseases, and so on. Typically, the worse the potential outcome, the more people try to prevent it. Therefore, health promoters try to motivate people by showing them how bad undesirable outcomes can be.

The dilemma is that while portraying some *conditions* as undesirable, promoters may stigmatize some *people* as undesirable. People may become so frightened of diseases that they avoid the people who have them. For instance, an image of a child with a disability may be frightening enough to make children observe safety rules, but how are they likely to feel about children with disabilities? The same dilemma applies to AIDS publicity. People may become so frightened that they overprotect themselves by avoiding people who have AIDS.

What Do You Think?

1. Should health promoters release information about potential health risks immediately or wait for more conclusive evidence?
   a. How long is it reasonable to wait?
   b. What constitutes conclusive evidence?
2. Can you think of a way to promote public health without seeming to place the blame on certain people or groups?
3. Do you think it is possible to warn people about health hazards without stigmatizing people who have already been affected? Why or why not?

---

who decides the best ways to accomplish that? When health promoters assume they have the answers to these questions, the result is often a paternalistic "I know what's best for you" mind-set. Actually, critical theorists argue, what is "best" is largely a matter of interpretation and value.

In the end, privileging one perspective, even if it seems to be "for people's own good," is an exercise in power and often serves to marginalize and alienate people who see the world differently. Mohan Dutta and Rebecca de Souza (2008) trace the history of health-promotion efforts, showing that the tradition has largely been for those "in the center" to assist those "in the margins." They write:

> This position was based on the assumption of the expertise of those at the center, who could examine an underdeveloped community, evaluate its needs based on scientific instruments, and propose solutions that would supposedly propel the community toward development; the category of the "underdeveloped" was fixed in its position as the object of interventions, its people portrayed as the "primitive" receivers of campaign messages who were incapable of development without the helping hand of the interventionists. (p. 327)

Such efforts have often been experienced as insulting and naive, and, despite (and perhaps partly because of) widespread health-promotion campaigns, the gap between the health rich and the health poor around the world continues to widen at a staggering pace (Dutta & de Souza, 2008).

One approach recommended by the critical-cultural perspective involves embracing the notion of "many realities," none more correct or dominant than another (Dutta-Bergman, 2005, p. 117). This means shedding the notion that health promoters should set the agenda. Instead, it requires that they immerse themselves in the communities they serve, acting as facilitators who support community members' efforts to decide for themselves what they consider important and how they can best attain their goals (Dutta-Bergman, 2005). Health experts can share what they know of science and theory, but it's important that they not presume (or behave as if) that information is more right or important than participants' own perspectives. In other words, knowledge is one of many resources to be shared, not a tool to be used in the process of controlling others (Dutta, 2008). The goal is an interactive, ongoing process in which "problems are configured and reconfigured; solutions are generated and worked on based on the needs of the community as defined by community members" (Dutta-Bergman, 2005, p. 116). One objective is to build social consciousness about health and to engender a sense of **collective efficacy**, a communal sense that positive change can be accomplished. Dutta-Bergman (2005) also emphasizes the necessity of **community capacity**, the resources needed for good health, such as healthy food and water, safe shelter, and medical care. These basics are lacking in many parts of the country and the world.

Considering our campus campaign, we might choose to work with people who are frequently "in the margins" of fitness efforts. For example, we might focus on students and employees with physical disabilities. To accomplish this, we will want to immerse ourselves, as best we can, in the concerns and viewpoints of the people in the focus community. (Even if you have a disability yourself, it is risky to make assumptions from your own perspective.) Perhaps there is an organization or support group at which people with disabilities openly discuss their goals and concerns. With permission, we might attend meetings, or, if such a format does not already exist, we might organize a series of meetings. The process of encouraging people with disabilities to talk about fitness goals may be powerful in itself. There is likely to be great diversity among the people who participate, but we might learn that they share some common goals and face some common barriers they would like to overcome. Perhaps they are already involved in fitness efforts we don't know much about. We may find that, like many other people, they dread feeling conspicuous at the gym. Or perhaps they require specialized equipment or space that is not currently available. Already, you can probably imagine how issues of collective efficacy and community capacity might emerge and how you might help. Also keep in mind that while it might seem patently audacious to tell people with disabilities how to behave if we don't understand their worldview, it can be equally as presumptuous to tell people from other cultures and communities how to think and act. Critical-cultural theory requires us to be respectful of "diverse realities" at every level.

The critical-cultural approach reminds us that nothing happens in isolation. What seem to be individual choices are often patterns of behavior shaped and reinforced by the systems in which they occur (Bohm, 1996; Senge, 2006). Ignoring the larger patterns can result in unproductive attempts at localized change. For example, health campaign designers frequently appeal to people to avoid or quit smoking, but they rarely tackle the larger issues of public policy and tobacco-industry standards (Dutta, 2008; Smith & Wakefield, 2006). Health promoters can help equalize disparities by advocating for community resources, public policies, and issues of social justice to help communities overcome their marginalized status.

Let's take this knowledge of theories and power differences back to our own campaign, as we discuss the three final stages: designing campaign messages, piloting and implementing the campaign, and evaluating and maintaining the effort.

Step 5: Designing Campaign Messages

As we discussed in Chapter 13, the first step in designing an effective campaign is to listen and ask questions. Experts recommend that campaign designers work closely with members of the focus community to determine what aspect of the problem is most important to them and then make that concern a focal point. Critical-cultural theory also behooves us to look at cultural values and the macro-level, systemic factors that affect the people we want to help.

It may turn out that our campaign does not involve the traditional step of creating messages that will be widely distributed to audience members. Instead, we might advocate for new hours at the fitness center, specialized fitness classes, more space or resources, skills training, or some other effort. Most campaigns, however, involve some degree of message creation and dissemination. Even if our principal effort is changing the structure, we will want to get the word out

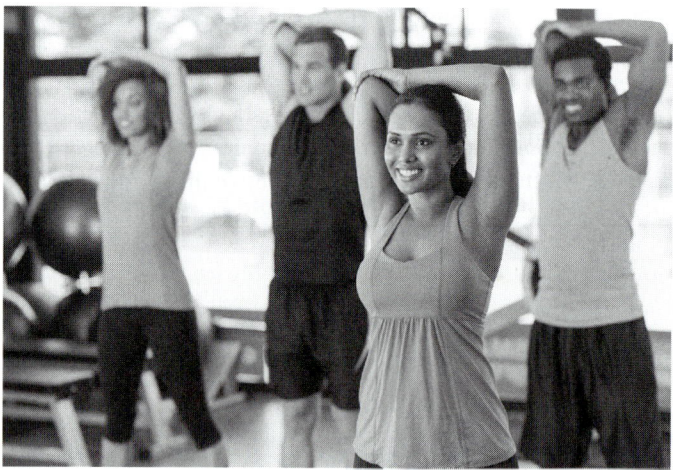

You might be a member of the target audience for the sports recreation campaign. Take a moment to reflect on your own characteristics as an audience member. Do you exercise frequently? Why or why not? How do your considerations match up with the theories in this chapter?

somehow. In this section we focus on the central principles of message design.

Choosing a Voice and/or Spokesperson

Campaign messages have a voice. The voice may seem masculine, feminine, young, old, friendly, casual, stern, or so on. Whatever its character, this voice embodies the mood and personality of the campaign. Here are some questions to consider in finding that voice.

- What is the campaign's personality and mood?
- Is it an authority figure or a friend?
- Is it a logical person or an emotional person?
- Is it the sort of person to whom the audience is likely to respond?

Even when words appear in print, the tone of the message gives the reader a sense of who is "talking" and what type of relationship the writer wishes to establish with the reader.

Of course, the source is even more apparent when the audience can see or hear a spokesperson deliver the message. Even the spokesperson's accent matters! Researchers conducted an experiment to see which accent—standard American English or Southern—would be more effective in getting residents of rural Appalachia to accept dental health messages (Dragojevic, Savage, Scott, & McGinnisa, 2018). Most listeners in the study bestowed the standard accent with a higher status, and, consequently, they agreed with those messages more than with messages recorded in a Southern accent. The lesson for health promoters is that subtle variations in the message, including "the accent in which the message is delivered," are important (Dragojevic et al., 2018, p. 8).

Generally, campaign messages have more impact when the target audience trusts the spokesperson and considers the person capable and attractive. Studies show that source credibility increases people's compliance with health recommendations (De Meulenaer, De Pelsmacker, & Dens, 2018). Credibility is determined by two factors: expertise and trustworthiness. Generally, the more knowledgeable and trustworthy the source (e.g., physician or medical expert), the more effective a health message is likely to be. But as De Meulenaer and colleagues (2018) found, sometimes source credibility can heighten perceived threat, which can actually lower compliance (this is likely because when people are too frightened or not confident they can perform the recommended behavior, they ignore the message and/or avoid the topic as a coping mechanism). The lesson for health promoters is valuable: *When source credibility is high, campaign designers should be wary of delivering highly threatening messages (De Meulenaer et al., 2018).*

Even when a health message and its source are credible, other factors sometimes muddy the waters. For example, when Ioannis Kareklas and colleagues studied vaccination PSAs that appeared online, they found that online comments about the PSAs contributed heavily to viewers' attitudes and intentions, especially when viewers considered the commenters to be highly credible (Kareklas, Muehling, & Weber, 2015). Thus, health promoters should take electronic feedback into account. If favorable, such feedback may reinforce a campaign's message. If not, it may deter people from taking the message seriously.

When it comes to choosing spokespersons, celebrities can sometimes fill the bill because they are often attractive, liked, and/or trusted. The *NO MORE Excuses* campaign to overcome domestic violence and sexual assault as well as the *got milk?* campaign feature dozens of recognizable artists, entertainers, athletes, and more. An evolving collection of famous spokespersons can attract regular attention, whether they are promoting healthy behavior or endorsing consumer goods, which is why companies often pay celebrities millions of dollars in endorsement deals.

Apart from the huge dollar amounts some celebrities command, there are sometimes other drawbacks to using well-known spokespersons. When cyclist Lance Armstrong admitted to using performance-enhancing drugs in 2013, his Livestrong charity to benefit cancer research took a hit as well. Megasponsors Nike and RadioShack pulled out, and individual contributions plummeted (Lapowsky, 2014).

Effective spokespersons don't have to be doctors or celebrities. There is considerable evidence that audiences often trust people who are similar to them, an effect called **source homophily** (Rogers, 1973). Not only do people pay more attention when a spokesperson who is similar to them describes a health risk, they feel more personally vulnerable to the risk (Rimal & Morrison, 2006). For example, when studying obesity PSAs, Joe Phua (2016) found that credible spokespersons who were similar to target audiences had a positive impact on audiences' diet and exercise self-efficacy. This may be partly because a sense of shared experiences engenders a sense of shared truths (Borkman, 1976). Audience members tend to feel more confident in their ability to lose weight after watching spokespersons who have struggled to lose weight themselves (Phua, 2016), such as Jennifer Hudson, Jessica Simpson, Oprah Winfrey, and DJ Kahled, to name just a few.

Shared experiential knowledge may also explain the success of 12-step programs, such as Alcoholics Anonymous and Overeaters Anonymous, in which meetings are led by (recovering) alcoholics and overeaters who share their insights and first-hand accounts of battling addiction (Noorani, Karlsson, & Borkman, 2019).

Capitalizing on source homophily is not always as simple as it sounds, however. In the study of audience reactions to standard and nonstandard accents that we mentioned earlier, Dragojevic and colleagues (2020) found that people tended to imbue standard accents with higher status, competence, and intelligence—even when those accents were different from their own. In that context, credibility might trump similarity. Of course, this may not be true for all audiences and all messages, which is why you should get to know your audience and test out message variables *before* launching a campaign.

As you can see, there is a lot to consider when deciding your campaign's voice and the type of spokesperson, if any, you will use. Next, we turn our attention to designing the actual message.

Designing the Message

In designing an effective health campaign message, it's important to consider community expectations and how logic, emotion, and novelty factor in. We begin this section by exploring the different ways that messages about the same health behavior can be framed. Then we talk about the art of matching messages to audience needs and emotions.

BOX 14.2 Career Opportunities

Health Campaign Design and Management

Campaign director
Communication director
Director of nonprofit organization
Media relations specialist
Professor/educator
Public relations specialist
Publication designer

Career Resources and Job Listings
- Chronicle of Philanthropy: philanthropy.com/jobs
- Wellness Council of America: welcoa.org
- American Journal of Health Promotion: healthpromotionjournal.com
- National Institutes of Health: nih.gov
- World Health Organization: who.int/employment/vacancies/en

THEORETICAL FOUNDATIONS: MESSAGE FRAMING

You are walking through the mall with a friend when you come upon a booth proclaiming "Free Health Screening." The health professionals staffing the booth say they can give you a relatively accurate cholesterol score. They just need a drop or two of blood from your finger. And they can tell your body-fat percentage by gently pinching and measuring the skin on your upper arm. One of you says, "Sure! What do I have to lose?" and steps up to participate. The other says, "No thanks," and backs away quickly. Why do you and your friend respond so differently?

Message-frame theorists are interested in the way people interpret health-related behaviors and in health promoters' efforts to affect those interpretations (Slater, 2006). A famous example involves smoking. For years, health promoters tried to get people to quit because it was bad for their health. But the real turning point occurred when researchers discovered the dangers of secondhand smoke. The issue was reframed from endangering self to endangering others (this idea informed the CATmageddon campaign that we discussed in Chapter 13). Whereas the personal risk seemed acceptable—even cool and rebellious to some—many people found it unacceptable to put others at risk. It was the same behavior, but framed differently.

As with most things health-related, effects are not simple or predictable. Men in the United States are still at particularly high risk for smoking and/or using smokeless tobacco products. One reason may be that advertisers have done a good job framing smoking in culturally masculine terms. In a study of smoking references in men's magazines, Mohan Dutta and Josh Boyd (2007) found that smoking was consistently framed as a sensual, independent, and mysterious, with ads set in powerful places, exotic lands, or appealing outdoor locations. Donald Helme and colleagues (2019) discovered that some young men, despite knowing that smokeless tobacco products were harmful, used the products because they felt that doing so demonstrated their masculinity to others. Researchers suggest that antismoking/smokeless tobacco campaigns might turn around the masculine appeal of these themes by framing campaign messages to resemble tobacco advertisements.

Messages may be framed in respect to potential gains, losses, and risks (Rothman & Salovey, 1997). A **gain-frame appeal** illustrates the advantages of performing the recommended behavior. For example, people might be persuaded that eating a low-carbohydrate diet will keep their weight down and help prevent diabetes and heart disease. In other words, they would gain something by following the diet. Conversely, a **loss-frame appeal** emphasizes the negative repercussions of not taking action. For example, cigarette labels might show the harmful effects of smoking either in words or in graphic photos (Nan, Zhao, Yang, & Iles, 2015), as we discussed in Chapter 13. Many cigarette warning labels, especially those in Europe, stress the long-term health problems associated with smoking in loss-framed appeals (e.g., developing lung cancer and increasing the chances of having a heart attack), but researchers have found that focusing on the short-term benefits of quitting smoking in gain-framed messages (e.g., lower blood pressure and heart rate, plus improved sense of smell and taste) is actually more successful at getting people to quit or decide that they should quit (Mollen, Engelen, Kessels, & van den Putte, 2017). At this point, you may be wondering: How do we know when to use a gain-frame appeal and when to use a loss-frame appeal?

Let's start with the research on gain-frames. Over several decades, researchers have amassed a good bit of evidence that suggests gain-frame appeals are more effective than loss-frame appeals at getting people to engage in preventive behaviors. Here are a few examples of recent studies:

- Researchers in the Netherlands found that messages about the heart-healthy benefits of eating fruits and vegetables increased people's intentions to eat them, especially when the messages were auditory versus written (Elbert & Ots, 2018). Negative-framed messages that stressed the higher risk of heart disease among people who eat too few fruits and vegetables were not as effective (Elbert & Ots, 2018).
- In another study, PSAs that showed the positive consequences of drinking responsibly were more effective with students than PSAs featuring the undesirable consequences of overdrinking (Park, Son, Lee, & Go, 2019, p. 8).
- Teens who admit to texting while driving responded more favorably to PSAs with gain-frame appeals than to those that stressed the dangers of distracted driving (Delgado et al., 2018).

Gain-frame appeals that encourage preventive behaviors are especially effective when message recipients know someone who has been adversely affected by the health issue in question. For example, women whose loved ones have experienced breast cancer tend to respond more favorably to gain-framed appeals and find loss-framed messages about breast cancer distressing, perhaps because their anxiety about the issue is already high (H. J. Kim, 2014).

In certain circumstances, however, loss-framed messages can be effective. The research is somewhat inconclusive, although it appears that loss-frames are *slightly* more effective at promoting certain detection behaviors. When Daniel O'Keefe and Jakob Jensen (2009) analyzed 53 studies about health messages encouraging procedures such as mammograms and colonoscopies, they found that loss-frames were more successful than gain-frames at encouraging breast cancer detection, but not at promoting other procedures.

Mixed results about the success of loss-appeals reflect a human dilemma. On the one hand, people are motivated to avoid undesirable outcomes, such as dying from breast cancer (O'Keefe & Jensen, 2009). On the other hand, the prospect of a disease such as breast cancer may be so frightening that people avoid thinking about it. The result is that people at highest risk for a condition may be most likely to engage in denial or avoidance when they are confronted with distressing information (Lipkis, Johnson, Amarasekara, Pan, & Updegraff, 2018).

Consider your own experiences. While you may willingly engage in protective behaviors, such as wearing sunscreen at the beach, what might you do if you notice a suspicious mole on your shoulder? If you are like most people, you will feel a range of complicated emotions. Seeking a diagnosis is emotionally risky. You might learn that you have cancer and will need treatment or surgery. It is emotionally self-protective to avoid what might be an anxiety-producing outcome. In fact, such avoidance can, and often does, last months or years.

But maybe something happens that shifts your thinking. You see an alarming PSA about the dangers of skin cancer or you hear about someone who has died of skin cancer. These are loss-frame messages, in that they highlight bad things that might happen if you don't take action. It's possible that your anxiety and the uncertainty will outweigh your desire to ignore the issue. Perhaps you make a doctor's appointment after all.

You may not be motivated to schedule the appointment because you think you have skin cancer—your motivation may be to confirm that you don't. That's what Isaac Lipkis and colleagues (2018) found when they studied messages urging colorectal cancer screening. People who read loss-frame messages were more likely to get screened if they believed that doing so would affirm their good health than if they thought it would reveal a problem (p. 268). Thus, presenting detection behaviors as a way to affirm good health may be a message tactic worth considering.

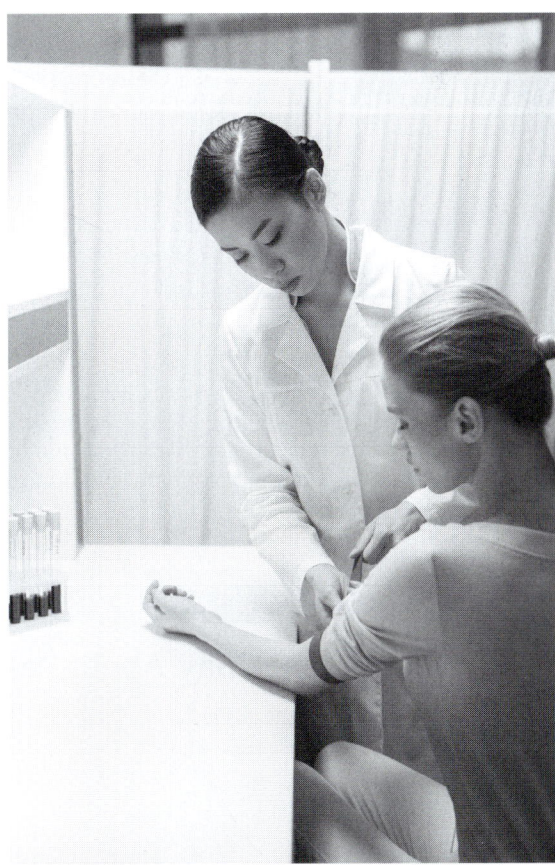

What factors might influence your decision to take part in a free health screening at the mall? What might you gain if you are tested? On the other hand, what unpleasant outcomes might result if you participate? What if the stakes were higher? If you suspected that you had been exposed to HIV, what factors would influence whether you got tested or not? Why?

COMMUNITY EXPECTATIONS

Health messages are only useful if people think the messages are relevant and meaningful. With that in mind, researchers interviewed a group of older African American women to see if they thought adding a spirituality component to messages about breast cancer screening would make the messages more helpful or relevant (Best, Spencer, Hall, Friedman, & Billings, 2015). The women suggested that such messages should reflect three themes—that one's body is a temple, that faith will help women cope if they find out they have breast cancer, and that consulting a physician is not inconsistent with having faith in God. As one woman put it, "You have to do your part so that God can do His part" (Best et al., 2015, p. 296). The women also suggested that messages should be spiritual without being "pushy" or specific to any one religion. By listening to the members of the target audience, researchers may be able to craft appeals that speak to the audience's beliefs, values, and concerns.

Shelia Mammen led a team of scholars who partnered with rural, low-income mothers to devise message strategies for improving the health and wellness of women and children living in rural communities. By using a participatory/collaborative approach, Mammen and colleagues (2019) learned that the women wanted face-to-face interventions, favored peers as sources of information about food security, and preferred medical experts' advice about dental health. One takeaway is that, without community members' involvement, health promoters can easily misread audience's needs and preferences. For that reason, the authors concluded:

> To ensure that such health information is appropriate, it is important to consider the input of the target population. Without their contribution to message creation, any attempt to promote health may not prove to be as effective; there has to be a partnership with and buy-in from the very population that experts claim to be helping. (Mammen, Sano, Braun, & Maring, 2019, p. 1148)

Another lesson is to beware of assumptions. For example, a good deal of research has focused on college students' alcohol consumption. There is consistent evidence that students who drink typically believe that alcohol frees their inhibitions and makes them less shy and more socially engaging (Sopory, 2005). That is a tough perception to overcome. And it's one reason students and health advocates often disagree about how much drinking is too much. Although researchers tend to define five or more drinks as "binge drinking," students typically perceive that five drinks are within the normal range for their peers (Lederman, Stewart, Goodhart, & Laitman, 2008). They define a binge in more extreme terms. Consequently, researchers who survey students about "binge drinking" may be measuring something different from what they think they are measuring. And students may feel that warnings about "binge drinking" do not apply to them because their behavior is within "normal" bounds (Lederman et al., 2008). (For more on social norms as the basis for safe-drinking campaigns, see Box 14.3.)

BOX 14.3 THEORETICAL FOUNDATIONS

What Does Science Say About Peer Pressure?

I think that alcohol is a huge part of adult life. It's like a rite of passage when you finally turn 21.

Every college student I know drinks.

College students love to party. It's tradition.

Thinking of your own undergraduate experience, you might find yourself nodding in agreement as you read these comments made by college students in Casper and colleagues' (2006) study (p. 295). Or you might shake your head in doubt. Experiences vary. And conventional wisdom suggests that your experience has a lot to do with the company you keep. It feels normal for partiers to party and nondrinkers not to drink. But in some instances, some people don't follow the crowd. What *does* science say about fitting in with the crowd?

On the one hand, there is ample evidence that people are more likely to engage in risky behaviors

continued

if their friends do. Having peers who smoke and approve of smoking is the single greatest predictor of a teen's decision to smoke cigarettes (Krosnick et al., 2006; Miller, Burgoon, Grandpre, & Alvaro, 2006). The same goes for kicking the habit. The overall decline in smoking has not occurred so much here and there as in distinct social clusters. In studying the issue, Nicholas Christakis and James Fowler (2008) found that smoking had persisted in some circles but that in others "whole groups of people were quitting in concert" (p. 2249).

One foundation for the RU SURE campaign that begins this chapter is **social norms theory,** which suggests that people base their behavior partly on what they consider appropriate and socially acceptable (Haines & Spear, 1996). The idea is that such campaigns may be especially influential in settings such as college campuses, where students are part of novel situations in which they are not immediately aware of cultural expectations. As you know, that campaign has had demonstrable success curbing student alcohol abuse.

But some social norm campaigns have been less successful. In a study of students at 37 colleges, Wechsler and colleagues (2003) found that drinking was the same on campuses with social norm campaigns as on those without them. In another study, 72.6% of college students surveyed disbelieved the assertion that "most students drink 0 to 4 drinks when they party" (Polonec, Major, & Atwood, 2006, p. 23). And Shelly Campo and Kenzie Cameron (2006) found that, after viewing social-norming messages, light drinkers were even more determined to keep their drinking within healthy bounds, but heavier drinkers often went the other way. Their drinking intentions were *more* intense after viewing the normative messages. Another challenge to the power of social norms is that, in some cases, people find nonconformity appealing. People of varying ages who rank high on individualism or rebellious tendencies are likely to go *against* the norm (Lapinski, Rimal, DeVries, & Lee, 2007; Lee & Bichard, 2006).

Rajiv Rimal and Kevin Real (2005) have sought to make sense of the complexity with their **theory of normative social behavior (TNSB).** The theory proposes that we *are* influenced by perceived social norms but that a variety of factors either strengthen or weaken how much those perceptions affect us. These include (1) how much we value the social approval to be gained from conforming, (2) the outcomes we expect from engaging in the behavior, (3) the degree to which we identify with the group, and (4) how confident we feel in our ability to say no to the behavior in question (Jang, Rimal, & Cho, 2013; Rimal & Real, 2005). In other words, if we like and value the group, we may want to "fit in" by acting in accordance with its norms, especially if the behavior offers rewards we like. However, our desire to fit in may be outweighed by other factors—as when the behavior seems inconsequential, we do not value or identify with the group very much, we enjoy being different, or we like the behavior so much that we are willing to buck convention to do it. There is evidence that college students drink if/when they perceive that the rewards (such as loss of social inhibitions) outweigh the potential for negative repercussions, such as getting in trouble or getting hurt. And this is particularly true if they also perceive that drinking is accepted and approved by their friends (Rimal & Real, 2005).

So back to the initial question: *Does believing that "most people drink" or "drink a lot" mean we are likely to do the same?* So far, the best answer is that it depends. For one, it depends on how we define "most people." The "norm" that researchers often use (as in "two of three college students stop at three or fewer drinks") is an aggregate statistic. It might change your mind about typical college student behavior. Or you might think, "They clearly haven't met *my* friends." Evidence suggests that, if the overall statistic seems different from what you perceive strongly within your own social network, you are likely to disbelieve or disregard it (Polonec et al., 2006; Yanovitzky, Stewart, & Lederman, 2006). A second consideration concerns the perceived value of the behavior (Rimal, 2008). Whereas a **descriptive norm** describes "what most people do," an **injunctive norm** characterizes the perception that people *should* do it based on particular values (Boer & Westhoff, 2006; Rimal, 2008). For example, even if you believe that most of your friends occasionally drink and drive, you may refuse to do so yourself because you consider it wrong or irresponsible. Finally, TNSB

continued

continued

suggests that norms affect us to the degree that it is socially and personally rewarding to live up to them. If any of a complex array of factors change (rewards, penalties, group membership, or so on), the power of the norm may change considerably.

Here are a few implications for health campaigns.

- *Correct misperceptions about descriptive norms.* Although descriptive norms do not tell the whole story, nearly everyone agrees that people who overestimate the prevalence of risky behaviors are more likely than others to feel that the behaviors are acceptable and even socially preferred.
- *Emphasize descriptive and injunctive norms.* For example, a sun-safety program was particularly effective when the health promoters presented both an injunctive norm (photos that showed undesirable skin damage) and a descriptive norm (information that most people now use sunscreen) (Mahler, Kulik, Butler, Gerrard, & Gibbons, 2008).
- *Do not rely solely on norming messages.* Norms sometimes take a backseat to other factors, such as personal enjoyment. College students in Cameron and Campo's (2006) study were most likely to smoke, exercise, and drink if they enjoyed those behaviors, even when there was no strong peer support for them. It may help to emphasize the negative repercussions of unhealthy behaviors as well as social norms.
- *Target social networks.* A common suggestion among social norm researchers is that campaigns treat alcohol abuse as a social network issue. This often involves developing partnerships with sororities and fraternities, sports teams, student governments, and other groups.

The debate continues to be lively and productive. The success of the RU SURE campaign at Rutgers may be based partly on its social norm foundation and partly on the integrated and multifaceted nature of the campaign itself. TNSB offers a rich, contextual understanding of the facets that figure into social norming, a concept that continues to evolve and to influence theorists as well as practitioners.

NARRATIVE MESSAGES

If history were taught in the form of stories, it would never be forgotten.

—Rudyard Kipling

Stories capture our imagination, hold our attention, and often affect us deeply. At least the good ones do. Narratives inspire a greater sense of realism, allow us to identify with characters, and engage us emotionally and cognitively more than many didactic approaches (Miller-Day & Hecht, 2013). They can transport us to scenarios we have not experienced personally and convey complex information in a way that is not overwhelming (Niederdeppe, Shapiro, Kim, Bartolo, & Porticella, 2014; Sanders-Jackson, 2014; Stavrositu & Kim, 2015).

For these reasons health promoters have increasingly begun to use stories to reach people, educate them, and persuade them to change their behaviors. And this approach seems to be working. A recent meta-analysis of narrative research shows that stories have statistically significant relationships with people's beliefs, attitudes, intentions, and behaviors (Braddock & Dillard, 2016).

A narrative's persuasiveness is usually measured along two dimensions: transportation and emotional response. **Transportation** describes a number of nuances, including how much attention people pay to the story, how involved they are with the story's characters, and how immersed they are in the story's imaginary world (Green & Brock, 2000). **Emotional response** describes how strongly the story affects people as well as people's emotional engagement with the story and/or characters (Dunlop, Wakefield, & Kashima, 2008). The more transported and emotionally affected people are by a story, the more likely they are to be persuaded by it.

Consider this example. Researchers in India wanted to know if exposure to a narrative message about domestic violence would increase bystander intervention. Could a story inspire someone who witnessed domestic violence to physically stop an abuser or call the police? To find out, Sidharth Muralidharan and Eunjin Kim (2019) recruited participants to read one of two PSAs about domestic violence—one a narrative PSA and the other an informational PSA. The participants then completed a survey that measured their attitudes about domestic violence, their emotional responses to the PSAs, and their behavioral intentions.

Compared to the informational PSA, the narrative PSA—a first-person account of a woman's experience being abused by her husband and later saved by an anonymous call to the police—elicited a stronger emotional response from study participants, which correlated with greater intentions to intervene in domestic violence situations.

Other studies have shown that narrative messages boost people's intentions to be screened for colon cancer (McQueen, Caburnay, Kreuter, & Sefko, 2019); increase empathy for people struggling with obesity, which, in turn, positively influences opinions about public policies to combat obesity (Sun, Lee, & Qian, 2019); and reduces the stigma surrounding opioid addiction, thus helping shift responsibility for the problem from individual sufferers to the larger social forces that helped create the opioid epidemic (Heley, Kennedy-Hendricks, Niederdeppe, & Barry, 2019).

LOGICAL APPEALS

A **logical appeal** attempts to demonstrate an evidentiary (demonstrable) link between a behavior and a result. For example, it may seem logical to eat less if it will result in greater health and a longer life. Logical appeals are often based on the results of scientific studies. Quoting science is not as clear cut as it sounds, however.

Daniel O'Keefe (2015) proposes that, to present evidence fairly and responsibly, health promoters should rely on data that are consistent across studies that involve a representative range of people and message types. He also urges health promoters to avoid unsupported generalizations by taking into account the effect of sizes (how strongly two or more variables are related) and confidence intervals (the likelihood that the results are accurate and consistent rather than the result of chance variations). Other theorists also stress that it is important to present clear and convincing evidence rather than "scientific flourishes" such as fancy words and irrelevant numbers (Hample & Hample, 2014).

As we have discussed, scientific evidence is not always the only, or even the most compelling, factor that people consider when making health choices. Community standards, emotions, and preferences play a role as well.

EMOTIONAL APPEALS

An **emotional appeal** (also called an *affect appeal*) suggests that people feel a certain way regarding their health and their behaviors. For example, they may be afraid to have unprotected sex, proud if they have quit smoking, or guilty if they are endangering others. Ellen Peters and colleagues (2006) propose that persuasive appeals that involve affect typically make one of four general claims:

- They campaign for particular interpretations, as when we think, "The people in that drug commercial look really happy; it must be a good medicine";
- They grab or hold our attention.
- They motivate us to think carefully or take action; and
- They link behaviors with community values, as when a message encourages us to recycle because it is good for the earth or to stop smoking because it puts our children in danger (Peters et al., 2006).

Although emotions occur along a complex continuum, Peters and colleagues observe that there are two basic "flavors"—positive and negative. For the most part, campaigns encourage people to strive for positive outcomes and to avoid negative ones. Research discussed in this section describes the usefulness and the limitations of various emotional appeals.

POSITIVE-AFFECT APPEALS. Campaigns may promote positive emotional rewards in the form of popularity, a sense of accomplishment, honor, fun, happiness, and so on. As we discussed in Chapter 11, pharmaceutical ads are famous for implying that people who take the advertised drugs are remarkably healthy, active, and attractive.

Campaigns may also inspire positive affect because the messages themselves are pleasant or entertaining. Let's consider the impact of funny messages. Research shows us that people are engaged by funny messages and, therefore, are often more motivated to pay attention and think about the messages. For example, Robin Nabi (2016) found that funny cancer prevention PSAs about breast and testicular self-exams increased people's motivation to process message content, which led to positive self-exam attitudes and intentions. And because people tend to pay more attention to funny messages, they often remember more about humorous appeals than other types of appeals (Blanc & Brigaud, 2014).

Funny messages are persuasive for other reasons as well. Exposure to humorous messages stimulates positive emotions, and people tend to associate the resulting "feel good vibes" with whatever the message is about, whether it's cancer prevention or a brand of beer. People also tend to talk more about funny messages, which reinforces positive attitudes about the messages' content. Hanneke Hendriks and Madelijn Strick (2019) discovered that beer ads work particularly well for this reason. When people were shown funny beer ads, they had more conversations about both the ads and alcohol, had longer conversations about alcohol, and had positive discussions about the ads. These conversations, in turn, led to more positive evaluations of the ads and of alcohol, which, as Hendriks and Strick (2019) cautioned, could lead to (more) positive drinking attitudes, social norms, and intentions.

Like advertisers, health promoters can use humor to stimulate conversations and shape attitudes, but Hanneke Hendriks and Loes Janssen (2018) suggest that the best tactic might be combining humor with fear—especially if the target audience is male. Hendricks and Janssen studied messages that discouraged excessive alcohol and caffeine consumption and they concluded that men were more likely than women to be persuaded by high threat messages that also contained humorous elements. We'll talk more about fear appeals below.

It's important to note that, while positive affect may be the honey that draws people to health messages they might otherwise ignore, it is no guarantee that the messages will be influential. Sometimes people pay attention to humor, graphics, or music, but they may not attend to a message's main information, especially if the issue is not one that concerns them very much.

NEGATIVE-AFFECT APPEALS. Some campaign designers attempt to motivate people by making them feel anxious, guilty, or fearful. The research on negative-affect appeals, however, is mixed. There is ample evidence that fearful appeals are effective at convincing people to be tested for AIDS and to take other health precautions (Green & Witte, 2006; Hullett, 2006). But there is also evidence that fear appeals don't work particularly well and can even be counterproductive (Kok, Peters, Kessel, Hoor, Ruiter, 2018).

Communication theorist Kim Witte, who has done a lot of work on fear appeals, explains that if people are not anxious about a health topic, then they probably are not motivated to learn about it or to take action. However, as we have said, if people are overly anxious or fearful, they may avoid the subject. Fear can be an effective motivator, but only under certain conditions.

Witte's **extended parallel process model** (EPPM) proposes that people evaluate a threatening or fearful message in two stages. First, they determine if they are personally at risk. Second, they judge whether they can prevent a harmful outcome based on the message's recommended behavior and on their ability to carry out the behavior. If people perceive a risk but do not feel they can avoid a bad outcome, perhaps because they lack self-efficacy, then they are likely to soothe their anxiety by avoiding the issue (Witte, 1997, 2008). But if self-efficacy is high, fear appeals can prompt behavior change (Kok et al., 2018). Some evidence suggests that a 1-to-1 ratio of threatening messages and confidence-building (efficacy) messages seems most effective (Carcioppolo et al., 2013). So, for every threat, a solution should also be presented. (A similar 1-to-1 approach is adopted in many risk communication models, as discussed in Chapter 12.)

Guilt, a feeling of remorse about having done something wrong, is a particularly strong emotion. Consequently, it's a popular tool for advertisers and health campaigners. People typically feel sorry or ashamed when they have behaved badly, especially when others are hurt by their actions. Messages that bring feelings of guilt to the surface often offer a way to make retribution or soothe one's conscience. On the flip side, people may behave in ways that prevent a guilty feeling in the first place. Evidence suggests that people are more likely to sign up as organ donors if they think that saying no will make them feel guilty (Wang, 2011).

Guilt appeals generally have a positive effect (Xu & Guo, 2018), but they can backfire. For instance, one meta-analysis found that guilt appeals that are highly explicit can actually stimulate anger in message recipients, making them less likely to change their behaviors (O'Keefe, 2000). Guilt can also trigger unhealthy eating habits and lower perceived behavioral control over eating (Kuijer, Boyce, & Marshall, 2015).

Overall, negative affect is a popular component of persuasive messages, but it must be used carefully. Health promoters have overshot the mark in some cases. Women in the United States now consistently overestimate their risk of breast cancer (Jones, Denham, & Springston, 2007). And it is not easy to reassure them. Amanda Dillard and colleagues found that it was just as difficult to reduce women's sense of breast cancer danger as it was to *stimulate* their concern about other health risks (Dillard, McCaul, Kelso, & Klein, 2006).

NOVEL AND SHOCKING MESSAGES

Novel messages tend to catch people's attention and stick in their memory (Parrott, 1995). Some messages are novel (new or different) without being **shocking** (intense or improper). For instance, London residents were surprised to find that the names of famous shops and landmarks had changed overnight as part of a National Health Service campaign (see Box 14.4). The novel approach was attention getting but not edgy enough to offend. At other times, novel messages may be shocking because they deal with topics not usually discussed in public or because they are purposefully controversial to attract attention. One difficulty about using novel images to attract attention is that novelty wears off. Keeping novelty alive may mean becoming ever more risqué. It's sometimes difficult to balance decorum with the need for public awareness.

One difficulty surrounding AIDS awareness is that health promoters must deal with delicate issues like premarital sex and anal intercourse. Even when promoters do not mean to be shocking, they often are. For instance, when AIDS first became a health concern, condoms and gay sex were not socially acceptable topics for mass-media campaigns. In the 1990s, controversy arose concerning a poster campaign in New York City.

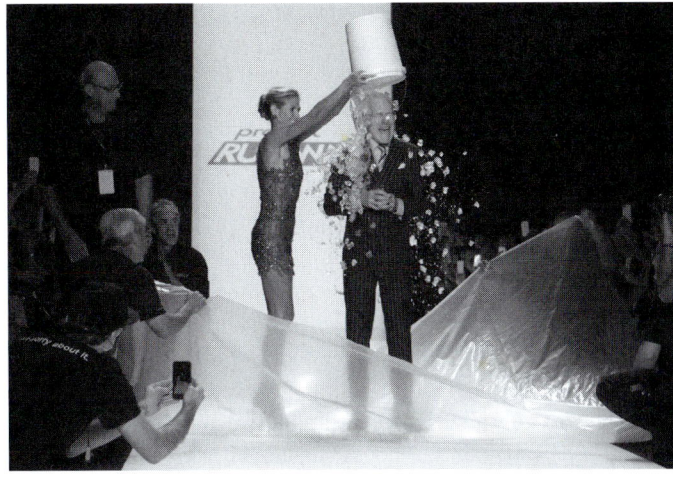

Heidi Klum obliges Tim Gunn with an Ice Bucket Challenge to raise awareness about amyotrophic lateral sclerosis (ALS). The challenge was to dump ice water over one's head or make a donation to the ALS Association. More than 3 million celebrities and everyday people took an ice bath for the cause, often capturing the experience on video and posting it online. The novel approach and publicity inspired donations as well, about $115 million worth within a few months (Tirrell, 2015).

The posters (which were hung in subway terminals) read "Young, Hot, Safe!" and showed images of same-sex couples kissing while holding condoms ("Controversy Heats Up," 1994). Some people felt the posters were indecent, while others argued that they communicated an important message to a high-risk group. (The poster campaign was discontinued soon thereafter.)

BOX 14.4

S-mething Is Missing

By Elizabeth McPherson

In June 2015, names of famous landmarks in the United Kingdom suddenly lost three important letters: A, O, and B. Overnight, world-renowned Downing Street became "D-wning Street" and the *Daily Mirror* became the "*D-ily M-rror*." In an online article, British Broadcasting Corporation (BBC) Newsbeat asked: "S- who is d-ing it, -nd why -re they d-ing it?" (BBC Newsbeat, 2015).

The missing letters, A, O, and B, all refer to blood groups in short supply. As part of a carefully crafted health campaign to raise awareness during the UK's National Blood Week, companies, individuals, and the media deleted the three letters on signs, messages, and headlines, then used the hashtag #missingtype to promote their activities on social media. Within days the campaign attracted international attention.

The high-profile campaign, started by the National Health Service (NHS), was designed to attract 204,000 new blood donors across England and North Wales (NHS, 2015). The NHS is funded through taxes. In return, all services—from preventive care to extensive medical procedures like transplants—are free to residents at the point of use (NHS, 2015).

LESSONS ABOUT EMOTIONAL APPEALS. Here are a few guidelines, suggested by theorists and researchers, about using emotional appeals.

- *Match the emotion to the goal.* Emotional appeals are most persuasive when they are appropriate to the desired response. For example, fear appeals can alert people to danger, disgust appeals can make unhealthy behaviors unappealing, hope appeals can convince people it is worth taking action, and so on (Dillard & Nabi, 2006).
- *Build empathy.* "It won't happen to me" is a common response to health messages, even when they are highly arousing. For example, we may feel concerned about intravenous drug users because they are at risk for AIDS but perceive our own risk to be negligible because we are not part of that group. We usually feel a sense of personal relevance only if we understand the message cognitively, the message effectively conveys feelings of vulnerability, and we perceive that those feelings are relevant to our own situations (Campbell & Babrow, 2004).
- *Don't overdo it.* Too much affect can be counterproductive and cause people to avoid the issue or to worry unnecessarily (Peters et al., 2006, p. S155).

Step 6: Piloting and Implementing the Campaign

It's important to pilot (pretest) a campaign before launching it full scale. **Piloting usually involves selecting members from the target audience to review the** campaign materials and comment on them. Salmon and Atkin (2003) state that early feedback is crucial:

> The feedback from the audience can reveal whether the tone is too righteous (admonishing unhealthy people about their incorrect behavior), the recommendations too extremist (rigidly advocating unpalatable ideas of healthy behavior), the execution too politically correct (staying within tightly prescribed boundaries of propriety to avoid offending overly sensitive authorities and interest groups), and the execution too self-indulgent (letting creativity and style overwhelm substance and substantive content). (p. 453)

Some questions to consider include the following:

- Are written messages easy to read and understand?
- Are recorded messages easy to understand?
- Do messages seem relevant and important?
- Are the messages appealing? Why or why not?
- Is the spokesperson effective?
- Does the information seem controversial or offensive?

It may be useful to survey people before and after they are exposed to campaign materials to see if there is any change in their knowledge, attitudes, and intentions. When possible, it is also advisable to survey people a week or a month after they were initially exposed to campaign materials to see how much they remember and whether message effects are still present. Remember to allow time to refine campaign messages based on the results of pretesting. Planning ahead will improve the campaign's likelihood of success.

Once campaign messages have been created, piloted, and refined, it's time to distribute them through chosen channels. In many cases (as with one-on-one communication, community presentations, online messages, and social media), health promoters have direct contact with community members and thus have control over what is conveyed. For some channels, however, health promoters must rely on others to share, and sometimes to edit, their messages. For instance, editors and news directors choose what PSAs to publicize and when, and what topics to cover in the news. On a social level, community opinion leaders focus on some issues more than others, affecting what the people around them think and believe. People in the media and the community who decide what information will be publicized and how are known as **gatekeepers**.

Good campaign designers employ a variety of communication channels to help ensure that messages make it to focus community members through one gate or another. Wise health promoters realize the importance of gatekeepers, include them in campaign planning, and consider their points of view. Media gatekeepers are bound by multiple pressures (e.g., operating budgets, community demands, and time constraints). The promoter who gets to know gatekeepers personally and makes it easy for them to pass along information has a better chance of getting messages to community members.

Step 7: Evaluating and Maintaining the Campaign

A campaign is not over when it has been released to the public. Effective health promotion requires that campaign managers evaluate the success of the project, help community members maintain any positive changes they may have made, and refine and develop future campaign messages.

Evaluation

The effects of a campaign may be evaluated in several ways. A **pretest–posttest design** means that campaigners survey people before the campaign is released and then survey them again afterward to see if their knowledge, intentions, or behaviors have changed. You might go about this in two different ways—by exposing people to campaign materials in a controlled environment such as a classroom or community center and evaluating their immediate responses (an **efficacy study**), or by studying campaign effects in the context of people's everyday lives (an **effectiveness study**) (Evans, Uhrig, Davis, & McCormack, 2009, p. 315). W. Douglas Evans and colleagues (2009) found that efficacy studies offer several advantages: (1) You can make sure the participants are exposed to your campaign messages before they respond to your questions, (2) you minimize the likelihood that responses have been affected by extraneous factors, and (3) you can expose

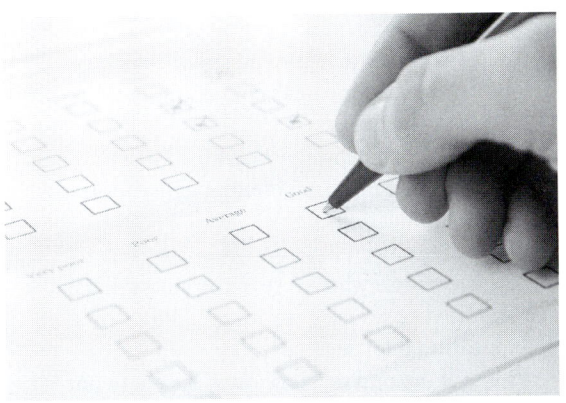

A pretest–posttest design involves surveying people before a campaign is released and then again afterward to see if their knowledge, intentions, or behaviors have changed.

Can you think of other ways to measure a campaign's success? How might you assess the effectiveness of our sports recreation campaign?

members of the target audience to multiple messages and see how their responses to messages differ. Of course, efficacy studies may not tell you how many people in the larger population are affected or how, so you may want to use both efficacy and effectiveness studies to evaluate your campaign. Keep in mind that if changes have occurred, they may or may not be the result of campaign exposure (e.g., the Montana Meth Project, which we discussed in Chapter 13).

Let's take a look at how the truth® campaign described in Chapter 13 was evaluated. Researchers conducted telephone surveys with 6,897 youth ages 12 to 17 before the campaign began (Farrelly, Healton, Davis, Messeri, & Haviland, 2002). The survey participants were chosen to represent teens in different ethnic and racial groups, urban and nonurban areas, and areas with and without other anti-tobacco campaigns. Researchers asked the youth to indicate their level of agreement or disagreement with statements about the tobacco industry, the social acceptability of smoking, and their intention to smoke within the next year. In follow-up interviews after the campaign's release, researchers asked 10,692 youth if they remembered seeing any anti-tobacco campaigns and, if so, what they remembered about them. They also asked about perceptions of the tobacco industry, the social acceptability of smoking, and the youths' intention to smoke in the next year. To factor out as many intervening variables as possible, researchers statistically controlled for such factors as the number of parents in the household, amount of television viewing, the presence of smokers in the household, and parental messages about smoking. With the data collected, researchers were able (1) to gauge the extent to which community members saw and remembered the campaign, and (2) to compare youth attitudes before and after the campaign.

Another way to evaluate a campaign's success is to study actual behavior changes, such as the number of people who sign up for gym memberships, or the number of hospital admissions, or calls to a hotline. These evaluation techniques are useful, but it's always difficult to know precisely what effects a campaign has had. For one thing, the campaign is not the only factor influencing people's attitudes and behavior. They may be affected by personal experiences, natural disasters, news stories, or other occurrences. Second, campaigns often have indirect effects. For instance, the campaign may have reached influential members of the community, who in turn spread the word to others. Thus, people who were not exposed to campaign messages directly may still be affected by them. Third, sometimes the success of a health campaign is reflected in what does *not* occur over the long run. For example, the coordinators of a drug-free program in elementary schools may not know if they have been successful until the children involved are adolescents or adults, by which time they will have been influenced by many other factors as well. When undesired behaviors do not occur, it's difficult to know how many people might have adopted those behaviors if not for the campaign.

For better or worse, sometimes the best that campaigners can do is evaluate the **reach** (number of people exposed to campaign messages) and **specificity** (the type of people exposed to the messages) of a campaign. For this purpose, promoters can survey community members and keep track of when and where campaign messages are publicized.

Maintenance

Maintaining behaviors that have been positively influenced by a campaign involves continued encouragement and skills training. Keep in mind that people are most likely to continue new behaviors if they fully understand the benefits of doing so. Because some people try new behaviors without taking this step, do not assume that people who begin a behavior are fully educated about it. Encouragement, incentives, and continued skills training can help people overcome setbacks they are likely to encounter.

Summary

Designing and Implementing Campaigns

- Many health-promotion efforts are based on social norms and social marketing.
- Social norms theory proposes that people base their behavior partly on what they consider to be normal among their peers.
- Social marketing is informed by the 4 Ps of marketing: price, product, promotion, and place.
- Social marketers conduct extensive audience analyses and strive to create messages with the same appeal as commercial messages.

Theories of Behavior Change

- Theories of behavior change explain the conditions under which people are likely to make lifestyle changes. The overall message is that behavior is influenced by a complex array of factors, both internal and external.
- Failing to consider these can lead to health campaigns that look good but have very little social value. In addition, campaign designers who fail to consider and accommodate audience members' beliefs and opportunities can alienate the people they hope to influence and can actually make things worse by promoting behaviors that people find offensive, puzzling, or even impossible to carry out.
- One alternative is for health advocates to serve as facilitators and enablers who help communities set their own agendas and build collective efficacy and social capacity.

Critical-Cultural Perspective

- In designing campaign messages, health promoters should consider ethical implications concerning timing, scapegoating, and stigmatizing, as well as audience needs, campaign goals, and benefits of the recommended behaviors.

Step 5: Designing Campaign Messages

- Campaign messages have different voices, ranging from stern to casual and friendly. Often, the spokesperson influences how the message is perceived.
- Research suggests that people typically respond most favorably to spokespersons who are similar to them, likable, and attractive.
- When it comes to health messages, source credibility increases people's compliance with recommended behaviors.
- The same behavior may be framed in a number of ways to emphasize potential gains, losses, or social implications.
- Narrative storytelling is a promising way to engage people who relate to the storytellers. Narratives are also a way to provide culturally appealing information.
- Some campaign messages also appeal to our logic and emotions. Messages may motivate people through positive affect, such as the promise of pleasure and happiness. Humorous appeals are particularly effective because they get attention, are memorable, stimulate discussion, and help shape attitudes. Negative-affect appeals may induce people to change by stirring up feelings of anxiety, fear, and guilt.

- According to the extended parallel process model, anxiety and fear are powerful motivators, except when the threat is so overwhelming that people would rather avoid the issue.
- Novel and shocking messages typically create interest, but they may be controversial and offensive to some people.

Step 6: Piloting and Implementing the Campaign

- Experts recommend that health promoters pilot new campaigns before implementing them. Testing campaign messages on sample community members can reveal unanticipated reactions and ambiguities so messages can be improved before they are publicly released.

Step 7: Evaluating and Maintaining the Campaign

- Health promoters should evaluate campaigns once they are released, apply what they have learned to future efforts, and compare the results with their goals.

Glossary

collective efficacy A communal sense that positive change can be accomplished. *See page 329.*

community capacity The resources needed for good health, such as healthy food and water, safe shelter, and medical care. *See page 329.*

critical-cultural approach Proposes that health is not merely the result of individual choices, but is intertwined with issues of culture, power, control, identity, and social consciousness. *See page 326.*

descriptive norm Typical patterns of behavior that describe what most people do. *See page 335.*

effectiveness study Involves studying campaign effects in the context of people's everyday lives. *See page 341.*

efficacy study Involves exposing people to campaign materials in a controlled environment such as a classroom or community center and evaluating their immediate responses. *See page 341.*

emotional appeal Suggests that people feel a certain way regarding their health and their behaviors. *See page 337.*

emotional response Describes how strongly a story affects people as well as people's emotional engagement with the story and/or characters. *See page 336.*

environmental factors Include social approval, physical environment, institutional rules, and the like. *See page 322.*

extended parallel process model (EPPM) Proposes that people evaluate a threatening or fearful message in two stages. First, they determine if they are personally at risk. Second, they judge whether they can prevent a harmful outcome based on the message's recommended behavior and on their ability to carry out the behavior. *See page 338.*

gain-frame appeal A message that illustrates the advantages of performing the recommended behavior. *See page 332.*

gatekeepers People in the media and the community who decide what information will be publicized and how. *See page 340.*

guilt Feeling of remorse about having done something wrong. *See page 338.*

health belief model Posits that people make behavioral choices based on six factors: perceived risk, severity of the risk, recommended actions, advantages of complying with recommendations, their belief in their ability to carry out recommendations, and specific cues to actions. *See page 321.*

injunctive norm Perceptions that people ought to engage in particular behaviors based on morals or values; the idea that certain behaviors are approved or disapproved. *See page 335.*

internal factors Include knowledge, skills, emotions, habits, and so on. *See page 322.*

loss-frame appeal A message that emphasizes the negative repercussions of not taking action. *See page 332.*

logical appeal Attempts to demonstrate an evidentiary (demonstrable) link between a behavior and a result. *See page 337.*

narrative message A message that uses a story to educate and/or persuade. *See page 336.*

novel messages Messages that are new or different. *See page 339.*

piloting Selecting members from the target audience to review the campaign materials and comment on them. *See page 340.*

pretest–posttest design Measurements taken both before and after exposure to campaign messages. Comparing the results determines if or how the audience's knowledge, intentions, or behaviors may have changed as a result of the campaign. *See page 341.*

reach The number of people exposed to campaign messages. *See page 342.*

scapegoat To blame one person or group for the whole problem. *See page 327.*

shocking messages Messages that are intense or improper. *See page 339.*

social marketing An approach wherein campaign designers apply principles of commercial advertising to prosocial campaigns, such as health-promotion efforts. *See page 320.*

social cognitive theory The proposition that people make decisions by considering the interplay of internal and environmental factors. *See page 322.*

source homophily Phenomenon whereby audiences place trust in people who are similar to them. *See page 331.*

social norms theory Suggests that people base their behavior partly on what they consider appropriate and socially acceptable. *See page 335.*

specificity The type of people exposed to campaign messages. *See page 342.*

theory of normative social behavior (TNSB) Theory proposing that we are influenced by perceived social norms, but that a variety of factors either strengthen or weaken how much those perceptions affect us: how much we value the social approval to be gained from conforming, the outcomes we expect from engaging in the behavior, the degree to which we identify with the group, and how confident we feel in our ability to say no to the behavior in question. *See page 335.*

theory of reasoned action (TRA) The theoretical assumption that people are rational decision makers who make decisions and deliberate choices based on two primary considerations: how strongly they believe a behavior will lead to positive outcomes and the perceived social implications of performing that behavior. *See page 323.*

theory of planned behavior Proposes that the difference between wanting to do something and actually doing it lies partly in the strength of a person's intentions, which are shaped by three main factors: the person's attitudes about the issue and behaviors, how socially rewarding and acceptable they consider it to be, and the extent to which they feel that they can carry out the behavior. *See page 323.*

transportation Describes how much attention people pay to a story, how involved they are with the story's characters, and how immersed they are in the story's imaginary world. *See page 336.*

transtheoretical model Proposes that change typically involves five stages: precontemplation, contemplation, preparation, action, and maintenance. *See page 324.*

Discussion Questions

1. What is the first health-related PSA or campaign that comes to your mind? Why do you think it is so memorable? What is your favorite PSA or campaign? Why? Do you think health campaigns influence the choices you make? Why or why not?
2. Identify several campaign messages.
    a. From the perspective of social marketing, what are the "costs" and rewards of the recommended behavior in each message?
    b. Analyze how the messages reflect components of the following theories: health belief model, social cognitive theory, theory of planned behavior, and transtheoretical model.
    c. Analyze the same messages from the critical-cultural perspective. Do they seem culturally inclusive and sensitive? What role do issues such as power, control, identity, and social consciousness play? Do the messages seem to build collective efficacy and/or community capacity? If so, how? How might you reframe these messages to reflect the goals and realities of a community with which you identify?
3. Think of a health-related behavior (e.g., drinking water, avoiding sweets, getting enough sleep). Brainstorm ways you can frame the behavior in terms of potential losses, gains, and risks. What do you think would be most effective? Why?
4. What do you think of the idea that health-promotion experts, although they mean well, often reinforce a group's marginal status by adopting a paternalistic "this is what you should do" mindset? Have you ever felt misunderstood or belittled by people who were trying to help you? If so, describe the experience.
5. In what circumstances are positive-affect messages usually effective? Negative-affect appeals? Think of as many examples as you can. Which type of appeal do you typically prefer, and why?
6. Explain the extended parallel process model as it relates to negative-affect appeals. Give an example from your own experience.

References

CHAPTER 1

Ashraf, A. A., Colakoglu, S., Nguyen, J. T., Anastasopulos, A. J., Ibrahim, A. M., Yueh, J. H., . . . Lee, B. T. (2013). Association for Academic Surgery: Patient involvement in the decision-making process improves satisfaction and quality of life in postmastectomy breast reconstruction. *Journal of Surgical Research*, *184*, 665–670.

Barnlund, D. (1970). A transactional model of communication. In K. K. Sereno & C. D. Mortensen (Eds.), *Foundations of communication theory* (pp. 83–102). New York: Harper.

Batra, N., Betts, D., & Davis, S. (2019). Forces of change: The future of health. Deloitte Insights. Retrieved from https://www2.deloitte.com/content/dam/Deloitte/ec/Documents/life-sciences-health-care/DI_Forces-of-change_Future-of-health%20(1).pdf

Birkeland, S., Murphy-Graham, E., & Weiss, C. (2005). Good reasons for ignoring good evaluation: The case of the drug abuse resistance education (D.A.R.E.) program. *Evaluation and Program Planning*, *28*, 247–256.

Clayton, M. F., Iacob, E., Reblin, M., & Ellington, L. (2019). Hospice nurse identification of comfortable and difficult discussion topics: Associations among self-perceived communication effectiveness, nursing stress, life events, and burnout. *Patient Education and Counseling*, *102*(10), 1793–1801.

Dutta, M. J., & de Souza, R. (2008). The past, present, and future of health development campaigns: Reflexivity and the critical-cultural approach. *Health Communication*, *23*, 326–339.

Dym, H. (2008). Risk management techniques for the general dentist and specialist. *Dental Clinics of North America*, *52*(3), 563–577.

Dyrbye, L. N., Varkey, P., Boone, S. L., Satele, D. V., Sloan, J. A., & Shanafelt, T. D. (2013). Physician satisfaction and burnout at different career stages. *Mayo Clinic Proceedings*, *88*(12), 1358–1367.

Fouad, A. M., Waheed, A., Gamal, A., Amer, S. A., Abdellah, R. F., & Shebl, F. M. (2017). Effect of chronic diseases on work productivity: A propensity score analysis. *Journal of Occupational and Environmental Medicine*, *59*(5), 480–485.

Friedman, D. B., Hooker, S. P., Wilcox, S., Burroughs, E. L., & Rheaume, C. E. (2012). African American men's perspectives on promoting physical activity: "We're not that difficult to figure out!" *Journal of Health Communication*, *17*, 1151–1170.

Gallagher, S., Phillips, A. C., Ferraro, A. J., Drayson, M. T., & Carroll, D. (2008). Social communication is positively associated with the immunoglobulin M response to vaccination with pneumococcal polysaccharides. *Biological Psychology*, *78*(2), 211–215.

Geertz, C. (1973). *The interpretation of cultures*. New York: Basic Books.

Health and economic costs of chronic diseases. (2019, February 11). Centers for Disease Control and Prevention and National Center for Chronic Disease Prevention and Health Promotion. Retrieved from https://www.cdc.gov/chronicdisease/about/costs/index.htm

Healthcare workers. (2017, January 13). Centers for Disease Control and Prevention and National Institute for Occupational Safety and Health. Retrieved from https://www.cdc.gov/niosh/topics/healthcare/default.html

Heart disease and stroke cost America nearly $1 billion a day in medical costs, lost productivity. (2015, April 19). CDC Foundation. Retrieved from https://www.cdcfoundation.org/pr/2015/heart-disease-and-stroke-cost-america-nearly-1-billion-day-medical-costs-lost-productivity

Hugin, R. J. (2018, February 14). How we can fix our broken health-care system. CNBC. Retrieved from https://www.cnbc.com/2018/02/13/how-we-can-fix-our-broken-health-care-system-commentary.html

Khullar, D., & Chokski, D. A. (2018, October 4). Health, income, & poverty: Where we are & what could help. *Health Affairs*. Retrieved from https://www.healthaffairs.org/do/10.1377/hpb20180817.901935/full/

Khvitsko, T. (2018, October 4). Being disabled or feeling disabled? Knit-Rite. Retrieved from https://blog.knitrite.com/2018/10/04/being-disabled-or-feeling-disabled/

Koch-Weser, S., Bradshaw, Y. S., Gualtieri, L., & Gallagher, S. S. (2010). The internet as a health information source: Findings from the 2007 Health Information National Trends Survey and implications for health communication. *Journal of Health Communication*, *15*, 279–293.

Kodjebacheva, G. D., Estrada, L. F., & Parker, S. (2017). Family-healthcare provider communication and reported health among children and adolescents in the United States: Results from the National Survey of Children's Health. *Californian Journal of Health Promotion*, *15*(1), 46–55.

Kreps, G. L. (2005). Disseminating relevant health information to underserved audiences: Implications of the Digital Divide Pilot Projects. *Journal of the Medical Library Association*, *93*(4S), S68–S73.

Kreps, G. L., Query, J. L., Jr., & Bonaguro, E. W. (2008). The interdisciplinary study of health communication and its relationship to communication science. In L. C. Lederman (Ed.), *Beyond these walls: Readings in health communication* (pp. 3–14). New York: Oxford University Press.

Kreps, G. L., & Thornton, B. C. (1992). *Health communication: Theory & practice* (2nd ed.). Prospect Heights, IL: Waveland Press.

Longino, C. F. (1997, December). Beyond the body: An emerging medical paradigm. *American Demographics*, *19*, 14–18.

Lovell, B., Moss, M., & Wetherell, M. A. (2011). Perceived stress, common health complaints and diurnal patterns of cortisol secretion in young, otherwise healthy individuals. *Hormones and Behavior, 60*, 301–305.

National Alliance on Mental Illness (NAMI). (2019, September). Mental health by the numbers. Retrieved from https://www.nami.org/learn-more/mental-health-by-the-numbers

National Diabetes Statistics Report. (2017). National Center for Chronic Disease Prevention and Health Promotion. Retrieved from https://www.cdc.gov/diabetes/pdfs/data/statistics/national-diabetes-statistics-report.pdf

National Health Council. (2014, July 29). *About chronic diseases*. Washington, DC: Author. Retrieved from https://www.nationalhealthcouncil.org/sites/default/files/AboutChronicDisease.pdf

Nemeth, S. A. (2000). Society, sexuality, and disabled/able bodied romantic relationships. In D. O. Braithwaite & T. L. Thompson (Eds.), *Handbook of communication and people with disabilities: Research and applications* (pp. 37–48). Mahwah, NJ: Lawrence Erlbaum.

Rains, S. A. (2008, June). Health at high speed: Broadband internet access, health communication, and the digital divide. *Communication Research, 35*(3), 283–297.

Rapaport, L. (2018, November 28). Untreated hearing loss linked to higher health costs, most hospitalizations. *Reuters*. Retrieved from https://www.reuters.com/article/us-health-costs-hearing-loss/untreated-hearing-loss-linked-to-higher-health-costs-more-hospitalizations-idUSKCN1NX2NV

Rogers, L. E., & Escudero, V. (2004). Theoretical foundations. In L. E. Rogers & V. Escudero (Eds.), *Relational communication: An interactional perspective to the study of process and form* (pp. 3–21). Mahwah, NJ: Lawrence Erlbaum.

Sanders, L. (2003). The ethics imperative. *Modern Healthcare, 33*(11), 46.

Senge, P. M. (2006). *The fifth discipline: The art and practice of the learning organization.* New York: Doubleday/Currency.

Smith, R. (2018, April 30). Hillsborough teen: Apple Watch saved my life. *ABC Action News*. Retrieved from https://www.abcactionnews.com/news/region-hillsborough/hillsborough-teen-apple-watch-saved-my-life

Stephens, N. M., Markus, H. R., & Fryberg, S. A. (2012). Social class disparities in health and education: Reducing inequality by applying a sociocultural self model of behavior. *Psychological Review, 119*, 723–744.

Street, J. R. L., Makoul, G., Arora, N. K., & Epstein, R. M. (2009). How does communication heal? Pathways linking clinician–patient communication to health outcomes. *Patient Education and Counseling, 74*(3), 295–301.

Suennen, L. (2015, February 15). My patient experience: At times comforted and other moments abandoned. *MedCity News*. Retrieved from https://medcitynews.com/2015/02/walked-patients-shoes-heres-good-bad-ugly/?rf=1

Thompson, T. L. (2014). *Encyclopedia of health communication*. Thousand Oaks, CA: Sage.

Thompson, T. L., Parrott, R., & Nussbaum, J. F. (2011). *The Routledge handbook of health communication.* New York: Taylor & Francis.

U.S. Bureau of Labor Statistics. (2019, September 4). Occupational handbook: Healthcare occupations. Retrieved from https://www.bls.gov/ooh/healthcare/home.htm

U.S. Department of Education. (2015). Digest of education: Statistics 2014, Table 507. Literacy skills of adults, by type of literacy, proficiency levels, and selected characteristics: 1992–2003. Retrieved from https://nces.ed.gov/fastfacts/display.asp?id=69

Vernon, J. A., Trujillo, A., Rosenbaum, S., & DeBuono, B. (2007). Low health literacy: Implications for national health policy. Retrieved from http://publichealth.gwu.edu/departments/healthpolicy/CHPR/downloads/LowHealthLiteracyReport10_4_07.pdf

von Bertalanffy, L. (1968). General system theory: Foundations, development, applications. New York: George Braziller.

Watzlawick, P., Beavin, J. H., & Jackson, D. D. (1967). *Pragmatics of human communication.* New York: W. W. Norton.

Wittenberg-Lyles, E., Washington, K., Demiris, G., Oliver, D. P., & Shaunfield, S. (2014). Understanding social support burden among family caregivers. *Health Communication, 29*, 901.

World Health Organization (WHO). (1948). *Preamble to the Constitution of the World Health Organization. Official records of the World Health Organization*, no. 2, p.100. Geneva, Switzerland: Author. Retrieved from www.who.int/about/definition/en

World Health Organization (WHO). (2002). Towards a common language for functioning, disability and health. *The International classification of functioning, disability, and health (ICF)*. Geneva, Switzerland: Author. Retrieved from https://www.who.int/classifications/icf/icfbeginnersguide.pdf

CHAPTER 2

Amadeo, K. (2019, June 25). Universal care in different countries, pros and cons of each. *The Balance*. Retrieved from https://www.thebalance.com/universal-health-care-4156211

American Medical Association. (2019). *2018 AMA prior authorization (PA) physician survey.* Washington, DC: Author. Retrieved from https://www.ama-assn.org/system/files/2019-02/prior-auth-2018.pdf

American Osteopathic Association. (2018, May 14). *Survey finds patients want to be friends with their physicians on social media.* Chicago, IL: Author. Retrieved from https://osteopathic.org/2018/05/14/survey-finds-patients-want-to-be-friends-with-their-physicians-on-social-media/

Bilicic, W. (n.d.). Spot-Aid [blog]. Retrieved from https://www.spot-aid.com/

Broderick, A., & Haque, F. (2015, May 13). Mobile health and patient engagement in the safety net: A survey of community health centers and clinics. *The Commonwealth Fund*. Retrieved from https://www.commonwealthfund.org/publications/issue-briefs/2015/may/mobile-health-and-patient-engagement-safety-net-survey-community?redirect_source=/publications/issue-briefs/2015/may/mobile-health-and-patient-engagement-in-the-safety-net

Brookhardt-Murray, J. (2005, September 1). Effectively navigating the healthcare system. *The Body*. Retrieved from https://www.thebody.com/article/effectively-navigating-healthcare-system

Catania, G., Bagnasco, A., Zanini, M., Aleo, G., & Sasso, L. (2016). The effect of nurse-led navigation programmes on cancer patients' outcomes. *Cancer Nursing Practice*, *15*(7), 32.

Center for Consumer Information and Insurance Oversight. (2011, November 16). Fighting unreasonable health insurance premium increases. Retrieved from https://www.cms.gov/CCIIO/Resources/Fact-Sheets-and-FAQs/ratereview05192011a.html

Centers for Disease Control and Prevention (CDC). (2019, February 11). *Health and economic costs of chronic diseases*. Washington, DC: Author. Retrieved from https://www.cdc.gov/chronicdisease/about/costs/index.htm

Chetty, R. (2016). The association between income and life expectancy in the United States, 2001–2014. *Journal of the American Medical Association*, *16*, 1750–1766.

Clark, S., Singer, D., Solway, E., Kirch, M., & Malani, P. (2018, June). *Logging in: Using patient portals to access health information*. University of Michigan National Poll on Healthy Aging. Retrieved from http://hdl.handle.net/2027.42/145683

Commonwealth Fund. (2013, September 18). *Health care in the two Americas: Findings for the scorecard on state health system performance for low-income populations, 2013*. New York: Author. Retrieved from http://www.commonwealthfund.org/publications/fund-reports/2013/sep/low-income-scorecard

Commonwealth Fund. (2015, March 16). *Washington health policy week in review*. New York: Author. Retrieved from http://www.commonwealthfund.org/publications/newsletters/washington-health-policy-in-review/2015/mar/mar-16-2015/many-households-lack-liquid-savings-to-pay-deductibles

Commonwealth Fund (2019, June 12). *State health care scorecard finds deaths from suicide, alcohol, drug are a regional epidemic; impact varies widely across states*. New York: Author. Retrieved from https://www.commonwealthfund.org/sites/default/files/2019-06/Radley_state_scorecard_2019_PRESS_RELEASE_final_06-12-2019_v2.pdf

Cozma, R. (2009, Fall). Online health communication: Source or eliminator of health myths? *Southwestern Mass Communication Journal*, *24*(2), 69–80.

Cubanksi, J. (2018, November 28). *Sources of supplemental coverage among Medicare beneficiaries in 2016*. Kaiser Family Foundation. Retrieved from https://www.kff.org/medicare/issue-brief/sources-of-supplemental-coverage-among-medicare-beneficiaries-in-2016/

Davis, K., Schoen, C., & Bandeali, F. (2015, April 30). *Medicare: 50 years of ensuring coverage and care*. Commonwealth Fund. Retrieved from https://www.commonwealthfund.org/publications/fund-reports/2015/apr/medicare-50-years-ensuring-coverage-and-care

Dorsey, J. L., & Berwick, D. M. (2008, February 27). Dirty words in healthcare. *Boston Globe*, Op-Ed, p. A9.

Economic Research Initiative on the Uninsured. (2005, December). Rising health care costs frustrate efforts to reduce uninsured rate. *ERIU Research Highlight* No. 10. Retrieved from eriu.sph.umich.edu/pdf/highlight-chernew.pdf

Fullman, N., Yearwood, J., Abay, S. M., Abbafati, C., Abd-Allah, F., Abdela, J., . . . & Lozano, R. (2018). Measuring performance on the Healthcare Access and Quality Index for 195 countries and territories and selected subnational locations: A systematic analysis from the Global Burden of Disease Study 2016. *The Lancet*, *391*(10136), 2236–2271.

Garfield, R., & Orgera, K. (2019, March 21). *The coverage gap: Uninsured poor adults in states that do not expand Medicaid*. Kaiser Family Foundation. Retrieved from https://www.kff.org/medicaid/issue-brief/the-coverage-gap-uninsured-poor-adults-in-states-that-do-not-expand-medicaid/

Health economics: Soaring healthcare premiums seen as threat to managed care. (2003, July 14). *Health & Medicine Week*, p. 56.

Hendrich, A., Chow, M., Skierczynski, B. A., & Lu, Z. (2008). A 36-hospital time and motion study: How do medical-surgical nurses spend their time? *The Permanente Journal*, *12*(3), 25–34.

Henry J. Kaiser Family Foundation. (2017, September 19). *2017 employer health benefits survey*. Menlo Park, CA: Author. Retrieved from https://www.kff.org/report-section/ehbs-2017-section-1-cost-of-health-insurance/

Henry J. Kaiser Family Foundation. (2018, October 3). *2018 employer health benefits survey*. Menlo Park, CA: Author. Retrieved from https://www.kff.org/report-section/2018-employer-health-benefits-survey-summary-of-findings/

Hsiao, W. C., Knight, A. G., Kappel, S., & Done, N. (2011). What other states can learn from Vermont's bold experiment: Embracing a single-payer health care financing system. *Health Affairs*, *30*, 1232–1241.

Hudson, A. P., Spooner, A. J., Booth, N., Penny, R. A., Gordon, L. G., Downer, T.-R., . . . Chan, R. J. (2019). Qualitative insights of patients and carers under the care of nurse navigators. *Collegian*, *26*(1), 110–117.

Jauhar, S. (2008). *Intern: A doctor's initiation*. New York: Farrar, Straus and Giroux.

Jiang, S., & Street, R. L. (2017). Factors influencing communication with doctors via the internet: A cross-sectional analysis of 2014 HINTS Survey. *Health Communication*, *32*(2), 180–188.

Kaiser Family Foundation. (2019, June 11). *Data note: American's challenges with health care costs*. Menlo Park, CA: Author. Retrieved from https://www.kff.org/health-costs/issue-brief/data-note-americans-challenges-health-care-costs/

Kern, L. M. (2018, October 9). *Whether fragmentation care is hazardous depends on how many chronic conditions a patient has*. The Commonwealth Fund. Retrieved from https://www.commonwealthfund

.org/publications/journal-article/2018/oct/fragmented-care-chronic-conditions-overuse-hospital

Key facts about the uninsured population. (2018, December 7). *Key facts about the uninsured population*. Kaiser Family Foundation. Retrieved from https://www.kff.org/uninsured/fact-sheet/key-facts-about-the-uninsured-population/

Khullar, D. (2018, September 23). Even as the U.S. grows more diverse, the medical profession is slow to follow. *The Washington Post*. Retrieved from https://www.washingtonpost.com/national/health-science/even-as-the-us-grows-more-diverse-the-medical-profession-is-slow-to-follow/2018/09/21/6e048d66-aba4-11e8-a8d7-0f63ab8b1370_story.html?utm_term=.4386ae93961a

Lefferts, D. (2018, November 2). The medicine maze. PW talks with Sana Goldberg. *Publishers Weekly*. Retrieved from https://www.publishersweekly.com/pw/by-topic/authors/interviews/article/78495-the-medicine-maze-pw-talks-with-sana-goldberg.html

Michelson, L. D. (2015). *The patient's playbook: How to save your life and the lives of those you love*. New York: Knopf Doubleday.

Organisation for Economic Co-Operation and Development (OECD). (2019a). *Health status: Life expectancy*. Paris: Author. Retrieved from https://stats.oecd.org/Index.aspx?DataSetCode=HEALTH_STAT

Organisation for Economic Co-Operation and Development (OECD). (2019b). *Health status: Perceived health status*. Paris: Author. Retrieved from https://stats.oecd.org/Index.aspx?DataSetCode=HEALTH_STAT

Organisation for Economic Co-Operation and Development (OECD). (2019c). *Health status: Cancer*. Paris: Author. Retrieved from https://stats.oecd.org/Index.aspx?DataSetCode=HEALTH_STAT

Peckham, C. (2013, March 28). *Physician lifestyles—linking to burnout*. Medscape. Retrieved from https://www.medscape.com/features/slideshow/lifestyle/2013/public

Rhiannon. (2018, February 8). How online community helped me. *Mind*. Retrieved from https://www.mind.org.uk/information-support/your-stories/how-online-community-helped-me/#.XQpGhtNKjlc

Roche, K. L., Angarita, A. M., Cristello, A., Lippitt, M., Haider, A. H., Bowie, J. V., . . . Tergas, A. I. (2016). "Little big things": A qualitative study of ovarian cancer survivors and their experiences with the health care system. *Journal of Oncology Practice*, *12*(12), e974–e980.

Rocque, G. B., Pisu, M., Jackson, B. E., Kvale, E. A., Demark-Wahnefried, W., Martin, M. Y., . . . Partridge, E. E. (2017). Resource use and Medicare costs during lay navigation for geriatric patients with cancer. *Journal of the American Medical Association Oncology*, *3*(6), 817–825.

Schneider, E., Abrams, M., Shah, A., Lewis, C., & Shah, T. (2018, October). *Health care in America: The experience of people with serious illnesses*. The Commonwealth Fund. Retrieved from https://www.commonwealthfund.org/sites/default/files/2018-10/Schneider_Health CareinAmerica.pdf

Sharmeen Shommu, N., Ahmed, S., Rumana, N., Barron, G. R. S., McBrien, K. A., & Chowdhury Turin, T. (2016). What is the scope of improving immigrant and ethnic minority healthcare using community navigators: A systematic scoping review. *International Journal for Equity in Health*, *15*, 1–12.

Should all Americans have the right (be entitled) to health care? (2019, February 14). *ProCon*. Retrieved from https://healthcare.procon.org

Tu, H. T. (2005, June). Medicare seniors much less willing to limit physician-hospital choice for lower costs. *Center for Studying Health System Change*, Issue Brief No. 96, nonpaginated. Retrieved from www.hschange.org/CONTENT/744

United Nations. (2019). *17 goals to change our world*. Geneva, Switzerland: Author. Retrieved from https://www.un.org/sustainabledevelopment/

U.S. Bureau of Labor Statistics. (2019, January 18). *Labor force statistics from the current population survey*. Washington, DC: Author. Retrieved from https://www.bls.gov/cps/cpsaat11.htm

U.S. Census Bureau. (2018, July 1). *Quick facts: Population estimates*. Washington, DC: Author. Retrieved from https://www.census.gov/quickfacts/fact/table/US#

Vespa, J., Armstrong, D. M., & Medina, L. (2018, March). *Demographic turning points for the United States: Population projections for 2020 to 2060*. U.S. Census Bureau. Retrieved from https://www.census.gov/content/dam/Census/library/publications/2018/demo/P25_1144.pdf

Walker, B. (2017, January 30). Insights on today's healthcare consumer. *C2B Solutions*. Retrieved from https://insights.c2bsolutions.com/blog/2-ways-improving-communication-for-underserved-patients

World Health Organization (WHO). (2011). *Fact file on health inequities. World Conference on Social Determinants of Health*. Geneva, Switzerland: Author. Retrieved from https://www.who.int/sdhconference/background/news/facts/en/

World Health Organization (WHO). (2015, June 10). *Ebola situation report*. Geneva, Switzerland: Author. Retrieved from http://apps.who.int/ebola/en/current-situation/ebola-situation-report-10-june-2015

World Health Organization (WHO). (2017). *Global health observatory (GHO) data. Life expectancy*. Geneva, Switzerland: Author. Retrieved from https://www.who.int/gho/mortality_burden_disease/life_tables/situation_trends_text/en/

World Health Organization (WHO). (2018a, February 8). *Ageing and health*. Geneva, Switzerland: Author. Retrieved from https://www.who.int/news-room/fact-sheets/detail/ageing-and-health

World Health Organization (WHO). (2018b). *Global expenditures database*. Geneva, Switzerland: Author. Retrieved from https://apps.who.int/nha/database/ViewData/Indicators/en

World Health Organization (WHO). (2018c, July 19). *HIV/AIDS. Data and statistics*. Geneva, Switzerland: Author. Retrieved from https://www.who.int/hiv/data/en/

World Health Organization (WHO). (2019a, January). *Migrants and refugees at higher risk of developing ill health than host populations, reveals first-ever WHO report on the health of displaced people in Europe*. Geneva,

Switzerland: Author. Retrieved from http://www.euro.who.int/en/media-centre/sections/press-releases/2019/migrants-and-refugees-at-higher-risk-of-developing-ill-health-than-host-populations-reveals-first-ever-who-report-on-the-health-of-displaced-people-in-europe

World Health Organization (WHO). (2019b). *Refugee and migrant health*. Geneva, Switzerland: Author. Retrieved from https://www.who.int/migrants/en/

World Health Organization (WHO). (2019c). *Ten threats to global health in 2019*. Author: Geneva, Switzerland. Retrieved from https://www.who.int/emergencies/ten-threats-to-global-health-in-2019

World Population Review. (2019). *Life expectancy by country 2019*. Walnut, CA: Author. Retrieved from http://worldpopulationreview.com/countries/life-expectancy/

CHAPTER 3

Adams, N., & Field, L. (2001). Pain management 1: Psychological and social aspects of pain. *British Journal of Nursing, 10*(14), 903–911.

Adams, R., Price, K., Tucker, G., Nguyen, A.-M., & Wilson, D. (2012). The doctor and the patient—How is a clinical encounter perceived? *Patient Education and Counseling, 86*(1), 127–133.

Anderson, P. M., & Hanna, R. (2019). Defining moments: Making time for virtual visits and catalyzing better cancer care. *Health Communication*. Online publication.

Arnetz, J. E., Zhdanova, L., & Arnetz, B. B. (2016). Patient involvement: A new source of stress in health care work? *Health Communication, 31*(12), 1566–1572.

Balint, J., & Shelton, W. (1996). Regaining the initiative: Forging a new model of the patient–physician relationship. *Journal of the American Medical Association, 275*, 887–892.

Barnes, R. K. (2018). Preliminaries to treatment recommendations in UK primary care: A vehicle for shared decision making? *Health Communication, 33*(11), 1366–1376.

Benjamin, J. M., Cox, E. D., Trapskin, P. J., Rajamanickam, V. P., Jorgenson, R. C., Weber, H. L., . . . Lubcke, N. L. (2015). Family-initiated dialogue about medications during family-centered rounds. *Pediatrics, 1*, 94.

Bethea, L. S., Travis, S. S., & Pecchioni, L. (2000). Family caregivers' use of humor in conveying information about caring for dependent older adults. *Health Communication, 12*(4), 361–376.

Blevins, C. E., Anderson, B. J., Caviness, C. M., Herman, D. S., & Stein, M. D. (2019). Emerging adults' discussion of substance use and sexual behavior with providers. *Journal of Health Communication, 2*, 121–128.

Bochner, S. (1983). Doctors, patients and their cultures. In D. Pendleton & J. Hasler (Eds.), *Doctor–patient communication* (pp. 127–138). London: Academic Press.

Bock, B. C., Becker, B. M., Niaura, R. S., Partridge, R., Fava, J. L., & Trask, P. (2008). Smoking cessation among patients in an emergency chest pain observation unit: Outcomes of the Chest Pain Smoking Study (CPSS). *Nicotine & Tobacco Research, 10*(10), 1523–1531.

Brady, M. J., & Cella, D. F. (1995, May 30). Helping patients live with their cancer. *Patient Care, 29*(10), 41–49.

Branch, W. T., Jr., & Malik, T. K. (1993). Using "windows of opportunities" in brief interviews to understand patients' concerns. *Journal of the American Medical Association, 269*, 1667–1668.

Britton, P. C., Williams, G. C., & Conner, K. R. (2008). Self-determination theory, motivational interviewing, and the treatment of clients with acute suicidal ideation. *Journal of Clinical Psychology, 64*(1), 52–66.

Broom, A. (2008). Virtually healthy: The impact of internet use on disease experience and the doctor–patient relationship. In L. C. Lederman (Ed.), *Beyond these walls: Readings in health communication* (pp. 92–109). New York: Oxford University Press.

Brown, J., & Addington-Hall, J. (2007). How people with motor neuron disease talk about living with illness: A narrative study. *Journal of Advanced Nursing, 62*(2), 200–208.

Brüggemann, A. J., Wijma, B., & Swahnberg, K. (2012, November). Patients' silence following healthcare staff's ethical transgressions. *Nursing Ethics, 19*(6), 750–763.

Buckley, L. M. (2008). *Talking with patients about the personal impact of illness: The doctor's role*. New York: Radcliffe.

Bundgaard, K., Sørensen, E. E., & Nielsen, K. B. (2011). The art of holding hands: A fieldwork study outlining the significance of physical touch in facilities for short-term stay. *International Journal for Human Caring, 15*(3), 34–41.

Cegala, D. J., Street, R. L., Jr., & Clinch, C. R. (2007). The impact of patient participation on physicians' information provision during a primary care medical interview. *Health Communication, 21*, 177–185.

Charon, R. (2006). *Narrative medicine: Honoring the stories of illness*. New York: Oxford University Press.

Charon, R. (2009a). Narrative medicine as witness for the self-telling body. *Journal of Applied Communication Research, 37*, 118–131.

Charon, R. (2009b). The polis of a discursive narrative medicine. *Journal of Applied Communication Research, 37*, 196–201.

Clayton, M. F., Iacob, E., Reblin, M., & Ellington, L. (in press). Hospice nurse identification of comfortable and difficult discussion topics: Associations among self-perceived communication effectiveness, nursing stress, life events, and burnout. *Patient Education and Counseling, 102*(10), 1793-1801.

Córdova, D., Lua, F. M., Ovadje, L., Fessler, K., Bauermeister, J. A., Salas-Wright, C. P., . . . Youth Leadership Council. (2018). Adolescent experiences of clinician–patient HIV/STI communication in primary care. *Health Communication, 33*(9), 1177–1183.

Coupland, N., Coupland, J., & Giles, H. (1991). *Language, society & the elderly*. Oxford: Blackwell.

Dervin, B. (1999, May). *Sense-making's theory of dialogue: A brief introduction*. Paper presented at a nondivisional workshop held at the meeting of the International Communication Association, San Francisco.

Dervin, B., & Frenette, M. (2001). Sense-making methodology: Communicating communicatively with campaign audiences. In R. Rice & C. Atkin (Eds.), *Public *communication campaigns* (3rd ed., pp. 69–87). Thousand Oaks, CA: Sage.

Dillon, P. J. (2012). Assessing the influence of patient participation in primary care medical interviews on recall of treatment recommendations. *Health Communication, 27,* 58–65.

Drugs facts. *Monitoring the future survey*: High school and youth trends. (2018, December). National Institute on Drug Abuse. Retrieved from https://www.drugabuse.gov/publications/drugfacts/monitoring-future-survey-high-school-youth-trends

du Pré, A. (1998). *Humor and the healing arts: Multimethod analysis of humor use in health care.* Mahwah, NJ: Lawrence Erlbaum.

Dym, H. (2008). Risk management techniques for the general dentist and specialist. *Dental Clinics of North America, 52*(3), 563–577.

Edgar, T. M., Satterfield, D. W., & Whaley, B. B. (2005). Explanations of illness: A bridge to understanding. In E. B. Ray (Ed.), *Health communication in practice: A case study approach* (pp. 95–109). Mahwah, NJ: Lawrence Erlbaum.

Eggly, S. (2002). Physician–patient co-construction of illness narratives in the medical interview. *Health Communication, 14,* 339–360.

Epstein, R. M., Fiscella, K., Lesser, C. S., & Stange, K. C. (2010). *Why the nation needs a policy push on patient-centered health care.* The Commonwealth Fund. Retrieved from http://www.commonwealthfund.org/Publications/In-the-Literature/2010/Aug/Why-the-Nation-Needs-a-Policy-Push.aspx

Eriksson, T. (2015). Evidence-based and pragmatic steps for pharmacists to improve patient adherence. *Integrated Pharmacy Research and Practice, 4,* 13–19.

Fahey, K. F., Rao, S. M., Douglas, M. K., Thomas, M. L., Elliott, J. E., & Miaskowski, C. (2008). Nurse coaching to explore and modify patient attitudinal barriers interfering with effective cancer pain management. *Oncology Nursing Forum, 35*(2), 234–240.

Farber, N. J., Novack, D. H., & O'Brien, M. K. (1997). Love, boundaries, and the patient–physician relationship. *Archives of Internal Medicine, 157,* 229–294.

Gade, C. J. (2007). Understanding and defining roles in the pharmacist–patient relationship. *Journal of Communication in Healthcare, 1,* 88–98.

Geist, P., & Dreyer, J. (1993). The demise of dialogue: A critique of medical encounter dialogue. *Western Journal of Communication, 57,* 233–246.

Geist, P., & Gates, L. (1996). The poetics and politics of recovering identities in health communication. *Communication Studies, 47,* 218–228.

Geller, G., Bernhardt, B. A., Carrese, J., Rushton, C. H., & Kolodner, K. (2008). What do clinicians derive from partnering with their patients? Reliable and valid measure of "personal meaning in patient care." *Patient Education and Counseling, 72,* 293–300.

Greene, K. (2009). An integrated model of health disclosure decision-making. In T. D. Afifi & W. A. Afifi (Eds.), *Uncertainty and information regulation in interpersonal contexts: Theories and applications* (pp. 226–253). New York: Routledge.

Greene, K., Magsamen-Conrad, K., Venetis, M. K., Checton, M. G., Bagdasarov, Z., & Banerjee, S. C. (2012). Assessing health diagnosis disclosure decisions in relationships: Testing the disclosure decision-making model. *Health Communication, 27,* 356–368.

Groopman, J. (2007). *How doctors think.* Boston: Houghton Mifflin.

Halkowski, T. (2006). Realizing the illness: Patients' narratives of symptom discovery. In J. Heritage & D. W. Maynard (Eds.), *Communication in medical care: Interactions between primary care physicians and patients* (pp. 86–114). Cambridge: Cambridge University Press.

Harres, A. (2008). "But basically you're feeling well, are you?" Tag questions in medical consultations. In L. C. Lederman (Ed.), *Beyond these walls: Readings in health communication* (pp. 49–57). New York: Oxford University Press.

Harter, L. M. (2009). Narratives as dialogic, contested, and aesthetic performances. *Journal of Applied Communication Research, 37,* 140–150.

He, X., Sun, Q., & Stetler, C. (2018). Warm communication style strengthens expectations and increases perceived improvement. *Health Communication, 33*(8), 939–945.

Heritage, J., & Robinson, J. D. (2006). The structure of patients' presenting concerns: Physicians' opening questions. *Health Communication, 19,* 89–102.

Hesson, A. M., Sarinopoulos, I., Frankel, R. M., & Smith, R. C. (2012). A linguistic study of patient-centered interviewing: Emergent interactional effects. *Patient Education and Counseling, 88,* 373–380.

Hummert, M. L., & Mazloff, D. C. (2001). Older adults' responses to patronizing advice. *Journal of Language & Social Psychology, 20*(1/2), 167–196.

Jacobsen, S. K., Bouchard, G. M., Emed, J., Lepage, K., & Cook, E. (2015). Experiences of "being known" by the healthcare team of young adult patients with cancer. *Oncology Nursing Forum, 42*(3), 250–257.

Jiang, S. (2017). Pathway linking patient-centered communication to emotional well-being: Taking into account patient satisfaction and emotion management. *Journal of Health Communication, 22*(3), 234–242.

Julliard, K., Vivar, J., Delgado, C., Cruz, E., Kabak, J., & Sabers, H. (2008). What Latina patients don't tell their doctors: A qualitative study. *Annals of Family Medicine, 6*(6), 543–549.

Kakai, H. (2002). A double standard in bioethical reasoning for disclosure of advanced cancer diagnosis in Japan. *Health Communication, 14,* 361–376.

Kaplan, R. M. (1997). Health outcomes and communication research. *Health Communication, 9,* 75–82.

Katz, J. (1984). *The silent world of doctor and patient.* New York: Free Press.

Koermer, C. D., & Kilbane, M. (2008). Physician sociality communication and its effect on patient satisfaction. *Communication Quarterly, 56,* 69–86.

Laine, C., & Davidoff, F. (1996). Patient-centered medicine: A professional evolution. *Journal of the American Medical Association, 275,* 152–155.

Lambert, B. L., Street, R. L., Cegala, D. J., Smith, D. H., Kurtz, S., & Schofield, T. (1997). Provider–patient communication, patient-centered care, and the mangle of practice. *Health Communication, 9*, 27–43.

Légaré, F., & Witteman, H. O. (2013). Shared decision making: examining key elements and barriers to adoption into routine clinical practice. *Health Affairs, 32*(2), 276–284.

Li, C.-C., Matthews, A. K., Dossaji, M., & Fullam, F. (2017). The relationship of patient–provider communication on quality of life among African-American and White cancer survivors. *Journal of Health Communication, 22*(7), 584–592.

Li, H. Z., Krysko, M., Desroches, N. G., & Deagle, G. (2004). Reconceptualizing interruptions in physician–patient interviews: Cooperative and intrusive. *Communication & Medicine, 1*(2), 145–157.

Lumma-Sellenthin, A. (2009). Talking with patients and peers: Medical students' difficulties with learning communication skills. *Medical Teacher, 31*, 528–534.

Maathuis, E. (2018, June 11). What to do if a doctor is being rude to you during an appointment. Quora. Retrieved from https://www.quora.com/What-do-you-do-if-a-doctor-is-being-rude-to-you-during-an-appointment

Magee, M., & D'Antonio, M. (2003). *The best medicine: Stories of doctors and patients who care for each other* (2nd ed.). New York: Spencer Books.

McBride, R. (2012, January 27). Talking to patients about sensitive topics: Communication and screening techniques for increasing the liability of patient self-report. MedEd Portal. Retrieved from https://www.mededportal.org/publication/9089/

McCall, C. (2018, May 22). Therapy completed changed my life—here's how. The Everygirl. Retrieved from http://theeverygirl.com/therapy-changed-my-life/

McCarley, P. (2009). Patient empowerment and motivational interviewing: Engaging patients to self-manage their own care. *Nephrology Nursing Journal, 36*(4), 409–413.

McCreaddie, M., & Payne, S. (2012). Humour in health-care interactions: A risk worth taking. *Health Expectations, 17*(3), 332–344.

Miller, W. R., & Rollnick, S. (2002). *Motivational interviewing: Preparing people for change.* New York: Guilford Press.

Morgan, S. E., Occa, A., Mouton, A., & Potter, J. (2017). The role of nonverbal communication behaviors in clinical trial and research study recruitment. *Health Communication, 32*(4), 461–469.

Nicolai, J., Demmel, R., & Farsch, K. (2010). Effects of mode of presentation on ratings of empathic communication in medical interviews. *Patient Education and Counseling, 80*, 76–79.

Nordby, H., & Nøhr, O. N. (2011). Care and empathy in ambulance services: Paramedics' experiences of communicative challenges in transports of patients with prolonged cancer. *Journal of Communication in Healthcare, 4*, 215–226.

Norling, G. R. (2005). Developing a theoretical model of rapport building: Implications for medical education and the physician–patient relationship. In M. Haider (Ed.), *Global public health communication* (pp. 407–414). Boston: Jones and Bartlett.

October, T. W., Dizon, Z. B., & Roter, D. L. (2018). Is it my turn to speak? An analysis of the dialogue in the family-physician intensive care unit conference. *Patient Education and Counseling, 101*(4), 647–652.

Palmer-Wackerly, A. L., Krieger, J. L., & Rhodes, N. D. (2017). The role of health care provider and partner decisional support in patients' cancer treatment decision-making satisfaction. *Journal of Health Communication, 22*, 10–19.

Pateet, J. R., Fremonta, L. M., & Miovic, M. K. (2011). Possibly impossible patients: Management of difficult behavior in oncology patients. *Journal of Oncology Practice, 7*, 242–246.

Patient-centered care continues to deliver on promise of better quality care a lower cost. (2015, August). Patient-Centered Primary Care Collaborative. Retrieved from https://www.pcpcc.org/resource/patient-centered-care-continues-deliver-promise-better-quality-care-lower-cost

Pelto-Piri, V., Engström, K., & Engström, I. (2013). Paternalism, autonomy and reciprocity: Ethical perspectives in encounters with patients in psychiatric in-patient care. *BMC [Biomed Central] Medical Ethics, 14*, 49.

Platt, F. W. (1995). *Conversation repair: Case studies in doctor–patient communication.* Boston: Little, Brown.

Rawlins, W. K. (1989). A dialectical analysis of the tensions, functions, and strategic challenges of communication in young adult friendships. *Communication Yearbook, 12*, 157–189.

Rawlins, W. K. (1992). *Friendship matters: Communication, dialectics, and the life course.* New York: Aldine De Gruyter.

Rawlins, W. K. (2009). Narrative medicine and the stories of friends. *Journal of Applied Communication Research, 37*, 167–173.

Reno, J. E., O'Leary, S., Garrett, K., Pyrzanowski, J., Lockhart, S., Campagna, E., . . . Dempsey, A. F. (2018). Improving provider communication about HPV vaccines for vaccine-hesitant parents through the use of motivational interviewing. *Journal of Health Communication, 23*(4), 313–320.

Riiser, K., Løndal, K., Ommundsen, Y., Småstuen, M. C., Misvær, N., & Helseth, S. (2014). The outcomes of a 12-week internet intervention aimed at improving fitness and health-related quality of life in overweight adolescents. *Plos ONE, 9*(12), 1–21.

Rollnick, S., & Miller, W. (1995). What is motivational interviewing? *Behavioural and Cognitive Psychotherapy, 23*, 325–334. Reprinted online. Retrieved from http://www.motivationalinterview.net/clinical/whatismi.html

Rosenberg, A., Starks, H., & Unguru, Y., Fuedtner, C., & Diekema, D. (2017, November). Truth telling in the setting of cultural differences and incurable pediatric illness: A review. *JAMA Pediatrics, 171*(11), 1113–1119.

Rosti, G. (2017). Role of narrative-based medicine in proper patient assessment. *Supportive Care in Cancer, 25*, 3–6.

Ruben, M. A., Meterko, M., & Bokhour, B. G. (2018, February). Do patient perceptions of provider communication relate to experiences of physical pain? *Patient Education & Counseling, 101*(2), 209–213.

Schmid Mast, M., Hall, J. A., & Roter, D. (2008). Caring and dominance affect participants' perceptions and behaviors during a virtual medical visit. *Journal of General Internal Medicine, 23*(5), 523–527.

Scholl, J. C. (2007). The use of humor to promote patient-centered care. *Journal of Applied Communication Research, 35*(2), 156–176.

Silvester, J., Patterson, F., Koczwara, A., & Ferguson, E. (2007). "Trust me . . .": Psychological and behavioral predictors or perceived physician empathy. *Journal of Applied Psychology, 92*(2), 519–527.

Sisk, B., Frankel, R., Kodish, E., & Harry Isaacson, J. (2016). The truth about truth-telling in American medicine: A brief history. *The Permanente Journal, 20*(3), 15–219. Retrieved from https://www.ncbi.nlm.nih.gov/pmc/articles/PMC4991917/

Small, D. (2019). Defining moments and healing emplotment: "I have cancer; it doesn't have me." *Health Communication, 34*(4), 515–517.

Smith, R. C., & Hoppe, R. B. (1991). The patient's story: Integrating the patient- and physician-centered approaches to interviewing. *Annals of Internal Medicine, 115*, 460–477.

Stepler, R. (2015, November 15). 4 facts about family caregivers. *Pew Research Center*. Retrieved from https://www.pewresearch.org/fact-tank/2015/11/18/5-facts-about-family-caregivers/

Stivers, T., Heritage, J., Barnes, R. K., McCabe, R., Thompson, L., & Toerien, M. (2018). Treatment recommendations as actions. *Health Communication, 33*(11), 1335–1344.

Street, R. L., Makoul, G., Arora, N. K., & Epstein, R. M. (2009). How does communication heal? Pathways linking clinician-patient communication to health outcomes. *Patient Education and Counseling, 74*(3), 295–301.

Suchman, A. L., Markakis, K., Beckman, H. B., & Frankel, R. (1997). A model of empathic communication in the medical interview. *Journal of the American Medical Association, 277*, 678–683.

Transue, E. R. (2004). *On call: A doctor's days and nights in residency*. New York: St. Martin's Griffin.

Ünal, S. (2012). Evaluating the effect of self-awareness and communication techniques on nurses' assertiveness and self-esteem. *Contemporary Nurse: A Journal for the Australian Nursing Profession, 43*(1), 90–98.

Underage drinking. (2017, February). National Institute on Alcohol Abuse and Alcoholism. Retrieved from https://www.niaaa.nih.gov/publications/brochures-and-fact-sheets/underage-drinking

van Zanten, M., Boulet, J. R., & McKinley, D. (2007). Using standardized patients to assess the interpersonal skills of physicians: Six years' experience with a high-stakes certification examination. *Health Communication, 22*(3), 195–205.

Walsh, K., Jordan, Z., & Apolloni, L. (2009). The problematic art of conversation: Communication and health practice evolution. *Practice Development in Health Care, 8*, 166–179.

Watson, T. J. (2014). What we have here is a failure to communicate! Communication mistakes account for 25 percent of malpractice claims at WILMIC and are among the most frequent grievances filed with the OLR; avoid communication breakdown with clients by following effective communication practices. *The Wisconsin Lawyer, 11*, 51.

Watzlawick, P., Beavin, J. H., & Jackson, D. D. (1967). *Pragmatics of human communication*. New York: W. W. Norton.

Weiss, G. G. (2008, June 20). The new doctor–patient paradigm: How the shift from the "physician as wise parent" model to one of more shared responsibility is playing out in the exam room. *Medical Economics, 85*(12), 48–52.

Welch, G., Rose, G., & Ernst, D. (2006). Motivational interviewing and diabetes: What is used, and does it work? *Diabetes Spectrum, 19*(1), 5–11.

Wynia, M. (2004, February). Invoking therapeutic privilege. *American Medical Association Journal of Ethics, 6*(2), 90–92. Retrieved from https://journalofethics.ama-assn.org/article/invoking-therapeutic-privilege/2004-02

Yang F., Zhang Q., Kong W., Shen H., Lu J., Ge, X., & Zhuang, Y. (2018). A qualitative study on the attitudes of patients with gastrointestinal cancer toward being informed of the truth. *Patient Preference and Adherence, 12*, 2283–2290.

Young, A., & Flower, L. (2002). Patients as partners, patients as problem-solvers. *Health Communication, 14*, 69–97.

Zaner, R. M. (2009). Narrative and decision. *Journal of Applied Communication Research, 37*, 174–187.

Zikmund-Fisher, B. J., Couper, M. P., Singer, E., Ziniel, S., Fowler, F., . . . Fagerlin, A. (2010) The DECISIONS study: A nationwide survey of U.S. adults regarding nine common medical decisions. *Medical Decision Making, 30*(5S), S20–S34.

Zisman-Ilani, Y., Roe, D., Elwyn, G., Kupermintz, H., Patya, N., Peleg, I., & Karnieli-Miller, O. (2019). Shared decision making for psychiatric rehabilitation services before discharge from psychiatric hospitals. *Health Communication, 34*(6), 631–637.

Zook, R. (1997, April). Handling inappropriate sexual behavior with confidence: Here are nine tips for keeping the boundaries clear. *Nursing, 27*, 65.

CHAPTER 4

Adams, J. R., Elwyn, G., Légaré, F., & Frosch, D. L. (2012). Communicating with physicians about medical decisions: A reluctance to disagree. *Archives of Internal Medicine, 172*(15), 1184–1186.

Ashley, B. M., & O'Rourke, K. D. (1997). *Health care ethics: A theological analysis* (4th ed.). Washington, DC: Georgetown University Press.

Bleustein, C., Valaitis, E., & Jones, R. (2010). Effect of wait room time on ambulatory patient satisfaction. *Otolaryngology—Head and Neck Surgery, 143*, P38–P39.

Brick, D. J., Scherr, K. A., & Ubel, P. A. (2019). The impact of cost conversations on the patient-physician relationship. *Health Communication, 34*(1), 65–73.

Brown, T. (2012, March 14). Hospitals aren't hotels. *The New York Times*. Retrieved from http://www.nytimes.com/2012/03/15/opinion/hospitals-must-first-hurt-to-heal.html

Burgoon, M. H., & Burgoon, J. K. (1990). Compliance-gaining and health care. In J. P. Dillard (Ed.), *Seeking compliance: The production of interpersonal influence messages* (pp. 161–188). Scottsdale, AZ: Gorsuch Scarisbrick.

Charmaz, K. (1987). Struggling for a self: Identity levels of the chronically ill. In J. Roth & P. Conrad (Eds.), *Research in the sociology of health care* (pp. 283–321). Greenwich, CT: JAI Press.

Chou, W.-Y., Wang, L. C., Finney Rutten, L. J., Moser, R. P., & Hesse, B. W. (2010). Factors associated with Americans' ratings of health care quality: What do they tell us about the raters and health care systems? *Journal of Health Communication*, *15*, 147–156.

Clements, B. (1996). Talk is cheaper than three extra office visits. *American Medical News*, *39*, 17–20.

Cortés, D. E., Drainoni, M.-L., Henault, L. E., & Paasche-Orlow, M. K. (2010). How to achieve informed consent for research from Spanish-speaking individuals with low literacy: A qualitative report. *Journal of Health Communication*, *15*, 172–182.

Cousin, G., Mast, M. S., Roter, D. L., & Hall, J. A. (2012). Concordance between physician communication style and patient attitudes predicts patient satisfaction. *Patient Education and Counseling*, *87*, 193–197.

Dahm, M. R. (2012). Tales of time, terms, and patient information-seeking behavior—An exploratory qualitative study. *Health Communication*, *27*, 682–689.

Defenbaugh, N. L. (2013). Revealing and concealing ill identity: A performance narrative of IBD disclosure. *Health Communication*, *28*, 159–169.

Deloitte. (2008). Reality check: 2008 survey of health care consumers. Retrieved from http://www.deloitte.com/dtt/article/0,1002,cid=192468,00.html

Egerton, J. (2007, September 21). 11 ways to keep your patients satisfied: Your front-desk staff can make the patient experience positive or turn them off. Here's how to make sure that all goes well. *Medical Economics*, *84*(18), 50–52.

Ellingson, L. L., & Borofka, K. G. E. (2018). Long-term cancer survivors' everyday embodiment. *Health Communication*, 1–12. Published online.

Emilsson, M., Gustafsson, P. A., Ohnstrom, G., & Marteinsdottir, I. (2017). Beliefs regarding medication and side effects influence treatment adherence in adolescents with attention deficit hyperactivity disorder. *European Child & Adolescent Psychiatry*, *26*(5), 559–571.

Fenton, J. J., Jerant, A. F., Bertakis, K. D., & Franks, P. (2012). The cost of satisfaction: A national study of patient satisfaction, health care utilization, expenditures, and mortality. *Archives of Internal Medicine*, *172*, 405–411. doi:10.1001/archinternmed.2011.1662

Fico, A. E., & Lagoe, C. (2018). Patients' perspectives of oral healthcare providers' communication: Considering the impact of message source and content. *Health Communication*, *33*(8), 1035–1044.

Field-Springer, K., & Margavio Striley, K. (2018). Managing meanings of embodied experiences theory: Toward a discursive understanding of becoming healthier. *Health Communication*, *33*(6), 700–709.

Frosch, D. L., May, S. G., Rendle, K. A. S., Tietbohl, C., & Elwyn, G. (2012). Authoritarian physicians and patients' fear of being labeled "difficult" among key obstacles to shared decision making. *Health Affairs*, *31*(5), 1030–1038.

Gillespie, S. R. (2001). The politics of breathing: Asthmatic Medicaid patients under managed care. *Journal of Applied Communication Research*, *29*(2), 97–116.

Gilotra, N. A., Shpigel, A., Okwuosa, I. S., Tamrat, R., Flowers, D., & Russell, S. D. (2017). Patients commonly believe their heart failure hospitalizations are preventable and identify worsening heart failure, nonadherence, and a knowledge gap as reasons for admission. *Journal of Cardiac Failure*, *23*(3), 252–256.

Goffman, E. (1971a). *The presentation of self in everyday life*. Garden City, NY: Doubleday.

Goffman, E. (1971b). *Relations in public*. New York: Basic Books.

Gordon, E. J., Leon, J. B., & Sehgal, A. R. (2003). Why are hemodialysis treatments shortened and skipped? Development of a taxonomy and relationship to patient subgroups. *Nephrology Nursing Journal*, *30*(2), 209–217.

Groopman, J. (2007). *How doctors think*. Boston: Houghton Mifflin.

Hall, I. J., Tangka, F. K. L., Sabatino, S. A., Thompson, T. D., Graubard, B. I., & Breen, N. (2018). Patterns and trends in cancer screening in the United States. *Preventing Chronic Disease*, *15*, E97.

Hamdidouche, I., Jullien, V., Boutouyrie, P., Billaud, E., Azizi, M., & Laurent, S. (2017). Drug adherence in hypertension: From methodological issues to cardiovascular outcomes. *Journal of Hypertension*, *35*(6), 1133–1144.

Harrington, N. G., Norling, G. R., Witte, F. M., Taylor, J., & Andrews, J. E. (2007). The effects of communication skills training on pediatricians' and parents' communication during "sick child" visits. *Health Communication*, *21*, 105–114.

Harwood, J., & Sparks, L. (2003). Social identity and health: An intergroup communication approach to cancer. *Health Communication*, *15*, 145–159.

Heath, C. (2006). Body work: The collaborative production of the clinical object. In J. Heritage & D. W. Maynard (Eds.), *Communication in medical care: Interactions between primary care physicians and patients* (pp. 184–213). Cambridge: Cambridge University Press.

Jadad, A. R., & Rizo, C. A. (2003). I am a good patient believe it or not. *British Medical Journal*, *326*(7402), 1293–1294.

Jangland, E., Gunningberg, L., & Carlsson, M. (2009). Patients' and relatives' complaints about encounters and communication in health care: Evidence for quality improvement. *Patient Education and Counseling*, *75*, 199–204.

Jauhar, S. (2008). *Intern: A doctor's initiation*. New York: Farrar, Straus and Giroux.

Jessica's story. (n.d.). Memorial Sloan Kettering Cancer Center. Retrieved from https://www.mskcc.org/experience/hear-from-patients/jessica-tar

Katz, J. (1995). Informed consent: Ethical and legal issues. In J. D. Arras & B. Steinbock (Eds.), *Ethical issues in modern medicine* (4th ed., pp. 87–97). Mountain View, CA: Mayfield.

Koszalinski, R. S., & Williams, C. (2012). Embodying identity in chemotherapy-induced alopecia. *Perspectives in Psychiatric Care, 48*, 116–121.

Kundrat, A. L., & Nussbaum, J. F. (2003). The impact of invisible illness on identity and contextual age. *Health Communication, 15*, 331–347.

The Lacks family [blog]. (2012). Retrieved from http://www.lacksfamily.net/.

Lo, M.-C. M. (2010). Cultural brokerage: Creating linkages between voices of lifeworld and medicine in cross-cultural clinical settings. *Health: An Interdisciplinary Journal for the Social Study of Health, Illness & Medicine, 14*(5), 484–504.

Mahomed, R., St. John, W., & Patterson, E. (2012). Understanding the process of patient satisfaction with nurse-led chronic disease management in general practice. *Journal of Advanced Nursing, 68*(11), 2538–2549.

Makarem, S. C., Smith, M. F., Mudambi, S. M., & Hunt, J. M. (2014). Why people do not always follow the doctor's orders: The role of hope and perceived control. *Journal of Consumer Affairs, 48*(3), 457–485.

Margonelli, L. (2010, February 5). Eternal life. Sunday book review. *The New York Times*. Retrieved from http://www.nytimes.com/2010/02/07/books/review/Margonelli-t.html?pagewanted=all&_r=0

Milika, R. M., & Trorey, G. M. (2008). Patients' expectations of the maintenance of their dignity. *Journal of Clinical Nursing, 17*, 2709–2717.

Mishler, E. G. (1981). The social construction of illness. In E. B. Mishler, L. R. Amarasingham, S. D. Osherson, S. T. Hauser, & R. Leim (Eds.), *Social contexts of health, illness, and patient care* (pp. 141–168). Cambridge: Cambridge University Press.

Mishler, E. G. (1984). *The discourse of medicine: Dialectics of medical interviews*. Norwood, NJ: Ablex.

Mizobe, M., & Fukuda, H. (2016). PHS130: Impact of patient nonadherence to diabetes treatment on complication risks and health care costs. *Value in Health, 19*(3), A32.

Neiman, A. B., Rupper, T., Ho, M., Garber, L., Weidle, P. J., Hong, Y., George, M. G., & Thorpe, P. G. (2017, November). CDC grand rounds: Improving medical adherence for chronic disease management—innovations and opportunities. *Centers for Disease Control and Prevention*. Retrieved from https://www.cdc.gov/mmwr/volumes/66/wr/mm6645a2.htm

Papi, A., Ryan, D., Soriano, J. B., Chrystyn, H., Bjermer, L., Rodríguez-Roisin, R., . . . Price, D. B. (2018). Relationship of inhaled corticosteroid adherence to asthma exacerbations in patients with moderate-to-severe asthma. *The Journal of Allergy and Clinical Immunology: In Practice, 6*(6), 1989–1998.

Silver, M. (2013, August 17). A new chapter in the immortal life of Henrietta Lacks. *National Geographic*. Retrieved from http://news.nationalgeographic.com/news/2013/08/130816-henrietta-lacks-immortal-life-hela-cells-genome-rebecca-skloot-nih/

Sugai, W. J. (2008, June 20). Taking a hard line with compliant patients. *Talk back. Letter to the editor. Medical Economics, 85*(12), 14.

Sutton, S. (2014, April 25). Stephen's story—when life gives you cancer [YouTube video]. Retrieved from https://www.youtube.com/watch?v=MvG3ifEd0t0

Tarrant, C., Windridge, K., Boulton, J., Baker, R., & Freeman, G. (2003, June 14). How important is personal care in general practice? *British Medical Journal (Clinical Research Edition), 326*, 1310.

Tsai, T. C., Orav, E. J., & Jha, A. K. (2015, January). Patient satisfaction and quality of surgical care in U.S. hospitals. *Annals of Surgery, 261*(1), 2–8.

United Health Foundation. (2015). *Preventable hospitalizations. United States*. Minnetonka, MN: Author. Retrieved from http://www.americashealthrankings.org/ALL/preventable

Waitzkin, H. (1991). *The politics of medical encounters: How patients and doctors deal with social problems*. New Haven, CT: Yale University Press.

Wanzer, M. B., Wojtaszczyk, A. M., Schimert, J., Missert, L., Baker, S., Baker, R., & Dunkle, B. (2010). Enhancing the "informed" in informed consent: A pilot test of a multimedia presentation. *Health Communication, 25*, 365–374.

Wright Nunes, J. A., Wallston, K. A., Eden, S. K., Shintani, A. K., Ikizler, T. A., & Cavanaugh, K. L. (2011). Associations among perceived and objective disease knowledge and satisfaction with physician communication in patients with chronic kidney disease. *Kidney International, 80*(12), 1344–1351.

Zhong, Z.-J., Nie, J., Xie, X., & Liu, K. (2019). How medic–patient communication and relationship influence Chinese patients' treatment adherence. *Journal of Health Communication, 24*(1), 29–37.

CHAPTER 5

Accreditation Council to Graduate Medical Education (ACGME). (2015). *Common program requirements*. Chicago: Author. Retrieved from http://www.acgme.org/acgmeweb/Portals/0/PFAssets/ProgramRequirements/CPRs_07012015_TCC.pdf

Adelman, S. A. (2008, January 4). Be careful what you promise. *Medical Economics, 85*(1), 14.

Allenbaugh, J., Corbelli, J., Rack, L., Rubio, D., & Spagnoletti, C. (2019). A brief communication curriculum improves resident and nurse communication skills and patient satisfaction. *Journal of General Internal Medicine, 34*(7), 1167–1173.

American Association of Medical Colleges. (2018, July). *Medical school graduation questionnaire: 2018 all schools summary report*. Washington DC: Author. Retrieved from https://www.aamc.org/download/490454/data/2018gqallschoolssummaryreport.pdf

Apker, J. (2001). Role development in the managed care era: A case in hospital-based nursing. *Journal of Applied Communication Research, 29*(2), 117–136.

Augusta Health. (n.d.). Pushing the limits: Two-time breast cancer survivor planning her next race. Retrieved from http://www.augustahealth.com/foundation/grateful-patient-stories/pushing-the-limits

Azevedo, D. (1996). Taking back health care: Doctors must work together. *Medical Economics, 73*, 156–162.

Banja, J. D. (2005). *Medical errors and medical narcissism*. Boston: Jones and Bartlett.

Banja, J. D., & Amori, G. (2005). The empathic disclosure of medical error. In *Medical errors and medical narcissism* (pp. 173-192). Boston: Jones and Bartlett.

Barnett, G. V., Hollister, L., & Hall, S. (2011). Use of the standardized patient to clarify interdisciplinary team roles. *Clinical Simulation in Nursing, 7*, e169–e173.

Beach, M. C., Roter, D., Korthuis, P. T., Epstein, R. M., Sharp, V., Ratanawongsa, N., . . . Saha, S. (2013). A multicenter study of physician mindfulness and health care quality. *Annals of Family Medicine, 11*(5), 421–428.

Bell, D. J., Bringman, J., Bush, A., & Phillips, O. P. (2006). Job satisfaction among obstetrician-gynecologists: A comparison between private practice physicians and academic physicians. *American Journal of Obstetrics and Gynecology, 195*(5), 1474–1478.

Berry, L. L., & Seltman, K. D. (2008). *Management lessons from Mayo Clinic: Inside one of the world's most admired service organizations*. New York: McGraw-Hill.

Bindler, R. C., Richardson, B., Daratha, K., & Wordell, D. (2012). Interdisciplinary health science research collaboration: Strengths, challenges, and case example. *Applied Nursing Research, 25*, 95–100.

Boodman, S. (1997, February 25). Silent doctors more likely to be sued; malpractice study suggests that physicians' manner affects patients' readiness to go to court. *Washington Post*, p. WH9.

Brett, A. L., Branstetter, J. E., & Wagner, P. D. (2014). Nurse educators' perceptions of caring attributes in current and ideal work environments. *Nursing Education Perspectives, 35*(6), 360–366.

Budzi, D., Lurie, S., Singh, K., & Hooker, R. (2010). Veterans' perceptions of care by nurse practitioners, physician assistants, and physicians: A comparison from satisfaction surveys. *Journal of the American Academy of Nurse Practitioners, 22*(3), 170–176.

Burda, D. (2008, April 28). The perfection injection; Not paying for "never events" is a slippery slope. *Modern Healthcare, 38*(17), 20.

Caldroney, R. D. (2008, March 21). Why we've never been sued: This doctor and his partners have stayed out of the courtroom for nearly 30 years. Learn how to follow their lead. *Medical Economics, 85*(6), 30–32.

Cassedy, J. H. (1991). *Medicine in America: A short history*. Baltimore: Johns Hopkins University Press.

Catlin, A., Armigo, C., Volat, D., Vale, E., Hadley, M. A., Gong, W., Bassir, R., & Anderson, K. (2008). Conscientious objection: A potential neonatal nursing response to care orders that cause suffering at the end of life? Study of a concept. *Neonatal Network, 27*(2), 101–108.

Chan, E. A., Jones, A., & Wong, K. (2013). The relationships between communication, care and time are intertwined: A narrative inquiry exploring the impact of time on registered nurses' work. *Journal of Advanced Nursing, 69*(9), 2020–2029.

Charlton, C. R., Dearing, K. S., Berry, J. A., & Johnson, M. J. (2008). Nurse practitioners' communication styles and their impact on patient outcomes: An integrated literature review. *Journal of the American Academy of Nurse Practitioners, 20*(7), 382–388.

Chung, M. P., Thang, C. K., Vermillion, M., Fried, J. M., & Uijtdehaage, S. (2018). Exploring medical students' barriers to reporting mistreatment during clerkships: A qualitative study. *Medical Education Online, 23*(1), 1–9.

Conrad, P. (1988). Learning to doctor: Reflections on recent accounts of the medical school years. *Journal of Health and Social Behavior, 29*, 323–332.

D'Agostino, T. A., Atkinson, T. M., Latella, L. E., Rogers, M., Morrissey, D., DeRosa, A. P., & Parker, P. A. (2017). Promoting patient participation in healthcare interactions through communication skills training: A systematic review. *Patient Education and Counseling, 100*(7), 1247–1257.

Dean, M., & Street, J. L. (2014). Review: A 3-stage model of patient-centered communication for addressing cancer patients' emotional distress. *Patient Education and Counseling, 94*, 143–148.

Defenbaugh, N., & Chikotas, N. E. (2015). The outcome of interprofessional education: Integrating communication studies into a standardized patient experience for advanced practice nursing students. *Nurse Education in Practice, 16*(1), 176–181.

Drucker, P. F. (1993). *Post-capitalistic society*. New York: HarperCollins.

Dube, S. P., Ghadlinge, M. S., Mungal, S. U., Saleem, B. T., & Kulkarni, M. B. (2014, May). Students' perception towards problem based learning. *IOSR Journal of Dental and Medical Sciences, 13*(5), 49–53.

Duggan, A. (2006). Understanding interpersonal communication processes across health contexts: Advances in the last decade and challenges for the next decade. *Journal of Health Communication, 11*, 93–108.

Ellingson, L. L. (2007). The performance of dialysis care: Routinization and adaptation on the floor. *Health Communication, 22*, 103–114.

Epstein, R. M. (1999). Mindful practice. *Journal of the American Medical Association, 282*(9), 833–839.

Epstein, R. M., Fiscella, K., Lesser, C. S., & Stange, K. C. (2010, August 3). Why the nation needs a policy push on patient-centered health care. The Commonwealth Fund. Retrieved from https://www.commonwealthfund.org/publications/journal-article/2010/aug/why-nation-needs-policy-push-patient-centered-health-care

Erickson, S. (2008, May 16). The day I received my final verdict: A lawsuit left the author with worries about his reputation, until a surprising visit took place. *Medical Economics, 85*(10), 32–33.

Fiabane, E., Giorgi, I., Sguazzin, C., & Argentero, P. (2013). Work engagement and occupational stress in nurses and other healthcare workers: The role of organisational and personal factors. *Journal of Clinical Nursing, 22*(17/18), 2614–2624.

Florida hospital surgeons mistakenly amputate wrong leg of patient. (1995, March 20). *Jet, 87*(1), 25

Fried, J. M., Vermillion, M., Parker, N. H., & Uijtdehaage, S. (2012). Eradicating medical student mistreatment: A longitudinal study of one institution's efforts. *Academic Medicine, 87*(9), 1191–1198.

Frustrated by bureaucracy of modern medicine, 1 in 5 physicians wants to reduce clinical hours. California Medical Association. (2017. December 4). Retrieved from https://www.cmadocs.org/newsroom/news/view/ArticleId/21186/Frustrated-by-bureaucracy-of-modern-medicin

Gelsema, T. I., van der Doef, M., Maes, S., Janssen, M., Akerboom, S., & Verhoeven, C. (2006). A longitudinal study of job stress in the nursing profession: Causes and consequences. *Journal of Nursing Management, 14*(4), 289–299.

Hagemeier, N. E., Hess, R., Jr., Hagen, K. S., & Sorah, E. L. (2014). Impact of an interprofessional communication course on nursing, medical, and pharmacy students' communication skill self-efficacy beliefs. *American Journal of Pharmaceutical Education, 78*(10), 1–10.

Halbesleben, J. R. (2006). Patient reciprocity and physician burnout: What do patients bring to the patient–physician relationship? *Health Services Management Research, 19*(4), 215–222.

Hall, L. H., Johnson, J., Watt, I., Tsipa, A., & O'Connor, D. B. (2016, July 8). Healthcare staff wellbeing, burnout, and patient safety: A systematic review. *PLoS ONE, 11*(7), 1–12.

Happell, B., Dwyer, T., Reid-Searl, K., Burke, K. J., Caperchione, C. M., & Gaskin, C. J. (2013). Nurses and stress: Recognizing causes and seeking solutions. *Journal of Nursing Management, 21*(4), 638–647.

Haskard, K. B., Williams, S. L., DiMatteo, R., Rosenthal, R., White, M. K., & Goldstein, M. G. (2008). Physician and patient communication training in primary care: Effects on participation and satisfaction. *Health Psychology, 27*(5), 513–522.

Henley, S. R., Horner, C. J., Wills-Smith, N., Paxtor, C., Perry, R., O'Cain, H., . . . Roseborough, B. (2018). An opinion on mistreatment faced by student nurses during clinical. *Journal of Psychosocial Nursing and Mental Health Services, 56*(10), 6–8.

Hirschmann, K. (2008). Blood, vomit, and communication: The days and nights of an intern on call. In L. C. Lederman (Ed.), *Beyond these walls: Readings in health communication* (pp. 58–73). New York: Oxford University Press.

Huang, K T. (2017). Day in the life—first year. American Student Dental Association. Retrieved from https://www.asdanet.org/index/get-into-dental-school/before-you-apply/a-day-in-the-life-of-a-dental-student/day-in-the-life-first-year

Janis, I. (1972). *Victims of groupthink* (2nd ed.). Boston: Houghton Mifflin.

Jauhar, S. (2008). *Intern: A doctor's initiation*. New York: Farrar, Straus and Giroux.

Jin, H. K., Park, S. H., Kang, J. E., Choi, K. S., Kim, H. A., Jeon, M. S., & Rhie, S. J. (2019). The influence of a patient counseling training session on pharmacy students' self-perceived communication skills, confidence levels, and attitudes about communication skills training. *BMC Medical Education, 19*(172), nonpaginated online version.

Johal, P. (2016, September 20) "It can be a tough profession"—a mental health social worker reflects. Think Ahead. Retrieved from https://thinkahead.org/news-item/can-tough-profession-mental-health-social-worker-reflects/

Joo, J. H., Jimenez, D. E., Xu, J., & Park, M. (2019). Perspectives on training needs for geriatric mental health providers: Preparing to serve a diverse older adult population. *The American Journal of Geriatric Psychiatry, 27*(7), 728–736.

Judd, D., & Sitzman, K. (2014). *A history of American nursing: Trends and eras* (2nd ed.). Burlington, MA: Jones & Bartlett.

Kenney, C. (2010). *Transforming health care: Virginia Mason Medical Center's pursuit of the perfect patient experience*. New York: Taylor & Francis.

Kisa, K., Kawabata, H., Itou, T., Nishimoto, N., & Maezawa, M. (2011). Survey of patient and physician satisfaction regarding patient-centered outpatient consultations in Japan. *Internal Medicine, 50*(13), 1403–1410.

Klass, P. (1987). *A not entirely benign procedure: Four years as a medical student*. New York: Penguin.

Kreps, G. L. (1988). Relational communication in health care. *Southern Speech Communication Journal, 53*, 344–359.

Kreps, G. L. (1990). Applied health communication research. In D. O'Hair & G. L. Kreps (Eds.), *Applied communication theory and research* (pp. 313–330). Hillsdale, NJ: Lawrence Erlbaum.

Lauer, C. S. (2008, March 10). The unwritten curriculum. Writer: Medical students learn from elders' cynicism. *Modern Healthcare, 38*(10), 50.

Lee, F. (2004). *If Disney ran your hospital: 9½ things you would do differently*. Bozeman, MT: Second River Healthcare Press.

Li, Y., Wang, X., Zhu, X., Zhu, Y., & Sun, J. (2019). Effectiveness of problem-based learning on the professional communication competencies of nursing students and nurses: A systematic review. *Nurse Education in Practice, 37*, 45–55.

Lief, H. L., & Fox, R. C. (1963). Training for "detached concern" in medical students. In J. I. Lief, V. F. Lief, & N. R. Lief (Eds., pp. 12–33), *The psychological basis of medical practice*. New York: Harper & Row.

MacLellan, D. L., & Lordly, D. (2008). The socialization of dietetic students: Influence of the preceptor role. *Journal of Allied Health, 37*(2), E81–E92.

Magee, M., & D'Antonio, M. (2003). *The best medicine: Stories of doctors and patients who care for each other* (2nd ed.). New York: Spencer Books.

Mars, R. (Producer). (2011, June 30). The blue yarn. *99% invisible* [podcast]. Distributed by Public Radio Exchange.

Maslach, C. (1982). *Burnout: The cost of caring*. Englewood Cliffs, NJ: Prentice Hall.

McKinley, C. J., & Perino, C. (2013). Examining communication competence as a contributing factor in health care workers' job satisfaction and tendency to report errors. *Journal of Communication in Healthcare, 6*(3), 158–165.

Mead, G. H. (1934). *Minds, self, and society*. Chicago: University of Chicago Press.

Micalizzi, D. A. (2008, March 3). The aftermath of a "never event": A child's unexplained death and a system seemingly designed to thwart justice. *Modern Healthcare, 38*(9), 24.

Miller, K. I., Birkholt, M., Scott, C., & Stage, C. (1995). Empathy and burnout in human service work: An extension of the communication model. *Communication Research, 22*, 123–147.

Miller, K. I., Stiff, J. B., & Ellis, B. H. (1988). Communication and empathy as precursors to burnout among human service workers. *Communication Monographs, 55*, 250–265.

Mishler, E. G. (1984). *The discourse of medicine: Dialectics of medical interviews*. Norwood, NJ: Ablex.

Morrell, B. L. M., Nichols, A. M., Voll, C. A., Hetzler, K. E., Toon, J., Moore, E. S., . . . Carmack, J. N. (2018). Care across campus: Athletic training, nursing, and occupational therapy student experiences in an interprofessional simulation. *Athletic Training Education Journal, 13*(4), 332–339.

Morris, D., & Matthews, J. (2014). Communication, respect, and leadership: Interprofessional collaboration in hospitals of rural Ontario. *Canadian Journal of Dietetic Practice & Research, 75*(4), 173–179.

Murray, D. (2007, November 2). Hospitals vow a better response. *Medical Economics, 85*(21), 18.

Novack, D. H., Suchman, A. L., Clark, W., Epstein, R. M., Najberg, G. E., & Kaplan, C. (1997). Calibrating the physician: Personal awareness and effective patient care. *Journal of the American Medical Association, 278*, 502–510.

Olson, K. D. (2017, November). Physician burnout—a leading indicator of health system performance? *Mayo Clinic Proceedings, 92*(11), 1608–1611. Retrieved from https://www.mayoclinicproceedings.org/article/S0025-6196(17)30690-0/fulltext

Olufowote, J. O., & Wang, G. E. (2017). Physician assimilation in medical schools: Dualisms of biomedical and biopsychosocial ideologies in the discourse of physician educators. *Health Communication, 6*, 676–684.

Ositelu, F. (2015, June 2). "Knowing is not enough": A lesson from my first patient interview. Pulse. Retrieved from https://www.linkedin.com/pulse/knowing-enough-lesson-from-my-first-patient-interview-fisayo/

Paris, M., & Hoge, M. A. (2010). Burnout in the mental health workforce: A review. *Journal of Behavioral Health Services and Research, 37*, 519–528.

Paterniti, D. A., Pan, R. J., Smith, L. F., Horan, N. M., & West, D. C. (2006). From physician-centered to community-centered perspectives on health care: Assessing the efficacy of community-based training. *Academic Medicine, 81*(4), 347–353.

Pham, J. C., Story, J. L., Hicks, R. W., Shore, A. D., Morlock, L. L., Cheung, D. S., . . . Pronovost, P. J. (2011). National study on the frequency, types, causes, and consequences of voluntarily reported emergency department medication errors. *Journal of Emergency Medicine, 40*, 485–492.

Pincus, C. R. (1995). Why medicine is driving doctors crazy. *Medical Economics, 72*, 40–44.

Platt, F. W., & Gordon, G. H. (2004). *Field guide to the difficult patient interview* (2nd ed.). Philadelphia: Lippincott Williams & Wilkins.

Plews-Ogan, M., Owens, J. E., & May, N. B. (2013). Medical errors: Wisdom through adversity: Learning and growing in the wake of an error. *Patient Education and Counseling, 91*, 236–242.

Query, J. L., Jr., & Kreps, G. L. (1996). Testing a relational model for health communication competence among caregivers for individuals with Alzheimer's disease. *Journal of Health Psychology, 1*, 335–351.

Reilly, P. (1987). *To do no harm: A journey through medical school*. Dover, MA: Auburn House.

Rodriguez, H. P., Anastario, M. P., Frankel, R. M., Odigie, E. G., Rogers, W. H., von Glahn, T., & Safran, D. G. (2008). Can teaching agenda-setting skills to physicians improve clinical interaction quality? A controlled intervention. *BMC Medical Education, 8*, 3–7.

Rosenstein, A. H., & O'Daniel, M. (2008). Managing disruptive physician behavior: Impact on staff relationships and patient care. *Neurology, 70*(17), 1564–1570.

Ross, S., Ryan, C., Duncan, E. M., Francis, J. J., Johnston, M., Ker, J. S., . . . Bond, C. (2013). Perceived causes of prescribing errors by junior doctors in hospital inpatients: A study from the PROTECT programme. *British Medical Journal Quality & Safety, 2*, 97.

Rudolph, J. (2008, March 7). Bonding with patients when time is scarce: Even the busiest physician can find time to convey caring and concern. *Medical Economics, 85*(5), 50–51.

Salas, E., Wilson, K. A., Murphy, C. E., King, H., & Salisbury, M. (2008, June). Communicating, coordinating, and cooperating when lives depend on it: Tips for teamwork. *Joint Commission Journal on Quality and Patient Safety, 34*, 333–341.

Saley, C. (2019, March 19). 2019 AAFP [American Academy of Family Physicians]/CompHealth physician happiness survey. CompHealth. Retrieved from https://comphealth.com/resources/physician-happiness-survey/

Schein, E. H. (1986). *Organizational culture and leadership*. San Francisco: Jossey-Bass.

Senge, P. M. (2006). *The fifth discipline: The art and practice of the learning organization*. New York: Doubleday/Currency.

Smith, T. M. (2017, February 7). Not your grandfather's med school: Changes trending in med ed. American Medical Association. Retrieved from https://www.ama-assn.org/education/accelerating-change-medical-education/not-your-grandfathers-med-school-changes-trending

Tellis-Nayak, V. (2005). Who will care for the caregivers? *Health Progress, 86*(6), 37–43.

10 facts on obesity. (2012, May). Geneva, Switzerland: World Health Organization. Retrieved from http://www.who.int/features/factfiles/obesity/en/

Tourangeau, A. E., & Cranley, L. A. (2005). Nurse intention to remain employed: Understanding and strengthening determinants. *Journal of Advanced Nursing, 55*(4), 497–509.

Transue, E. R. (2004). *On call: A doctor's days and nights in residency.* New York: St. Martin's Griffin.

Trujillo, J. M., & Hardy, Y. (2009). A nutrition journal and diabetes shopping experience to improve pharmacy students' empathy and cultural competence. *American Journal of Pharmaceutical Education, 73*(2), 1–10.

Twaddle, A. C., & Hessler, R. M. (1987). *A sociology of health* (2nd ed.). New York: Macmillan.

UC Davis Health. (2002, June 18). *UC Davis Children's Hospital launches unique program* [Press release]. https://www.newswise.com//articles/uc-davis-childrens-hospital-launches-unique-program

Unsworth, C. (1996). Team decision-making in rehabilitation. *American Journal of Physical Medicine & Rehabilitation, 75,* 483–486.

U.S. Bureau of Labor Statistics. (2019). Healthcare occupations. Washington, DC: Author. Retrieved from https://www.bls.gov/ooh/healthcare/home.htm

van der Riet, P., Rossiter, R., Kirby, D., Dluzewska, T., & Harmon, C. (2015). Piloting a stress management and mindfulness program for undergraduate nursing students: Student feedback and lessons learned. *Nurse Education Today, 35*(1), 44–49.

Wang, H., Kline, J. A., Jackson, B. E., Laureano-Phillips, J., Robinson, R. D., Cowden, C. D., . . . Zenarosa, N. R. (2018). Association between emergency physician self-reported empathy and patient satisfaction. *PLoS ONE, 13*(9), 1–12.

Weinberg, D. (2011, May 2). U.S. hospitals turn to Toyota for management inspiration. Voice of America. Retrieved from https://www.voanews.com/usa/us-hospitals-turn-toyota-management-inspiration

Weir, K. (2013, November). *Feel like a fraud?* American Psychological Association. Retrieved from http://www.apa.org/gradpsych/2013/11/fraud.aspx

Weisman, E. (n.d.). Hi! I'm Dr. Errin Weisman, and I'm so glad you're here. Truth Prescriptions. Retrieved from http://www.truthrxs.com/aboutme

West, C. P., Dyrbye, L. N., Rabatin, J. T., Call, T. G., Davidson, J. H., Multari, A., . . . Shanafelt, T. D. (2014). Intervention to promote physician well-being, job satisfaction, and professionalism: A randomized clinical trial. *Journal of the American Medical Association Internal Medicine, 174*(4), 527–533.

Weston, W. W., & Lipkin, M., Jr. (1989). Doctors learning communication skills: Developmental issues. In M. Stewart & D. Roter (Eds.), *Communicating with medical patients. Vol. 9. Interpersonal communication* (pp. 43–57). Newbury Park, CA: Sage.

Wicks, R. J. (2008). *The resilient clinician.* Oxford: Oxford University Press.

Williams, B., Brown, T., Boyle, M., McKenna, L., Palermo, C., & Etherington, J. (2014). Levels of empathy in undergraduate emergency health, nursing, and midwifery students: A longitudinal study. *Advances in Medical Education & Practice, 5,* 299–306.

World Health Organization. (2013). Interprofessional collaborative practice in primary health care: Nursing and midwifery perspectives. Geneva, Switzerland: Author. Retrieved from http://www.who.int/hrh/resources/IPE_SixCaseStudies.pdf

Zakrzewski, P. A., Ho, A. L., & Braga-Mele, R. (2008). Should ophthalmologists receive communication skills training in breaking bad news? *Canadian Journal of Ophthalmology, 43*(4), 419–424.

CHAPTER 6

Adams, R. J., & Parrott, R. (1994, February). Pediatric nurses' communication of role expectations to parents of hospitalized children. *Journal of Applied Communication Research, 22,* 36–47.

Alegría, M., Roter, D. L., Valentine, A., Chen, C., Li, X., Lin, J., . . . Shrout, P. E. (2013). Patient–clinician ethnic concordance and communication in mental health intake visits. *Patient Education and Counseling, 93*(2), 188–196.

American Medical Association (AMA). (2003). Low literacy has a high impact on patients' ability to follow doctors' orders. Retrieved from www.ama-assn.org/ama/pub/print/article/4197-7395.html

American Medical Association (AMA). (2005, April). Quality health care for minorities: Understanding physicians' experience. Retrieved from http://www.ama-assn.org/ama/pub/physician-resources/public-health/eliminating-health-disparities/commission-end-health-care-disparities/quality-health-care-minorities-understanding-physicians.page

Anderson, M., & Perrin, A. (2017, May 17). Technology use among seniors. Pew Research Center. Retrieved from https://www.pewinternet.org/2017/05/17/technology-use-among-seniors/

Arendt, F., & Karadas, N. (2019). Ethnic concordance in patient–physician communication: Experimental evidence from Germany. *Journal of Health Communication, 24*(1), 1–8.

Armstrong, K., Putt, M., Halbert, C., Grande, D., Schwartz, J., Liao, K., . . . Shea, J. (2013). Prior experiences of racial discrimination and racial differences in health care system distrust. *Medical Care, 51*(2), 144–150.

Arpey, N. C., Gaglioti, A. H., & Rosenbaum, M. E. (2017). How socioeconomic status affects patient perceptions of health care: A qualitative study. *Journal of Primary Care & Community Health, 8,* 169–175.

Artiga, S., & Orgera, K. (2019, February 13). *Changes in health coverage by race and ethnicity since implementation of the ACA, 2013–2017.* Henry J. Kaiser Family Foundation. Retrieved from https://www.kff.org/disparities-policy/issue-brief/changes-in-health-coverage-by-race-and-ethnicity-since-implementation-of-the-aca-2013-2017/

Ask Me 3. (n.d.). American Medical Association and National Patient Safety Foundation. Retrieved from http://www.npsf.org/?page=askme3

Atherly, A., Kane, R. L., & Smith, M. A. (2004). Older adults' satisfaction with integrated capitated health and long-term care. *The Gerontologist, 44*(3), 348–357.

Baltes, M. M., & Wahl, H.-W. (1996). Patterns of communication in old age: The dependence-support and independence-ignore script. *Health Communication, 8,* 217–231.

Bao, Y., Fox, S. A., & Escarce, J. J. (2007). Socioeconomic and racial/ethnic differences in the discussion of cancer screening: "Between-" versus "within-" physician differences. *Health Services Research, 42*(3), 950–970.

Batalova, J., & Alperin, E. (2018, July 10). Immigrants in the U.S. states with the fastest-growing foreign-born populations. Migration Policy Institute. Retrieved from https://www.migrationpolicy.org/article/immigrants-us-states-fastest-growing-foreign-born-populations#Languages

Bauer, G. R. (2014). Incorporating intersectionality theory into population health research methodology: Challenges and the potential to advance health equity. *Social Science & Medicine, 110*, 10–17.

Berkman, N. D., Sheridan, S. L., Donahue, K. E., Halpern, D. J., Viera, A., . . . Viswanathan, M. (2011, March). Health literacy interventions and outcomes: A systematic review. AHRQ Evidence Report/Technology Assessment No. 199. AHRQ Publication No. 11-E006. Retrieved from http://www.ncbi.nlm.nih.gov/books/NBK82434/?report=reader

Bernheim, S. M., Ross, J. S., Krumholz, H. M., & Bradley, E. H. (2008). Influence of patients' socioeconomic status on clinical management decisions: A qualitative study. *Annals of Family Medicine, 6*(1), 53–59.

Bibace, R., & Walsh, M. E. (1981). Children's conceptualizations of illness. In R. Bibace & M. E. Walsh (Eds.), *Children's conceptualizations of health, illness, and bodily functions* (pp. 31–48). San Francisco: Jossey-Bass.

Blair, J., Glaysher, K., & Cooper, S. (2010). *Intellectual disability and health: Passport to health*. University of Hertfordshire. Retrieved from http://www.intellectualdisability.info/historic-articles/articles/passport-to-health

Boodman, S. G. (2011, February 28). Many Americans have poor health literacy. *The Washington Post*. Retrieved from http://www.washingtonpost.com/wp-dyn/content/article/2011/02/28/AR2011022805957.html

Bowleg, L. (2008). When black + lesbian + woman ≠ black lesbian woman: The methodological challenges of qualitative and quantitative intersectionality research. *Sex Roles, 59*(5/6), 312–325.

Bowleg, L. (2012). The problem with the phrase women and minorities: Intersectionality—an important theoretical framework for public health. *American Journal of Public Health, 102*(7), 1267–1273.

Braithwaite, D. O., & Harter, L. M. (2000). Communication and the management of dialectic tensions in the personal relationships of people with disabilities. In D. O. Braithwaite & T. L. Thompson (Eds.), *Handbook of communication and people with disabilities: Research and applications* (pp. 17–36). Mahwah, NJ: Lawrence Erlbaum.

Braithwaite, D. O., & Thompson, T. L. (Eds.). (2000). *Handbook of communication and people with disabilities: Research and applications*. Mahwah, NJ: Lawrence Erlbaum.

Braveman, P. (2006). Health disparities and health equity: Concepts and measurement. *Annual Review of Public Health, 27*, 167–194.

Buchholz, B. (1992, January–February). Psyching yourself: How to prepare for medical procedures. *Arthritis Today, 6*(1), 20–24.

Butler, J. (1999). *Gender trouble: Feminism and the subversity of identity* (2nd ed.). New York: Routledge.

Candib, L. M. (1994). Reconsidering power in the clinical relationship. In E. S. More & M. A. Milligan (Eds.), *The empathic practitioner: Empathy, gender, and medicine* (pp. 135–155). New Brunswick, NJ: Rutgers University Press.

Cavallaro, F., Seilhamer, M. F., Chee, Y. T. F., & Ng, B. C. (2016). Overaccommodation in a Singapore eldercare facility. *Journal of Multilingual & Multicultural Development, 37*(8), 817–831.

Centers for Disease Control and Prevention (CDC). (2014, March 13). Vital signs: Preventable deaths from heart disease and stroke. Atlanta, GA: Author. Retrieved from https://www.cdc.gov/dhdsp/vital_signs.htm

Centers for Disease Control and Prevention (CDC). (2015, May). Vital signs: Hispanic health. Atlanta, GA: Author. Retrieved from https://www.cdc.gov/vitalsigns/hispanic-health/index.html

Centers for Disease Control and Prevention (CDC). (2018, March 7). Hispanics/Latinos and tobacco use. Atlanta, GA: Author. Retrieved from https://www.cdc.gov/tobacco/disparities/hispanics-latinos/index.htm

Chen, N. N.-T., Moran, M. B., Frank, L. B., Ball-Rokeach, S. J., & Murphy, S. T. (2018). Understanding cervical cancer screening among Latinas through the lens of structure, culture, psychology and communication. *Journal of Health Communication, 23*(7), 661–669.

Chetty, R., Stepner, M., & Abraham, S. (2016). The association between income and life expectancy in the United States, 2001–2014. *Journal of the American Medical Association, 315*(16), 1750–1766.

Christmas, C., Park, E., Schmaltz, H., Gozu, A., & Durso, S. C. (2008). A model intensive course in geriatric teaching for non-geriatric educators. *Journal of General Internal Medicine, 23*(7), 1048–1052.

Clark-Hitt, R., Smith, S. W., & Broderick, J. S. (2012). Help a buddy take a knee: Creating persuasive messages for military service members to encourage others to seek mental health help. *Health Communication, 27*, 429–438. doi:10.1080/10410236.2011.606525

Clarke, L. H., & Griffin, M. (2008). Visible and invisible ageing: Beauty work as a response to ageism. *Aging & Society, 28*(5), 653–674.

Collins, S. R., Rasmussen, P. W., Doty, M. M., & Beutel, S. (2015). The rise in health care coverage and affordability since health care reform took effect—Findings from the Commonwealth Fund Biennial Health Insurance Survey, 2014. Retrieved from http://www.commonwealthfund.org/publications/issue-briefs/2015/jan/biennial-health-insurance-survey

Columnist, off the charts. (n.d.). *STAT*. Retrieved from https://www.statnews.com/staff/jennifer-okwerekwu/

Commonwealth Fund. (2008, July). Doctor–patient communication by race/ethnicity, family income, insurance, and residence, 2004. Results of the National Scorecard on U.S. Health System Performance, 2008: Chartpack.

New York: Commonwealth Fund, Commission on a High Performance Health System, p. 48. Retrieved from https://www.commonwealthfund.org/sites/default/files/documents/___media_files_publications_fund_report_2008_jul_why_not_the_best__results_from_the_national_scorecard_on_u_s__health_system_performance__2008_scorecard_chartpack_2008_pdf.

Coupland, N., Coupland, J., & Giles, H. (1991). *Language, society & the elderly*. Oxford: Blackwell.

Crenshaw, K. (1989). Demarginalizing the intersection of race and sex: A black feminist critique of antidiscrimination doctrine, feminist theory and antiracist politics. *University of Chicago Legal Forum*, 1989, 139–167.

Crenshaw, K. (1991). Mapping the margins: Intersectionality, identity politics, and violence against women of color. *Stanford Law Review*, 6, 1241–1299.

Cruz, G. G. (2014). Oral health disparities: Opportunities and challenges for policy communication. *Journal of Communication in Healthcare*, 7(2), 74–76. doi:10.1179/1753807614Y.0000000049

Dilger, D. (2013, November 16). The emotional health literacy block. KevinMD.com. Retrieved from http://www.kevinmd.com/blog/2013/11/emotional-health-literacy-block.html

Dinwiddie, G. Y., Zambrana, R. E., & Garza, M. A. (2014). Exploring risk factors in Latino cardiovascular disease: The role of education, nativity, and gender. *American Journal of Public Health*, 104(9), 1742–1750.

Do, T.-P., & Geist, P. (2000). Embodiment and disembodiment: Identity transformation and persons with physical disabilities. In D. O. Braithwaite & T. L. Thompson (Eds.), *Handbook of communication and people with disabilities: Research and applications* (pp. 49–65). Mahwah, NJ: Lawrence Erlbaum.

Duggan, A., Bradshaw, Y. S., Carroll, S. E., Rattigan, S. H., & Altman, W. (2009). What can I learn from this interaction? A qualitative analysis of medical student self-reflection and learning in a standardized patient exercise about disability. *Journal of Health Communication*, 14, 797–811. doi:10.1080/10810730903295526

Ferguson, B., Lowman, S. G., & DeWalt, D. A. (2011). Assessing literacy in clinical and community settings: The patient perspective. *Journal of Health Communication*, 16, 124–134. doi:10.1080/10810730.2010.535113

Finkelstein, A., Carmel, S., & Bachner, Y. G. (2015). Physicians' communication styles as correlates of elderly cancer patients' satisfaction with their doctors. *European Journal of Cancer Care*, 26(1), nonpaginated. Retrieved from https://www.researchgate.net/publication/283293604_Physicians'_communication_styles_as_correlates_of_elderly_cancer_patients'_satisfaction_with_their_doctors

Fisher, Y. (n.d.). 16 expressions medical interpreters should know. Interpreter Training Programs. Retrieved from http://interpretertrain.com/16-expressions-medical-interpreters-should-know/

Fleming, M. D., Shim, J. K., Yen, I. H., Thompson-Lastad, A., Rubin, S., Van Natta, M., & Burke, N. J. (2017). Patient engagement at the margins: Health care providers' assessments of engagement and the structural determinants of health in the safety-net. *Social Science & Medicine*, 183, 11–18.

Fowler, B. A. (2006). Claiming health: Mammography screening decision making of African American women. *Oncology Nursing Forum*, 33(5), 969–975.

Fowler, C., & Nussbaum, J. (2008). Communicating with the aging patient. In K. B. Wright & S. D. Moore (Eds.), *Applied health communication* (pp. 159–178). Cresskill, NJ: Hampton Press.

Gamlin, R. (1999). Sexuality: A challenge for nursing practice. *Nursing Times*, 95(7), 48–50.

Garfield, R., & Orgera, K. (2019, January 25). The uninsured and the ACA: A primer—key facts about health insurance and the uninsured amidst changes to the Affordable Care Act. Henry J. Kaiser Family Foundation. Retrieved from https://www.kff.org/report-section/the-uninsured-and-the-aca-a-primer-key-facts-about-health-insurance-and-the-uninsured-amidst-changes-to-the-affordable-care-act-how-many-people-are-uninsured/

Garret, P. W., Dickson, H. G., Young, L., & Klinken Whelan, A. (2008). "The happy migrant effect": Perceptions of negative experiences of healthcare by patients with little or no English: A qualitative study across seven language groups. *Quality & Safety in Health Care*, 17(2), 101–103.

Giles, H., Ballard, D., & McCann, R. M. (2002). Perceptions of intergenerational communication across cultures: An Italian case. *Perceptual and Motor Skills*, 95, 583–591.

Ginossar, T. (2014). Disparities and antecedents to cancer prevention information seeking among cancer patients and caregivers attending a minority-serving cancer center. (2014). *Journal of Communication in Healthcare*, 7(2), 93–105.

Goins, E. S., & Pye, D. (2013). Check the box that best describes you: Reflexively managing theory and praxis in LGBTQ health communication research. *Health Communication*, 28, 397–407. doi:10.1080/10410236.2012.690505

Grady, M., & Edgar, T. (2003). Racial disparities in healthcare: Highlights from focus group findings. In. B. D. Smedley, A. Y. Stith, & A. R. Nelson (Eds.), *Unequal treatment: Confronting racial and ethnic disparities in health care* (pp. 392–405). Washington, DC: Board on Health Sciences Policy, Institute of Medicine. Retrieved from http://books.nap.edu/openbook.php?isbn=030908265X

Groopman, J. (2007). *How doctors think*. Boston: Houghton Mifflin.

Hankivsky, O. (2012). Women's health, men's health, and gender and health: Implications of intersectionality. *Social Science & Medicine*, 74, 1712–1720. doi:10.1016/j.socscimed.2011.11.029

Hankivsky, O., Grace, D., Hunting, G., Giesbrecht, M., Fridkin, A., Rudrum, S., . . . Clark, N. (2014). An intersectionality-based policy analysis framework: Critical reflections on a methodology for advancing equity. *International Journal for Equity in Health*, 13(1), 50–78. doi:10.1186/s12939-014-0119-x

Haskell, H., Mannix, M. E., James, J. T., & Mayer, D. (2012). Parents and families as partners in the care of pediatric cardiology patients. *Progress in Pediatric Cardiology*, 33, 67–72.

Heifetz, M., & Lunsky, Y. (2018). Implementation and evaluation of health passport communication tools in emergency departments. *Research in Developmental Disabilities*, 72, 23–32.

Henry J. Kaiser Family Foundation. (2018, December 7). Key facts about the uninsured population. Menlo Park, CA: Author. Retrieved from https://www.kff.org/uninsured/fact-sheet/key-facts-about-the-uninsured-population/

Horowitz, A. M., Wang, M. Q., & Kleinman, D. V. (2012). Opinions of Maryland adults regarding communication practices of dentists and staff. *Journal of Health Communication*, 17(10), 1204–1214.

Hovick, S. R., Liang, M., & Kahlor, L. (2014). Predicting cancer risk knowledge and information seeking: The role of social and cognitive factors. *Health Communication*, 29, 656. doi:10.1080/10410236.2012.763204

Howe, N. (2018, March 16). The graying of wealth. *Forbes*. Retrieved from https://www.forbes.com/sites/neilhowe/2018/03/16/the-graying-of-wealth/#6dbe168e302d

Human Genome Project Information Archive. (2008). Website sponsored by the U.S. Department of Energy Office of Science, Office of Biological and Environmental Research, & Human Genome Program. Retrieved from http://www.ornl.gov/sci/techresources/Human_Genome/home.shtml

Hummert, M. L., & Shaner, J. L. (1994). Patronizing speech to the elderly as a function of stereotyping. *Communication Studies*, 45, 145–158.

Hwang, S. S., Rybin, D. V., Kerr, S. M., Heeren, T. C., Colson, E. R., & Corwin, M. J. (2017). Predictors of maternal trust in doctors about advice on infant care practices: The SAFE study. *Academic Pediatrics*, 17(7), 762–769.

Improving Americans' health literacy. (2011, January). T. H. Chan School of Public Health at Harvard University. Retrieved from http://www.hsph.harvard.edu/news/multimedia-article/healthliteracy/

Jenkins, H. S. (2008, February 15). Patients love my broken Spanish: This determined ER physician taught himself a second language so he could communicate with all his patients. *Medical Economics*, 85(4), 42–43.

Jensen, J. D., King, A. J., Guntzviller, L. M., & Davis, L. A. (2010). Patient–provider communication and low-income adults: Age, race, literacy, and optimism predict communication satisfaction. *Patient Education and Counseling*, 79, 30–35.

Jones, D., Gill, P., Harrison, R., Meakin, R., & Wallace, P. (2003). An exploratory study of language interpretation services provided by videoconferencing. *Journal of Telemedicine and Telecare*, 9(1), 51–56.

Juckett, G., & Unger, K. (2014, October 1). Appropriate use of medical interpreters. *American Family Physician*, 90(7), 470–480.

Kaufman, J. S., Dolman, L., Rushani, D., & Cooper, R. S. (2015). The contribution of genomic research to explaining racial disparities in cardiovascular disease: A systematic review. *American Journal of Epidemiology*, 181(7), 464–472.

Kopfman, J. E., & Ray, E. B. (2005). Talking to children about illness. In E. B. Ray (Ed.), *Health communication in practice: A case study approach* (pp. 111–119). Mahwah, NJ: Lawrence Erlbaum.

Koven, S. (2012, June 29). Marriage equality, in sickness and in health. BostonGlobe.com. Retrieved from https://www.bostonglobe.com/lifestyle/health-wellness/2012/06/24/marriage-equality-sickness-and-health/H9whMdY9Bi53vrCvdAZ6QI/story.html

Kundrat, A. L., & Nussbaum, J. F. (2003). The impact of invisible illness on identity and contextual age. *Health Communication*, 15, 331–347.

Lansdale, D. (2002). Touching lives: Opening doors for elders in retirement communities through e-mail and the Internet. In R. W. Morrell (Ed.), *Older adults, health information, and the World Wide Web* (pp. 133–151). Mahwah, NJ: Lawrence Erlbaum.

Lee, C., Ramírez, A. S., Lewis, N., Gray, S. W., & Hornik, R. C. (2012). Looking beyond the Internet: Examining socioeconomic inequalities in cancer information seeking among cancer patients. *Health Communication*, 27, 806–817. doi:10.1080/10410236.2011.647621

Levine, D. A. (2013). Office-based care for lesbian, gay, bisexual, transgender, and questioning youth. *Pediatrics*, 132(1), 198–203. doi:10.1542/peds.2013-1282

Levinsky, N. (1995). The doctor's master. In J. D. Arras & B. Steinbock (Eds.), *Ethical issues in modern medicine* (4th ed., pp. 116–119). Mountain View, CA: Mayfield.

Levy, B. R., Chung, P. H., Bedford, T., & Navrazhina, K. (2014). Facebook as a site for negative age stereotypes. *Gerontologist*, 54(2), 172–176.

Lewis, C., Abrams, M. K., & Seervia, S. (2017, December 1). Listening to low-income patients: Obstacles to the care we need, when we need it. Commonwealth Fund. Retrieved from https://www.commonwealthfund.org/blog/2017/listening-low-income-patients-obstacles-care-we-need-when-we-need-it

Lindberg, D. A. B. (2002). Older Americans, health information, and the Internet. In R. W. Morrell (Ed.), *Older adults, health information, and the World Wide Web* (pp. 13–19). Mahwah, NJ: Lawrence Erlbaum.

Lindley, L. L., Friedman, D. B., & Struble, C. (2012). Becoming visible: Assessing the availability of online sexual health information for lesbians. *Health Promotion Practice*, 13(4), 472. doi:10.1177/1524839910390314

Macias, W., & McMillan, S. (2008). The return of the house call: The role of Internet-based interactivity in bringing health information home to older adults. *Health Communication*, 23, 34–44.

Mackert, M., Donovan, E. E., Mabry, A., Guadagno, M., & Stout, P. A. (2014). Stigma and health literacy: An agenda for advancing research and practice. *American Journal of Health Behavior*, 38(5), 690–698. doi:10.5993/AJHB.38.5.6

Maertens, J. A., Jimenez-Zambrano, A. M., Albright, K., & Dempsey, A. F. (2017). Using community engagement to develop a web-based intervention for Latinos about the HPV vaccine. *Journal of Health Communication*, 22(4), 285–293.

Manfredi, C., Kaiser, K., Matthews, A. K., & Johnson, T. P. (2010). Are racial differences in patient-physician cancer communication and information explained by background, predisposing, and enabling factors? *Journal of Health Communication*, *15*, 272–292. doi: 10.1080/10810731003686598

Marion, G., Hildebrandt, C., Davis, S., Marin, A., & Crandall, S. (2008). Working effectively with interpreters: A model curriculum for physician assistant students. *Medical Teacher*, *30*(6), 612–617.

McCague, J. J. (2001, May 21). On today's older patients. *Medical Economics*, *78*(10), 104.

McConatha, D. (2002). Aging online: Toward a theory of e-equality. In R. W. Morrell (Ed.), *Older adults, health information, and the World Wide Web* (pp. 21–41). Mahwah, NJ: Lawrence Erlbaum.

Meredith, L. S., Eisenman, D. P., Rhodes, H., Ryan, G., & Long, A. (2007, April–May). Trust influences response to public health messages during a bioterrorist event. *Journal of Health Communication*, *12*, 217–232.

Moffatt, L. (n.d.). 29 genius Japanese idioms that all learners should know. FluentU. Retrieved from https://www.fluentu.com/blog/japanese/japanese-idioms-2/

Moore, L. W., & Miller, M. (2003). Older men's experiences of living with severe visual impairment. *Journal of Advanced Nursing*, *43*(1), 10–18.

Moyse, E. (2014). Age estimate from faces and voices: A review. *Psychologica Belgica*, *54*(3), 255–265.

Mulac, A., & Giles, H. (1996). "You're only as old as you sound": Perceived vocal age and social meanings. *Health Communication*, *8*, 199–215.

National Assessment of Adult Literacy. (2014). Fast facts. National Center for Education Statistics. Retrieved from http://nces.ed.gov/fastfacts/display.asp?id=69

National Center for Health Statistics. (2012). Health, United States, 2011: With special features on socioeconomic status and health. Hyattsville, MD: U.S. Department of Health and Human Services. Retrieved from http://www.cdc.gov/nchs/data/hus/hus11.pdf

Nemeth, S. A. (2000). Society, sexuality, and disabled/able bodied romantic relationships. In D. O. Braithwaite & T. L. Thompson (Eds.), *Handbook of communication and people with disabilities: Research and applications* (pp. 37–48). Mahwah, NJ: Lawrence Erlbaum.

Nussbaum, J. F. (2007). Presidential address: Life span communication and quality of life. *Journal of Communication*, *57*, 1–7.

Nussbaum, J. F., Pecchioni, L., Grant, J. A., & Folwell, A. (2000). Explaining illness to older adults: The complexities of the provider–patient interaction as we age. In B. B. Whaley (Ed.), *Explaining illness* (pp. 171–194). Mahwah, NJ: Lawrence Erlbaum.

Nussbaum, J. F., Ragan, S., & Whaley, B. (2003). Children, older adults, and women: Impact on provider–patient interaction. In T. L. Thompson, A. M. Dorsey, K. I. Miller, & R. Parrott (Eds.), *Handbook of health communication* (pp. 183–204). Mahwah, NJ: Lawrence Erlbaum.

O'Reilly, K. B. (2012, March 19). The ABCs of health literacy. *American Medical News*. Retrieved from http://www.amednews.com/article/20120319/profession/303199949/4/

Okwerekwu, J. A. (2016, April 11). The patient called me "colored girl." The senior doctor training me said nothing. *STAT*. Retrieved from https://www.statnews.com/2016/04/11/racism-medical-education/

Okwerekwu, J. A. (2017, August 16). The sting of everyday racism. *Boston Globe*. Retrieved from https://www.bostonglobe.com/opinion/columns/2017/08/16/the-sting-everyday-racism/mhZuZXUehBXwfJm9km50wM/story.html

Older adults: Health and age-related changes. Reality or myth: Which is it? (n.d.). American Psychological Association. Retrieved from http://www.apa.org/pi/aging/resources/guides/older-adults.pdf

Ortman, J. M., Velkoff, V. A., & Hogan, H. (2014, May). An aging nation: The older population in the United States. U.S. Census Bureau. Retrieved from http://www.census.gov/prod/2014pubs/p25-1140.pdf

Overton, B. C., du Pré, A., & Pecchioni, L. L. (2015). Media portrayals of aging: Women's sexuality concealed and revealed. In N. Jones & B. Batchelor (Eds.), *Aging heroes: Growing old in popular culture* (pp. 181–197). New York: Rowman & Littlefield.

Page-Reeves, J., Niforatos, J., Mishra, S., Regino, L., Gingrich, A., & Bulten, J. (2013). Health disparity and structural violence: How fear undermines health among immigrants at risk for diabetes. *Journal of Health Disparities Research & Practice*, *6*(2), 30–47.

Peretti-Watel, P., Seror, V., Verger, P., Guignard, R., Legleye, S., & Beck, F. (2014). Smokers' risk perception, socioeconomic status and source of information on cancer. *Addictive Behaviors*, *39*(9), 1304–1310. doi:10.1016/j.addbeh.2014.04.016

Piñeiro, B., Díaz, D. R., Monsalve, L. M., Martínez, Ú., Meade, C. D., Meltzer, L. R., . . . Simmons, V. N. (2018). Systematic transcreation of self-help smoking cessation materials for Hispanic/Latino smokers: Improving cultural relevance and acceptability. *Journal of Health Communication*, *23*(4), 350–359.

Potter, J. E. (2002). Do ask, do tell. *Annals of Internal Medicine*, *137*(5), 341–343.

Redfern, J. S., & Sinclair, B. (2014). Improving health care encounters and communication with transgender patients. *Journal of Communication in Healthcare*, *7*(1), 25–40. doi:10.1179/1753807614Y.0000000045

Reducing disparities to improve the quality of care for racial and ethnic minorities. (2014). Robert Wood Johnson Foundation. Retrieved from https://www.rwjf.org/en/library/research/2014/06/reducing-disparities-to-improve-care-for-racial-and-ethnic-minorities.html

Rhodes, S. D., Yee, L. J., & Hergenrather, K. C. (2003). Hepatitis A vaccination among young African American men who have sex with men in the Deep South: Psychosocial predictors. *Journal of the American Medical Association*, *95*(4), 31S–36S.

Robinson, T., Callister, M., Magoffin, D., & Moore, J. (2006). The portrayal of older characters in Disney animated films. *Journal of Aging Studies*, *21*, 203–213.

Rose, I. D., & Friedman, D. B. (2013). We need health information too: A systematic review of studies examining the health information seeking and communication practices of sexual minority youth. *Health Education Journal*, 72(4), 417–430.

Ross, K. A., & Castle Bell, G. (2017). A culture-centered approach to improving healthy trans-patient–practitioner communication: Recommendations for practitioners communicating with trans individuals. *Health Communication*, 32(6), 730–740.

Ryan, E. B., Anas, A. P., & Vuckovich, M. (2007). The effects of age, hearing loss, and communication difficulty on first impressions. *Communication Research Reports*, 24(1), 13–19.

Ryan, E. B., & Butler, R. N. (1996). Communication, aging, and health: Toward understanding health provider relationships with older clients. *Health Communication*, 8, 191–197.

Ryan, L., Logsdon, M. C., McGill, S., Stikes, R., Senior, B., Helinger, B., . . . Davis, D. W. (2014). Evaluation of printed health education materials for use by low-education families. *Journal of Nursing Scholarship*, 46(4), 218–228. doi:10.1111/jnu.12076

Ryan-Wenger, N., & Gardner, W. (2012). Hospitalized children's perspectives on the quality and equity of their nursing care. *Journal of Nursing Care Quality*, 27(1), 35–42.

Saadi, A. (2016, February 7). A Muslim-American doctor on the racism in our hospitals. KevinMD.com. Retrieved from https://www.kevinmd.com/blog/2016/02/muslim-american-doctor-racism-hospitals.html

Saha, S., Guiton, G., Wimmers, P. F., & Wilkerson, L. (2008). Student body racial and ethnic composition and diversity-related outcomes in U.S. medical schools. *Journal of the American Medical Association*, 300(10), 1135–1145.

Salamon, J. (2008, May 26). My year inside Maimonides: A hospital with a polyglot patient body learns the importance of communication. *Modern Healthcare*, 38(21), 24.

Schulman, K. A., Berlin, J. A., Harless, W., Kerner, J. F., Sistrunk, S., Gersh, B. J., . . . Escarce, J. J. (1999). The effect of face and sex on physicians' recommendations for cardiac catheterization. *New England Journal of Medicine*, 340, 618–626.

Schur, L. (director and producer), & Thompson, L. (producer). (2008). *Greedy for life*. Arlington, VA: Schur Schot Productions.

Schur, L. (director and producer), & Thompson, L. (producer). (2012). *The beauty of aging*. Arlington, VA: Schur Schot Productions.

Seervai, S. (2018a, January 19). Listening to low-income patients: Where we live matters to our health. The Commonwealth Fund. Retrieved from https://www.commonwealthfund.org/publications/other-publication/2018/jan/listening-low-income-patients-where-we-live-matters-our

Seervai, S. (2018b, December 5). "Why I love my job": Listening to primary care physicians for low-income patients. The Commonwealth Fund. Retrieved from https://www.commonwealthfund.org/publications/2018/dec/why-i-love-my-job-listening-primary-care-physicians-low-income-patients

Sentell, T., & Braun, K. L. (2012). Low health literacy, limited English proficiency, and health status in Asians, Latinos, and other racial/ethnic groups in California. *Journal of Health Communication*, 17, 82–99. doi:10.1080/10810730.2012.712621

Seo, M., & Matsaganis, M. D. (2013). How interpersonal communication mediates the relationship of multichannel communication connections to health-enhancing and health-threatening behaviors. *Journal of Health Communication*, 18(8), 1002–1020. doi:10.1080/10810730.2013.768726

Singh, S., Evans, N., Williams, M., Sezginis, N., & Baryeh, N. A. K. (2018). Influences of socio-demographic factors and health utilization factors on patient-centered provider communication. *Health Communication*, 33(7), 917–923.

6 tips for communicating with non-English speaking patients. (2016, April 12). Morningside Translations. Retrieved from https://www.morningtrans.com/6-tips-for-communicating-with-non-english-speaking-patients/

Smith, S. G., Wolf, M. S., & Wagner, C. V. (2010). Socioeconomic status, statistical confidence, and patient-provider communication: An analysis of the Health Information National Trends Survey (HINTS 2007). *Journal of Health Communication*, 15, 169–185. doi:10.1080/10810730.2010.522690

Soule, K. P, & Roloff, M. E. (2000). Help between persons with and without disabilities from a resource theory perspective. In D. O. Braithwaite & T. L. Thompson (Eds.), *Handbook of communication and people with disabilities: Research and applications* (pp. 67–83). Mahwah, NJ: Lawrence Erlbaum.

Squires, A. (2018). Strategies for overcoming language barriers in healthcare. *Nursing Management*, 49(4), 20–27.

Szanton, S., Rifkind, J., Mohanty, J., Miller, E., Thorpe, R., Nagababu, E., . . . Evans, M. (2012). Racial discrimination is associated with a measure of red blood cell oxidative stress: A potential pathway for racial health disparities. *International Journal of Behavioral Medicine*, 19(4), 489–495.

Turpin, T. P. (2013). Unintended consequences of a segmentation strategy: Exploring constraint recognition among black women targeted in HIV/AIDS campaigns. *Public Relations Journal*, 7(2), 96–127.

U.S. Bureau of Labor Statistics. (2014). Employed persons by detailed occupation, sex, race, and Hispanic or Latino ethnicity. Washington, DC: Author. Retrieved from http://www.bls.gov/cps/cpsaat11.pdf

U.S. Bureau of Labor Statistics. (2019, January 18). Labor force statistics from the current population survey. Washington, DC: Author. Retrieved from https://www.bls.gov/cps/cpsaat11.htm

U.S. Census Bureau. (2011, November). *The older population: 2010*. Washington, DC: Author. Retrieved from http://www.census.gov/prod/cen2010/briefs/c2010br-09.pdf

U.S. Census Bureau. (2014). Population estimates. Washington, DC: Author. Retrieved from http://www.census.gov/popest/data/national/asrh/2014/index.html

U.S. Census Bureau News. (2018, July 1). Quick facts: United States. Washington, DC: Author. Retrieved from https://www.census.gov/quickfacts/fact/table/US/IPE120218

USDA defines food deserts. (2011, Spring). *Nutrition Digest*, *38*(2), nonpaginated. Retrieved from http://americannutritionassociation.org/newsletter/usda-defines-food-deserts

U.S. Department of Education. (2015). Digest of education: Statistics 2014, Table 507. Literacy skills of adults, by type of literacy, proficiency levels, and selected characteristics: 1992–2003. Retrieved from https://nces.ed.gov/fastfacts/display.asp?id=69

U.S. Department of Health & Human Services (USDHHS). (n.d.-a). America's health literacy: Why we need accessible health information. Office of Disease Prevention and Health Promotion. Washington, DC: Author. Retrieved from https://health.gov/communication/literacy/issuebrief/

U.S. Department of Health & Human Services (USDHHS). (n.d.-b). Civil rights: Limited English proficiency. Washington, DC: Author. Retrieved from https://www.hhs.gov/civil-rights/for-individuals/special-topics/limited-english-proficiency/index.html

U.S. Department of Health & Human Services (DHHS). (2016). 2016 national healthcare quality and disparities report. Agency for Healthcare Research and Quality. Washington, DC: Author. Retrieved from https://www.ahrq.gov/research/findings/nhqrdr/nhqdr16/summary.html#Key

U.S. Department of Health and Human Services (DHHS). (2017). A profile of older Americans. Administration on Aging and Administration for Community Living. Washington, DC: Author. Retrieved from https://acl.gov/sites/default/files/Aging%20and%20Disability%20in%20America/2017OlderAmericansProfile.pdf

Vangeest, J. B., Welch, V. L., & Weiner, S. J. (2010). Patients' perceptions of screening for health literacy: Reactions to the newest vital sign. *Journal of Health Communication*, *15*, 402–412.

Vardeman-Winter, J. (2017). The framing of women and health disparities: A critical look at race, gender, and class from the perspectives of grassroots health communicators. *Health Communication*, *32*(5), 629–638.

Venetis, M. K., Meyerson, B. E., Friley, L. B., Gillespie, A., Ohmit, A., & Shields, C. G. (2017). Characterizing sexual orientation disclosure to health care providers: Lesbian, gay, and bisexual perspectives. *Health Communication*, *32*(5), 578–586.

Venkatesh, A. K., Chou, S.-C., Li, S.-X., Choi, J., Ross, J. S., D'Onofrio, G., . . . Dharmarajan, K. (2019). Association between insurance status and access to hospital care in emergency department disposition. *JAMA Internal Medicine*, *179*(5), 686–693.

Verlinde, E., De Laender, N., De Maesschalck, S., Deveugele, M., & Willems, S. (2012). The social gradient in doctor-patient communication. *International Journal for Equity in Health*, *11*(1), 12–25. doi:10.1186/1475-9276-11-12

Vernon, J. A., Trujillo, A., Rosenbaum, S., & DeBuono, B. (2007). Low health literacy: Implications for national health policy. Retrieved from http://publichealth.gwu.edu/departments/healthpolicy/CHPR/downloads/LowHealthLiteracyReport10_4_07.pdf

Vickers, C., & Goble, R. (2011). Well, now, okey dokey: English discourse markers in Spanish-language medical consultations. *The Canadian Modern Language Review*, *67*, 536–567.

Whaley, B. B. (1999). Explaining illness to children: Advancing theory and research by determining message content. *Health Communication*, *11*, 185–193.

Whaley, B. B. (2000). Explaining illness to children: Theory, strategies, and future inquiry. In B. B. Whaley (Ed.), *Explaining illness* (pp. 195–207). Mahwah, NJ: Lawrence Erlbaum.

Whaley, B. B., & Edgar, T. (2008). Explaining illness to children. In K. B. Wright & S. D. Moore (Eds.), *Applied health communication* (pp. 145–158). Cresskill, NJ: Hampton Press.

Willems, S. J., Swinnen, W., & De Maeseneer, J. M. (2005). The GP's perception of poverty: A qualitative study. *Family Practice*, *22*(2), 177–183.

Wolf, M. S., Williams, M. V., Parker, R. M., Parikh, N. S., Nowlan, A. W., & Baker, D. W. (2007). Patients' shame and attitudes toward discussing the results of literacy screening. *Journal of Health Communication*, *12*, 721–732.

World Health Organization (WHO). (1998). Health promotion glossary. Geneva, Switzerland: Author. Retrieved from www.who.int/hpr/ncp/support.documents.shtml

World Health Organization (WHO). (2002). Towards a common language for functioning, disability and health. The International Classification of Functioning, Disability, and Health (ICF). Geneva, Switzerland: Author. Retrieved from https://www.who.int/classifications/icf/icfbeginnersguide.pdf

World Health Organization (WHO). (2017, April). 10 facts on health inequities and their causes. Geneva, Switzerland: Author. Retrieved from https://www.who.int/features/factfiles/health_inequities/en/

Yeon-Hwan, P., & HeeKyung, C. (2014). Effect of a health coaching self-management program for older adults with multimorbidity in nursing homes. *Patient Preference & Adherence*, *8*, 959–970. doi:10.2147/PPA.S62411

CHAPTER 7

Ahmad, N. N. (2004, April 15). Arab-American culture and health care. Retrieved from https://web.archive.org/web/20160515131135/http://www.case.edu/med/epidbio/mphp439/Arab-Americans.htm

Alden, D. L., Merz, M. Y., & Thi, L. M. (2010). Patient decision-making preference and physician decision-making style for contraceptive method choice in an Asian culture: Does concordance matter? *Health Communication*, *25*, 718–725.

Baglia, J. (2005). *The Viagra ad venture*. New York: Peter Lang.

Barnes, L. (n.d.). I am not a victim of breast cancer. Great Inspirational Quotes. Retrieved from http://www.great-inspirational-quotes.com/i-am-not-a-victim-of-breast-cancer.html

Bealieu-Volk, D. (2014). Motivating patients with diabetes. *Medical Economics*, *91*(10), 36–39.

Bias, S. (2014, November 7). Self acceptance vs. self esteem [Blog post]. Retrieved from http://stacybias.net/2014/11/self-acceptance-vs-self-esteem/

Bias, S. (2015, January 20). I stood up to a fat-shaming bully on a train because I'm tired of fighting for the right to exist. *xoJane*. Retrieved from https://web.archive.org/web/20170831042508/http://www.xojane.com/issues/fat-shaming-train-bully

Bohm, D. (1980). *Wholeness and the implicate order*. London: Routledge & Kegan Paul.

Bonsteel, A. (1997, March–April). Behind the white coat. *The Humanist, 57*, 15–19.

Borkhoff, C. M., Hawker, G. A., Kreder, H. J., Glazier, R. H., Mahomed, N. N., & Wright, J. G. (2013). Influence of patients' gender on informed decision making regarding total knee arthroplasty. *Arthritis Care & Research, 65*(8), 1281. doi:10.1002/acr.21970

Boyd, J. E., Adler, E. P., Otilingam, P. G., & Peters, T. (2014). Internalized stigma of mental illness (ISMI) scale: A multinational review. *Comprehensive Psychiatry, 55*, 221–231. doi:10.1016/j.comppsych.2013.06.005

Byck, R. (1986). *The encyclopedia of psychoactive drugs: Treating mental illness*. New York: Chelsea House.

Caba, J. (2016, February 24). Gigantism and acromegaly explained: Why taller people die earlier than most. *Medical Daily*. Retrieved from http://www.medicaldaily.com/gigantism-acromegaly-why-tall-people-die-374890

Capriotti, T. (1999, February 1). Exploring the "herbal jungle." *MedSurg Nursing, 8*, 53.

Carcioppolo, N., Jensen, J. D., Wilson, S. R., Collins, W. B., Carrion, M., & Linnemeier, G. (2013). Examining HPV threat-to-efficacy ratios in the Extended Parallel Process Model. *Health Communication, 28*, 20–28.

Cassell, E. J. (1991). *The nature of suffering*. New York: Oxford University Press.

Centers for Disease Control and Prevention (CDC). (2012). Suicide: Facts at a glance. Atlanta, GA: Author. Retrieved from http://www.cdc.gov/violenceprevention/pdf/Suicide-DataSheet-a.pdf

Centers for Disease Control and Prevention (CDC). (2013). Deaths. Final data for 2013. Table 12, number of deaths from 113 selected causes. Atlanta, GA: Author. Retrieved from http://www.cdc.gov/nchs/fastats/homicide.htm

Centers for Disease Control and Prevention (CDC). (2014). The national intimate partner and sexual violence survey. Atlanta, GA: Author. Retrieved from http://www.cdc.gov/violenceprevention/NISVS/index.html

Centers for Disease Control and Prevention (CDC). (2015). Leading causes of death in females United States, 2011. Atlanta, GA: Author. Retrieved from https://web.archive.org/web/20190615082659/http://www.cdc.gov/Women/lcod/2011/index.htm

Chang, L., & Lim, J. C. J. (2019). Traditional Chinese medicine physicians' insights into interprofessional tensions between traditional Chinese medicine and biomedicine: A critical perspective. *Health Communication, 34*(2), 238–247.

Chen, H., Tu, H., & Ho, C. (2013). Understanding biophilia leisure as facilitating well-being and the environment: An examination of participants' attitudes toward horticultural activity. *Leisure Sciences, 35*(4), 301–319.

Cho, S.-H., Lee, J.-S., Thabane, L., & Lee, J. (2009). Acupuncture for obesity: A systematic review and meta-analysis. *International Journal of Obesity, 33*, 183–196.

Christian Science Board of Directors. (n.d.). A closer look at health: The next breakthrough is here. Retrieved 2017 from http://christianscience.com/what-is-christian-science/a-closer-look-at-health

Clarke, J. N., & Binns, J. (2006). The portrayal of heart disease in mass print magazines, 1991–2001. *Health Communication, 19*, 39–48.

Coleman, K. (2009). Personal and communal reactions to cancer: An interpretative phenomenological analysis of the beliefs held by charedi Jewish breast cancer patients. *At the Interface/Probing the Boundaries, 55*, 75–97.

Crowder, M. K., & Kemmelmeier, M. (2014). Untreated depression predicts higher suicide rates in U.S. honor cultures. *Journal of Cross-Cultural Psychology, 45*(7), 1145–1161.

Dalgliesh, J., & Nutt, K. (2013). Treating men with eating disorders in the NHS. *Nursing Standard, 27*(35), 42–46.

de Souza, R. (2009, November). Women living with HIV/AIDS: Stories of power and powerlessness. Presented at the conference of the National Communication Association. Chicago, IL.

Dharmananda, S. (2010). FENG: The meaning of wind in Chinese medicine. Institute of Traditional Medicine. Portland, OR: Author. Retrieved from http://www.itmonline.org/articles/feng/feng.htm

Douki, S., Zineb, S. B., Nacef, F., & Halbreich, U. (2007). Women's mental health in the Muslim world: Cultural, religious, and social issues. *Journal of Affective Disorders, 102*(1–3), 177–189.

Duggleby, W. (2003). Helping Hispanic/Latino home health patients manage their pain. *Home Healthcare Nurse, 21*(3), 174–179.

Duke, A. (2014, August 12). Robin Williams dead; family, friends, and fans are "totally devastated." CNN Online. Retrieved from http://www.cnn.com/2014/08/11/showbiz/robin-williams-dead/

Durà-Vilà, G., & Hodes, M. (2012). Cross-cultural study of idioms of distress among Spanish nationals and Hispanic American migrants: *Susto, nervios* and *ataque de nervios*. *Social Psychiatry & Psychiatric Epidemiology, 47*(10), 1627–1637. doi:10.1007/s00127–011–0468–3

Dutta, M. J. (2009). Cultural theories of health communication. In *Encyclopedia of Communication Theory, 1*, 273–276.

Dutta, M. J., Mandal, I., Kaur, S., Pitaloka, D., Pandi, A., Tan, N., . . . Sastry, S. (2016). Culture-centered method: The nuts and bolts of co-creating communication infrastructures of listening in communities. Care White Paper Series, *Vol. 2*. Retrieved from https://www.researchgate.net/publication/321005848_Culture-Centered_Method_The_nuts_and_bolts_of_co-creating_communication_infrastructures_of_listening_in_communities

Emanuel, E. J., & Emanuel, L. L. (1995). Four models of the physician–patient relationship. In J. D. Arras & B.

Steinbock (Eds.), *Ethical issues in modern medicine* (4th ed., pp. 67–76). Mountain View, CA: Mayfield.

Evans, B. C., & Ume, E. (2012). Psychosocial, cultural, and spiritual health disparities in end-of-life and palliative care: Where we are and where we need to go. *Nursing Outlook, 60* (Special Issue: State of the Science: Palliative Care and End of Life), 370–375.

Evans, W. D., Uhrig, J., Davis, K., & McCormack, L. (2009). Efficacy methods to evaluate health communication and marketing campaigns. *Journal of Health Communication, 14*, 315–330.

Fadiman, A. (1997). *The spirit catches you and you fall down: A Hmong child, her American doctors, and the collision of two cultures*. New York: Farrar, Straus and Giroux.

Fertility acupuncture: Fear and discovery. (2012, May 23). Path to Fertility [Blog post]. Retrieved from http://fertility-news.rmact.com/Path-To-Fertility-Blog/bid/105392/Fertility-Acupuncture-My-Personal-Experience-with-RMACT-Experts

Fisher, J. A. (1994). *The plague makers*. New York: Simon & Schuster.

Flood-Grady, E., & Koenig Kellas, J. (2019). Sense-making, socialization, and stigma: Exploring narratives told in families about mental illness. *Health Communication, 34*(6), 607–617.

Friedman, H. S., & DiMatteo, M. R. (1979). Health care as an interpersonal process. *Journal of Social Issues, 35*, 1–11.

Fuller, J. (2003). Intercultural health care as reflective negotiated practice. *Western Journal of Nursing Research, 25*(7), 781-797.

Galanti, G.-A. (2014). *Caring for patients from different cultures* (5th ed.). Philadelphia, PA: University of Pennsylvania Press.

Gao, H., Dutta, M., & Okoror, T. (2016). Listening to Chinese immigrant restaurant workers in the Midwest: Application of the culture-centered approach (CCA) to explore perceptions of health and health care. *Health Communication, 31*(6), 726–737.

Geist-Martin, P., & Bell, K. K. (2009). "Open your heart first of all": Perspectives of holistic providers in Costa Rica about communication in the provision of health care. *Health Communication, 24*, 631–646.

Glass, R. M. (1996). The patient–physician relationship: JAMA focuses on the center of medicine. *Journal of the American Medical Association, 275*, 147–148.

Goffman, E. (1963). *Stigma: Notes on the management of spoiled identity*. Englewood Cliffs, NJ: Prentice Hall.

Goode, E. E. (1993, February 15). The cultures of illness. *U.S. News & World Report, 114*, 74–76.

Gupta, V. (2010). Impact of culture on healthcare seeking behavior of Asian Indians. *Journal of Cultural Diversity, 17*(1), 13–19.

Gustavo, S. A., Parsons-Perez, C., Goltz, S., Bhadelia, A., Durstine, A., Knaul, F., . . . Lu, R. (2013). Recommendations towards an integrated life-course approach to women's health in the post-2015 agenda. *Bulletin of the World Health Organization, 91*, 704–706.

Hain, D. J., & Sandy, D. (2013). Partners in care: Patient empowerment through shared decision-making. *Nephrology Nursing Journal, 40*(2), 153–157.

Haines, M. P., & Spear, S. F. (1996). Changing the perceptions of the norm: A strategy to decrease binge drinking among college students. *Journal of American College Health, 45*, 134–140.

Hall, A. (2014, November 13). Eco advocates for a 20 percent increase in green space by 2020. USA News.com.

Ho, E. Y. (2006). Behold the power of *Qi*: The importance of *Qi* in the discourse of acupuncture. *Research on Language and Social Interaction, 39*(4), 411–440.

Ho, E. Y., & Bylund, C. L. (2008). Models of health and models of interaction in the practitioner–client relationship in acupuncture. *Health Communication, 23*, 506–515.

Hofstede, G. (2001). *Culture's consequences: Comparing values, behaviors, institutions, and organizations across nations* (2nd ed.). Thousand Oaks, CA: Sage.

Holland, J. C., & Zittoun, R. (1990). Psychosocial issues in oncology: A historical perspective. In J. C. Holland & R. Zittoun (Eds.), *Psychosocial aspects of oncology* (pp. 1–10). New York: Springer-Verlag.

Hrisanfow, E., & Hägglund, D. (2013). Impact of cough and urinary incontinence on quality of life in women and men with chronic obstructive pulmonary disease. *Journal of Clinical Nursing, 22*(1/2), 97–105.

Hufford, D. J. (1997). Gender, culture and experience: A painful case. *Southern Folklore, 54*, 114–123.

Hutch, R. (2013). Health and healing: Spiritual, pharmaceutical, and mechanical medicine. *Journal of Religion & Health, 52*(3), 955–965.

Kean, S. (2012). *The violinist's thumb: And other lost tales of love, war, and genius, as written by our genetic code*. New York: Back Bay Books.

Kearney, M. (1978). Spiritualistic healing in Mexico. In P. Morley & R. Wallis (Eds.), *Culture and curing* (pp. 19–39). Pittsburgh: University of Pittsburgh Press.

Kennedy, J., Chi-Chuan, W., & Wu, C.-H. (2007, May 17). Patient disclosure about herb and supplement use and adults in the US. *eCam*, pp. 1–6.

Kirkham, S. R. (2003). The politics of belonging and intercultural health care. *Western Journal of Nursing Research, 7*, 762.

Kleinman, A., Eisenberg, L., & Good, B. (1978). Culture, illness, and care: Clinical lessons from anthropological and cross-cultural research. *Annals of Internal Medicine, 88*, 251–258.

Knight-Agarwal, C. R., Kaur, M., Williams, L. T., Davey, R., & Davis, D. (2014). The views and attitudes of health professionals providing antenatal care to women with a high BMI: A qualitative research study. *Women and Birth, 27*, 138–144.

Komaroff, A. L., & Fagioli, J. (1996). *Medical assessment of fatigue and chronic fatigue syndrome: An integrative approach to evaluation and treatment* (pp. 154–181). New York: Guilford Press.

Krajewski, L. A., & Beach Slatten, T. (2013). The changing roles of Japanese women in the Japanese business world. *Business Studies Journal, 5*(1), 29–41.

Kreps, G. L. (1990). Applied health communication research. In D. O'Hair & G. L. Kreps (Eds.), *Applied communication theory and research* (pp. 313–330). Hillsdale, NJ: Lawrence Erlbaum.

Kumar, R., Warnke, J. H., & Karabenick, S. A. (2014). Arab-American male identity negotiations: Caught in the crossroads of ethnicity, religion, nationality and current contexts. *Social Identities*, *20*(1), 22–41.

Lowrey, W., & Anderson, W. B. (2006). The impact of Internet use on the public perception of physicians: A perspective from the sociology of professions literature. *Health Communication*, *19*, 125–131.

MacDonald, M. (1981). *Mystical bedlam: Madness, anxiety, and healing in seventeenth-century England*. Cambridge: Cambridge University Press.

Marantz, P. R. (1990). Blaming the victim: The negative consequences of preventive medicine. *American Journal of Public Health*, *80*, 1186–1187.

Marwick, C. (1997). Proponents gather to discuss evidence-based medicine. *Journal of the American Medical Association*, *278*, 531–532.

McCune, S. K., Beck, A. M., & Johnson, R. A. (2011). *The health benefits of dog walking for people and pets: Evidence and case studies*. West Lafayette, IN: Purdue University Press.

McGregor, D. (1960). *The human side of organization*. New York: McGraw-Hill.

McWhinney, I. (1989). The need for a transformed clinical method. In M. Stewart & D. Roter (Eds.), *Communicating with medical patients: Vol. 9. Interpersonal communication* (pp. 25–40). Newbury Park, CA: Sage.

Mead, E. L., Doorenbos, A. Z., Javid, S. H., Haozous, E. A., Arviso Alvord, L., Flum, D. R., & Morris, A. M. (2013). Shared decision-making for cancer care among racial and ethnic minorities: A systematic review. *American Journal of Public Health*, *103*(12), e15–e29.

Mendenhall, E., Fernandez, A., Adler, N., & Jacobs, E. (2012). Susto, coraje, and abuse: Depression and beliefs about diabetes. *Culture, Medicine & Psychiatry*, *36*(3), 480–492. doi:10.1007/s11013-012-9267-x

Moore, L. G., Van Arsdale, P. W., Glittenberg, J. E., & Aldrich, R. A. (1987). *The biocultural basis of health: Expanding views of medical anthropology*. Prospect Heights, IL: Waveland Press.

Morris, J. L., Lippman, S. A., Philip, S., Bernstein, K., Neilands, T. B., & Lightfoot, M. (2014). Sexually transmitted infection related stigma and shame among African American male youth: Implications for testing practices, partner notification, and treatment. *AIDS Patient Care & STDs*, *28*(9), 499–506.

Murgatroyd, C. (2015). Disease and sport. *Power of the gene (blog)*. Retrieved from https://web.archive.org/web/20170201120810/http://powerofthegene.com/joomla/index.php/conversational-genetics/genetics-in-sport

Naeem, A. G. (2003). The role of culture and religion in the management of diabetes: A study of Kashmiri men in Leeds. *Journal of the Royal Society of Health*, *123*(2), 110–116.

Napier, A. D., Ancarno, C., Butler, B., Calabrese, J., Chater, A., Chatterjee, H., . . . Tyler, N. (2014). Culture and health. *Lancet*, *384*(9954), 1607–1639.

National Center for Complementary and Alternative Medicine at the National Institutes of Health. (2012). The use of complementary and alternative medicine in the United States. Washington, DC: Author. Retrieved from http://nccam.nih.gov/news/camstats/2007/camsurvey_fs1.htm#use

National Eating Disorders Association. (2015). *Statistics on eating disorders*. New York: Author. Retrieved from http://www.nationaleatingdisorders.org/general-statistics

National Institute of Medicine. U.S. Committee on the Use of Complementary and Alternative Medicine by the American Public. (2005). *Complementary and alternative medicine in the United States. Prevalence, cost, and patterns of CAM use*. Washington, DC: Author. National Academies Press. Retrieved from http://www.ncbi.nlm.nih.gov/books/NBK83794/

Native American religions: Balance and harmony. (2010, October 4). Native American Netroots. Retrieved from http://nativeamericannetroots.net/diary/705

Neihardt, J. G. (1932). *Black Elk speaks: Being the life story of a holy man of the Oglala Sioux*. New York: Morrow.

Nelkin, D., & Gilman, S. L. (1991). Placing blame for devastating disease. In A. Mack (Ed.), *In time of plague: The history and social consequences of lethal epidemic disease* (pp. 39–56). New York: New York University Press.

Newman, M. A. (1986). *Health as expanding consciousness*. St. Louis, MO: C. V. Mosby.

Newman, M. A. (2000). *Health as expanding consciousness* (2nd ed.). Boston: Jones & Bartlett.

Padela, A., Killawi, A., Forman, J., DeMonner, S., & Heisler, M. (2012). American Muslim perceptions of healing: Key agents in healing, and their roles. *Qualitative Health Research*, *22*(6), 846–858.

Patel, S., Schnall, R., Little, V., Lewis-Fernández, R., & Pincus, H. (2014). Primary care professionals' perspectives on treatment decision making for depression with African Americans and Latinos in primary care practice. *Journal of Immigrant & Minority Health*, *16*(6), 1262. doi:10.1007/s10903-013-9903-8

Peate, I. (2012). Breaking the silence: Helping men with erectile dysfunction. *British Journal of Community Nursing*, *17*(7), 310–317.

Pendleton, D., Schofield, T., Tate, P., & Havelock, P. (1984). *The consultant: An approach to learning and teaching*. Oxford: Oxford University Press.

Puhl, R., & Heuer, C. (2010). Obesity stigma: Important considerations for public health. *American Journal of Public Health*, *100*(6), 1019–1028.

Purnell, L. D. (2008, February). Traditional Vietnamese health and healing. *Urologic Nursing*, *28*(1), 63–67.

Raffel, M. W., & Raffel, N. K. (1989). *The U.S. health system: Origins and functions* (3rd ed.). New York: John Wiley & Sons.

Rampell, C. (2014, November 6). Many more men say they want to be stay-at-home dads than actually are. *The Washington Post*. Retrieved from http://www.washingtonpost.com/news/rampage/wp/2014/11/06/many-more-men-say-they-want-to-be-stay-at-home-dads-than-actually-are/

Reducing health disparities in Asian American and Pacific Islander populations: Communicating across cultures. (2005). Management Sciences of Health. Office of Minority Health and Bureau of Primary Health Care. Retrieved from https://web.archive.org/web/20160625234659/http://erc.msh.org/aapi/ca6.html

Rohde, J. A., Wang, Y., Cutino, C. M., Dickson, B. K., Bernal, M. C., Bronda, S., . . . Farraye, F. A. (2018). Impact of disease disclosure on stigma: An experimental investigation of college students' reactions to inflammatory bowel disease. *Journal of Health Communication*, 23(1), 91–97.

Rossiter, C. M., Jr. (1975). Defining "therapeutic communication." *Journal of Communication*, 25(3), 127–130.

Rubenstein, A., & Macías-González, V. M. (2012). *Masculinity and sexuality in Modern Mexico*. Albuquerque, NM: University of New Mexico Press.

Samovar, L. A., & Porter, R. E. (2007). *Communication between cultures* (6th ed.). Belmont, CA: Wadsworth.

Schreiber, L. (2005). The importance of precision in language: Communication research and (so-called) alternative medicine. *Health Communication*, 17, 173–190.

Shepard, D. S., & Rabinowitz, F. E. (2013). The power of shame in men who are depressed: Implications for counselors. *Journal of Counseling & Development*, 91(4), 451–457.

Skluth, M. (2007, September 7). Get patients involved. *Medical Economics*, 84(17), 16.

Slack, P. (1991). Responses to plague in early modern Europe: The implications of public health. In A. Mack (Ed.), *In time of plague: The history and social consequences of lethal epidemic disease* (pp. 111–132). New York: New York University Press.

Sobo, E. J., & Loustaunau, M. O. (2010). *The cultural context of health, illness, and medicine*. Santa Barbara, CA: Praeger.

Studts, C. T., Tarasenko, Y. Y., & Schoenberg, N. (2013). Barriers to cervical cancer screening among middle-aged and older rural Appalachian women. *Journal of Community Health*, 38(3), 500–512.

Swazey, J. P., & Reeds, K. (1978). *Today's medicine, tomorrow's science: Essays on paths of discovery in the biomedical sciences*. U.S. Department of Health, Education, and Welfare. Washington, DC: Author. Retrieved from https://web.archive.org/web/20160501165838/http://www.baruch.cuny.edu/library/alumni/online_exhibits/digital/2001/swazey_reeds_1978/default.htm

Swiderski, R. M. (1976). The idiom of diagnosis. *Communication Quarterly*, 24, 3–11.

Taha, H., Al-Qutob, R., Nyström, L., Wahlström, R., & Berggren, V. (2013). "Would a man smell a rose then throw it away?" Jordanian men's perspectives on women's breast cancer and breast health. *BMC Women's Health*, 13(1), 1–21.

Tauber, M. (2014, August 13). How Robin Williams fought, and lost, his battles with addiction and depression. *People*. Retrieved from http://www.people.com/article/robin-williams-dies-depression-addiciton-struggles

Tough, E. A., & White, A. R. (2011). Effectiveness of acupuncture/dry needling for myofascial trigger point pain. *Physical Therapy Reviews*, 16, 147–154.

Tovey, P., & Broom, A. (2007). Oncologists' and specialist cancer nurses' approaches to complementary and alternative medicine and their impact on patient action. *Social Science & Medicine*, 64, 2550–2564.

Twaddle, A. C., & Hessler, R. M. (1987). *A sociology of health* (2nd ed.). New York: Macmillan.

Uba, L. (1992). Cultural barriers to health care for Southeast Asian refugees. *Public Health Reports*, 107, 544–548.

U.S. Bureau of Labor Statistics. (2019, September 4). *Chiropractors. Occupational outlook handbook*. Washington, DC: Author. Retrieved from https://www.bls.gov/ooh/healthcare/chiropractors.htm

U.S. Food and Drug Administration (FDA). (2008). Beware of online cancer fraud. Washington, DC: Author. Retrieved from http://www.fda.gov/ForConsumers/ConsumerUpdates/ucm048383.htm

Usta, J., Antoun, J., Ambuel, B., & Khawaja, M. (2012). Involving the health care system in domestic violence: What women want. *Annals of Family Medicine*, 10(3), 213–220.

Veatch, R. M. (1983). The physician as stranger: The ethics of the anonymous patient–physician relationship. In E. E. Shelp (Ed.), *The clinical encounter: The moral fabric of the patient–physician relationship* (pp. 187–207). Dordrecht, The Netherlands: D. Reidel.

Vogt, D. (2013). Research on women, trauma and PTSD. Washington, DC: National Center for PTSD. Retrieved from https://www.ptsd.va.gov/professional/treat/specific/ptsd_research_women.asp

Warren-Jeanpiere, L., Miller, K. S., & Warren, A. M. (2010). African American women's retrospective perceptions of the intergenerational transfer of gynecological health care information received from mothers: Implications for families and providers. *Journal of Family Communication*, 10(2), 81–98.

White, A. D. (1925). *A history of the warfare of science with theology in Christendom* (vol. 2). New York: D. Appleton (originally published in 1896).

Wilson, K. (2003). Therapeutic landscapes and the First Nations people: An exploration of culture, health and place. *Health & Place*, 9(2), 83–93.

Winkelman, M. (2009). *Culture and health: Applying medical anthropology*. San Francisco: Jossey-Bass.

Woodyard, C. (2011). Exploring the therapeutic effects of yoga and its ability to increase quality of life. *International Journal of Yoga*, 4(2), 49–54. doi:10.4103/0973-6131.85485

World Health Organization (WHO). (1948). Preamble to the Constitution of the World Health Organization. Official records of the World Health Organization, no. 2, p. 100. Retrieved from www.who.int/about/definition/en

World Health Organization. (2003, June 18). Epidemic and pandemic alert and response (EPR). Update 83. One hundred days into the outbreak. Geneva, Switzerland: Author. Retrieved from http://www.who.int/csr/don/2003_06_18/en/index.html

World Health Organization. (2008). Traditional medicine. Geneva, Switzerland: Author. Retrieved 2017 from https://web.archive.org/web/20081222030204/http://www.who.int/mediacentre/factsheets/fs134/en/

World Health Organization (WHO). (2014, May). The top ten causes of death. Geneva, Switzerland: Author.

Retrieved from http://www.who.int/mediacentre/factsheets/fs310/en/

Zhang, Z.-J., Chen, H.-Y., Yip, K.-C., Ng, R., & Wong, V. T. (2010). The effectiveness and safety of acupuncture therapy in depressive disorders: Systematic review and meta-analysis. *Journal of Affective Disorders, 124,* 9–21. doi: 10.1016/j.jad.2009.07.005

Zimmerman, B., & Zimmerman, D. (2002). *Killer germs: Microbes and diseases that threaten humanity.* New York: McGraw-Hill.

Zoucha, R., & Broome, B. (2008, April). The significance of culture in nursing: Examples from the Mexican-American culture and knowing the unknown. *Urologic Nursing, 28*(2), 140–142.

CHAPTER 8

Al-Janabi, H., Coast, J., & Flynn, T. N. (2008). What do people value when they provide unpaid care for an older person? A meta-ethnography with interview follow-up. *Social Science & Medicine, 67,* 111–121.

Alam, R., Barrera, M., D'Agostino, N., Nicholas, D. B., & Schneiderman, G. (2012). Bereavement experiences of mothers and fathers over time after the death of a child due to cancer. *Death Studies, 36,* 1–22. doi:10.1080/07481187.2011.553312

Albrecht, T. L., & Adelman, M. B. (1987). Communicating social support: A theoretical perspective. In T. L. Albrecht & M. B. Adelman (Eds.), *Communicating social support* (pp. 18–39). Newbury Park, CA: Sage.

Allen, K. A., Blascovich, J., & Mendes, W. B. (2002). Cardiovascular reactivity and the presence of pets, friends, and spouses: The truth about cats and dogs. *Psychosomatic Medicine, 64,* 727–739.

Alston, S. (2007). Nothing to laugh at: Humour as a means of coping with pain and stress. *Australian Journal of Communication, 34*(1), 77–89.

American Transplant Foundation. (2019). Facts: Did you know? Retrieved from https://www.americantransplantfoundation.org/about-transplant/facts-and-myths/

Anderson, J. O., & Geist-Martin, P. (2003). Narratives and healing: Exploring one family's stories of cancer survivorship. *Health Communication, 15*(2), 133–143.

Babrow, A. S. (1992). Communication and problematic integration: Understanding diverging probability and value, ambiguity, ambivalence, and impossibility. *Communication Theory, 2,* 95–130.

Babrow, A. S. (2001). Uncertainty, value, communication, and problematic integration. *Journal of Communication, 51*(3), 553–573.

Bandura, A. (1986). *Social foundations of thought and action: A social cognitive approach.* Englewood Cliffs, NJ: Prentice Hall.

Barker, S. A., & Dawson, K. S. (1998). The effects of animal-assisted therapy on anxiety ratings of hospitalized psychiatric patients. *Psychiatric Services, 49,* 797–801.

Barnes, M. K., & Duck, S. (1994). Everyday communicative contexts for social support. In B. R. Burleson, T. L. Albrecht, & I. G. Sarason (Eds.), *Communication of social support: Messages, interactions, relationships, and community* (pp. 175–194). Thousand Oaks, CA: Sage.

Baxter, L. A. (1988). A dialectic perspective of communication strategies in relationship development. In S. Duck (Ed.), *Handbook of personal relationships* (pp. 257–273). New York: Wiley.

Baxter, L. A., & Montgomery, B. M. (1996). *Relating: Dialogues and dialectics.* New York: Guilford Press.

Beach, W. A. (2002). Between dad and son: Initiating, delivering, and assimilating bad cancer news. *Health Communication, 14*(3), 271–298.

Berger, P., & Luckmann, T. (1966). *The social construction of reality.* New York: Doubleday.

Bergstrom, M. J., & Holmes, M. E. (2000). Lay theories of successful aging after the death of a spouse: A network text analysis of bereavement advice. *Health Communication, 12*(4), 377–406.

Bernhard, T. (2019, April 29). 7 things I've come to appreciate due to chronic illness. *Psychology Today.* Retrieved from https://www.psychologytoday.com/us/blog/turning-straw-gold/201904/7-things-i-ve-come-appreciate-due-chronic-illness

Bevan, J. L., Rogers, K. E., Andrews, N. F., & Sparks, L. (2012). Topic avoidance and negative health perceptions in the distant family caregiving context. *Journal of Family Communication, 12*(4), 300–314.

Block, S. D. (2001). Psychological considerations, growth, and transcendence at the end of life. *Journal of the American Medical Association, 285*(22), 2898–2905.

Booth-Butterfield, M., Anderson, R., & Booth-Butterfield, S. (2000). Adolescents' use of tobacco, health locus of control, and self-monitoring. *Health Communication, 12,* 137–148.

Borreani, C., Brunelli, C., Miccinesi, G., Morino, P., Piazza, M., Piva, L., & Tamburini, M. (2008). Eliciting individual preferences about death: Development of the End-of-Life Preferences Interview. *Journal of Pain and Symptom Management, 36*(4), 335–350.

Botta, R. A., & Dumlao, R. (2002). How do conflict and communication patterns between fathers and daughters contribute to or offset eating disorders? *Health Communication, 14,* 199–219.

Boylstein, C., Rittman, M., & Hinojosa, R. (2007). Metaphor shifts in stroke recovery. *Health Communication, 21,* 279–287.

Braithwaite, D. O. (1996). "Persons first": Expanding communicative choices by persons with disabilities. In E. B. Ray (Ed.), *Communication and disenfranchisement: Social health issues and implications* (pp. 449–464). Mahwah, NJ: Lawrence Erlbaum.

Branch, W. T., Jr., Levinson, W., & Platt, F. W. (1996). Diagnostic interviewing: Make the most of your time. *Patient Care, 30*(12), 68–76.

Brann, M., Himes, K. L., Dillow, M. R., & Weber, K. (2010). Dialectic tensions in stroke survivor relationships. *Health Communication, 25,* 323–332.

Brashers, D. E., & Babrow, A. S. (1996). Theorizing health communication. *Communication Studies, 47,* 237–251.

Brett, R. (2003, February 21). Life's great, say area survivors. *The Plain Dealer,* p. B1.

Burleson, B. R. (1990). Comforting as social support: Relational consequences of supportive behaviors. In S. Duck

& R. C. Silver (Eds.), *Personal relationships and social support* (pp. 66–82). London: Sage.

Burleson, B. R. (1994). Comforting messages: Significance, approaches, and effects. In B. R. Burleson, T. L. Albrecht, & I. G. Sarason (Eds.), *Communication of social support: Messages, interactions, relationships, and community* (pp. 175–194). Thousand Oaks, CA: Sage.

Bute, J. J., Donovan-Kicken, E., & Martins, N. (2007). Effects of communication-debilitating illnesses and injuries on close relationships: A relational maintenance perspective. *Health communication*, *21*(3), 235–246.

Caplan, S. E., Haslett, B. J., & Burleson, B. R. (2005). Telling it like it is: The adaptive function of narratives in coping with loss in later life. *Health Communication*, *17*, 233–251.

Caregiving in the U.S. (2009). National Alliance of Caregiving and the American Association of Retired Persons. Retrieved from http://www.caregiving.org/data/Caregiving_in_the_US_2009_full_report.pdf

Carpiac-Claver, M. L., & Levy-Storms, L. (2007). In a manner of speaking: Communication between nurse aides and older adults in long-term care settings. *Health Communication*, *22*, 59–67.

Charchuk, M., & Simpson, C. (2005). Hope, disclosure, and control in the neonatal intensive care unit. *Health Communication*, *17*, 191–203.

Chesler, M. A., & Barbarin, O. A. (1984). Difficulties of providing help in a crisis: Relationships between parents of children with cancer and their friends. *Journal of Social Issues*, *40*, 113–134.

Chia, H. L. (2009). Exploring facets of a social network to explicate the status of social support and its effects on stress. *Social Behavior & Personality: An International Journal*, *37*(5), 701–710.

Cohen, S., & Wills, T. A. (1985). Stress, social support, and buffering hypothesis. *Psychological Bulletin*, *98*, 310–357.

Cowart, D., & Burt, R. (1998). Confronting death: Who chooses, who controls? *The Hastings Center Report*, *28*, 14–24.

Cutrona, C. E., & Suhr, J. A. (1994). Social support communication in the context of marriage: An analysis of couples' supportive interactions. In B. R. Burleson, T. L. Albrecht, & I. G. Sarason (Eds.), *Communication of social support: Messages, interactions, relationships, and community* (pp. 113–135). Thousand Oaks, CA: Sage.

DeLucia, M. (2011, December 14). Dogs offer patient care that cannot be matched. Fox5 News, Las Vegas, Nevada. Retrieved from https://web.archive.org/web/20140621124200/http://www.fox5vegas.com/story/16157761/pets-overcome-adversity-to-help-sunrise-patients-dogs-vegas-sunrise-hospital

Dennis, M. R. (2006). Compliance and intimacy: Young adults' attempts to motivate health-promoting behaviors for romantic partners. *Health Communication*, *19*, 259–267.

du Pré, A., & Ray, E. B. (2008). Comforting episodes: Transcendent experiences of cancer survivors. In L. Sparks, H. D. O'Hair, & G. L. Kreps (Eds.), *Cancer, communication and aging* (pp. 99–114). Cresskill, NJ: Hampton Press.

Dyer, J. (1996). *In a tangled wood: An Alzheimer's journey*. Dallas: Southern Methodist University Press.

Edwards, H., & Noller, P. (1998). Factors influencing caregiver–care receiver communication and the impact on the well-being of older care receivers. *Health Communication*, *10*, 317–342.

Egbert, N., Koch, L., Coeling, H., & Ayers, D. (2006). The role of social support in the family and community integration of right-hemisphere stroke survivors. *Health Communication*, *20*, 45–55.

Egbert, N., Sparks, L., Kreps, G. L., & du Pré, A. (2008). Finding meaning in the journey: Methods of spiritual coping for aging patients with cancer. In L. Sparks, H. D. O'Hair, & G. L. Kreps (Eds.), *Cancer, communication and aging* (pp. 277–291). Cresskill, NJ: Hampton Press.

Emanuel, E. J., & Emanuel, L. L. (1998, May 16). The promise of a good death. *The Lancet*, *351*, S21–S29.

English, J., Wilson, K., & Keller-Olaman, S. (2008). Health, healing and recovery: Therapeutic landscapes and the everyday lives of breast cancer survivors. *Social Science & Medicine*, *67*, 68–78.

Erdman, L. (1993). Laughter therapy for patients with cancer. *Journal of Psychosocial Oncology*, *11*, 55–67.

Family Caregiver Alliance. (2019, April 17). Caregiver statistics: Demographics. Retrieved from https://www.caregiver.org/caregiver-statistics-demographics

Floyd, K., Hesse, C., & Haynes, M. T. (2007, January). Human affection exchange: SV. Metabolic and cardiovascular correlates of trait expressed affection. *Communication Quarterly*, *55*(1), 79–94.

Flynn, J. J., Hollenstein, T., & Mackey, A. (2010). The effect of suppressing and not accepting emotions on depressive symptoms: Is suppression different for men and women? *Personality and Individual Differences*, *49*, 49582–49586. doi:10.1016/j.paid.2010.05.022

Ford, L. A., Babrow, A. S., & Stohl, C. (1996). Social support messages and the management of uncertainty in the experience of breast cancer: An application of problematic integration theory. *Communication Monographs*, *63*, 189–208.

Forsythe, L. P., Alfano, C. M., Kent, E. E., Weaver, K. E., Bellizzi, K., Arora, N., . . . Rowland, J. H. (2014). Social support, self-efficacy for decision-making, and follow-up care use in long-term cancer survivors. *Psycho-Oncology*, *23*(7), 788–796.

Foster, E. (2007). *Communicating at the end of life: Finding magic in the mundane*. Mahwah, NJ: Lawrence Erlbaum.

Frankl, V. E. (1959). *Man's search for meaning*. Boston: Beacon Press.

Frates, J., Bohrer, G. G., & Thomas, D. (2006). Promoting organ donation to Hispanics: The role of the media and medicine. *Journal of Health Communication*, *11*(7), 683–698.

Friedmann, E., & Thomas, S. A. (1995). Pet ownership, social support, and one-year survival after acute myocardial infarction in the cardiac arrhythmia suppression trial. *American Journal of Cardiology*, *76*, 1213–1217.

Fry, R. B., & Prentice-Dunn, S. (2005). Effects of coping information and value affirmation on responses to a perceived health threat. *Health Communication, 17*, 133–147.

Giles, L. C., Glonek, G. F., Luszcz, M. A., & Andrews, G. R. (2005, July). Effect of social networks on 10-year survival in very old Australians: The Australian longitudinal study of aging. *Journal of Epidemiology & Community Health, 59*(7), 574–579.

Gill, E. A., & Babrow, A. S. (2007). To hope or to know: Coping with uncertainty and ambivalence in women's magazine breast cancer articles. *Journal of Applied Communication Research, 35*(2), 133–155.

Gilstrap, C. M., & White, Z. M. (2015). Interactional communication challenges in end-of-life care: dialectical tensions and management strategies experienced by home hospice nurses. *Health Communication, 30*, 525–535.

Green, F. (2003, June 20). Booze ads target Black teens, report finds. *San-Diego Union-Tribune*, p. C1.

Green, R. (1999). *The Nicholas Effect: A boy's gift to the world*. Cambridge, MA: O'Reilly.

Han, J. Y., Hou, J., Kim, E., & Gustafson, D. H. (2014). Lurking as an active participation process: A longitudinal investigation of engagement with an online cancer support group. *Health Communication, 29*, 911–923.

Han, J. Y., Shah, D. V., Kim, E., Namkoong, K., Lee, S.-Y., Moon, J., . . . Gustafson, D. H. (2011). Empathic exchanges in online cancer support groups: Distinguishing message expression and reception effects. *Health Communication, 26*, 185–197.

Hawkley, L. C., Masi, C. M., Berry, J. D., & Cacioppo, J. T. (2006). Loneliness is a unique predictor of age-related differences in systolic blood pressure. *Psychology and Aging, 21*(1), 152–164.

Hegedus, K., Zana, Á., & Szabó, B. (2008). Effect of end-of-life education on medical students' and health care workers' death attitude. *Palliative Medicine, 22*, 264–269.

Hines, S. C. (2001). Coping with uncertainties in advance care planning. *Journal of Communication, 51*(3), 498–513.

Hospice care in America. (2012). Alexandria, VA: National Hospice and Palliative Care Organization. Retrieved from https://web.archive.org/web/20160827213230/http://www.nhpco.org/sites/default/files/public/Statistics_Research/2011_Facts_Figures.pdf

Jeong, S.-H. (2007). Effects of news about genetics and obesity on controllability attribution and helping behavior. *Health Communication, 22*, 221–228.

Keeley, M. P. (2004). Final conversations: Survivors' memorable messages concerning religious faith and spirituality. *Health Communication, 16*, 87–104.

Kramer, H., & Kramer, K. Conversations at midnight. (1993, March–April). *Psychology Today, 26*, 26–27.

Krug, P. (1998). Where does physician-assisted suicide stand today? *Association of Operating Room Nurses Journal, 68*, 869.

Kübler-Ross, E. (1969). *On death and dying*. New York: Macmillan.

Laframboise, D. (1998). When home is the hospital. *Chatelaine, 71*, 26–31.

Lehman, D. R., Ellard, J. H., & Wortman, C. B. (1986). Social support for the bereaved: Recipients' and providers' perspectives on what is helpful. *Journal of Consulting and Clinical Psychology, 54*, 438–446.

"Life interrupted" by cancer diagnosis at 22. (2012, May 15). National Public Radio. *Talk of the Nation* broadcast. Transcript retrieved at http://www.npr.org/2012/05/16/152840031/life-interrupted-by-cancer-diagnosis-at-22

Living with cancer. (1997, September). *Harvard Health Letter, 22*, 4–5.

Lockwood, N. L., & Yoshimura, S. M. (2014). The heart of the matter: The effects of humor on well-being during recovery from cardiovascular disease. *Health Communication, 29*, 410–420.

Malis, R. S., & Roloff, M. E. (2007). The effect of legitimacy and intimacy on peer interventions into alcohol abuse. *Western Journal of Communication, 71*(1), 49–68.

Maynard, D. W., & Frankel, R. M. (2006). On diagnostic rationality: Bad news, good news, and the symptoms residue. In J. Heritage & D. W. Maynard (Eds.), *Communication in medical care: Interactions between primary care physicians and patients* (pp. 248–278). Cambridge: Cambridge University Press.

McCormick, T. R., & Conley, B. J. (1995). Patients' perspectives on dying and the care of dying patients. *Western Journal of Medicine, 163*, 236–243.

McCue, J. D. (1995). The naturalness of dying. *Journal of the American Medical Association, 273*, 1039–1044.

Metts, S., & Manns, H. (1996). Coping with HIV and AIDS: The social and personal challenges. In E. B. Ray (Ed.), *Communication and disenfranchisement: Social issues and implications* (pp. 347–364). Mahwah, NJ: Lawrence Erlbaum.

Miller, L. E. (2014). Uncertainty management and information seeking in cancer survivorship. *Health Communication, 29*, 233–243.

Miller-Day, M., & Marks, J. (2006). Perceptions of parental communication orientation, perfectionism, and disordered eating behaviors of sons and daughters. *Health Communication, 19*, 153–163.

Mills, C. B. (2005). Catching up with Down syndrome: Parents' experiences in dealing with the medical and therapeutic communities. In E. B. Ray (Ed.), *Health communication in practice: A case study approach* (pp. 195–210). Mahwah, NJ: Lawrence Erlbaum.

Morgan, L. A., & Brazda, M. A. (2013). Transferring control to others: Process and meaning for older adults in assisted living. *Journal of Applied Gerontology, 32*(6), 651.

Morgan, S. E., Harrison, T. R., Afifi, W. A., Long, S. D., & Stephenson, M. T. (2008). In their own words: The reasons why people will (not) sign an organ donor card. *Health Communication, 23*, 23–33.

Muskin, P. R. (1998). The request to die: Role for a psychodynamic perspective on physician-assisted suicide. *Journal of the American Medical Association, 279*, 323–328.

National Cancer Institute (NCI). (2019, June 17). A new normal. Author: Bethesda, MD. Retrieved from https://www.cancer.gov/about-cancer/coping/survivorship/new-normal

Nussbaum, J. F., Baringer, D., Fisher, C. L., & Kundrat, A. L. (2008). Connecting health, communication, and aging. In L. Sparks, H. D. O'Hair, & G. L. Kreps (Eds.), *Cancer, communication and aging* (pp. 67–76). Cresskill, NJ: Hampton Press.

Organ donation: Don't let these myths confuse you. (2008). Rochester, MN: Mayo Clinic. Retrieved from http://www.mayoclinic.com/health/organ-donation/FL00077

Ortman, J. M., Velkoff, V. A., & Hogan, H. (2014, May). An aging nation: The older population in the United States. Washington, DC: U.S. Census Bureau. Retrieved from http://www.census.gov/prod/2014pubs/p25-1140.pdf

Parkes, C. M. (1998). The dying adult. *British Medical Journal, 316*, 1313–1315.

Perry, B. (2002, November). Growth and satisfaction: "I became a nurse because I wanted to help others." *Canadian Business and Current Affairs, 98*(10), nonpaginated.

Pet Partners video: The health benefits of pets. (n.d.). Bellevue, WA: Author. Retrieved from http://www.deltasociety.org/page.aspx?pid=642

Peterson, B. L. (2019). Dialectical tensions associated with health advocacy. *Health Communication* [online], 1–4.

Pighin, S., & Bonnefon, J.-F. (2011). Facework and uncertain reasoning in health communication. *Patient Education and Counseling, 85*, 169–172.

Platt, F. W. (1995). *Conversation repair: Case studies in doctor–patient communication*. Boston: Little, Brown.

Potter, E. (n.d.). We used to love to travel and eat out . . . now, nothing. Caregiver stories. Family Caregiver Alliance. Retrieved from https://caregiver.org/we-used-love-travel-and-eat-out-now-nothing

Ragan, S. L., & Goldsmith, J. (2008). End-of-life communication: The drama of pretense in the talk of dying patients and their M.D. In K. B. Wright & S. D. Moore (Eds.), *Applied health communication* (pp. 207–227). Cresskill, NJ: Hampton Press.

Ragan, S. L., Wittenberg, E., & Hall, H. T. (2003). The communication of palliative care for the elderly cancer patient. *Health Communication, 15*(2), 219–226.

Ragan, S. L., Wittenberg-Lyles, E. W., Goldsmith, J., & Sanchez-Reilly, S. (2008). *Communication as comfort: Multiple voices in palliative care*. New York: Routledge.

Ramanadhan, S., & Viswanath, K. (2006). Health and the information nonseeker: A profile. *Health Communication, 20*, 131–139.

Rao, J. K., Anderson, L. A., Lin, F., & Laux, J. P. (2014). Completion of advance directives among U.S. consumers. *American Journal of Preventive Medicine, 46*, 65–70. doi:10.1016/j.amepre.2013.09.008

Rawlins, W. K. (1989). A dialectical analysis of the tensions, functions, and strategic challenges of communication in young adult friendships. *Communication Yearbook, 12*, 157–189.

Reinhardt, J. P., Boerner, K., & Horowitz, A. (2006). Good to have but not to use: Differential impact of perceived and received support on well-being. *Journal of Social and Personal Relationships, 23*(1), 117–129.

Rimal, R. (2000). Closing the knowledge–behavior gap in health promotion: The mediating role of self-efficacy. *Health Communication, 12*, 219–238.

Robertson, T. (1999, March 26). Michigan jury gets Kevorkian case: Defendant cites civil rights leaders. *Boston Globe*, p. A3.

Robinson, J. D., & Tian, Y. (2009). Cancer patients and the provision of informational social support. *Health Communication, 24*, 381–390. doi:10.1080/10410230903023261

Ruppert, R. A. (1996, March). Caring for the lay caregiver. *American Journal of Nursing, 96*, 40–46.

Russell, L. D., & Babrow, A. S. (2011). Risk in the making: Narrative, problematic integration, and the social construction of risk. *Communication Theory, 21*(3), 239–260. doi:10.1111/j.1468-2885.2011.01386.x

Salander, P. (2002). Bad news from the patient's perspective: An analysis of the written narratives of newly diagnosed cancer patients. *Social Science & Medicine, 55*, 721–732.

Sastre, M. T. M., Sorum, P. C., & Mullet, E. (2011). Breaking bad news: The patient's viewpoint. *Health Communication, 26*, 649–655.

Segrin, C., & Domschke, T. (2011). Social support, loneliness, recuperative processes, and their direct and indirect effects on health. *Health Communication, 26*, 221–232. doi:10.1080/10410236.2010.546771

Segrin, C., & Passalacqua, S. A. (2010). Functions of loneliness, social support, health behaviors, and stress in association with poor health. *Health Communication, 25*, 312–322.

Sharf, B. (2010). The day Patrick Swayze died. *Health Communication, 25*, 628–631.

Shuler, S. (2011). Social support without strings attached. *Health Communication, 26*, 198–201.

Siegel, J. T., Alvaro, E. M., Crano, W. D., Lienemann, B. A., Hohman, Z. P., & O'Brien, E. (2012). Increasing social support for depressed individuals: A cross-cultural assessment of an affect-expectancy approach. *Journal of Health Communication, 17*(6), 713–732.

Sparks, L., Villagran, M. M., Parker-Raley, J., & Cunningham, C. B. (2007). A patient-centered approach to breaking bad news: Communication guidelines for health care providers. *Journal of Applied Communication, 35*(2), 177–196.

Stepler, R. (2015, November 18). 5 facts about family caregivers. Pew Research Center. Retrieved from https://www.pewresearch.org/fact-tank/2015/11/18/5-facts-about-family-caregivers/

Sudore, R. L., Schillinger, D., Knight, S. J., & Fried, T. R. (2010). Uncertainty about advance care planning treatment preferences among diverse older adults. *Journal of Health Communication, 15*, 159–171.

Tardy, C. H. (1994). Counteracting task-induced stress: Studies of instrumental and emotional support in problem-solving contexts. In B. R. Burleson, T. L. Albrecht, & I. G. Sarason (Eds.), *Communication of social support: Messages, interactions, relationships, and community* (pp. 71–87). Thousand Oaks, CA: Sage.

Thompson, T. L. (2011). Hope and the act of informed dialogue: A delicate balance at the end of life. *Journal of Language and Social Psychology, 30*, 177–192.

Thompson, T. L., & Gillotti, C. (2005). Staying out of the line of fire: A medical student learns about bad news delivery. In E. B. Ray (Ed.), *Health communication in practice: A case study approach* (pp. 11–25). Mahwah, NJ: Lawrence Erlbaum.

Thomsen, T., Rydahl-Hansen, S., & Wagner, L. (2010). A review of potential factors relevant to coping in patients with advanced cancer. *Journal of Clinical Nursing, 19*, 3410–3426. doi:10.1111/j.1365-2702.2009.03154.x

Thomtén, J., Soares, J., & Sundin, Ö. (2011). The role of psychosocial factors in the course of pain: A 1-year follow-up study among women living in Sweden. *Archives of Women's Mental Health, 14*, 493–503. doi:10.1007/s00737-011-0244-0

Tiedtke, C., de Rijk, A., Donceel, P., Christiaens, M., & Dierckx de Casterl, B. (2012). Survived but feeling vulnerable and insecure: A qualitative study of the mental preparation for RTW after breast cancer treatment. *BMC Public Health, 12*(1), 538–550.

Troth, A., & Peterson, C. C. (2000). Factors predicting safe-sex talk and condom use in early sexual relationships. *Health Communication, 12*, 195–218.

U.S. Census Bureau. (2009, June 23). Census Bureau reports world's older population projected to triple by 2050. Washington, DC: Author. Retrieved from https://web.archive.org/web/20151005004506/https://www.census.gov/newsroom/releases/archives/international_population/cb09-97.html

Venetis, M. K., Robinson, J. D., & Kearney, T. (2015). Breast-cancer patients' participation behavior and coping during presurgical consultations: A pilot study. *Health Communication, 30*(1), 19–25.

Vilhauer, R. P. (2011). "Them" and "us": The experiences of women with metastatic disease in mixed-stage versus stage-specific breast cancer support groups. *Psychology & Health, 26*(6), 781–797.

Wanzer, M. B., Sparks, L., & Frymier, A. B. (2009). Humorous communication within the lives of older adults: The relationships among humor, coping efficacy, age, and life satisfaction. *Health Communication, 24*, 128–136.

Wells, D. L. (2009). The effects of animals on human health and well-being. *Journal of Social Issues, 65*, 1540–1560.

White, A., Philogene, G., Fine, L., & Sinha, S. (2009). Social support and self-reported health status of older adults in the United States. *American Journal of Public Health, 99*(10), 1872–1878.

Willing, R. (1999, April 14). Kevorkian sentenced to 10-25 years. *USA Today*, p. 1A.

World Population Review. (2019). Life expectancy by country, 2019. Retrieved from http://worldpopulationreview.com/countries/life-expectancy-by-country/

Wright, K. (2002). Social support within an on-line cancer community: An assessment of emotional support, perceptions of advantages and disadvantages, and motives for using the community from a communication perspective. *Journal of Applied Communication Research, 31*(3), 195–209.

Wright, K. B., & Rains, S. A. (2014). Weak tie support preference and preferred coping styles as predictors of perceived credibility within health-related computer-mediated support groups. *Health Communication, 29*, 281–287.

Zook, E. (1993). Diagnosis HIV/AIDS: Caregiver communication in the crisis of terminal illness. In E. B. Ray (Ed.), *Case studies in health communication* (pp. 113–128). Hillsdale, NJ: Lawrence Erlbaum.

CHAPTER 9

Abroms, L. C., Ahuja, M., Kodl, Y., Thaweethai, L., Sims, J., Winickoff, J. P., & Windsor, R. A. (2012). Text2Quit: Results from a pilot test of a personalized, interactive mobile health smoking cessation program. *Journal of Health Communication, 17*, 44–53.

Afifi, W. A., & Weiner, J. L. (2004). Toward a theory of motivated information management. *Communication Theory, 14*, 167–190.

American Heart Association. (2019). *All about heart rate (pulse)*. Retrieved from https://www.heart.org/en/health-topics/high-blood-pressure/the-facts-about-high-blood-pressure/all-about-heart-rate-pulse

Anderson, M. (2019). *Mobile technology and home broadband 2019. Pew Research Center*. Retrieved from https://www.pewresearch.org/internet/2019/06/13/mobile-technology-and-home-broadband-2019/

Anderson, M., Perrin, A. Jiang, J. & Kumar, M. (2019). *10% of Americans don't use the internet. Who are they? Pew Research Center*. Retrieved from https://www.pewresearch.org/fact-tank/2019/04/22/some-americans-dont-use-the-internet-who-are-they/

Barnes, D. (2015, May 1). TeleMIND brings specialty health care to rural clinic. *The University of Mississippi Medical Center*. Retrieved from https://www.umc.edu/news/News_Articles/2015/May/TeleMIND-brings-specialty-health-care-to-rural-clinic.html

Basu, A., & Dutta, M. J. (2008). The relationship between health information seeking and community participation: The roles of health information orientation and efficacy. *Health Communication, 23*(1), 70–79.

Beach, W. A. (2002). Between dad and son: Initiating, delivering, and assimilating bad cancer news. *Health Communication, 14*(3), 271–298.

Berry, L. L., & Seltman, K. D. (2008). *Management lessons from Mayo Clinic: Inside one of the world's most admired service organizations*. New York: McGraw-Hill.

Brown, V. A., Parker, P. A., Furber, L., & Thomas, A. L. (2011). Patient preferences for the delivery of bad news—The experience of a UK Cancer Centre. *European Journal of Cancer Care, 20*(1), 56–61.

Bull, S., & Ezeanochie, N. (2016). From Foucault to Freire through Facebook: Toward an integrated theory of mHealth. *Health Education and Behavior, 43*(4), 399–411.

Chaiken, S. (1980). Heuristic versus systematic information processing and the use of source versus message cues in persuasion. *Journal of Personality and Social Psychology, 39*, 752–766.

Chaiken, S., Giner-Sorolla, R., & Chen, S. (1996). Beyond accuracy: Defense and impression motives in heuristic and systematic information processing. In P. M. Gollwitzer & J. A. Bargh (Eds.), *The psychology of action: Linking cognition and motivation to behavior* (pp. 553–578). New York: Guilford.

Chamberlain, M. A. (1994). New technologies in health communication: Progress or panacea? *American Behavioral Scientist, 38*, 271–285.

Chen, R., Jankovic, F., Marinsek, N., Foschini, L., Kourtis, L., Signorini, A., . . . Trister, A. (2019). Developing measures of cognitive impairment in the real world from consumer-grade multimodal sensor streams. *Proceeding KDD '19 Proceedings of the 25th ACM SIGKDD International Conference on Knowledge Discovery & Data Mining, USA*, 2145–2155.

Chesser, A., Burke, A., Reyes, J., & Rohrberg, T. (2016). Navigating the digital divide: A systematic review of eHealth literacy in underserved populations in the United States. *Informatics for Health and Social Care, 41*, 1–19.

COPD Foundation. (n.d.). *What is COPD?* Washington, DC: Author. Retrieved from http://www.copdfoundation.org/

Coughlin, S., Stewart, J., Young, L., Heboyan, V., & Da Leo, G. (2018). Health literacy and patient web portals. *International Journal of Medical Informatics, 113*, 43–48.

Definitive Healthcare. (2015, April 14). Controversy over telemedicine in Texas. Retrieved from https://web.archive.org/web/20150629212314/http://www.definitivehc.com/news/2015/04/14/controversy-over-telemedicine-texas-medical-board-votes-to-restrict-and-limit-telemedicine-practices/

Duplaga, M. (2015). A cross-sectional study assessing determinants of the attitude to the introduction of eHealth services among patients suffering from chronic conditions. *BMC Medical Informatics & Decision Making, 15*(1), 1–15.

Dutta, M. J., Bodie, G. D., & Basu, A. (2008). Health disparity and the racial divide among the nation's youth: Internet as a site for change? In A. Everett (Ed.), *Learning race and ethnicity: Youth and the digital media* (pp. 175–198). Cambridge, MA: MIT Press.

The e-mail advantage. (2007, September 7). *Medical Economics, 84*(17), 28.

Emme, C., Rydahl-Hansen, S., Østergaard, B., Schou, L., Svarre Jakobsen, A., & Phanareth, K. (2014). How virtual admission affects coping—telemedicine for patients with chronic obstructive pulmonary disease. *Journal of Clinical Nursing, 23*(9/10), 1445–1458.

Esmaeilzadeh, P. (2019). The effects of public concern for information privacy on the adoption of health information exchanges (HIEs) by healthcare entities. *Health Communication, 34*(10), 1202–1211.

Farahani, B. Firouzi, F., Chang, V., Badaroglu, M., Constant, N., & Mankodiya, K. (2018). Towards fog-driven IoT eHealth: Promises and challenges of IoT in medicine and healthcare. *Future Generation Computer Systems, 78*(2), 659–676.

Fathi, J., Modin, H., & Scott, J. (2017, May). Nurses advancing telehealth services in the era of healthcare reform. *Online Journal of Issues in Nursing, 22*(2). Retrieved from http://ojin.nursingworld.org/MainMenuCategories/ANAMarketplace/ANAPeriodicals/OJIN/TableofContents/

Freimuth, V. S., Stein, J. A., & Kean, T. J. (1989). *Searching for health information: The cancer information service model.* Philadelphia: University of Pennsylvania Press.

Goodyear, V., Armour, K., & Wood, H. (2019). Young people learning about health: The role of apps and wearable devices. *Journal Learning, Media and Technology 44*(2), 193–210.

Granja, C., Janssen, W., & Johansen, M. (2018). Factors determining the success and failure of eHealth interventions: Systematic review of the literature. *Journal of Medical Internet Research, 20*(5), e10235.

Griffin, R. J., Dunwoody, S., & Neuwirth, K. (1999). Information insufficiency and risk communication. *Media Psychology, 6*, 23–61.

Hall, A. K., Bernhardt, J. M., Dodd, V., & Vollrath, M. W. (2015). The digital health divide: Evaluating online health information access and use among older adults. *Health Education & Behavior, 42*(2), 202.

Handley, L. (2019, January 24). Nearly three quarters of the world will use just their smartphones to access the internet by 2025. *CNBC News.* Retrieved from https://www.cnbc.com/2019/01/24/smartphones-72percent-of-people-will-use-only-mobile-for-internet-by-2025.html

Hartzband, P., & Groopman, J. (2008). Off the record: Avoiding the pitfalls of going electronic. *New England Journal of Medicine, 358*(16), 1656.

Health care delivery, quality and transformation. (2015). American Telemedicine Association. Retrieved from https://web.archive.org/web/20150323123819/http://www.americantelemed.org/ata-2015/ata-2015-awards

Hermann, J. (2010, August 24). Giz explains: How blind people see the Internet. *Gizmodo.* Retrieved from http://gizmodo.com/5620079/giz-explains-how-blind-people-see-the-internet

Hinton, L., Kurinczuk, J. J., & Ziebland, S. (2010). Infertility; isolation and the internet: A qualitative interview study. *Patient Education and Counseling, 81*, 436–441.

Holst, A. (2019, August 22). Share of households with a computer at home worldwide from 2005 to 2018. *Statista.* Retrieved from https://www.statista.com/statistics/748551/worldwide-households-with-computer/

Hong, S. G., Kim, D. W., Trimi, S., & Hyun, J. H. (2015). A Delphi study of factors hindering web accessibility for persons with disabilities. *Journal of Computer Information Systems, 55*(4), 28–34.

Horvath, K. J., Harwood, E. M., Courtenay-Quirk, C., McFarlane, M., Fisher, H., Dickenson, T., . . . Simon Rosser, B. R. (2010). Online resources for persons recently diagnosed with HIV/AIDS: An analysis of HIV-related webpages. *Journal of Health Communication, 15*, 516–531.

Hou, J., & Shim, M. (2010). The role of provider-patient communication and trust in online sources in Internet use of health-related activities. *Journal of Health Communication, 15*, 186–199.

Huston, L. (2019, March 15). Beware the hype over the Apple Watch heart app. The device could do more harm than good. *STAT*. Retrieved from https://www.statnews.com/2019/03/15/apple-watch-atrial-fibrillation/

Imes, R. S., Bylund, C. L., Sabee, C. M., Routsong, T. R., & Sanford, A. A. (2008). Patients' reasons for refraining from discussing Internet health information with their healthcare providers. *Health Communication, 23*, 538–547.

Jacobs, J. (2019, March 9). Doctor on video screen told a man he was near death, leaving relatives aghast. *The New York Times*. Retrieved from https://www.nytimes.com/2019/03/09/science/telemedicine-ethical-issues.html

Jiang, S. (2018). How does online patient–provider communication heal? Examining the role of patient satisfaction and communication experience in China. *Health Communication 34*(13), 1637–1644.

Johnson, K., & Kalkbrenner, M. (2017). The utilization of technological innovations to support college student mental health: Mobile health communication. *Journal of Technology in Human Services, 35*(4), 314–339.

Johnson, L. J. (2007, August 3). Patient e-mail perils. *Medical Economics, 84*(15), 30.

Jones, R. K., & Biddlecom, A. E. (2011). Is the internet filling the sexual health information gap for teens? An exploratory study. *Journal of Health Communication, 16*, 112–123.

Kane, C., & Gillis, K. (2018). The use of telemedicine by physicians: Still the exception rather than the rule. *Health Affairs, 37*(10). Abstract retrieved from https://www.healthaffairs.org/doi/full/10.1377/hlthaff.2018.05077

Karcher, N., & Presser, N. (2016). Ethical and legal issues addressing the use of mobile health (mHealth) as an adjunct to psychotherapy. *Ethics and Behavior, 28*(1), 1–22.

Katz, E., Blumler, J., & Gurevitch, M. (1974). Uses of mass communication by the individual. In J. G. Blumler & E. Katz (Eds.), *The uses of mass communication* (pp. 19–32). Newbury Park, CA: Sage.

Kealey, E., & Berkman, C. S. (2010). The relationship between health information sources and mental models of cancer: Findings of the 2005 Health Information National Trends Survey. *Journal of Health Communication, 15*, 236–251.

Kim, H. (2011). Pharmaceutical companies as a source of health information: A pilot study of the effects of source, web site interactivity, and involvement. *Health Marketing Quarterly, 28*, 57–85.

Kim, K., & Kwon, N. (2010). Profile of e-patients: Analysis of their cancer information-seeking from a national survey. *Journal of Health Communication, 15*, 712–733.

Koch-Weser, S., Bradshaw, Y, S., Gualtieri, L., & Gallagher, S. S. (2010). The internet as a health information source: Findings from the 2007 Health Information National Trends Survey and implications for health communication. *Journal of Health Communication, 15*, 279–293.

Kowalski, K. M. (1997, October). On guard against health rip-off. *Current Health, 24*, 6–11.

Kulhánek, A., Gabrhelík, R., Novák, D., Burda, V., & Brendryen, H., (2018). eHealth intervention for smoking cessation for Czech tobacco smokers: Pilot study of user acceptance. *Adiktologie, 18*(2), 81–85.

Lafata, J., Miller, C., Shires, D., Dyer, K., Ratliff, S., & Schreiber, M. (2018). Patients' adoption of and feature access within electronic patient portals. *American Journal of Managed Care, 24*(11), e352–e357. Retrieved from https://www.ncbi.nlm.nih.gov/pubmed/30452203

Larkin, M. (2014, October 27). Dr. Eric Topol: Digital healthcare will put the patient in charge. *ElsevierConnect*. Retrieved from http://www.elsevier.com/connect/Dr-Eric-Topol-Digital-healthcare-will-put-the-patient-in-charge

Lee, H., & Cho, J. (2019). Social media use and well-being in people with physical disabilities: Influence of SNS and online community uses on social support, depression, and psychological disposition. *Health Communication, 34*(9), 1043–1052.

Lee, J. Y., & Sundar, S. S. (2013). To tweet or to retweet? That is the question for health professionals on Twitter. *Health Communication, 28*, 509–524.

Lee, S. Y., & Hawkins, R. (2010). Why do patients seek an alternative channel? The effects of unmet needs on patients' health-related internet use. *Journal of Health Communication, 15*, 152–166.

Lee, S., & Lin, J. (2019). The influence of offline and online intrinsic motivations on online health information seeking. *Health Communication*. Advance online publication. doi:10.1080/10410236.2019.1620088

Lee, Y. J., Park, J., & Widdows, R. (2009). Exploring antecedents of consumer satisfaction and repeated search behavior on e-health information. *Journal of Health Communication, 14*, 160–173.

Li, N., Orrange, S., Kravitz, R. L., & Bell, R. A. (2014). Reasons for and predictors of patients' online health information seeking following a medical appointment. *Family Practice, 31*, 550–556.

Lui, X., Sawada, Y., Takizawa, T., Sato, H., Sato, M., Sakamoto, H., . . . Sakamaki, T. (2007). Doctor-patient communication: A comparison between telemedicine consultation and face-to-face consultation. *Internal Medicine, 46*, 227–232.

Magsamen-Conrad, K., Dillon, J. M., Bilotte Verhoff, C., & Faulkner, S. L. (2019a). Online health-information seeking among older populations: Family influences and the role of the medical professional. *Health Communication 34*(8), 859–871.

Magsamen-Conrad, K., Wang, F., Tetteh, D., & Lee, Y. (2019b). Using technology adoption theory and a lifespan approach to develop a theoretical framework for ehealth literacy: Extending UTAUT. *Health Communication*. Advance online publication. doi:10.1080/10410236.2019.1641395

Modahl, M., Tompsett, L., & Moorhead, T. (2011, September). Doctors, patients and social media. Study conducted by the Care Continuum Alliance. Retrieved from http://www.quantiamd.com/q-qcp/doctorspatientssocialmedia.pdf

Modave, F., Shokar, N. K., Peñaranda, E., & Nguyen, N. (2014). Analysis of the accuracy of weight loss information search engine results on the internet. *American Journal of Public Health, 104*(10), 1971–1978.

Moldovan-Johnson, M., Tan, A. S. L., & Hornik, R. C. (2014). Navigating the cancer information environment: The reciprocal relationship between patient-clinician information engagement and information seeking from nonmedical sources. *Health Communication, 29,* 974–983.

Moore, G., Wilding, H., Gray, K., & Castle, D. (2019). Participatory methods to engage health service users in the development of electronic health resources: Systematic review. *Journal of Participatory Medicine, 11*(1), e11474.

Morozov, S. & Vladzymyrsky, A. (2019). The use of telemedicine in radiodiagnosis in the 1920–1980s. *History of Medicine, 6*(2), 81–87.

Murray, E., Burns, J., May, C., Finch, T., O'Donnell, C., Wallace, P., & Mair, F. (2011). Why is it difficult to implement e-health initiatives? A qualitative study. *Implementation Science, 6*(6), nonpaginated. Retrieved from http://www.implementationscience.com/content/6/1/6

National Institute on Aging. (2018). *How is Alzheimer's disease treated?* Retrieved from https://www.nia.nih.gov/health/how-alzheimers-disease-treated

Niederdeppe, J., Davis, K. C., Farrelly, M. C., & Yarsevich, J. (2007). Stylistic features, need for sensation, and confirmed recall of national smoking prevention advertisements. *Journal of Communication, 57,* 272–292.

Oeldorf-Hirsch, A., High, A., & Christensen, J. (2019). Count your calories and share them: Health benefits of sharing mHealth information on social networking sites. *Health Communication, 34*(10), 1130–1140.

Office of the National Coordinator for Health Information Technology. (2018). *Quick stats.* Retrieved from https://dashboard.healthit.gov/quickstats/quickstats.php.

Overton, B. C. (2020). *Unintended consequences of electronic medical records systems: An emergency room ethnography.* Lanham, MD: Lexington Books.

Palmer, S. (2017). Swipe right for health care: How the state may decide the future of the mHealth app industry in the wake of FDA uncertainty. *Journal of Legal Medicine, 37,* 249–263.

Palokangas, M. (2017). *CeHRes Roadmap utilization in development of eHealth Technology solutions: A Scoping review.* (Unpublished master's thesis). University of Oulu, Oulu, Finland.

Pennic, J. (2015, March 4). Mayo Clinic, Gentag partner to develop wearable biosensors for obesity and diabetes. *Health Information Technology.* Retrieved from http://hitconsultant.net/2015/03/04/mayo-clinic-gentag-partner-to-develop-wireless-sensors/

Perrin, A. (2019). *Digital gap between rural and nonrural America persists. Pew Research Center's Digital Divide Series.* Retrieved from https://www.pewresearch.org/fact-tank/2019/05/31/digital-gap-between-rural-and-nonrural-america-persists/

Perrin, A., & Kumar, M. (2019). *About three-in-ten U.S. adults say they are "almost constantly" online. Pew Research Center.* Retrieved from https://www.pewresearch.org/fact-tank/2019/07/25/americans-going-online-almost-constantly/

Pew Research Center. (2019). *Internet/broadband fact sheet.* Retrieved from https://www.pewresearch.org/internet/fact-sheet/internet-broadband/

Pratt, M. (2018, July 3). The future of patient portals. *Medical Economics, 95*(13). Retrieved from https://www.medicaleconomics.com/business/future-patient-portals

Qiang, J. K., & Marras, C. (2015). Short communication: Telemedicine in Parkinson's disease: A patient perspective at a tertiary care centre. *Parkinsonism and Related Disorders, 21,* 525–528.

Quant, C., Altieri, L., Torres, J., & Craft, N. (2016). The self-perception and usage of medical apps amongst medical students in the United States: A cross-sectional survey. *International Journal of Telemedicine and Applications,* 2016, 1–5. doi: 10.1155/2016/3929741

Reese, S. (2008, April 18). Pick up the mouse, put down the phone: Trading e-mails with patients is easier than playing phone tag, and you may even get paid for it. *Medical Economics, 85*(8), 24–28.

Research 2 Guidance. (2016). *mHealth app developer economics 2016: The current status and trends of the mHealth app market.* Retrieved from https://research2guidance.com/product/mhealth-app-developer-economics-2016/

Research 2 Guidance. (2018). *mHealth developer economics: How mHealth app publishers are monetizing their apps.* Retrieved from https://research2guidance.com/product/mhealth-economics-how-mhealth-app-publishers-are-monetizing-their-apps/

Rideout, V., Fox, S., & Well Being Trust (2018). *Digital health practices, social media use, and mental well-being among teens and young adults in the U.S.* (Research Report No. 1093). Retrieved from https://digitalcommons.psjhealth.org/publications/1093

Roberts, J. A., Luc Honore Petnji, Y., & Manolis, C. (2014). The invisible addiction: Cell-phone activities and addiction among male and female college students. *Journal of Behavioral Addictions, 3*(4), 254–265.

Robinson, J. D., Turner, J. W., & Levine, Y. (2011). Expanding the walls of the health care encounter: Support and outcomes for patients online. *Health Communication, 26,* 125–134.

Roter, D. L., Larson, S., Sands, D. Z., Ford, D. E., & Houston, T. (2008). Can e-mail messages between patients and physicians be patient-centered? *Health Communication, 23,* 80–86.

Sachdeva, N., Tuikka, A., Kimppa, K. K., & Suomi, R. (2015). Digital disability divide in information society. *Journal of Information, Communication & Ethics in Society, 13*(3/4), 283.

Saeed, N., Manzoor, M., & Khosravi, P. (2019). An exploration of usability issues in telecare monitoring systems and possible solutions: A systematic literature review. *Disability and Rehabilitation: Assistive Technology.* Advance online publication. doi: 10.1080/17483107.2019.1578998

Seo, M., Kim, J., & Yang, H. (2016). Frequent interaction and fast feedback predict perceived social support: Using crawled and self-reported data of Facebook users. *Journal of Computer-Mediated Communication, 21,* 282–297.

Seymour, B., Getman, R., Saraf, A., Zhang, L. H., & Kalenderian, E. (2015). When advocacy obscures accuracy online: Digital pandemics of public health misinformation through an antifluoride case study. *American Journal of Public Health, 105*(3), 517–523.

Shortsleeve, C. (2018). This Apple watch feature helped save a man's life. *Men's Journal*. Retrieved from https://www.mensjournal.com/health-fitness/how-this-apple-watch-feature-saved-a-mans-life/

Silver, L., Huang, C., & Taylor, K. (2019). *In emerging economies, smartphone and social media users have broader social networks*. Pew Research Center. Retrieved from https://www.pewresearch.org/internet/2019/08/22/in-emerging-economies-smartphone-and-social-media-users-have-broader-social-networks/

Smith, D. (2011). Health care consumer's use of trust and health information sources. *Journal of Communication in Healthcare*, *4*, 200–209.

Smith, R. (2018, April 30). Hillsborough teen: Apple watch saved my life. *ABC News*. Retrieved from https://www.abcactionnews.com/news/region-hillsborough/hillsborough-teen-apple-watch-saved-my-life

Smith-McLallen, A., Fishbein, M., & Hornik, R. C. (2011). Psychosocial determinants of cancer-related information seeking among cancer patients. *Journal of Health Communication*, *16*, 212–225.

Snowden, W. (2016, March 17). Apple watch saved Alberta man's life, makes international headlines. *CBC News*. Retrieved from https://www.cbc.ca/news/canada/edmonton/apple-watch-saved-alberta-man-s-life-makesinternational-headlines-1.3495397

Stanford University. (2019, March 16). Apple heart study demonstrates ability of wearable technology to detect atrial fibrillation. Retrieved from https://med.stanford.edu/news/all-news/2019/03/apple-heart-study-demonstrates-ability-of-wearable-technology.html

Stevens, W., van der Sande, R., Beijer, L., Gerritsen, M., & Assendelft, W. (2019). eHealth apps replacing or complementing health care contacts: Scoping review on adverse effects. *Journal of Medical Internet Research*, *21*(3), e10736.

Taylor, K., & Silver, L. (2019). *Smartphone ownership is growing rapidly around the world, but not always equally*. Pew Research Center. Retrieved from https://www.pewresearch.org/global/2019/02/05/smartphone-ownership-is-growing-rapidly-around-the-world-but-not-always-equally/

Thubron, R. (2019, February 5). Apple watch's fall detection feature saves man's life. *Techspot*. Retrieved from https://www.techspot.com/news/78581-apple-watch-fall-detection-feature-probably-saved-man.html

Topol, E. (2015). *The patient will see you now: The future of medicine is in your hands*. New York: Basic Books.

Tustin, N. (2010). The role of patient satisfaction in online health information seeking. *Journal of Health Communication*, *15*, 3–17.

United States Census Bureau. (2017). New American community survey statistics for income, poverty and health insurance available for states and local areas. Washington, D.C. Author. Retrieved from https://www.census.gov/newsroom/press-releases/2017/acs-single-year.html?CID=CBSM+ACS16

Uscher-Pines, L., & Mehrotra, A. (2014). Analysis of Teladoc use seems to indicate expanded access to care for patients without prior connection to a provider. *Health Affairs*, *33*(2), 258–264.

U.S. Food & Drug Administration (FDA). (2008). *Beware of online cancer fraud*. Washington, DC: Author. Retrieved from http://www.fda.gov/ForConsumers/ConsumerUpdates/ucm048383.htm

van Gemert-Pijnen, J., Nijland, N., van Limburg, M., Ossebaard, H., Kelders, S., Eysenbach, G., & Seydel, E. (2011). A holistic framework to improve the uptake and impact of eHealth technologies. *Journal of Medical Internet Research*, *13*(4), e111.

Venkatesh, V., Morris, M. G., Davis, G. B., & Davis, F. D. (2003). User acceptance of information technology: Toward a unified view. *MIS Quarterly*, *27*, 425–478.

Venkatesh, V., Thong, J. Y., & Xu, X. (2012). Consumer acceptance and use of information technology: Extending the unified theory of acceptance and use of technology. *MIS Quarterly*, *36*, 157–178.

Wallace, S., Clark, M., & White, J. (2012). "It's on my iPhone": attitudes to the use of mobile computing devices in medical education, a mixed-methods study. *British Medical Journal Open* 2012(2), e00109.

Walsh, S. (2018, July 31). *Smart watch saves man's life*. 9 News. Retrieved from https://www.9news.com.au/national/apple-watch-smart-watch-savesmans-life/d6a279e2-dfc4-4cf9-bf32-21a59b308ef5

Walters, E. (2015, February 12). Virtual doctors making medical board really nervous. *WeeksMD*. Retrieved from http://weeksmd.com/2015/02/virtual-medicine-vs-standard-care/

Wartella, E., Rideout, V., Montague, H., Beaudoin-Ryan, L. & Lauricella, A. (2016). Teens, health and technology: A national survey. *Media and Communication 4*(3), 13–23.

Weaver, J. (2013, July 16). More people search for health information online. *NBC News*. Retrieved from http://www.nbcnews.com/id/3077086/t/more-people-search-health-online/#.Xc7vrS2ZNZg

Welch, B., Harvey, J., O'Connell, N., & McElligott, J. (2017). Patient preferences for direct-to-consumer telemedicine services: A nationwide survey. *BMC Health Services Research*, *17*, 1–7.

Wernhart, A., Gahbauer, S., & Haluza, D. (2019). eHealth and telemedicine: Practices and beliefs among healthcare professionals and medical students at a medical university. *PLoS ONE 14*(2): e0213067.

Whitten, P., Sypher, B. D., & Patterson, J. D., III. (2000). Transcending the technology of telemedicine: An analysis of telemedicine in North Carolina. *Health Communication*, *12*, 109–135.

World Health Organization. (2010a). Telemedicine: Opportunities and developments in member states. *Global Observatory for eHealth series. Volume 2*. Geneva, Switzerland: Author. Retrieved from http://www.who.int/goe/publications/ehealth_series_vol3/en/index.html

World Health Organization. (2010b). *The world health report. Executive summary*. Geneva, Switzerland: Author. Retrieved from http://www.who.int/whr/2010/10_summary_en.pdf

World Health Organization. (2011). *Compendium of new and emerging health technologies*. Geneva, Switzerland: Author. Retrieved from http://www.who.int/goe/call2012/en/index.html

Yazdi, D. (2019, January 8). The Apple Watch 4 is an iffy atrial fibrillation detector in those under age 55. *STAT*. Retrieved from https://www.statnews.com/2019/01/08/apple-watch-iffy-atrial-fibrillation-detector/

Ye, J., Rust, G., Fry-Johnson, Y., & Strothers, H. (2010). E-mail in patient-provider communication: A systematic review. *Patient Education and Counseling, 80*, 266–273.

Youn, S. (2018, December 11). An Apple watch told a 46-year-old man he had an irregular heartbeat. It was right. *ABC News*. Retrieved from https://abcnews.go.com/Health/apple-watch-told-46-year-man-irregular-heartbeat/story?id=59726093

CHAPTER 10

All about my job: Working in healthcare PR. (2016, September 28). Veronika's Blushing [blog]. Retrieved from https://www.veronikasblushing.com/2016/09/all-about-my-job-working-in-healthcare.html

Amelung, D., Whitaker, K. L., Lennard, D., Ogden, M., Sheringham, J., Zhou, Y., . . . & Black, G. (2019). Influence of doctor-patient conversations on behaviours of patients presenting to primary care with new or persistent symptoms: A video observation study. *British Medical Journal Quality & Safety*. Advance online publication.

American Association of Colleges of Nursing. (2015). 2014–2015 enrollment and graduations in baccalaureate and graduate programs in nursing. Washington, DC: Author. Retrieved from http://www.aacn.nche.edu/research-data/standard-data-reports

American Hospital Association (AHA). (2008, March). Hospital facts to know. Washington, DC: Author. Retrieved from http://www.aha.org/aha/content/2008/pdf/08-issue-facts-to-know-.pdf

Americans' experience with medical errors and views on patient safety. (2017, September). Institute for Healthcare Improvement and National Opinion Research Center. Retrieved from http://www.ihi.org/about/news/Documents/IHI_NPSF_Patient_Safety_Survey_Fact_Sheets_2017.pdf

Becoming a hospital human resource manager. (2011). HealthcareAdministration.com. Retrieved from http://www.healthcareadministration.com/what-is-the-function-of-hospital-human-resource-management/

Berkowitz, E. N. (2007). The evolution of public relations and the use of the internet: The implications for health care organizations. *Health Marketing Quarterly, 24*(3–4), 117–130.

Berry, L. L., & Seltman, K. D. (2008). *Management lessons from Mayo Clinic: Inside one of the world's most admired service organizations*. New York: McGraw-Hill.

Bliss, W. G. (2012, January 24). Cost of employee turnover. *Small Business Advisor*. Retrieved from http://www.hermangroup.com/store/bliss_article.html

Brohi, N. A., Jantan, A. H., Qureshi, M. A., Jaffar, A. R. Bin, Ali, J. Bin, & Hamid, K. B. A. (2018). The impact of servant leadership on employees attitudinal and behavioural outcomes. *Cogent Business & Management, 1*(1), 1–15.

Budden, J. S., Zhong, E. H., Moulton, P., & Cimiotti, J. P. (2013, July). Highlights of the National Workforce Survey of Registered Nurses. *Journal of Nursing Regulation, 4*(2), 5–14.

Carter, J., Ward, C., Wexler, D., & Donelan, K. (2018). The association between patient experience factors and likelihood of 30-day readmission: A prospective cohort study. *British Medical Journal Quality & Safety, 27*(9), 683–690.

Chang, L.-C., Shih, C.-H., & Lin, S.-M. (2010). The mediating role of psychological empowerment and organizational commitment for school health nurses: A cross-sectional questionnaire survey. *International Journal on Nursing Studies, 47*, 427–433.

Cohen, C. (2009, February 17). Surgeons send "tweets" from operating room. *CNN.com/technology*. Retrieved from http://www.cnn.com/2009/TECH/02/17/twitter.surgery/index.html

Collins, J. C. (2001a). Good to great (article). *Fast Company*. Retrieved from http://www.jimcollins.com/article_topics/articles/good-to-great.html

Collins, J. C. (2001b). *Good to great: Why some companies make the leap . . . and others don't*. New York: HarperCollins.

Cornwall, L. (2018, December 12). RNnetwork 2018 portrait of a modern nurse survey. *RN Network*. Retrieved from https://rnnetwork.com/blog/rnnetwork-2018-portrait-of-a-modern-nurse-survey/

Crisis emergency risk communication manual. (2014). U.S. Department of Health and Human Services. Retrieved from https://emergency.cdc.gov/cerc/ppt/CERC_Crisis_Communication_Plans.pdf

Crosby, L. A. (2011, Spring). Healthy relationships: Think relationship management when it comes to solving the health care crisis. *Marketing Management, 20*(1), 12–13.

Currie, D. (2009). *Special report: Crisis communication and social media. Expert roundtable on social media and risk communication during times of crisis: Strategic challenges and opportunities*. Sponsored by American Public Health Association, the George Washington University School of Public Health and Health Services, International Association of Emergency Managers, and National Association of Government Communicators. Retrieved from https://web.archive.org/web/20160214094038/http://www.boozallen.com/content/dam/boozallen/media/file/Risk_Communications_Times_of_Crisis.pdf

Dall, T., & West, T. (2015). The complexities of physician supply and demand: Projections from 2013 to 2025. Association of American Medical Colleges. Retrieved from https://web.archive.org/web/20150925143749/https://www.aamc.org/download/426242/data/ihsreportdownload.pdf?cm_mmc=AAMC-_-ScientificAffairs-_-PDF-_-ihsreport

de Charms, R. (1968). *Personal causation: The internal effective determinants of behavior*. New York: Academic Press.

de Charms, R. (1977). Students need not be pawns. *Theory Into Practice, 16*(4), 296–301.

Dill, M. J., & Salsberg, E. S. (2008, November). The complexities of physician supply and demand projections through 2025. Center for Workforce Studies, American

Association of Medical Colleges. Retrieved from http://www.innovationlabs.com/pa_future/1/background_docs/AAMC%20Complexities%20of%20physician%20demand,%202008.pdf

D'Innocenzo, L., Luciano, M. M., Mathieu, J. E., Maynard, M. T., & Chen, G. (2016). Empowered to perform: A multilevel investigation of the influence of empowerment on performance in hospital units. *Academy of Management Journal, 59*(4), 1290–1307.

Donahue, M. O., Piazza, I. M., Griffin, M. Q., Dykes, P. C., & Fitzpatrick, J. J. (2008). The relationship between nurses' perceptions of empowerment and patient satisfaction. *Applied Nursing Research, 21*, 2–7.

du Pré, A. (2005). Making empowerment work: Medical center soars in satisfaction ratings. In E. B. Ray (Ed.), *Health communication in practice: A case study approach* (pp. 311–322). Mahwah, NJ: Lawrence Erlbaum.

Dwyer, F. R., Schurr, P. H., & Oh, S. (1987). Developing buyer-seller relationships. *Journal of Marketing, 51*(2), 11–27.

Engaging with tomorrow's patients: The new health care customer. (n.d.). Deloitte. Retrieved from https://www2.deloitte.com/content/dam/Deloitte/us/Documents/life-sciences-health-care/us-lshc-the-new-health-care-customer.pdf

Fearn-Banks, K. (1996). *Crisis communication: A casebook approach*. Mahwah, NJ: Lawrence Erlbaum.

Fernandez, S., & Moldogaziev, T. (2013). Employee empowerment, employee attitudes, and performance: Testing a causal model. *Public Administration Review, 73*(3), 490–506.

5 statistics that show you how to attract quality new patients. (2018, January 26). BlueIQ. Retrieved from http://getblueiq.com/how-to-attract-new-patients/

Green, K. C. (1988, January). Who wants to be a nurse? *American Demographics, 10*, 46–49.

Grunig, J. E. (Ed.). (1992). *Excellence in public relations and communication management*. Hillsdale, NJ: Lawrence Erlbaum.

Grunig, L. A., Grunig, J. E., & Dozier, D. M. (2002). *Excellent public relations and effective organizations: A study of communication management in three countries*. Mahwah, NJ: Lawrence Erlbaum.

Guy, B., Williams, D. R., Aldridge, A., & Roggenkamp, S. D. (2007). Approaches to organizing public relations functions in healthcare. *Health Marketing Quarterly, 24*(3–4), 1–18. doi: 10.1080/07359680802118969.

Herzberg, F. (1968, January/February). One more time: How do you motivate employees again? *Harvard Business Review, 46*, 53–62.

Herzberg, F., Mausner, B., & Snyderman, B. B. (1959). *The motivation to work*. New York: Wiley.

Hoy, W. (2003). Shared decision making: The Hoy-Tarter Simplified Model. PowerPoint available at http://www.waynekhoy.com/shared_dm_model.html

Hoy, W. K., & Tarter, C. J. (2008). *Administrators solving the problems of practice: Decision-making cases, concepts, and consequence* (3rd ed.). Boston: Allyn & Bacon.

Jackson, K. T. (2004). *Building reputational capital: Strategies for integrity and fair play that improve the bottom line*. Oxford: Oxford University Press.

Jobes, M., & Steinbinder, A. (1996). Transitions in nursing leadership roles. *Nursing Administration Quarterly, 20*, 80–84.

Kaldjian, L. C. (2017). Concepts of health, ethics, and communication in shared decision making. *Communication & Medicine, 14*(1), 83–95.

Lee, F. (2004). *If Disney ran your hospital: 9½ things you would do differently*. Bozeman, MT: Second River Healthcare Press.

Mayer, T. A., & Cates, R. J. (2004). *Leadership for great customer service: Satisfied patients, satisfied employees*. Chicago: Health Administration Press.

McGregor, D. (1960). *The human side of organization*. New York: McGraw-Hill.

Mills, A. W. (1939). *Hospital public relations*. Chicago: Physicians Record Company.

Morgan, R. M., & Hunt, S. D. (1994). The commitment-trust theory of relationship marketing. *Journal of Marketing, 58*(3), 20–38.

National nursing workforce study. (2018). National Council of State Boards of Nursing. Retrieved from https://www.ncsbn.org/workforce.htm

Okunrintemi, V., Spatz, E. S., Di Capua, P., Salami, J. A., Valero-Elizondo, J., Warraich, H., . . . Nasir, K. (2017). Patient-provider communication and health outcomes among individuals with atherosclerotic cardiovascular disease in the United States: Medical Expenditure Panel Survey 2010 to 2013. *Circulation: Cardiovascular Quality and Outcomes, 10*(4), e003635. doi: 10.1161/CIRCOUTCOMES.117.003635

Pascale, R. T. (1999). Leading from a different place: Applying complexity theory to tap potential. In J. A. Conger, G. M. Spreitzer, & E. E. Lawler, III (Eds.), *The leader's change handbook: An essential guide to setting direction and taking action* (pp. 195–220). San Francisco: Jossey-Bass.

Patterson, J. (2012, March 4). Social media linking Las Vegas doctors, patients. *Las Vegas Review-Journal*. Retrieved from http://www.lvrj.com/health/social-media-linking-las-vegas-doctors-patients-141389473.html

Pepicello, J. A., & Murphy, E. C. (1996). Integrating medical and operational management. *Physician Executive, 22*, 4–9.

The Physicians Foundation. (2018). 2018 survey of America's physicians: Practice patterns & perspectives. Retrieved from https://physiciansfoundation.org/wp-content/uploads/2018/09/physicians-survey-results-final-2018.pdf

Press, I. (2002). *Patient satisfaction: Defining, measuring, and improving the experience of care*. Chicago: Health Administration Press.

Schuyler, S. (n.d.). How I got my job and where I'm going. Khan Academy. Retrieved from https://www.khanacademy.org/college-careers-more/career-content/manage-people-and-processes/manage-population-health-director/v/sarah-population-health-director-how-i-got-my-job-and-where-im-going

Seltzer, T., Gardner, E., Bichard, S., & Callison, C. (2012). PR in the ER: Managing internal organization-public relationships in a hospital emergency department. *Public Relations Review, 38*, 128–136.

Stamp, B. (2019, February 26). How better communication can improve patient outcomes and lower readmission rates. *Health Business and Technology*. Retrieved from http://www.healthcarebusinesstech.com/how-better-communication-can-improve-patient-outcomes-and-lower-readmission-rates/

Studer, Q. (2003). *Hardwiring excellence: Purpose, worthwhile work, making a difference*. Gulf Breeze, FL: Fire Starter.

Sutton, B. (2007, May 22). "15 Things I Believe" Work Matters [blog]. Retrieved from https://bobsutton.typepad.com/my_weblog/2007/05/brazen_careeris.html

Sutton, R. L. (2007). *The no asshole rule: Building a civilized workplace and surviving one that isn't*. New York: Warner Business.

U.S. Bureau of Labor Statistics. (2012a, February 1). *Employment projections 2010–2020*. Washington, DC: Author. Retrieved from http://bls.gov/news.release/ecopro.nr0.htm

U.S. Bureau of Labor Statistics. (2012b). *Occupational outlook handbook*. Washington, DC: Author. Retrieved from http://www.bls.gov/ooh/Healthcare/Registered-nurses.htm

U.S. Bureau of Labor Statistics. (2019a, September 4). *Medical and health services managers. Occupational outlook handbook*. Washington, D.C.: Author. Retrieved from https://www.bls.gov/ooh/management/medical-and-health-services-managers.htm

U.S. Bureau of Labor Statistics. (2019b, September 4). *Registered nurses*. Washington, D.C.: Author. Retrieved from https://www.bls.gov/ooh/healthcare/registered-nurses.htm

U.S. Census Bureau News. (2008, August 14). An older and more diverse nation by midcentury. Washington, DC: Author. Retrieved from https://web.archive.org/web/20080814174733/http://www.census.gov/Press-Release/www/releases/archives/population/012496.html

Vaughan, C. (2012, March 8). 4 social media strategies to build patient loyalty. *HealthLeaders Media*. Retrieved from http://www.healthleadersmedia.com/page-1/MAR-277456/4-Social-Media-Strategies-to-Build-Patient-Loyalty

What's right in health care: 365 stories of purpose, worthwhile work, and making a difference. (2007). Compiled by Studer Group. Gulf Breeze, FL: Fire Starter.

Wise, K. (2007). The organization and implementation of relationship management. *Health Marketing Quarterly*, 24(3–4), 151–166.

Zusman, E. E. (2012, August). HCAHPS replaces Press Ganey survey as quality measure for patient hospital experience. *Neurosurgery*, 71(2), N21–N24. Retrieved from https://academic.oup.com/neurosurgery/article/71/2/N21/2595747

CHAPTER 11

Alliance for Eating Disorders Awareness. (2019). *What are eating disorders?* Retrieved from https://www.allianceforeatingdisorders.com/eating-disorders/

Alter, C. (2014, February 6). In defense of Barbie: Why she might be the most feminist doll around. *Time*. Retrieved from http://time.com/4597/in-defense-of-barbie-why-she-might-be-a-feminist-doll-after-all/

Angell, M. (2004). *The truth about drug companies*. New York: Random House.

Aslam, S. (2019, September 6). Instagram by the numbers: Stats, demographics & fun facts. *Omnicore*. Retrieved from https://www.omnicoreagency.com/instagram-statistics/

Association of Health Care Journalists. (2015). Main web page. Retrieved from http://healthjournalism.org/

Austin, E. W. (1993). Exploring the effects of active parental mediation of television content. *Journal of Broadcasting & Electronic Media*, 37, 147–158.

Austin, E. W. (1995). Reaching young audiences: Developmental considerations in designing health messages. In E. Maibach & R. L. Parrott (Eds.), *Designing health messages* (pp. 114–144). Thousand Oaks, CA: Sage.

Austin, E. W., & Meili, H. K. (1994). Effects of interpretations of televised alcohol portrayals on children's alcohol beliefs. *Journal of Broadcasting & Electronic Media*, 38, 417–435.

Austin, E. W., Roberts, D. F., & Nass, C. I. (1990). Influences of family communication on children's television-interpretation process. *Communication Research*, 17, 545–564.

Bae, H.-S., & Kang, S. (2008). The influence of viewing an entertainment-education program on cornea donation intention: A test of the theory of planned behavior. *Health Communication*, 23(1), 87–95.

Baek, T., & Mayer, M. (2010). Sexual imagery in cigarette advertising before and after the Master Settlement Agreement. *Health Communication*, 25, 747–757. doi:10.1080/10410236.2010.521917

Baglia, J. (2005). *The Viagra ad venture*. New York: Peter Lang.

Baker, K. (2016, June 3). Here's the powerful letter the Stanford victim read to her attacker. *BuzzFeed News*. Retrieved from https://www.buzzfeednews.com/article/katiejmbaker/heres-the-powerful-letter-the-stanford-victim-read-to-her-ra

Baker, M. (2007). Is there a critic in the house? Poking holes in TV medical dramas—and loving it. *Sandford Medicine Magazine*. Retrieved from http://sm.stanford.edu/archive/stanmed/2007fall/med-tv.html

Ball, J., Liang, A., & Wei-Na, L. (2009). Representation of African Americans in direct-to-consumer pharmaceutical commercials: A content analysis with implications for health disparities. *Health Marketing Quarterly*, 26, 372–390. doi:10.1080/07359680903304328

Bandura, A. (1977). *Social learning theory*. Oxford, England: Prentice-Hall.

Banerjee, S. C., & Greene, K. (2006). Analysis versus production: Adolescent cognitive and attitudinal responses to antismoking interventions. *Journal of Communication*, 56, 773–794.

Barbie. [Barbie]. (2014, February 1). Be YOU. Be bold. Be #Unapologetic [Tweet]. Retrieved from https://twitter.com/barbie/status/429673457127657472

Barclay, E. (2016, January 29). Scientists are building a case for how food ads make us overeat. *National Public Radio*. Retrieved from https://www

.npr.org/sections/thesalt/2016/01/29/462838153/food-ads-make-us-eat-more-and-should-be-regulated

Barlett, C., Kowalewski, D., Kramer, S., & Helmstetter, K. (2019). Testing the relationship between media violence exposure and cyberbullying perpetration. *Psychology of Popular Media Culture*, *8*(3), 280–286.

Basow, S. A., & O'Neil, K. (2014). Men's body depilation: An exploratory study of United States college students' preferences, attitudes, and practices. *Body Image*, *11*, 409–417.

Beautiful people, beautiful products. (2011, July 2). Psysociety. Retrieved from https://psysociety.wordpress.com/2011/07/02/beautiful-people-beautiful-products/

Bechara, A., Casabé, A., De Bonis, W., Hellen, A., & Bertolino, M. V. (2010). Recreational use of phosphodiesterase type 5 inhibitors by healthy young men. *The Journal of Sexual Medicine*, *7*, 3736–3742.

Beer commercials among favorite Super Bowl ads for teens. (2009, February 5). Alexandria, VA: Drug-Free Action Alliance. Retrieved from http://50-201-129-166-static.hfc.comcastbusiness.net/resources/detail/beer-commercials-among-favorite-super-bowl-ads-teens

Bender, P., Plante, C., & Gentile, D. (2019). The effects of violent media content on aggression. *Current Opinion in Psychology*, *19*, 104–108.

Betts, K. (2002, March 31). The tyranny of skinny, fashion's insider secret. *New York Times*. Retrieved from http://www.nytimes.com/2002/03/31/style/the-tyranny-of-skinny-fashion-s-insider-secret.html?pagewanted=all

Bilmes, A. (2014, October 8). When did male body hair become a bad thing? *The Guardian*. Retrieved from http://www.theguardian.com/fashion/shortcuts/2014/oct/08/when-did-male-body-hair-become-such-a-bad-thing

Boden, W. E., & Diamond, G. A. (2008, May 22). DTCA for PTCA—Crossing the line in consumer health education? *The New England Journal of Medicine*, *358*(21), 2197.

Bond, B. (2015). Portrayals of sex and sexuality in gay- and lesbian-oriented media: A quantitative content analysis. *Sexuality & Culture*, *19*(1), 37–56.

Boris, C. (2014, October 20). TV viewers would rather skim social media than watch TV commercials. *Marketing Pilgrim*. Retrieved from https://web.archive.org/web/20150730225930/http://www.marketingpilgrim.com/2014/10/tv-viewers-would-rather-skim-social-media-than-watch-tv-commercials.html

Bose, N. (2019, September 20). UPDATE 3—Walmart to stop sales of e-cigarettes in U.S. stores—company memo. *CNBC News*. Retrieved from https://www.cnbc.com/2019/09/20/reuters-america-update-3-walmart-to-stop-sales-of-e-cigarettes-in-u-s-stores-company-memo.html?&qsearchterm=UPDATE%203-Walmart%20to%20stop%20sales%20of%20e-cigarettes%20in%20U.S.%20stores%20-company%20memo

Bosman, J., & Richtel, M. (2019, September 15). Vaping bad: Were 2 Wisconsin brothers the Walter Whites of THC oils? *The New York Times*. Retrieved from https://www.nytimes.com/2019/09/15/health/vaping-thc-wisconsin.html

Boswell, R., & Kober, H. (2016). Food cue reactivity and craving predict eating and weight gain: A meta-analytic review. *Obesity Reviews*, *17*(2), 159–177. doi: 10.1111/obr.12354

Boyce Rogers, K., Hust, S., Willoughby, J., Wheeler, J., & Li, J. (2019). Adolescents' sex-related alcohol expectancies and alcohol advertisements in magazines: The role of wishful identification, realism, and beliefs about women's enjoyment of sexualization. *Journal of Health Communication*, *24*(4), 395–404.

Boyland, E., Nolan, S., Kelly, B., Tudur-Smith, C., Jones, A., Halford, J., & Robinson, E. (2016). Advertising as a cue to consume: A systematic review and meta-analysis of the effects of acute exposure to unhealthy food and nonalcoholic beverage advertising on intake in children and adults. *American Journal of Clinical Nutrition*, *103*(2), 519–533.

Braithwaite, S. R., Coulson, G., Keddington, K., & Fincham, F. D. (2015). The influence of pornography on sexual scripts and hooking up among emerging adults in college. *Archives of Sexual Behavior*, *44*(1), 111–123.

Bulik, B. S. (2014, September 2). Mattel pushes Barbie as model of empowerment for young girls. *Advertising Age*. Retrieved from http://adage.com/article/news/mattel-pushes-barbie-model-empowerment-young-girls/294755/

Cacioli, J., & Mussap, A. J. (2014). Avatar body dimensions and men's body image. *Body Image*, *11*(2), 146–155.

Carlisle, M. (2019, September 17). Seventh person to die from vaping-related illness in U.S. dies in California. *Time*. Retrieved from https://time.com/5679005/vaping-death/

Centers for Disease Control and Prevention (CDC). (2015, June 2). *Measles cases and outbreaks*. Atlanta, GA: Author. Retrieved from http://www.cdc.gov/measles/cases-outbreaks.html

Centers for Disease Control and Prevention (CDC). (2019). *Smoking and tobacco use*. Retrieved from https://www.cdc.gov/tobacco/

Chen, Y.-C. (2013). The effectiveness of different approaches to media literacy in modifying adolescents' responses to alcohol. *Journal of Health Communication*, *18*, 723–739.

Cho, S. (2006). Network news coverage of breast cancer. *Journalism and Mass Communication*, *83*(1), 116–130.

Cho, Y. Thrasher, J., Reid, J., Hitchman, S. & Hammond, D. (2019). Youth self-reported exposure to and perceptions of vaping advertisements: Findings from the 2017 International Tobacco Control Youth Tobacco and Vaping Survey. *Science Direct*. Advance online publication. doi: 10.1016/j.ypmed.2019.105775

Clarke, C. E., Dixon, G. N., Holton, A., & McKeever, B. W. (2015). Including "evidentiary balance" in news media coverage of vaccine risk. *Health Communication*, *30*, 461–472.

Cline, R. J. W., & Young, H. N. (2004). Marketing drugs, marketing health care relationships: A content analysis of visual cues in direct-to-consumer prescription drug advertising. *Health Communication*, *16*, 131–157.

Cohen, J. (1997). The media's love affair with AIDS research: Hope vs. hype. *Science*, *275*, 289–299.

CollegeHumor. (2014, March 11). *Photoshop has gone too far [Video]*. YouTube. Retrieved from https://www.youtube.com/watch?v=Hnvoz91k8hc

Conley, M. (2012, April 23). The real-life Ukrainian Barbie doll. Retrieved from http://abcnews.go.com/blogs/health/2012/04/23/the-real-life-ukrainian-barbie-doll/

Conlin, L., & Bissell, K. (2014). Beauty ideals in the checkout aisle: Health-related messages in women's fashion and fitness magazines. *Journal of Magazine & New Media Research, 15*(2), 1–19.

Cornwell, T. B., McAlister, A. R., & Polmear-Swendris, N. (2014). Research report: Children's knowledge of packaged and fast food brands and their BMI. Why the relationship matters for policy makers. *Appetite, 81,* 277–283.

Corriea, A. R. (2015, May 12). *Assassin's Creed Syndicate story, characters, and setting breakdown. Two heads are better than one*. E3. Retrieved from http://www.gamespot.com/articles/assassin-s-creed-syndicate-story-characters-and-se/1100-6427217/

Data Resource Center for Child and Adolescent Health. (2017). *2017 national survey of children's health (NSCH) data query*. Retrieved from https://www.childhealthdata.org/browse/survey?s=2&y=28&r=1

Davis, J. (2007). The effect of qualifying language on perceptions of drug appeal, drug experience, and estimates of side-effect incidence in DTC advertising. *Journal of Health Communication, 12,* 617–622.

Davison, W. P. (1983). The third-person effect in communication. *Public Opinion Quarterly, 47,* 1–13.

Deary, I. J., Whiteman, M. C., & Fowkes, F. G. R. (1998). Medical research and the popular media. *The Lancet, 351,* 1726–1727.

de Droog, S. M., Valkenburg, P. M., & Buijzen, M. (2011). Using brand characters to promote young children's liking of and purchase requests for fruit. *Journal of Health Communication, 16,* 79–89. doi:10.1080/10810730.2010.529487

DeFrank, J., Berkman, N., Kahwati, L., Cullen, K., Aikin, K. & Sullivan, H. (2019). Direct-to-consumer advertising of prescription drugs and the patient–prescriber encounter: A systematic review. *Health Communication*. Advance online publication. doi: 10.1080/10410236.2019.1584781

DeMatteo, D., Galloway, M., Arnold, S., & Patel, U. (2015). Sexual assault on college campuses: A 50-state survey of criminal sexual assault statutes and their relevance to campus sexual assault. *Psychology, Public Policy, and Law, 21*(3), 227.

Desrochers, D. M., & Holt, D. J. (2007). Children's exposure to television advertising: Implications for childhood obesity. *Journal of Public Policy & Marketing, 26*(2), 182–201.

Diem, S., Lantos, J., & Tulsky, J. (1996). Cardiopulmonary resuscitation on television: Miracles and misinformation. *The New England Journal of Medicine, 334*(24), 1578–1582.

DiFranza, J. R., Richard, J. W., Paulman, P. M., Wolf-Gillespie, N., Fletcher, C., Jaffe, R. D., & Murray, D. (1991). RJR Nabisco's cartoon camel promotes Camel cigarettes to children. *Journal of the American Medical Association, 266,* 3149–3153.

Dreisbach, S. (2014). How do you feel about your body? *Glamour*. Retrieved from http://www.glamour.com/health-fitness/2014/10/body-image-how-do-you-feel-about-your-body

Duewald, M. (2003, June 22). Body and image; one size definitely does not fit all. *The New York Times*. Retrieved from https://www.nytimes.com/2003/06/22/health/body-and-image-one-size-definitely-does-not-fit-all.html

Dutta, M. J. (2006). Theoretical approaches to entertainment education campaigns: A subaltern critique. *Health Communication, 20,* 221–231.

Entertainomercials. (1996, November 4). *Forbes, 158,* 322–323.

Erdelyi, M. H., & Zizak, D. M. (2004). Beyond gizmo subliminality. In L. J. Shrum (Ed.), *The psychology of entertainment media: Blurring the lines between entertainment and persuasion* (pp. 13–44). Mahwah, NJ: Lawrence Erlbaum.

Espinoza, P., Penelo, E., & Raich, R. M. (2013). Prevention programme for eating disturbances in adolescents. Is their effect on body image maintained at 30 months later? *Body Image, 10,* 175–181.

Fallon, E. A., Harris, B. S., & Johnson, P. (2014). Prevalence of body dissatisfaction among a United States adult sample. *Eating Behaviors, 15*(1), 151–158.

Fardouly, J., & Holland, E. (2018). Social media is not real life: The effect of attaching disclaimer-type labels to idealized social media images on women's body image and mood. *News Media & Society, 20*(11), 4311–4328.

Farrar, K. M., Krcmar, M., & Nowak, K. L. (2006). Contextual features of violent video games, mental models, and aggression. *Journal of Communication, 56,* 387–405.

Fawcett, K. (2015, April 16). How mental illness is represented in the media. *US News & World Report*. Retrieved from http://health.usnews.com/health-news/health-wellness/articles/2015/04/16/how-mental-illness-is-misrepresented-in-the-media

Fertig, N., & Owermohl, S. (2019, September 14). Trump responds to one vaping crisis by attacking another. *Politico*. Retrieved from https://www.politico.com/story/2019/09/14/donald-trump-vaping-crisis-marijuana-1733703

Festinger, L. (1957). *A theory of cognitive dissonance*. Stanford, CA: Stanford University Press.

Fischer, P. M., Schwartz, M. P., Richard, J. W., & Goldstein, A. O. (1991). Brand logo recognition by children aged 3 to 6 years: Mickey Mouse and Old Joe the Camel. *Journal of the American Medical Association, 266,* 3154–3158.

Forman-Brunell, M. (n.d.). What Barbie dolls have to say about postwar American culture. *Smithsonian Center for Education and Museum Studies*. Retrieved from http://www.smithsonianeducation.org/idealabs/ap/essays/barbie.htm

Fox, M., & Connor, T. (2015, February 7). Think the U.S. has a measles problem? Just look at Europe. *NBC News*. Retrieved from http://www.nbcnews.com/storyline/measles-outbreak/think-u-s-has-measles-problem-just-look-europe-n301726

Frank, L., & Nagel, S. (2017). Addiction and moralization: The role of the underlying model of addiction. *Neuroethics, 10*(1), 129–139.

Freytag, J., & Ramasubramanian, S. (2019). Are television deaths good deaths? A narrative analysis of hospital death and dying in popular medical dramas. *Health Communication, 34*(7), 747–754.

Gallagher, J. (2019, May 28). Fertility paradox in male beauty quest. *BBC News*. Retrieved from https://www.bbc.com/news/health-48396071

Gerbner, G. (1996, Fall). TV violence and what to do about it. *Nieman Reports, 50*, 10–12.

Gerbner, G., Gross, L., Morgan, M., & Signorielli, N. (1980). The "mainstreaming" of America: Violence profile no. 11. *Journal of Communication, 30*(3), 10–29.

Gerbner, G., Gross, L., Morgan, M., & Signorelli, N. (1994). *Living with television: The dynamics of the cultivation process*. In J. Bryant & D. Zillmann (Eds.), *Perspectives on media effects* (pp. 17–40). Hillsdale, NJ: Lawrence Erlbaum.

Gjorgievska, A., & Rothman, L. (2014, July 10.). Laverne Cox is the first transgender person nominated for an Emmy—she explains why that matters. *Time*. Retrieved from https://time.com/2973497/laverne-cox-emmy/

Green, C. E., Mojtabai, R., Cullen, B. A., Spivak, A., Mitchell, M., & Spivak, S. (2017). Exposure to direct-to-consumer pharmaceutical advertising and medication nonadherence among patients with serious mental illness. *Psychiatric Services, 68*(12), 1299–1302.

Gubler, J., Herrick, S., Price, R., & Wood, D. (2018). Violence, aggression, and ethics: the link between exposure to human violence and unethical behavior. *Journal of Business Ethics, 147*(1), 25–34.

Gunther, A. C., Bolt, D., Borzekowski, D. L. G., Liebhart, J. L., & Dillard, J. P. (2006). Presumed influence on peer norms: How mass media indirectly affect adolescent smoking. *Journal of Communication, 56*, 52–68.

Hales, C., Carroll, M., Fryar, C., & Ogden, C. (2017). Prevalence of obesity among adults and youth: United States, 2015–2016. (Research Report No. 288). Retrieved from the U.S. Department of Health and Human Services website, https://stacks.cdc.gov/view/cdc/49223

Harkness, E. L., Mullan, B. M., & Blaszczynski, A. (2015). Association between pornography use and sexual risk behaviors in adult consumers: A systematic review. *Cyberpsychology, Behavior and Social Networking, 18*(2), 59–71.

Harrison, K. (2005). Is "fat free" good for me? A panel study of television viewing and children's nutritional knowledge and reasoning. *Health Communication, 17*, 117–132.

Heldman, C. (2014, Feburary 9). The sexy lie. TEDxYouth. Retrieved from http://everydayfeminism.com/2014/02/the-sexy-lie/

Hennessy, M., Romer, D., Valois, R. F., Vanable, P., Carey, M. P., Stanton, B., . . . Salazar, L. F. (2013). Safer sex media messages and adolescent sexual behavior: 3-year follow-up results from project iMPPACS. *American Journal of Public Health, 103*(1), 134–140.

Henry J. Kaiser Family Foundation. (2010, January 20). *Generation M2: Media in the lives of 8- to 18-year-olds.* Author: Menlo Park, CA. Retrieved from http://kff.org/other/event/generation-m2-media-in-the-lives-of/

Hetsroni, A. (2009). If you must be hospitalized, television is not the place: Diagnoses, survival rates and demographic characteristics of patients in TV hospital dramas. *Communication Research Reports, 26*, 311–322.

Hilgard, J., Englehardt, C., Rouder, J., Segert, I., & Bartholow, B. (2019). Null effects of game violence, game difficulty, and 2D:4D digit ratio on aggressive behavior. *Psychological Science, 30*(4), 606–616.

Hill, D. (2016). *Why to avoid TV for infants & toddlers*. Retrieved from the Health Children website, https://www.healthychildren.org/English/family-life/Media/Pages/Why-to-Avoid-TV-Before-Age-2.aspx

Hills, R. (2015a, August 4). I failed at being a "sex object"—and became something so much hotter. The Blog. Retrieved from http://www.huffingtonpost.com/rachel-hills/failed-at-being-a-sex-object-and-became-something-hotter_b_7933376.html

Hills, R. (2015b). *The sex myth: The gap between our fantasies and reality*. New York: Simon & Schuster.

Hines, D. A., Armstrong, J. L., Reed, K. P., & Cameron, A. Y. (2012). Gender differences in sexual assault victimization among college students. *Violence and Victims, 27*(6), 922–940.

Hinkelbein, J., Spelten, O., Marks, J., Hellmich, M., Böttiger, B. W., & Wetsch, W. A. (2014). Simulation and education: An assessment of resuscitation quality in the television drama emergency room: Guideline non-compliance and low-quality cardiopulmonary resuscitation lead to a favorable outcome? *Resuscitation, 85*, 1106–1110.

Hust, S., Boyce Rogers, K., Cameron, N., & Li, J. (2019). Viewers' perceptions of objectified images of women in alcohol advertisements and their intentions to intervene in alcohol-facilitated sexual assault situations. *Journal of Health Communication, 24*(3), 328–338.

Hust, S. J. T., Brown, J. D., & L'Engle, K. L. (2008). Boys will be boys and girls better be prepared: An analysis of the rare sexual health messages in young adolescents' media. *Mass Communication and Society, 11*(1), 3–23.

Iati, M. (2019, September 5). Her name is Chanel Miller, not "unconscious intoxicated woman" in Stanford assault case. *The Washington Post*. Retrieved from https://www.washingtonpost.com/nation/2019/09/05/her-name-is-chanel-miller-not-unconsciousintoxicated-woman-stanford-assault-case/

James, S. D. (2011, June 9). Honeymoon with Viagra could be over. *ABC News*. Retrieved from http://abcnews.go.com/Health/viagra-prescription-sales-sexual-expectations/story?id=13794726#.T_by6BzHSCA

Jamieson, P. E., & Romer, D. (2014). Violence in popular U.S. prime time TV dramas and the cultivation of fear: A time series analysis. *Media and Communication, 2*, 31–41.

Jang, S. A., Rimal, R. N., & Cho, N. (2013). Normative influences and alcohol consumption: The role of drinking refusal self-efficacy. *Health Communication, 28*, 443–451.

Jensen, J. D., Moriarty, C. M., Hurley, R. J., & Stryker, J. (2010). Making sense of cancer news coverage trends:

A comparison of three comprehensive content analyses. *Journal of Health Communication, 15*, 136–151. doi:10.1080/10810730903528025

Jerit, J., Zhao, Y., Tan, M. & Wheeler, M. (2018). Differences between national and local media in news coverage of the Zika virus. *Health Communication, 34*(14), 1816–1823.

Jung, J., Forbes, G. B., & Chan, P. (2010). Global body and muscle satisfaction among college men in the United States and Hong Kong-China. *Sex Roles, 63*, 104–117.

Kang, H., & Lee, M. (2017). Designing anti-binge drinking prevention messages: Message framing vs. evidence type. *Health Communication, 22*(12), 1494–1502.

Kean, L. G., & Prividera, L. C. (2007). Communicating about race and health: A content analysis of print advertisements in African American and general readership magazines. *Health Communication, 21*, 289–297.

Kilbourne, J. (2000). *Killing us softly 3: Advertising's image of women*. North Hampton, MA: Media Education Foundation.

Kim, M., Popova, L., Halpern-Felsher, B., & Ling, P. (2019). Effects of e-cigarette advertisements on adolescents' perceptions of cigarettes. *Health Communication, 34*(3), 290–297.

Kim, S., & Baek, Y. (2019). Medical drama viewing and healthy lifestyle behaviors: Understanding the role of health locus of control beliefs and education level. *Health Communication, 34*(4), 392–401.

Kinsler, J., Glik, D., Buffington, S., Malan, H., Nadjat-Haiem, C., Wainwright, N., & Papp-Green, M. (2019) A content analysis of how sexual behavior and reproductive health are being portrayed on primetime television shows being watched by teens and young adults. *Health Communication, 34*(6), 644–651.

Kirsch, A. C., & Murnen, S. K. (2015). "Hot" girls and "cool dudes": Examining the prevalence of the heterosexual script in American children's television media. *Psychology of Popular Media Culture, 4*(1), 18–30.

Kleemans, M., Daalmans, S., Carbaat, I., & Anschütz, D. (2018). Picture perfect: The direct effect of manipulated Instagram photos on body image in adolescent girls. *Media Psychology, 21*(1), 93–110.

Krantz-Kent, R. (2018). Television, capturing America's attention at prime time and beyond. Retrieved from https://www.bls.gov/opub/btn/volume-7/pdf/television-capturing-americas-attention.pdf

Kyrrestad Strøm, H., Adolfsen, F., Fossum, S., Kaiser, S., & Martinussen, M. (2014). Effectiveness of school-based preventive interventions on adolescent alcohol use: A meta-analysis of randomized controlled trials. *Substance Abuse Treatment, Prevention & Policy, 9*(1), no pagination specified.

Landsverk, G. (2019, September 17). People are protesting the Weight Watchers "healthy eating" app for kids, citing toxic diet culture and experiences with disordered eating. *Business Insider*. Retrieved from https://www.businessinsider.com/weight-watchers-kurbo-app-for-kids-diet-culture-2019-9

Larasi, I. (2013, September 2). Why do music videos portray black women as exotic sex objects? *The Guardian*. Retrieved from http://www.theguardian.com/lifeandstyle/the-womens-blog-with-jane-martinson/2013/sep/02/music-video-black-women-sex-objects

LaVail, K. H. (2010). Coverage of older adults and HIV/AIDS: Risk information for an invisible population. *Communication Quarterly, 58*, 170–187.

Lee, S.-J. (2013). Parental restrictive mediation of children's Internet use: Effective for what and for whom? *New Media & Society, 15*(4), 466.

Levin, D. E., & Kilbourne, K. (2008). *So sexy so soon: The new sexualized childhood and what parents can do to protect their kids*. New York: Ballantine Books.

Lim, R. Tham, D., Cheung, O., Adaikan, P., & Wong, M. (2019) A public health communication intervention using edutainment and communication technology to promote safer sex among heterosexual men patronizing entertainment establishments. *Journal of Health Communication, 24*(1), 47–64.

Lowe, G., & Costabile, R. A. (2012). 10-year analysis of adverse event reports to the Food and Drug Administration for phosphodiesterase type-5 inhibitors. *Journal of Sexual Medicine, 9*, 265–270. doi: 10.1111/j.1743-6109.2011.02537

Ludtke, M., & Trost, C. (1998). Covering children's health. *American Journalism Review, 20*, 81–88.

Lyon, A. (2007, November). "Putting patients first": Systematically distorted communication and Merck's marketing of Vioxx. *Journal of Applied Communication Research, 35*(4), 376–398.

Macias, W., Pashupati, K., & Lewis, L. S. (2007). A wonderful life or diarrhea and dry mouth? Policy issues of direct-to-consumer drug advertising on television. *Health Communication, 22*, 241–252.

Madanikia, Y., & Bartholomew, K. (2014). Themes of lust and love in popular music lyrics from 1971 to 2011. *Sage Open*. Retrieved from sgo.sagepub.com/content/spsgo/4/3/2158244014547179.full.pdf

Maier, J. A., Gentile, D. A., Vogel, D. L., & Kaplan, S. A. (2014). Media influences on self-stigma of seeking psychological services: The importance of media portrayals and person perception. *Psychology of Popular Media Culture, 3*(4), 239–256.

Mastin, T., Andsager, J. L., Choi, J., & Lee, K. (2007). Health disparities and direct-to-consumer prescription drug advertising: A content analysis of targeted magazine genres, 1992–2002. *Health Communication, 22*, 49–58.

Mazur, A., Caroli, M., Radziewicz-Winnicki, I., Nowicka, P., Weghuber, D., Neubauer, D., . . . & Hadjipanayis, A. (2018). Reviewing and addressing the link between mass media and the increase in obesity among European children: The European Academy of Paediatrics (EAP) and The European Childhood Obesity Group (ECOG) consensus statement. *Acta Pædiatrica, 107*(4), 568–576.

Meerkerk, G., & van Straaten, B. (2019). Alcohol marketing and underage drinking: Which subgroups are most susceptible to alcohol advertisements? *Substance Use & Misuse, 54*(5), 737–746.

Melki, J. P., Hitti, E. A., Oghia, M. J., & Mufarrij, A. A. (2015). Media exposure, mediated social comparison to idealized images of muscularity, and anabolic steroid use. *Health Communication, 30*(5), 473–484.

Moonhee, Y., & Roskos-Ewoldsen, D. R. (2007). The effectiveness of brand placements in the movies: Levels of placements, explicit and implicit memory, and brand-choice behavior. *Journal of Communication, 57*, 469–489.

Morgan, S. E., Harrison, T. R., Chewning, L., Davis, L., & DiCorcia, M. (2007). Entertainment (mis)education: The framing of organ donation in entertainment television. *Health Communication, 22*, 143–151.

Moss, M. (2011). *The media and the models of masculinity*. Lanham, MD: Lexington Books.

Nathanson, A. I., & Yang, M.-S. (2003, January). The effects of mediation content and form on children's responses to violent television. *Human Communication Research, 29*, 111–134.

National Center for Health Statistics. (2012). *Health, United States, 2011: with special features on socioeconomic status and health*. Hyattsville, MD: U.S. Department of Health and Human Services. Retrieved from http://www.cdc.gov/nchs/data/hus/hus11.pdf

National Eating Disorders Association. (2015). *Statistics on eating disorders*. New York: Author. Retrieved from http://www.nationaleatingdisorders.org/general-statistics

National Institute on Alcohol Abuse and Alcoholism. (2018). *Alcohol facts and statistics*. Retrieved from https://www.niaaa.nih.gov/publications/brochures-and-fact-sheets/alcohol-facts-and-statistics

National Institute on Drug Abuse (NIDA). (2007, December). *InfoFacts: High school and youth trends*. Bethesda, MD: Author. Retrieved from http://www.drugabuse.gov/infofacts/hsyouthtrends.html

National Institute on Drug Abuse. (2018). *Monitoring the future study: Trends in prevalence of various drugs*. Retrieved from https://www.drugabuse.gov/trends-statistics/monitoring-future/monitoring-future-study-trends-in-prevalence-various-drugs

Nestle, M. (1997, March–April). Alcohol guidelines for chronic disease prevention: From prohibition to moderation. *Nutrition Today, 32*, 86–92.

Nicksic, N., Brosnan, P., Chowdhury, N., Barnes, A., & Cobb, C. (2019). "Think it. Mix it. Vape it.": A content analysis on e-cigarette radio advertisements. *Substance Use & Misuse, 54*(8), 1355-1364.

Niederdeppe, J., Fowler, E. F., Goldstein, K., & Pribble, J. (2010). Does local television news coverage cultivate fatalistic beliefs about cancer prevention? *Journal of Communication, 60*, 230–253.

Nielsen Company. (2019). *The Nielsen total audience report*. Retrieved from https://web.archive.org/web/20190823182100/https://www.rbr.com/wp-content/uploads/Q1-2019-Nielsen-Total-Audience-Report-FINAL.pdf

Ogden, C. L., Carroll, M. D., Kit, B. K., Flegal, K. M. (2014). Prevalence of childhood and adult obesity in the United States, 2011-2012. *Journal of the American Medical Association, 311*, 806–814.

Olds, T. (2014, June 1). You're not Barbie and I'm not GI Joe, so what is a normal body? *The Conversation*. Retrieved from http://theconversation.com/youre-not-barbie-and-im-not-gi-joe-so-what-is-a-normal-body-14567

Ophir, Y. & Jamieson, K. (2018). The effects of Zika virus risk coverage on familiarity, knowledge and behavior in the U.S.—A time series analysis combining content analysis and a nationally representative survey. *Health Communication*. doi: 10.1080/10410236.2018.1536958

Padon, A., Maloney, E., & Cappella, J. (2017). Youth-targeted e-cigarette marketing in the US. *Tobacco Regulatory Science, 3*, 95–101.

Pan, W., & Peña, J. (2019). Looking down on others to feel good about the self: The exposure effects of online model pictures on men's self-esteem. *Health Communication*. Advance online publication. doi: 10.1080/10410236.2019.1584780

Parker-Pope, T. (2002, November 11). Viagra is misunderstood despite name recognition. *Wall Street Journal*, online. Retrieved December 23, 2008, from http://www.usrf.org/breakingnews/bn_111202_viagra/bn_111202_viagra.html

Peeke, P. (2011, March 29). Reality shows abut the obese: Empowering or exploitative? *Everyday Fitness (blog)*. Retrieved from https://web.archive.org/web/20110504055043/http://blogs.webmd.com/pamela-peeke-md/2011/03/reality-shows-about-the-obese-empowering-or-exploitative.html

Peters, L. (2014, March 12). "Photoshop has gone too far" video reveals what the program is really capable of. *Bustle*. Retrieved from https://www.bustle.com/articles/17916-photoshop-has-gone-too-far-video-reveals-what-the-program-is-really-capable-of

Pinkleton, B. E., Austin, E. W., Cohen, M., Miller, A., & Fitzgerald, E. (2007). A statewide evaluation of the effectiveness of media literacy training to prevent tobacco use among adolescents. *Health Communication, 21*, 23–34.

Piotrow, P. T., Rimon, J. G., II, Payne Merritt, A., & Saffitz, G. (2003). *Advancing health communication: The PCS experience in the field*. Center Publication 103. Baltimore: Johns Hopkins Bloomberg School of Public Health/Center for Communication Programs. Retrieved from http://pdf.usaid.gov/pdf_docs/Pnact765.pdf

Potter, W. J. (1998). Media literacy. Thousand Oaks, CA: Sage.

Quenqua, D. (2014, August 1). Tell me what you see, even if it hurts me. *The New York Times*. Retrieved from http://www.nytimes.com/2014/08/03/fashion/am-i-pretty-videos-posed-to-the-internet-raise-questions.html

Quesada, A., & Summers, S. L. (1998, January). Literacy in the cyberage: Teaching kids to be media savvy. *Technology & Learning, 18*, 30–36.

Quintero Johnson, J. M., Harrison, K., & Quick, B. L. (2013). Understanding the effectiveness of the entertainment-education strategy: An investigation of how audience involvement, message processing, and message design influence health information recall. *Journal of Health Communication, 18*, 160–178.

Ra, C., Cho, J., Stone, M., De La Cerda, J., Goldenson, N., Moroney, E., . . . Leventhal, A. (2018). Association of digital media use with subsequent symptoms of attention-deficit/hyperactivity disorder among adolescents. *Journal of the American Medical Association*, *320*(3), 255–263.

Radesky, J. (2017). *Kids and digital media*. Retrieved from the C.S. Mott Children's Hospital website: https://www.mottchildren.org/posts/your-child/kids-and-digital-media

Reinhardt, J. D., Pennycott, A., & Fellinghauer, B. G. (2014). Impact of a film portrayal of a police officer with spinal cord injury on attitudes towards disability: A media effects experiment. *Disability & Rehabilitation*, *36*(4), 289–294.

Renwick, R., Schormans, A. F., & Shore, D. (2014). Hollywood takes on intellectual/developmental disability: Cinematic representations of occupational participation. *Occupation, Participation and Health*, *34*(1), 20–31.

Rey-Lopez, J. P., Ruiz, J. R., Vicente-Rodriguez. G., Gracia-Marco, L., Manios, Y., Sjostrom, M., De Bourdeaudhuij, I., & Moreno, L. A. (2012). Physical activity does not attenuate the obesity risk of TV viewing in youth. *Pediatric Obesity*, *7*, 240–250.

Rhoades, E., & Jernigan, D. H. (2013). Risky messages in alcohol advertising, 2003–2007: Results from content analysis. *Journal of Adolescent Health*, *52*(1), 116–121.

Rodgers, R., O'Flynn, J., & McLean, S. (2019). Media and eating disorders. In R. Hobbs & P. Mihailidis (Eds.), *The International Encyclopedia of Media Literacy*. Retrieved from https://onlinelibrary.wiley.com/doi/pdf/10.1002/9781118978238.iem10060

Rodgers, S., & Hust, S. (2018). Sexual objectification in music videos and acceptance of potentially offensive sexual behaviors. *Psychology of Popular Media Culture*, *7*(4), 413–428.

Russell, C. A., & Buhrau, D. (2015). Research report: The role of television viewing and direct experience in predicting adolescents' beliefs about the health risks of fast-food consumption. *Appetite*, *92*, 200–206.

Santa Cruz, J. (2014, March 10). Body-image pressure increasingly affects boys. *The Atlantic*. Retrieved from http://www.theatlantic.com/health/archive/2014/03/body-image-pressure-increasingly-affects-boys/283897/

Schwartz, L., & Woloshin, S. (2019). Medical marketing in the United States, 1997–2016. *Journal of the American Medical Association*, *32*(1), 80–96.

Semaan, R., Kocher, B., & Gould, S. (2018). How well will this brand work? The ironic impact of advertising disclosure of body-image retouching on brand attitudes. *Psychology & Marketing*, *35*(10), 766–777.

Silberner, J. (1997, August 8). Rx Ads. *National Public Radio*. Retrieved from https://www.npr.org/templates/story/story.php?storyId=1038711

Singer, D. G., & Singer, J. L. (1998). Developing critical viewing skills and media literacy in children. *Annals of the American Academy of Political and Social Science*, *557*, 164–179.

Sismondo, S. (2008). How pharmaceutical industry funding affects trial outcomes: Causal structures and responses. *Social Science & Medicine*, *66*(9), 1909–1914.

Skinner, A., Ravanbakht, S., Skelton, J., Perrin, E., & Armstrong, S. (2018). Prevalence of obesity and severe obesity in US children, 1999–2016. *Pediatrics*, *141*(3), e20173459.

Smedema, S. M., Ebener, D., & Grist-Gordon, V. (2012). The impact of humorous media on attitudes toward persons with disabilities. *Disability & Rehabilitation*, *34*(17), 1431–1437.

Smith, R. A., Downs, E., & Witte, K. (2007, June). Drama theory and entertainment education: Exploring the effects of a radio drama on behavioral intentions to limit HIV transmission in Ethiopia. *Communication Monographs*, *74*(2), 133–153.

Sterling, W. (2019, September 14). New Weight Watchers diet app puts kids at risk for eating disorders and body shaming. *NBC News*. Retrieved from https://www.nbcnews.com/think/opinion/new-weight-watchers-diet-app-puts-kids-risk-eating-disorders-ncna1053391

Sumner, P., Vivian-Griffiths, S., Boivin, J., Williams, A., Venetis, C. A., Davies, A., . . . Chambers, C. D. (2014). The association between exaggeration in health related science news and academic press releases: Retrospective observational study. *BMJ (Clinical Research Ed.)*, *349*, g7015.

Swanson, A. (2015, February 11). Big pharmaceutical companies are spending far more on marketing than research. *Washington Post*. Retrieved from http://www.washingtonpost.com/blogs/wonkblog/wp/2015/02/11/big-pharmaceutical-companies-are-spending-far-more-on-marketing-than-research/

Tanner, A. H., Friedman, D. B., & Zheng, Y. (2015). Influences on the construction of health news: The reporting practices of local television news health journalists. *Journal of Broadcasting & Electronic Media*, *59*(2), 359–376.

Taubes, G. (1998). Telling time by the second hand. *Technology Review*, *101*, 76–78.

Thomas, K. (2012, March 6). AARP study says price of popular drugs rose 26%. *The New York Times* reprints online, n.p. Retrieved from http://www.nytimes.com/2012/03/07/business/aarp-study-says-price-of-popular-drugs-rose-26.html

Thomas, S. (2019). The alarming increase in vaping among youth. *Issues in Mental Health Nursing*, *40*(4), 287–288.

Tian, Y., & Yoo, J. (2018). Medical drama viewing and medical trust: A moderated mediation approach. *Health Communication*, *35*(1), 46–55.

Tiggemann, M., Brown, Z., & Anderberg, I. (2019). Effect of digital alteration information and disclaimer labels attached to fashion magazine advertisements on women's body dissatisfaction. *Body Image*, *30*, 221–227.

Turner, J. T. (2011). Sex and the spectacle of music videos: An examination of the portrayal of race and sexuality in music videos. *Sex Roles*, *64*(3/4), 173–191.

Uwujaren, J. (2012, December 9). Mental illness: How the media contributes to its stigma. *Everyday Feminism*. Retrieved from http://everydayfeminism.com/2012/12/mental-illness-stigma/

Van Ouytsel, J., Ponnet, K., & Walrave, M. (2014). The associations between adolescents' consumption of pornography and music videos and their sexting behavior. *Cyberpsychology, Behavior and Social Networking*, *17*(12), 772–778.

Vardigan, B. (2015, March 11). Fear of illness is the illness itself, and health information on the Internet is fueling the phobia. *Health Day*. Retrieved from http://

consumer.healthday.com/encyclopedia/diseases-and-conditions-15/misc-diseases-and-conditions-news-203/hypochondria-647704.html

Vest, J. (1997, July 21). Joe Camel walks his last mile. *U.S. News & World Report, 123*, 56.

Viagra (2019)

Wakefield, J. (2018, March 27). Children spend six hours or more a day on screens. *BBC News*. Retrieved from https://www.bbc.com/news/technology-32067158

Wang, Z., & Gantz, W. (2010). Health content in local television news: A current appraisal. *Health Communication, 25*, 230–237. doi:10.1080/10410231003698903

Watson, A. (2018, December 17). Media use–statistics & facts. *Statista*. Retrieved from https://www.statista.com/topics/1536/media-use/

Webb, T., Jenkins, L., Browne, N., Abdelmonen, A. A., & Kraus, J. (2007). Violent entertainment pitched to adolescents: An analysis of PG-13 films. *Pediatrics, 119*(6), e1219–e1229.

Williams, D. E. (2015). Take a deep breath: Marijuana product placement is on the way. *Health Business Blog*. Retrieved from http://healthbusinessblog.com/2014/09/17/take-a-deep-breath-marijuana-product-placement-is-on-the-way/

Wood, J. (1999). *Gendered lives* (33rd ed.). Belmont, CA: Wadsworth.

World Health Organization. (2019). *New measles surveillance data*. Retrieved from https://www.who.int/immunization/newsroom/new-measles-data-august-2019/en/

Yang, F., Salmon, C. T., Pang, J. S., & Cheng, W. J. (2015). Media exposure and smoking intention in adolescents: A moderated mediation analysis from a cultivation perspective. *Journal of Health Psychology, 20*(2), 188–197.

Youth exposure to alcohol advertising on television, 2001–2009. (2010, December 15). Baltimore, MD: Johns Hopkins University and the Center on Alcohol Marketing and Youth. Retrieved from https://web.archive.org/web/20110905023856/http://www.camy.org/bin/u/r/CAMYReport2001_2009.pdf

Zhang, L., & Haller, B. (2013). Consuming image: How mass media impact the identity of people with disabilities. *Communication Quarterly, 61*(3), 319–334.

Zimmerman, F. J. (2008, June). *Children's media use and sleep problems: Issues and unanswered questions*. Prepaid for the Henry J. Kaiser Family Foundation. Retrieved from http://www.kff.org/entmedia/upload/7674.pdf

CHAPTER 12

About us. (2012). truth® website. Washington, DC: American Legacy Foundation. Retrieved from https://www.thetruth.com/about-truth

Ali, S. (2019, September 4). After Dorian's destruction in Bahamas, relief efforts start trickling in. *NBC News*. Retrieved from https://www.nbcnews.com/news/world/after-dorian-s-destruction-bahamas-relief-efforts-start-trickling-n1049836

Anderson, K. B., Thomas, S. J., & Endy, T. P. (2016). The emergence of Zika virus: A narrative review. *Annals of Internal Medicine, 165*, 175–183.

Appenzeller, T. (2005, October). Tracing the next killer flu. *National Geographic, 208*(4), 2–31.

Bellafante, G. (2014, October 10). Fear of vaccines goes viral. *The New York Times*. Retrieved from http://www.nytimes.com/2014/10/12/nyregion/fear-of-vaccines-goes-viral.html

Bennett, C. (2015, April 27). Don't rush to Nepal to help. Read this first. *The Guardian*. Retrieved from http://www.theguardian.com/commentisfree/2015/apr/27/earthquake-nepal-dont-rush-help-volunteers-aid

Bernstein, S. (2015, May 14). California Senate votes to end beliefs waiver for school vaccinations. *Reuters*. Retrieved from http://www.reuters.com/article/us-usa-measles-vaccinations-idUSKBN0O003320150515

Broome, B. (2018, April 28). Amid the opioid epidemic, white means victim, black means addict. *The Guardian*. Retrieved from https://www.theguardian.com/us-news/2018/apr/28/opioid-epidemic-selects-white-victim-black-addict

Broussard, C., Shapiro-Mendoza, C., Peacock, G., Rasmussen, S., Mai, C., Petersen, E., . . . Moore, C. (2018). Public health approach to addressing the needs of children affected by congenital Zika syndrome. [Supplement]. *Pediatrics, 141*(S2), s137–s145.

Cajun Navy Relief. (2019). *About the Cajun Navy relief*. Retrieved from https://www.cajunnavyrelief.com/about-us-2/

Centers for Disease Control and Prevention (CDC). (2005, May 3). Frequently asked questions about SARS. Atlanta: Author. Retrieved from http://www.cdc.gov/sars/about/faq.html

Centers for Disease Control and Prevention (CDC). (2008, July 1). Overview of crisis & emergency risk communication. Atlanta: Author. Retrieved from http://emergency.cdc.gov/cerc

Centers for Disease Control and Prevention. (2014). *CERC: Crisis communication plans*. Retrieved from https://emergency.cdc.gov/cerc/ppt/CERC_Crisis_Communication_Plans.pdf

Centers for Disease Control and Prevention (CDC). (2015a, February 17). Complications of measles. Atlanta, GA: Author. Retrieved from http://www.cdc.gov/measles/about/complications.html

Centers for Disease Control and Prevention (CDC). (2015b, March 24). Outbreaks chronology: Ebola virus disease. Atlanta, GA: Author. Retrieved from http://www.cdc.gov/vhf/ebola/outbreaks/history/chronology.html

Centers for Disease Control and Prevention. (2018). *Opioid overdose: Understanding the epidemic*. Retrieved from https://www.cdc.gov/drugoverdose/epidemic/index.html

Centers for Disease Control and Prevention. (2019). *PrEP*. Retrieved from https://www.cdc.gov/hiv/basics/prep.html

Chen, S., Xu, Q., Buchenberger, J., Bagavathi, A., Fair, G., Shaikh, S., & Krishnan, S. (2018). Dynamics of health agency response and public engagement in public health emergency: A case study of CDC tweeting patterns during the 2016 Zika epidemic. *JMIR Public Health and Surveillance, 4*(4), e10827.

Citroner, G. (2018, July 11). Cost of HIV prevention drug discouraging people from doing PrEP therapy. *Healthline*. Retrieved from https://www.healthline.com/health-news/cost-of-hiv-prevention-drug-discouraging-people-from-doing-prep-therapy#1

Clarke, L. (2002, Fall). Panic: Myth or reality? *Contexts, 1*(3), 21–26.

Covello, V. T. (2003). Best practices in public health risk and crisis communication. *Journal of Health Communication, 8*, 5–8.

Cruz, D. (2015). Kristen Bell: No vaccines? You can't hold my children. *Parenting*. Retrieved 2017 from http://www.parenting.com/news-break/kristen-bell-no-vaccines-you-cant-hold-my-children

Damhewage, G. M. (2014). Complex, confused, and challenging: Communicating risk in the modern world. *Journal of Communication in Healthcare, 7*(4), 252–254. doi:10.1179/1753806814Z.00000000094

Durkin, E. (2018, September 11). September 11: Nearly 10,000 people affected by "cesspool of cancer." *The Guardian*. Retrieved from https://www.theguardian.com/us-news/2018/sep/10/911-attack-ground-zero-manhattan-cancer

Eckert, S., Sopory, P., Day, S., Wilkins, L., Padgett, D., Novak, J., . . . Gamhewage, G. (2018). Health-related disaster communication and social media: Mixed-method systematic review. *Health Communication, 33*(12), 1389–1400.

Elam-Evans, L. D., Yankey, D., Singleton, J. A., Kolasa, M. (2014, August 29). National, state, and selected local area vaccination coverage among children aged 19–35 months—United States, 2013. *Morbidity and Mortality Weekly Report 63*(34), 741–748. Retrieved from http://www.cdc.gov/mmwr/preview/mmwrhtml/mm6334a1.htm

Epidemiology of measles—United States, 1998. (1999, September 3). *Morbidity and Mortality Weekly Reports, 48*(34), 749–753. Retrieved from http://www.cdc.gov/mmwr/preview/mmwrhtml/mm4834a1.htm

Eriksson, M. (2018). Lessons for crisis communication on social media: A systematic review of what research tells the practice. *International Journal of Strategic Communication, 12*(5), 526–551.

Food and Drug Administration. (2018). *H5N1 influenza virus vaccine, manufactured by Sanofi Pasteur, Inc. Questions and answers*. Retrieved from https://www.fda.gov/vaccines-blood-biologics/vaccines/h5n1-influenza-virus-vaccine-manufactured-sanofi-pasteur-inc-questions-and-answers

Fox, M., & Connor, T. (2015, February 7). Think the U.S. has a measles problem? Just look at Europe. *NBC News*. Retrieved from http://www.nbcnews.com/storyline/measles-outbreak/think-u-s-has-measles-problem-just-look-europe-n301726

Frank, L., & Nagel, S. (2017). Addiction and moralization: The role of the underlying model of addiction. *Neuroethics, 10*(1), 129–139.

Freimuth, V. S. (2006). Order out of chaos: The self-organization of communication following the anthrax attacks. *Health Communication, 20*, 141–148.

Friedersdorf, C. (2015, February 3). Should anti-vaxxers by shamed or persuaded? The backlash to a measles outbreak—and a case against politicizing it. *The Atlantic*. Retrieved from http://www.theatlantic.com/politics/archive/2015/02/should-anti-vaxxers-be-shamed-or-persuaded/385109/

Frizell, S. (2014, October 18). Obama on Ebola: "We can't give in to hysteria." *Time*. Retrieved from http://time.com/3520341/obama-ebola-fear/

Glik, D. C. (2007, April). Risk communication for public health emergencies. *Annual Review of Public Health, 28*, 33–54.

Guidry, J., Meganck, S., Lovari, A., Messner, M., Medina-Messner, V., Sherman, S., & Adams, J. (2019, May 26). Tweeting about #diseases and #publichealth: Communicating global health issues across nations. *Health Communication*. Advance online publication. doi:10.1080/10410236.2019.1620089

Hendrix, K. S. (2015, March 9). What doctors should tell parents who are afraid of vaccines. *The Washington Post*. Retrieved from https://www.washingtonpost.com/posteverything/wp/2015/03/09/what-doctors-should-tell-parents-who-are-afraid-of-vaccines/

Hillier, D. (2006). *Communicating health risks to the public: A global perspective*. Burlington, VT: Gower.

History of public health. (2002). *Encyclopedia of public health*. Farmington Hills, MI: Gale Cengage.

HIV.gov. (2019). *The global HIV/AIDS epidemic*. Retrieved from https://www.hiv.gov/hiv-basics/overview/data-and-trends/global-statistics

Hutchinson, A. (2019, April 24). Facebook reaches 2.38 billion users, beats revenue estimates in latest update. *Social Media Today*. Retrieved from https://www.socialmediatoday.com/news/facebook-reaches-238-billion-users-beats-revenue-estimates-in-latest-upda/553403/

In her own words. (2004). Commentary about *The most dangerous woman in America* [video documentary], Nancy Porter (Writer/Director). NOVA in association with WGBH/Boston. Retrieved from http://www.pbs.org/wgbh/nova/typhoid

Jerit, J., Zhao, Y., Tan, M. & Wheeler, M. (2018). Differences between national and local media in news coverage of the Zika virus. *Health Communication, 34*(14), 1816–1823.

Johnson, C., & Mulvihill, G. (2019, October 6). Victims gain a voice to help guide Purdue Pharma bankruptcy. *AP News*. Retrieved from https://apnews.com/03c831fe7bd94f02b0fea51d2e9f81ed

Johnson, D. (2006, November.) Risk communication in the fog of disaster. Lessons from Ground Zero. *Industrial Safety & Hygiene News, 40*(11), 58, 60, 62.

Jones, J., Banks, L., Plotkin, I., Chanthavongsa, S., & Walker, N. (2015). Profile of the public health workforce: Registered TRAIN learners in the United States. [Supplement]. *American Journal of Public Health, 105*(S2), e30–e36.

Kean, J. (2013, November 27). Why the US fails at treating addiction. *Live Science*. Retrieved from https://www.livescience.com/41557-why-america-fails-at-addiction-treatment.html

Lwin, M., Lu, J., Sheldenkar, A., & Schulz, P. (2018). Strategic uses of Facebook in Zika outbreak communication: Implications for the crisis and emergency risk communication model. *International Journal of Environmental Research and Public Health, 15*(9), 1974–1993.

Lyapustina, T., & Alexander, G. C. (2015, June 11). The prescription opioid addiction and abuse epidemic: How it happened and what we can do about it. *The Pharmaceutical Journal*. Retrieved from https://www.pharmaceutical-journal.com/news-and-analysis/opinion/comment/the-prescription-opioid-addiction-and-abuse-epidemic-how-it-happened-and-what-we-can-do-about-it/20068579.article

Mad cows and the minister. (1990, May 24). *Nature, 345*, 277–278.

Margesson, R., & Sullivan, M. (2019). Bahamas: Response to Hurricane Dorian. *Congressional Research Service*. Retrieved from https://crsreports.congress.gov/product/pdf/IN/IN11171

Maxmen, A. (2015, January 30). How the fight against Ebola tested a culture's traditions. *National Geographic*. Retrieved from http://news.nationalgeographic.com/2015/01/150130-ebola-virus-outbreak-epidemic-sierra-leone-funerals/

McCarthy, T. (2019, September 3). Hurricane Dorian: "Historic tragedy" prompts worldwide call for aid for Bahamas. *The Guardian*. Retrieved from https://www.theguardian.com/world/2019/sep/03/hurricanedorian-us-un-bahamas

McComas, K. A. (2006). Defining moments in risk communication research: 1996–2005. *Journal of Health Communication, 11*, 75–91.

McDonald, P., & Holden, W. (2018). Zika and public health: Understanding the epidemiology and information environment. [Supplement]. *Pediatrics, 141*(S2), s137–s145.

Measles outbreak traced to Disneyland is declared over. (2015, April 17). *NBC News*. Retrieved from http://www.nbcnews.com/storyline/measles-outbreak/measles-outbreak-traced-disneyland-declared-over-n343686

The most dangerous woman in America [video documentary]. (2004). Nancy Porter (Writer/Director). NOVA in association with WGBH/Boston. Retrieved from http://www.pbs.org/wgbh/nova/typhoid/about.html

Mugo, N., Ngure, K., Kiragu, M., Irungu, E., & Kilonzo, N. (2016). PrEP for Africa: What we have learnt and what is needed to move to program implementation. *Current Opinion in HIV and AIDS, 11*(1), 80–86.

National Association of City & County Health Officials. (2015). About NACCHO. Washington, DC: Author. Retrieved from http://www.naccho.org/about/

National Institute on Drug Abuse. (2019). *Opioid overdose crisis*. Retrieved from https://www.drugabuse.gov/drugs-abuse/opioids/opioid-overdose-crisis

National Research Council. (1989). *Improving risk communication*. Washington, DC: National Academy Press. Retrieved from http://www.nap.edu/openbook.php?isbn=0309039436

Nolan, D. (2016, February 26). How bad is the opioid epidemic? *Frontline*. Received from https://www.pbs.org/wgbh/frontline/article/how-bad-is-the-opioid-epidemic/

Nyhan, B., Reifler, J., Richey, S., & Freed, G. L. (2014). Effective messages in vaccine promotion: A randomized trial. *Pediatrics, 133*(4). doi:10.1542/peds.2013-2365

Ophir, Y. (2018). Coverage of epidemics in American newspapers through the lens of the crisis and emergency risk communication framework. *Health Security, 16*(3), 147–157.

Ophir, Y. (2019). The effects of news coverage of epidemics on public support for and compliance with the CDC—An experimental study. *Journal of Health Communication, 24*(5), 547–558.

Ophir, Y., & Jamieson, K. H. (2018). The effects of Zika virus risk coverage on familiarity, knowledge and behavior in the U.S.—A time series analysis combining content analysis and a nationally representative survey. *Health Communication, 35*(1), 35–45.

Parmer, J., Baur, C., Eroglu, D., Lubell, K., Prue, C., Reynolds, B., & Weaver, J. (2016). Crisis and emergency risk messaging in mass media news stories: Is the public getting the information they need to protect their health? *Health Communication, 31*(10), 1215–1222.

Patel, D. S. (2005). Social mobilization as a tool for outreach programs in the HIV/AIDS crisis. In M. Haider (Ed.), *Global public health communication: Challenges, perspectives, and strategies* (pp. 91–102). Boston: Jones and Bartlett.

Petroff, A., & Rooney, B. (2015, April 28). Nepal earthquake donations: Who's sending what. *CNN Money*. Retrieved from http://money.cnn.com/2015/04/27/news/nepal-earthquake-donations/

Philpott, A., Knerr, W., & Maher, D. (2006). Promoting protection and pleasure: Amplifying the effectiveness of barriers against sexually transmitted infections and pregnancy: Viewpoint. *The Lancet, 368*, pp. 1–4. Retrieved from http://www.thelancet.com/journals/lancet/article/PIIS0140673606698103/abstract

Plane passengers sue TB patient. (2007, July 13). CNN.com/health. Retrieved from http://www.cnn.com/2007/HEALTH/conditions/07/12/tb.suit/index.html

Ratzan, S., & Meltzer, W. (2005). State of the art in crisis communication: Past lessons and principles of practice. In M. Haider (Ed.), *Global public health communication: Challenges, perspectives, and strategies* (pp. 321–347). Boston: Jones and Bartlett.

Ratzan, S. C., & Moritsugu, K. P. (2014). Ebola crisis-communication chaos we can avoid. *Journal of Health Communication, 19*(11), 1213–1215.

Reynolds, B. (2006, August). Response to best practices. *Journal of Applied Communication Research, 34*(4), 249–252.

Rifkin, L. (2008, March 21). Still a privilege to be a doctor: Though not immune to the hassles and hardships of practice, this physician tells why he experiences the joy of medicine. *Medical Economics, 85*(6), 28–29.

Rosenstock, I. M. (1960). What research in motivation suggests for public health. *American Journal of Public Health, 50*, 295–301.

Rubyan-Ling, D. (2015). *Briefing paper: Diaspora communications and health seeking behavior in the time of Ebola: Findings from the Sierra Leonean community in London.* Retrieved from http://www.ebola-anthropology.net/wp-content/uploads/2015/11/Diaspora-communication-and-health-seeking-behaviour1.pdf

Sandman, P. M. (2006a, August). Crisis communication best practices: Some quibbles and additions. *Journal of Applied Communication Research, 34*(3), 257–262.

Sandman, P. M. (2006b). Telling 9/11 emergency responders to wear their masks. In Comments and questions (and some answers). The Peter Sandman Risk Communication Website. Retrieved from http://www.psandman.com/gst2006.htm

Schneider, M.-J. (2006). *Introduction to public health* (2nd ed.). Boston: Jones and Bartlett.

Secretary of Agriculture: Bird flu poses "no health issue" to humans. (2015, May 31). *NPR.* Retrieved from http://www.npr.org/2015/05/31/410924073/secretary-of-agriculture-bird-flu-poses-no-health-issue-to-humans

Seeger, M. W. (2006, August). Best practices in crisis communication: An expert panel process. *Journal of Applied Communication Research, 34*(3), 232–244.

Sellnow, D., Lane, D., Sellnow, T., & Littlefield, R. (2017). The IDEA model as a best practice for effective instructional risk and crisis communication. *Communication Studies, 68,* 552–567.

Sellnow, D., & Sellnow, T. (2014). Risk communication: Instructional principles. In T. Thompson (Ed.), *Encyclopedia of health communication* (pp. 1181–1184). Thousand Oaks, CA: Sage.

Sellnow-Richmond, D., George, A., & Sellnow, D. (2018). An IDEA model analysis of instructional risk communication in the time of Ebola. *Journal of International Crisis and Risk Communication Research, 1*(1), 135–166.

Skolnick, P. (2018). The opioid epidemic: Crisis and solutions. *The Annual Review of Pharmacology and Toxicology, 58,* 143–159.

Stretcher, V. J., & Rosenstock, I. M. (1997). The health belief model. In K. Glanz, F. M. Lewis, & B. K. Rimer (Eds.), *Health behavior and health education* (pp. 41–59). San Francisco: Jossey-Bass.

Sugg, C. (2016). *Coming of age: Communication's role in powering global health.* Retrieved from http://downloads.bbc.co.uk/mediaaction/policybriefing/role-of-communication-in-global-health-report.pdf

Tai, Z., & Sun, T. (2007, December). Media dependencies in a changing media environment: The case of the 2003 SARS epidemic in China. *New Media & Society, 9*(6), 987–1009.

Thompson, D. (2014, July 2). Ebola's deadly spread in African driven by public health failures, cultural beliefs. *National Geographic.* Retrieved from http://news.nationalgeographic.com/news/2014/07/140702-ebola-epidemic-fever-world-health-guinea-sierra-leone-liberia/

Toppenberg-Pejcic, D., Noyes, J., Allen, T., Alexander, N., Vanderford, M. & Gamhewage, G. (2019). Emergency risk communication: Lessons learned from a rapid review of recent gray literature on Ebola, Zika, and yellow fever. *Health Communication, 34*(4), 437–455.

Turner, A. (2019, July 10). Merck's Ebola vaccine helps combat deadly outbreak in the Congo as the virus spreads. *CNBC.* Retrieved from https://www.cnbc.com/2019/07/09/mercks-ebola-vaccine-helps-combat-deadly-outbreak-in-the-congo.html

Ulmer, R. R., Seeger, M. W., & Sellnow, T. L. (2007, June). Post-crisis communication and renewal: Expanding the parameters of post-crisis discourse. *Public Relations Review, 33*(2), 130–134.

U.S. Agency for International Development. (2019, September 6). *4 ways USAID is responding to Hurricane Dorian in the Bahamas.* Retrieved from https://medium.com/usaid-2030/4-ways-usaid-is-responding-to-hurricane-dorian-in-the-bahamas-e7c4a7e1b8ec

U.S. Department of Health and Human Services. (2017). *HHS acting secretary declares public health emergency to address national opioid crisis.* Retrieved from https://www.hhs.gov/about/news/2017/10/26/hhs-acting-secretary-declares-public-health-emergency-address-national-opioid-crisis.html

Wakefield, A. J., Murch, S. H., Anthony, A., Linnell, J., Casson, D. M., Malik, M., . . . Walker-Smith, J. A. (1998). Ileal-lymphoid-nodular hyperplasia, non-specific colitis, and pervasive developmental disorder in children. *The Lancet, 351,* 637–641. [Retracted]

Wax-Thibodeaux, E. (2017, August 28). "Cajun Navy" races from Louisiana to Texas, using boats to pay it forward. *The Washington Post.* Retrieved from https://www.washingtonpost.com/national/cajun-navy-races-from-louisiana-to-texas-using-boats-to-pay-it-forward/2017/08/28/1a010c8a-8c1f-11e7-84c0-02cc069f2c37_story.html

Willingham, E., & Helft, L. (2014, September 5). The autism-vaccine myth. NOVA. Retrieved from http://www.pbs.org/wgbh/nova/body/autism-vaccine-myth.html

Winslow, C.-E. A. (1923). *The evolution and significance of the modern public health campaign.* New Haven, CT: Yale University Press.

World Health Organization. (2003a, June 18). Epidemic and pandemic alert and response (EPR). Update 83. One hundred days into the outbreak. Geneva, Switzerland: Author. Retrieved from http://www.who.int/csr/don/2003_06_18/en/index.html

World Health Organization. (2003b, March 16). Epidemic and pandemic alert and response (EPR). Severe acute respiratory syndrome (SARS). Multi-country outbreak. Update. Geneva, Switzerland: Author. Retrieved from http://www.who.int/csr/don/2003_03_16/en/index.html

World Health Organization. (2007, October). Interim protocol: Rapid operations to contain the initial emergence of pandemic influenza. Geneva, Switzerland: Author. Retrieved from http://www.who.int/influenza/resources/documents/RapidContProtOct15.pdf

World Health Organization (WHO). (2008). World health statistics. Part 2. Global health indicators. Global health indicators. Geneva, Switzerland: Author. Retrieved from www.who.int/whosis/whostat/EN_WHS08_Table4_HSR.pdf

World Health Organization (WHO). (2015a, June 10). Ebola situation report. Geneva, Switzerland: Author. Retrieved

from http://apps.who.int/ebola/en/current-situation/ebola-situation-report-10-june-2015
World Health Organization (WHO). (2015b, April). Ebola virus disease. Geneva, Switzerland: Author. Retrieved from http://www.who.int/mediacentre/factsheets/fs103/en/
World Health Organization. (2018a). Communicating risk in public health emergencies. Retrieved from https://www.who.int/risk-communication/guidance/download/en/
World Health Organization. (2018b). Global health observatory data on HIV/AIDS. Retrieved from https://www.who.int/gho/hiv/en/
World Health Organization. (2019, September 27). Cumulative number of confirmed human cases of avian influenza A(H5N1) reported to WHO. Retrieved from https://www.who.int/influenza/human_animal_interface/H5N1_cumulative_table_archives/en/
World Health Report, 2007. (2007). *A safer future: Global public health security in the 21st century*. Geneva, Switzerland: World Health Organization. Retrieved from http://www.who.int/whr/2007/en/index.html
Zillmann, D. (1999). Exemplification theory: Judging the whole by some of its parts. *Media Psychology*, *1*, 69–94.

CHAPTER 13

Ahn, S. J. (2015). Incorporating immersive virtual environments in health promotion campaigns: A construal level theory approach. *Health Communication*, *30*(6), 545–556.

Anderson, D. M. (2010). Does information matter? The effect of the Meth Project on meth use among youths. *Journal of Health Economics*, *29*(5), 732–742.

Anghelcev, G., & Sar, S. (2011). The influence of pre-existing audience and message relevance on the effective of health PSAs: Differential effects by message type. *Journal and Mass Communication Quarterly*, *88*, 481–501.

Arasaratnam, L. A., & Banerjee, S. C. (2011). Sensation seeking and intercultural communication competence: A model test. *International Journal of Intercultural Relations*, *35*, 226–233. doi:10.1016/j.ijintrel.2010.07.003.

Austin, E. W. (1995). Reaching young audiences: Developmental considerations in designing health messages. In E. Maibach & R. L. Parrott (Eds.), *Designing health messages* (pp. 114–144). Thousand Oaks, CA: Sage.

Backer, T. E., & Rogers, E. M. (1993). Introduction. In T. E. Backer & E. M. Rogers (Eds.), *Organizational aspects of health communication campaigns: What works?* (pp. 1–9). Newbury Park, CA: Sage.

Balbale, S. N., Schwingel, A., Wojtek, C., & Huhman, M. (2014). Visual and participatory research methods for the development of health messages for underserved populations. *Health Communication*, *29*(7), 728–740.

Beaudoin, C. E., & Thorson, E. (2006). The social capital of Blacks and Whites: Differing effects of the mass media in the United States. *Human Communication Research*, *32*, 157–177.

Brehm, J. W. (1966). *A theory of psychological reactance*. New York: Academic Press.

Brennan, P. F., & Fink, S. V. (1997). Health promotion, social support, and computer networks. In R. L. Street, Jr., W. R. Gold, & T. Manning (Eds.), *Health promotion and interactive technology: Theoretical implications and future directions* (pp. 157–169). Mahwah, NJ: Lawrence Erlbaum.

Briñol, P., & Petty, R. E. (2006). Fundamental processes leading to attitude change: Implications for career prevention communications. *Journal of Communication*, *56*, S81–S104.

Brosius, H., & Weimann, G. (1996). Who sets the agenda? Agenda-setting as a two-step flow. *Communication Research*, *23*, 561–580.

Casper, M. F., Child, J. T., Gilmour, D., McIntyre, K. A., & Pearson, J. C. (2006). Healthy research perspectives: Incorporating college student experiences with alcohol. *Health Communication*, *20*, 289–298.

Centers for Disease Control and Prevention (CDC). (2011, March 21). Tobacco-related mortality. Atlanta: Author. Retrieved from http://www.cdc.gov/tobacco/data_statistics/fact_sheets/health_effects/tobacco_related_mortality/

Centers for Disease Control and Prevention (CDC). (2015). Chronic disease prevention and health promotion. Atlanta, GA: Author. Retrieved from http://www.cdc.gov/chronicdisease/

Chen, L., & Yang, X. (2019). Using EPPM to evaluate the effectiveness of fear appeal messages across different media outlets to increase the intention of breast self-examination among Chinese women. *Health Communication*, *34*(11), 1369–1376.

Cheong, P. H. (2007). Health communication resources for uninsured and insured Hispanics. *Health Communication*, *21*, 153–163.

Clark-Hitt, R., Smith, S. W., & Broderick, J. S. (2012). Help a buddy take a knee: Creating persuasive messages for military service members to encourage others to seek mental health help. *Health Communication*, *27*, 429–438. doi:10.1080/10410236.2011.606525

Designated driving statistics. (2020). DesignatedDriving.net. Retrieved http://www.designateddriving.net/designateddrivingstatistics.html

Donohew, L., Palmgreen, P., & Duncan, J. (1980). An activation model of information exposure. *Communication Monographs*, *47*, 295–303.

D'Silva, M. U., & Palmgreen, P. (2007). Individual differences and context: Mediating recall of anti-drug public service announcements. *Health Communication*, *21*, 65–71.

Dutta, M., Collins, W., Sastry, S., Dillard, S., Anaele, A., Kumar, R., . . . Bonu, T. (2019). A culture-centered community-grounded approach to disseminating health information among African Americans. *Health Communication*, *34*(10), 1075–1084.

Dutta-Bergman, M. J. (2005). Theory and practice in health communication campaigns: A critical interrogation. *Health Communication*, *18*, 103–122.

Edgar, T., Freimuth, V., & Hammond, S. L. (2003). Lessons learned from the field on prevention and health campaigns. In T. L. Thompson, A. M. Dorsey, K. I. Miller, &

R. Parrott (Eds.), *Handbook of health communication* (pp. 625–636). Mahwah, NJ: Lawrence Erlbaum.

Effertz, T., Franke, M., & Teichert, T. (2014). Adolescents' assessments of advertisements for unhealthy food: An example of warning labels for soft drinks. *Journal of Consumer Policy*, *2*, 279–299.

Erceg-Hurn, D. (2008). Drugs, money, and graphic ads: A critical review of the Montana meth project. *Prevention Science*, *9*(4), 256–263.

Everett, M. W., & Palmgreen, P. (1995). Influences of sensation seeking, message sensation value, and program context on effectiveness of anticocaine public service announcement. *Health Communication*, *7*, 225–248.

Farrelly, M. C., Healton, C. G., Davis, K. C., Messeri, P., & Haviland, M. L. (2002, June). Getting to the truth: Evaluating national tobacco countermarketing campaigns. *American Journal of Public Health*, *92*(6), 901–907.

Frey, L. R., Botan, C. H., Friedman, P. G., & Kreps, G. (1999). *Investigating communication: An introduction to research methods* (2nd ed.). New York: Pearson.

Friederichs, S. H., Oenema, A., Bolman, C., Guyaux, J., van Keulen, H. M., & Lechner, L. (2014). I Move: Systematic development of a web-based computer tailored physical activity intervention, based on motivational interviewing and self-determination theory. *BMC Public Health*, *14*(1), 1–29.

Helme, D. W., Donohew, R. L., Baier, M., & Zittleman, L. (2007). A classroom-administered simulation of a television campaign on adolescent smoking: Testing an activation model of information exposure. *Journal of Health Communication*, *12*, 399–415.

Helms, S. W., Choukas-Bradley, S., Widman, L., Giletta, M., Cohen, G. L., & Prinstein, M. J. (2014). Adolescents misperceive and are influenced by high-status peers' health risk, deviant, and adaptive behavior. *Developmental Psychology*, *50*, 2697–2714.

Holland, J. J. (2014, September 16). Blacks, Hispanics have doubts about media accuracy. *AP*. Retrieved from http://apnorc.org/news-media/Pages/News+Media/Blacks-Hispanics-have-doubts-about-media-accuracy.aspx

Holliday, J., Audrey, S., Campbell, R., & Moore, L. (2016). Identifying well-connected opinion leaders for informal health promotion: The example of the ASSIST smoking prevention program. *Health Communication*, *31*(8), 946–953.

Hubbell, A. P. (2006). Mexican American women in a rural area and barriers to their ability to enact protective behaviors against breast cancer. *Health Communication*, *20*, 35–44.

Inbar, M. (2009). Is PSA about driving while texting too graphic? *NBCNews*. Retrieved from http://www.today.com/id/32551351/ns/today-money/t/psa-about-texting-while-driving-too-graphic/#.VZL0gxNViko

Johnston, L. D., O'Malley, P. M., Miech, R. A., Bachman, J. G., & Schulenberg, J. E. (2014). Monitoring the future national results on drug use: 1975–2013: Overview, key findings on adolescent drug use. Institute for Social Research at the University of Michigan. Retrieved from http://www.monitoringthefuture.org/pubs/monographs/mtf-overview2013.pdf

Junghans, A. F., Cheung, T. L., & De Ridder, D. T. (2015). Under consumers' scrutiny—An investigation into consumers' attitudes and concerns about nudging in the realm of health behavior. *BMC Public Health*, *15*(1), 1–13.

Kim, S.-H., & Willis, L. A. (2007, June). Talking about obesity: News framing of who is responsible for causing and fixing the problem. *Journal of Health Communication*, *12*, 359–376.

Kreps, G. L. (2005). Narrowing the digital divide to overcome disparities in care. In E. B. Ray (Ed.), *Health communication in practice: A case study approach* (pp. 357–364). Mahwah, NJ: Lawrence Erlbaum.

Lang, A. (2006). Using the limited-capacity model of motivated mediated message processing to design effective cancer communication messages. *Journal of Communication*, *56*, S57–S80.

Lang, A., Chung, Y., Lee, S., & Zhao, X. (2005). It's the product: Do risky products compel attention and elicit arousal in media users? *Health Communication*, *17*, 283–300.

Lang, A., Schwartz, N., Lee, S., & Angelini, J. R. (2007, September). Processing radio PSAs: Production pacing, arousing content, and age. *Journal of Health Communication*, *12*, 581–599.

Lavoie, N. R., & Quick, B. L. (2013). What is the truth? An application of the extended parallel process model to televised truth® ads. *Health Communication*, *28*, 53–62.

Lazarsfeld, P., Burleson, B., & Gaudet, H. (1948). *The people's choice*. New York: Columbia University Press.

Ledlow, G. R., Johnson, J. A., & Hakoyama, M. (2008). Social marketing and organizational efficacy. In K. B. Wright & S. D. Moore (Eds.), *Applied health communication* (pp. 85–103). Cresskill, NJ: Hampton Press.

Lee, M. J. (2010). The effects of self-efficacy statements in humorous anti-alcohol abuse messages targeting college students: Who is in charge? *Health Communication*, *25*, 638–646. doi:10.1080/10410236.2010.521908

Lefebvre, R. C., Doner, L., Johnston, D., Loughrey, K., Balch, G. I., & Sutton, S. M. (1995). Use of database marketing and consumer-based health communication in message design: An example for the Office of Cancer Communications' "5 a Day for Better Health" program. In E. Maibach & R. L. Parrott (Eds.), *Designing health messages: Approaches from communication theory and public health practice* (pp. 217–246). Thousand Oaks, CA: Sage.

Lim, R. Tham, D., Cheung, O., Adaikan, P. & Wong, M. (2019). A public health communication intervention using edutainment and communication technology to promote safer sex among heterosexual men patronizing entertainment establishments. *Journal of Health Communication*, *24*(1), 47–64.

Lustria, M. A., Noar, S. M., Cortese, J., Van Stee, S. K., Glueckauf, R. L., & Lee, J. (2013). A meta-analysis of web-delivered tailored health behavior change interventions. *Journal of Health Communication*, *18*, 1039–1069.

Maibach, E. W., & Parrott, R. L. (Eds.). (1995). *Designing health messages*. Thousand Oaks, CA: Sage.

Matsaganis, M. D., Golden, A. G., & Scott, M. E. (2014). Communication infrastructure theory and reproductive health disparities: Enhancing storytelling network integration by developing interstitial actors. *International Journal of Communication*, 1495–1515.

Meth Project named third most effective philanthropy. (2010, December 6). *Barron's Magazine*. Retrieved from http://www.siebelscholars.com/news/meth-project-named-third-most-effective-philanthropy-world-barrons-magazine

Miller, C. H., Lane, L. T., Deatrick, L. M., Young, A. M., & Potts, K. A. (2007). Psychological reactance and promotional health messages: The effects of controlling language, lexical concreteness, and the restoration of freedom. *Human Communication Research*, 33, 219–240.

Moran, M. B., & Sussman, S. (2014). Translating the link between social identity and health behavior into effective health communication strategies: An experimental application using antismoking advertisements. *Health Communication*, 29, 1057-1066.

Mosavel, M., & El-Shaarawi, N. (2007, December). "I have never heard of that one": Young girls' knowledge and perception of cervical cancer. *Journal of Health Communication*, 12, 707–719.

Niederdeppe, J., Davis, K. C., Farrelly, M. C., & Yarsevich, J. (2007). Stylistic features, need for sensation, and confirmed recall of national smoking prevention advertisements. *Journal of Communication*, 57, 272–292.

Noar, S. M., Zimmerman, R. S., Palmgreen, P., Lustria, M., & Horosewski, M. L. (2006). Integrating personality and psychosocial theoretical approaches to understanding safer sexual behavior: Implications for message design. *Health Communication*, 19(2), 165–174.

Paek, H.-J. (2008). Mechanisms through which adolescents attend and respond to antismoking media campaigns. *Journal of Communication*, 58, 84–105.

Parrott, R., & Polonec, L. (2008). Preventing green tobacco sickness in farming youth: A behavioral adaptation to health communication in health campaigns. In K. B. Wright & S. D. Moore (Eds.), *Applied health communication* (pp. 341–359). Cresskill, NJ: Hampton Press.

Petty, R. E., & Cacioppo, J. T. (1981). *Attitudes and persuasion: Classic and contemporary approaches*. Dubuque, IA: Wm. C. Brown.

Pilling, V. K., & Brannon, L. A. (2007). Assessing college students' attitudes toward responsible drinking messages to identify promising binge drinking intervention strategies. *Health Communication*, 22, 265–276.

Rains, S. A. (2008a, June). Health at high speed: Broadband internet access, health communication, and the digital divide. *Communication Research*, 35(3), 283–297.

Rains, S. A. (2008b, January/March). Seeking health information in the information age: The role of internet self-efficacy. *Western Journal of Communication*, 72(1), 1–18.

Rains, S. A., & Turner, M. M. (2007). Psychological reactance and persuasive health communication: A test and extension of the intertwined model. *Human Communication Research*, 33(2), 241–269.

Richards, A. S., & Banas, J. A. (2015). Inoculating against reactance to persuasive health messages. *Health Communication*, 30, 451–460.

Roberto, A. J., Zimmerman, R. S., Carlyle, K. E., Abner, E. L., Cupp, P. K., & Hansen, G. L. (2007). The effects of computer-based pregnancy, STD, and HIV prevention intervention: A nine-school trial. *Health Communication*, 21, 115–124.

Rogers, E. M. (1983). *Diffusion of innovations* (3rd ed.). New York: The Free Press.

Rucinski, D. (2004, August). Community boundedness, personal relevance, and the knowledge gap. *Communication Research*, 31(4), 472–495.

Sacks, R. J., Copas, A. J., Wilkinson, D. M., & Robinson, A. J. (2014). Uptake of the HPV vaccination programme in England: A cross-sectional survey of young women attending sexual health services. *Sexually Transmitted Infections*, 90(4), 315–321.

Sanders-Jackson, A., Clayton, R., Tan, A., & Yie, K. (2019). Testing the effect of vapor in ends public service announcements on current smokers and ENDS users' psychophysiological responses and smoking and vaping urge. *Journal of Health Communication*, 24(4), 413–421.

Scarpaci, J., & Burke, C. (2016). Tailoring but not targeting: A critical analysis of "the Meth Project" aimed at Hispanic youth. *International Journal of Nonprofit and Voluntary Sector Marketing*, 21(3), 168–179.

Schooler, C., Chaffee, S. H., Flora, J. A., & Roser, C. (1998). Health campaign channels: Tradeoffs among reach, specificity, and impact. *Health Communication Research*, 24, 410–432.

Shi, J., & Salmon, C. (2018). Identifying opinion leaders to promote organ donation on social media: Network study. *Journal of Medical Internet Research*, 21(1), e7.

Shorty Awards. (2017). *#CATmageddon: About this entry*. Retrieved from https://shortyawards.com/9th/catmageddon

Smith, R. (2007, April/May). Media depictions of health topics: Challenge and stigma formats. *Journal of Health Communication*, 12, 233–249.

thetruth.com. (2015). Legacy Foundation. Retrieved from http://www.thetruth.com/?video=LvgUUeSu9tA&gclid=CJfStovwtcYCFY89gQodNnYMFg

Tichenor, P. J., Donohue, G. A., & Olien, C. N. (1970). Mass media flow and differential growth in knowledge. *Public Opinion Quarterly*, 34, 159–170.

Torres-Ruiz, M., Robinson-Ector, K., Attinson, D., Trotter, J., Anise, A., & Clauser, S. (2018). A portfolio analysis of culturally tailored trials to address health and healthcare disparities. *International Journal of Environmental Research and Public Health*, 15(9), 1859–1873.

Truth Initiative. (2019). *Why the FDA needs to regulate e-cigarettes now*. Retrieved from https://truthinitiative.org/research-resources/emerging-tobacco-products/why-fda-needs-regulate-e-cigarettes-now

truth® named one of the top 15 ad campaigns of 21st century. (2015, January 12). *PR Newswire*.

Wang, B., Deveaux, L., Li, X., Marshall, S., Chen, X., & Stanton, B. (2014). The impact of youth, family, peer and neighborhood risk factors on developmental trajectories of risk involvement from early through middle adolescence. *Social Science & Medicine*, 106, 43–52.

Wikler, D. (1987). Who should be blamed for being sick? *Health Education Quarterly*, *14*, 11–25.

Winsten, J. (2010, March 18). The Designated Driver Campaign: Why it worked. *Huffington Post*. Retrieved from http://www.huffingtonpost.com/jay-winston/designated-driver-campaig_b_405249.html

World Health Organization. (2012, May). Tobacco. Geneva, Switzerland: Author. Retrieved from http://www.who.int/mediacentre/factsheets/fs339/en/index.html

Zuckerman, M. (1994). *Behavioral expressions and biosocial bases of sensation seeking*. Cambridge: Cambridge University Press.

CHAPTER 14

Ajzen, I. (1985). From intentions to actions: A theory of planned behavior. In J. Kuhl & J. Beckman (Eds.), *Action control: From cognition to behavior* (pp. 11–39). Heidelberg: Springer.

Ajzen, I. (1991). The theory of planned behavior. *Organizational Behavior and Human Decision Processes*, *50*, 179–211.

Ajzen, I., & Fishbein, M. (1980). *Understanding attitudes and predicting behavior*. Englewood Cliffs, NJ: Prentice Hall.

Andrews, K. R., Silk, K. S., & Eneli, I. U. (2010). Parents as health promoters: A theory of planned behavior perspective on the prevention of childhood obesity. *Journal of Health Communication*, *15*, 95–107. doi:10.1080/10810730903460567

Bandura, A. (1986). *Social foundations of thought and action: A social cognitive approach*. Englewood Cliffs, NJ: Prentice Hall.

Bandura, A. (1994). Social cognitive theory of mass communication. In J. Bryant & D. Zillman (Eds.), *Media effects: Advances in theory and research* (pp. 61–90). Hillsdale, NJ: Lawrence Erlbaum.

BBC Newsbeat. (2015, June 8). The letters A, O & B are vanishing around the UK. Why? *BBC Newsbeat*. Retrieved from http://www.bbc.co.uk/newsbeat/article/33046805/the-letters-a-o--b-are-vanishing-around-the-uk-why?ocid=socialflow_facebook

Best, A. L., Spencer, M., Hall, I. J., Friedman, D. B., & Billings, D. (2015). Developing spiritually framed breast cancer screening messages in consultation with African American women. *Health Communication*, *30*(3), 290–300.

Blanc, N., & Brigaud, E. (2014). Humor in print health advertisements: Enhanced attention, privileged recognition, and persuasiveness of preventive messages. *Health Communication*, *29*, 669–677.

Boer, H., & Westhoff, Y. (2006, February). The role of positive and negative signaling communication by strong and weak ties in the shaping of safe sex subjective norms of adolescents in South Africa. *Communication Theory*, *16*(1), 75–90.

Bohm, D. (1996). *On dialogue*. L. Nichol (Ed.). London: Routledge & Kegan Paul.

Booms, B. H., & Bitner, M. J. (1981). Marketing strategies and organization structures for service firms. In J. H. Donnelly & W. R. George (Eds.), *Marketing of services* (pp. 47–51). Chicago: American Marketing Association.

Borden, N. H. (1964). The concept of the marketing mix. *Journal of Advertising Research*, *4*(2), 2–7.

Borkman, T. (1976). Experiential knowledge: A new concept for the analysis of self-help groups. *Social Service Review*, *50*, 445–456.

Braddock, K., & Dillard, J. (2016). Meta-analytic evidence for the persuasive effect of narratives on beliefs, attitudes, intentions, and behaviors. *Communication Monographs*, *83*(4), 446–467.

Cameron, K. A., & Campo, S. (2006). Stepping back from social norms campaigns: Comparing normative influences to other predictors of health behaviors. *Health Communication*, *20*, 277–288.

Campbell, R. G., & Babrow, A. S. (2004). The role of empathy in responses to persuasive risk communication: Overcoming resistance to HIV prevention messages. *Health Communication*, *16*, 159–182.

Campo, S., & Cameron, K. A. (2006). Differential effects of exposure to social norm campaigns: A cause for concern. *Health Communication*, *19*, 209–219.

Carcioppolo, N., Jensen, J. D., Wilson, S. R., Collins, W. B., Carrion, M., & Linnemeier, G. (2013). Examining HPV threat-to-efficacy ratios in the Extended Parallel Process Model. *Health Communication*, *28*, 20–28.

Casper, M. F., Child, J. T., Gilmour, D., McIntyre, K. A., & Pearson, J. C. (2006). Healthy research perspectives: Incorporating college student experiences with alcohol. *Health Communication*, *20*, 289–298.

Cho, H., & Salmon, C. T. (2007). Unintended effects of health communication campaigns. *Journal of Communication*, *57*, 293–317.

Christakis, N. A., & Fowler, J. H. (2008, May 22). The collective dynamics of smoking in a large social network. *New England Journal of Medicine*, *358*, 2249.

Cohen, E. L., Head, K. J., McGladrey, M. J., Hoover, A. G., Vanderpool, R. C., Bridger, C., . . . Winterbauer, N. (2015). Designing for dissemination: Lessons in message design from "1-2-3 Pap." *Health Communication*, *30*, 196–207.

Controversy heats up over subway's safer sex ads. (1994, February 7). *AIDS Weekly*, *9*, 9–10.

Delgado, M., McDonald, C., Winston, F., Halpern, S., Buttenheim, A., Setubal, C., . . . Lee, Y. (2018). Attitudes on technological, social, and behavioral economic strategies to reduce cellphone use among teens while driving. *Traffic Injury Prevention*, *19*(6), 569–576.

De Meulenaer, S., De Pelsmacker, P., & Dens, N. (2018) Power distance, uncertainty avoidance, and the effects of source credibility on health risk message compliance. *Health Communication*, *33*(3), 291–298.

Dillard, A. J., McCaul, K. D., Kelso, P. D., & Klein, W. M. P. (2006). Resisting good news: Reactions to breast cancer risk communication. *Health Communication*, *19*, 115–123.

Dillard, J. P., & Nabi, R. L. (2006). The persuasive influence of emotion in cancer prevention and detection messages. *Journal of Communication*, *56*, S123–S139.

Dragojevic, M., Savage, M., Scott, A., & McGinnis, T. (2018). Promoting oral health in Appalachia: Effects of threat label and source accent on message acceptance. *Health Communication*. Advance online publication. doi: 10.1080/10410236.2018.1560581

Dunlop, S., Wakefield, M., & Kashima, Y. (2008). Can you feel it? Negative emotion, risk, and narrative in health communication. *Media Psychology, 11*(1), 52–75.

Dutta, M. J. (2008). *Communicating health: A culture-centered approach*. Cambridge, MA: Polity Press.

Dutta, M. J., & Boyd, J. (2007). Turning "smoking man" images around: Portrayals of smoking in men's magazines as a blueprint for smoking cessation campaigns. *Health Communication, 22*, 253–263.

Dutta, M. J., & de Souza, R. (2008). The past, present, and future of health development campaigns: Reflexivity and the critical-cultural approach. *Health Communication, 23*, 326–339.

Dutta-Bergman, M. J. (2005). Theory and practice in health communication campaigns: A critical interrogation. *Health Communication, 18*, 103–122.

Elbert, S., & Ots, P. (2018) Reading or listening to a gain- or loss-framed health message: Effects of message framing and communication mode in the context of fruit and vegetable intake. *Journal of Health Communication, 23*(6), 573–580.

Evans, W. D., Uhrig, J., Davis, K., & McCormack, L. (2009). Efficacy methods to evaluate health communication and marketing campaigns. *Journal of Health Communication, 14*, 315–330. doi:10.1080/10810730902872234

Faden, R. R. (1987). Ethical issues in government sponsored public health campaigns. *Health Education Quarterly, 14*, 27–37.

Farrelly, M. C., Healton, C. G., Davis, K. C., Messeri, P., & Haviland, M. L. (2002, June). Getting to the truth: Evaluating national tobacco countermarketing campaigns. *American Journal of Public Health, 92*(6), 901–907.

Gordon, R. (2012). Re-thinking and re-tooling the social marketing mix. *Australasian Marketing Journal, 20*, 122–126.

Gothe, N. (2018). Correlates of physical activity in urban African American adults and older adults: Testing the social cognitive theory. *Annals of Behavioral Medicine, 52*, 743–751.

Goyal Wasan, P., & Tripathi, G. (2014). Revisiting social marketing mix: A socio-cultural perspective. *Journal of Services Research, 14*(2), 127–144.

Green, E. C., & Witte, K. (2006). Can fear arousal in public health campaigns contribute to the decline of HIV prevalence? *Journal of Health Communication, 11*(3), 245–259.

Green, M. C., & Brock, T. C. (2000). The role of transportation in the persuasiveness of public narratives. *Journal of Personality and Social Psychology, 79*(5), 701–721.

Grönroos, C. (1994). From marketing mix to relationship marketing: Towards a paradigm shift in marketing. *Management Decision, 32*(2), 4–20.

Haines, M. P., & Spear, S. F. (1996). Changing the perceptions of the norm: A strategy to decrease binge drinking among college students. *Journal of American College Health, 45*, 134–140.

Hample, D., & Hample, J. M. (2014). Persuasion about health risks: Evidence, credibility, scientific flourishes, and risk perceptions. *Argumentation & Advocacy, 51*(1), 17–29.

Heley, K., Kennedy-Hendricks, A., Niederdeppe, J., & Barry, C. (2019). Reducing health-related stigma through narrative messages. *Health Communication*. Advance online publication.

Helme, D., Oser, C., Knudsen, H., Morris, E., Serna, A., & Zelaya, C. (2019). Smokeless tobacco and the rural teen: How culture and masculinity contribute to adolescent use. *Journal of Health Communication, 24*(3), 311–318.

Hendriks, H., & Janssen, L. (2018). Frightfully funny: Combining threat and humour in health messages for men and women. *Psychology & Health, 33*, 594–613.

Hendriks, H., & Strick, M. (2019). A laughing matter? How humor in alcohol ads influences interpersonal communication and persuasion. *Health Communication*. Advance online publication. doi:10.1080/10410236.2019.1663587

Holtgrave, D. R., Tinsley, B. J., & Kay, L. S. (1995). Encouraging risk reduction: A decision-making approach to message design. In E. Maibach & R. L. Parrott (Eds.), *Designing health messages: Approaches from communication theory and public health practice* (pp. 24–40). Thousand Oaks, CA: Sage.

Hullett, C. R. (2006). Using functional theory to promote HIV testing: The impact of value-expressive messages, uncertainty, and fear. *Health Communication, 20*, 57–67.

Jang, S. A., Rimal, R. N., & Cho, N. (2013). Normative influences and alcohol consumption: The role of drinking refusal self-efficacy. *Health Communication, 28*, 443–451.

Jenkins, M. (2012, May 31). "Pink ribbons," tied up with more than hope. National Public Radio. Retrieved from http://www.npr.org/2012/05/31/153912165/pink-ribbons-tied-up-with-more-than-hope

Jones, C., Jensen, J., Scherr, C., Brown, N., Christy, K., & Weaver, J. (2015). The health belief model as an explanatory framework in communication research: Exploring parallel, serial, and moderated mediation. *Health Communication, 30*(6), 566–576.

Jones, K. O., Denham, B. E., & Springston, J. K. (2007). Differing effects of mass and interpersonal communication on breast cancer risk estimates: An exploratory study of college students and their mothers. *Health Communication, 21*, 165–175.

Kareklas, I., Muehling, D., & Weber, T. (2015). Reexamining health messages in the digital age: A fresh look at source credibility effects. *Journal of Advertising, 44*(2), 88–104.

Kim, H. J. (2014). The impacts of vicarious illness experience on response to gain- versus loss-framed breast cancer screening (BCS) messages. *Health Communication, 29*, 854–865.

Kok, G., Peters, G., Kessels, L., Hoor, G., & Ruiter, R. (2018). Ignoring theory and misinterpreting evidence: The false belief in fear appeals. *Health Psychology Review, 12*(2), 111–125.

Kotler, P., & Zaltman, G. (1971). Social marketing: An approach to planned social change. *Journal of Marketing, 35*(3), 3–12.

Krosnick, J. A., Chang, L., Sherman, S. J., Chassin, L., & Presson, C. (2006). The effects of beliefs about the health consequences of cigarette smoking on smoking onset. *Journal of Communication*, *56*, S18–S37.

Kuijer, R., Boyce, J., & Marshall, E., (2015). Associating a prototypical forbidden food item with guilt or celebration: Relationships with indicators of (un)healthy eating and the moderating role of stress and depressive symptoms. *Psychology & Health*, *30*(2), 203–217.

Lapinski, M. K., Rimal, R. N., DeVries, R., & Lee, E. L. (2007). The role of group orientation and descriptive norms on water conservation and behaviors. *Health Communication*, *22*, 133–142.

Lapowsky, I. (2014, April 1). Livestrong without Lance. *Moneybox*. http://www.slate.com/blogs/moneybox/2014/04/01/lance_armstrong_livestrong_how_the_charity_came_back_from_the_scandal.html

Lederman, L. C., & Stewart, L. P. (2005). *Changing the culture of college drinking: A socially situated health communication campaign*. Cresskill, NJ: Hampton Press.

Lederman, L. C., Stewart, L. P., Barr, S. L., Powell, R. L., Laitman, L., & Goodhart, F. W. (2001). Using communication theory to reduce dangerous drinking on a college campus. In R. E. Rice & C. K. Atkin (Eds.), *Public communication campaigns* (3rd ed., pp. 295–299). Thousand Oaks, CA: Sage.

Lederman, L. C., Stewart, L. P., Goodhart, F. W., & Laitman, L. (2008). A case against "binge" as the term of choice. In L. C. Lederman (Ed.), *Beyond these walls: Readings in health communication* (pp. 292–303). New York: Oxford University Press.

Lederman, L. C., Stewart, L. P., & Russ, T. L. (2007). Addressing college drinking through curriculum infusion: A study of the use of experience-based learning in the communication classroom. *Communication Education*, *56*(4), 476–494.

Lee, M. J., & Bichard, S. L. (2006). Effective message design targeting college students for the prevention of binge-drinking: Basing design on rebellious risk-taking tendency. *Health Communication*, *20*, 299–308.

Lefebvre, R. C., & Flora, J. A. (1988). Social marketing and public health intervention. *Health Education Quarterly*, *15*, 299–315.

Lipkis, I., Johnson, C., Amarasekara, S., Pan, W., & Updegraff, J. (2018). Reactions to online colorectal cancer risk estimates among a nationally representative sample of adults who have never been screened. *Journal of Behavioral Medicine*, *41*(3), 289–298.

Mahler, H. I. M., Kulik, J. A., Butler, H. A., Gerrard, M., & Gibbons, F. X. (2008). Social norms information enhances the efficacy of an appearance-based sun protection intervention. *Social Science & Medicine*, *67*, 321–329.

Mammen, S., Sano, Y., Braun, B., & Maring, E. (2019). Shaping core health messages: Rural, low-income mothers speak through participatory action research. *Health Communication*, *34*(10), 1141–1149.

McQueen, A., Caburnay, C., Kreuter, M., & Sefko, J. (2019) Improving adherence to colorectal cancer screening: A randomized intervention to compare screener vs. survivor narratives. *Journal of Health Communication*, *24*(2), 141–155.

Menegatos, L., Lederman, L. C., & Hess, A. (2010). Friends don't let Jane hook up drunk: A qualitative analysis of participation in a simulation of college drinking-related decisions. *Communication Education*, *59*(3), 374–388.

Miller, C. H., Burgoon, M., Grandpre, J. R., & Alvaro, E. M. (2006). Identifying principal risk factors for the initiation of adolescent smoking behaviors: The significance of psychological reactance. *Health Communication*, *19*, 241–252.

Miller-Day, M., & Hecht, M. L. (2013). Narrative means to preventative ends: A narrative engagement framework for designing prevention interventions. *Health Communication*, *28*, 657–670.

Mollen, S., Engelen, S., Kessels, L., & Putte, B. (2017). Short and sweet: The persuasive effects of message framing and temporal context in antismoking warning labels. *Journal of Health Communication*, *22*(1), 20–28.

Muralidharan, S., & Kim, E. (2019): Can empathy offset low bystander efficacy? Effectiveness of domestic violence prevention narratives in India. *Health Communication*. Advance online publication. doi: 10.1080/10410236.2019.1623645

Nabi, R. L. (2016). Laughing in the face of fear (of disease detection): Using humor to promote cancer self-examination behavior. *Health Communication*, *31*, 873–883.

Nan, X., Zhao, X., Yang, B., & Iles, I. (2015). Effectiveness of cigarette warning labels: Examining the impact of graphics, message framing, and temporal framing. *Health Communication*, *30*, 81–89.

National Health Service (NHS). (2015). National Blood Week #Missing Type. Retrieved from http://www.blood.co.uk/news-media/campaigns/national-blood-week/

Niederdeppe, J., Shapiro, M. A., Kim, H. Y., Bartolo, D., & Porticella, N. (2014). Narrative persuasion, causality, complex integration, and support for obesity policy. *Health Communication*, *29*, 431–444.

Noar, S. M., Myrick, J. G., Zeitany, A., Kelley, D., Morales-Pico, B., & Thomas, N. E. (2015). Testing a social cognitive theory-based model of indoor tanning: Implications for skin cancer prevention messages. *Health Communication*, *30*, 164–174.

Noar, S. M., Zimmerman, R. S., Palmgreen, P., Lustria, M., & Horosewski, M. L. (2006). Integrating personality and psychosocial theoretical approaches to understanding safer sexual behavior: Implications for message design. *Health Communication*, *19*(2), 165–174.

Noorani, T., Karlsson, M., and Borkman, T. (2019) Deep experiential knowledge: Reflections from mutual aid groups for evidence-based practice. *Evidence & Policy*, *15*(2), 217–234.

O'Keefe, D. J. (2000). Guilt and social influence. *Annals of the International Communication Association*, *23*, 67–101.

O'Keefe, D. J. (2015). Message generalizations that support evidence-based persuasive message design: Specifying the evidentiary requirements. *Health Communication, 20*, 106–113.

O'Keefe, D., & Jensen, J. (2009). The relative persuasiveness of gain-framed and loss-framed messages for encouraging disease detection behaviors: A meta-analytic review. *Journal of Communication, 59*, 296–316.

Park, S., Son, H., Lee, J., & Go, E. (2019): Moderating effects of social norms and alcohol consumption on message framing in responsible drinking campaigns: Value from deviance regulation theory. *Health Communication*. Advance online publication. doi: 10.1080/10410236.2019.1593077

Parrott, R. (1995). Motivation to attend to health messages: Presentation of content and linguistic considerations. In E. Maibach & R. L. Parrott (Eds.), *Designing health messages: Approaches from communication theory and public health practice* (pp. 7–23). Thousand Oaks, CA: Sage.

Peters, E., Lipkus, I., & Diefenbach, M. A. (2006). The functions of affect in health communications and in the construction of health preferences. *Journal of Communication, 56*, S140–S162.

Phua, J. (2016). The effects of similarity, parasocial identification, and source credibility in obesity public service announcements on diet and exercise self-efficacy. *Journal of Health Psychology, 21*(5), 699–708.

Polonec, L. D., Major, A. M., & Atwood, L. E. (2006). Evaluating the believability and effectiveness of the social norms message. "Most students drink 0 to 4 drinks when they party." *Health Communication, 20*, 23–34.

Prochaska, J. O., & DiClemente, C. C. (1983). Stages and processes of self-change of smoking: Toward an integrative model of change. *Journal of Consulting and Clinical Psychology, 51*, 390–395.

Prochaska, J. O., DiClemente, C. C., & Norcross, J. C. (1992). In search of how people change applications to the addictive behaviors. *American Psychologist, 47*, 1102–1114.

Prochaska, J. O., Johnson, S., & Lee, P. (1998). The transtheoretical model of behavior change. In S. A. Shumaker, E. B. Schron, J. K. Ockene, & W. L. McBee (Eds.), *The handbook of behavior change* (2nd ed., pp. 59–84). New York: Springer-Verlag.

Rimal, R. N. (2008, March/April). Modeling the relationship between descriptive norms and behaviors: A test and extension of the theory of normative social behavior (TNSB). *Health Communication, 23*, 103–116.

Rimal, R. N., & Morrison, D. (2006). A uniqueness to personal threat (UPT) hypothesis: How similarity affects perceptions of susceptibility and severity in risk assessment. *Health Communication, 20*, 209–219.

Rimal, R. N., & Real, K. (2005, June). How behaviors are influenced by perceived norms: A test of the theory of normative social behavior. *Communication Research, 32*, 389–414.

Rogers, E. M. (1973). *Communication strategies for family planning*. New York: Free Press.

Rogers, E. M. (1983). *Diffusion of innovations* (3rd ed.). New York: The Free Press.

Romain, A. J., Bortolon, C., Gourlan, M., Carayol, M., Decker, E., Lareyre, O., . . . Bernard, P. (2018). Matched or nonmatched interventions based on the transtheoretical model to promote physical activity. A meta-analysis of randomized controlled trials. *Journal of Sport and Health Science, 7*, 50–57.

Romain, A. J., Horwath, C., & Bernard, P. (2018). Prediction of physical activity level using processes of change from the transtheoretical model: Experiential, behavioral, or an interaction effect? *American Journal of Health Promotion, 32*(1), 16–23.

Rosenstock, I. M. (1960). What research in motivation suggests for public health. *American Journal of Public Health, 50*, 295–301.

Rothman, A. J., & Salovey, P. (1997). Shaping perceptions to motivate healthy behavior: The role of message framing. *Psychological Bulletin, 121*, 3–19.

RU SURE. (2019). Rutgers University Center for Communication and Health Studies. Retrieved from http://www.chi.rutgers.edu/rusure

Salmon, C. T., & Atkin, C. (2003). Using media campaigns for health promotion. In T. L. Thompson, A. M. Dorsey, K. I. Miller, & R. Parrott (Eds.), *Handbook of health communication* (pp. 449–472). Mahwah, NJ: Lawrence Erlbaum.

Sanders-Jackson, A. (2014). Rated measures of narrative structure for written smoking-cessation texts. *Health Communication, 29*, 1009–1019.

Sarbazi, E., Moradi, F., Ghafari-Fam, S., Mirzaeian, K., & Babazadeh, T. (2019). Cognitive predictors of physical activity behaviors among rural patients with type 2 diabetes: Applicability of the extended theory of reasoned action (ETRA). *Journal of Multidisciplinary Healthcare, 12*, 429–436.

Scruggs, S., Mama, S., Carmack, C., Douglas, T., Diamond, P., & Basen-Engquist, K. (2018). Randomized trial of a lifestyle physical activity intervention for breast cancer survivors: Effects on transtheoretical model variables. *Health Promotion Practice, 19*(1), 134–144.

Senge, P. M. (2006). *The fifth discipline: The art and practice of the learning organization*. New York: Doubleday/Currency.

Silk, K. J., Bigsby, E., Volkman, J., Kingsley, C., Atkin, C., Ferrara, M., & Goins, L.-A. (2006). Formative research on adolescent and adult perceptions of risk factors for breast cancer. *Social Science & Medicine, 63*, 3124–3136.

Slater, M. D. (2006). Specification and misspecification of theoretical foundations and logic models for health communication campaigns. *Health Communication, 20*, 149–158.

Smith, K. C., & Wakefield, M. (2006). Newspaper coverage of youth and tobacco: Implications for public health. *Health Communication, 19*, 19–28.

Sopory, P. (2005). Metaphor in formative evaluation and message design: An application to relationship and alcohol use. *Health Communication, 17*, 149–172.

Stavrositu, C. D., & Kim, J. (2015). All blogs are not created equal: The role of narrative formats and user-generated comments in health prevention. *Health Communication, 30*, 485–495.

Stewart, L. P., Lederman, L. C., Golubow, M., Cattafesta, J. L., Godhart, F. W., Powell, R. L., & Laitman, L. (2002, Winter). Applying communication theories to prevent dangerous drinking among college students: The RU SURE campaign. *Communication Studies, 53*(4), 381–399.

Stretcher, V. J., & Rosenstock, I. M. (1997). The health belief model. In K. Glanz, F. M. Lewis, & B. K. Rimer (Eds.), *Health behavior and health education* (pp. 41–59). San Francisco: Jossey-Bass.

Sun, Y., Lee, T., & Qian, S. (2019). Beyond personal responsibility: Examining the effects of narrative engagement on communicative and civic actions. *Journal of Health Communication, 24*(6), 603–614.

Tirrell, M. (2015, February 9). Ice Bucket Challenge: 6 months later. *CNBC*. Retrieved from http://www.cnbc.com/id/102405889

Wang, X. (2011). The role of anticipated guilt in intentions to register as organ donors and to discuss organ donation with family. *Health Communication, 26*, 683–690. doi:10.1080/10410236.2011.563350

Wechsler, H., Nelson, T. F., Lee, J. E., Seibring, M., Lewis, C., & Keeling, R. P. (2003, July). Perception and reality: A national evaluation of social norms marketing interventions to reduce college students' heavy alcohol use. *Journal of Studies on Alcohol, 64*(4), 484–494.

Witte, K. (1997). Preventing teen pregnancy through persuasive communications: Realities, myths, and hard-fact truths. *Journal of Community Health, 22*, 137–154.

Witte, K. (2008). Putting the fear back into fear appeals: The extended parallel process model. In L. C. Lederman (Ed.), *Beyond these walls: Readings in health communication* (pp. 273–291). New York: Oxford University Press.

Xu, Z., & Guo, H. (2018). A meta-analysis of the effectiveness of guilt on health-related attitudes and intentions. *Health Communication, 33*(5), 519–525.

Yanovitzky, I., Stewart, L. P., & Lederman, L. C. (2006). Social distance, perceived drinking by peers, and alcohol use by college students. *Health Communication, 19*, 1–10.

Yee, A., Lwin., M. & Lau, J. (2019). Parental guidance and children's healthy food consumption: Integrating the theory of planned behavior with interpersonal communication antecedents. *Journal of Health Communication, 24*(2), 183–194.

Credits

CHAPTER 1
Page 4, AleksandarNakic/iStock.com; page 5, Neustockimages/iStock.com; page 9, SeventyFour/iStock.com; page 13, monkeybusinessimages/iStock.com; page 15, monkeybusinessimages/iStock

CHAPTER 2
Page 22, tiero/iStock.com; page 25, monkeybusinessimages/iStock.com; page 27, designer491/iStock.com; page 34, © Richard Levine/Alamy Stock Photo

CHAPTER 3
Page 42, Dmytro Zinkevych/123RF; page 45, OcusFocus/iStock.com; page 48, Dinis Tolipov/123RF; page 51, ra2studio/123RF; page 56, Prostock-Studio/iStock.com

CHAPTER 4
Page 65, mark adams/123RF; page 66, Photo by Vivien Killilea/Getty Images; page 68, Andrea Obzerova/123RF; page 71, Katarzyna Białasiewicz/123RF; page 73, belchonock/123RF; page 74, ©iStockphoto/zhudifeng

CHAPTER 5
Page 81, angellodeco/123RF; page 84, david tiberio/123RF; page 87, Sergii Gnatiuk/123RF; page 88, KatarzynaBialasiewicz/iStock.com; page 92, michaeljung/Shutterstock.com; page 93, wavebreakmedia/Shutterstock.com; page 97, Rido/Shutterstock.com

CHAPTER 6
Page 106, Dinis Tolipov/123RF page 107, Courtesy of Public Health – Seattle & King County; page 110, teolazarev/123RF; page 111, tuan_azizi/iStock.com; page 117, AP Photo/The Spokesan-Review, Colin Mulvany; Page 121, Rawf8/iStock.com; page 126, © EdStock/iStock.com

CHAPTER 7
Page 133, joserpizarro/123RF; pg 135, marino bocelli/123RF; page 140, Courtesy of Stacy Bias; page 143, Dean Drobot/123RF; page 145, yupiramos/123RF; page 147, Chakrapong Trakulrattananon/Alamy Stock Photo; page 150, tobkatrina/iStock.com; page 152, © TongRo Images/Alamy Stock Photo

CHAPTER 8
Page 160, rawpixel/123RF; page 163, froxx/123RF; page 168, Cathy Yeulet/123RF; page 175, Akhararat Wathanasing/123RF; page 178, Владимир Константинов/123RF

CHAPTER 9
Page 188, guteksk7/Shutterstock.com; NEERAZ CHATURVEDI/Shutterstock.com; page 190, SolStock/iStock.com; page 191, LightFieldStudios/iStock.com; page 192, AJ_Watt/iStock.com; page 195, monkeybusinessimages/iStock.com; page 197, Drazen Zigic/iStock.com; page 198, Vlad Teodor/Shutterstock.com; page 200, New Africa/Shutterstock.com; page 203, Syda Productions/Shutterstock.com; page 205, © Phanie/Alamy Stock Photo; page 209, Virgiliu Obada/Shutterstock.com

CHAPTER 10
Page 217, Courtesy of Veronika Javor; page 222, Rawpixel/Shutterstock.com; page 223, Syda Productions/Shutterstock.com; page 225, Wavebreak Media Ltd/123RF; page 230, iuphotos/123RF; page 231, ©iStockphoto/Dean Mitchell

CHAPTER 11
Page 238, Khosrork/iStock.com; page 239, Syda Productions/Shutterstock.com; page 241, alphaspirit/Shutterstock.com; page 243, AP Photo/Diane Bondareff; page 244, ammentorp/123RF; page 247, one photo/Shutterstock.com; page 250, KLH49/iStock.com; page 252, Vincenzo Lombardo/Getty Images Entertainment/Getty Images; page 254, Hannes Magerstaedt/Getty Images Entertainment/Getty Images; page 255, ©iStockphoto/Brendan Hunter; page 257, Photo by Diane Bondareff/Invision/AP; page 260, Featureflash Photo Agency/Shutterstock.com; page 262, little star/Shutterstock.com; page 264, ©iStockphoto/Imgorthand

CHAPTER 12
Page 270, Zerbor/Shutterstock.com; page 271, Jay Directo/AFP/Getty Images; page 272, VitaminCo/Shutterstock.com; page 274, Sean Locke/123RF; page 279, vm/iStock.com; page 282, Tommy E Trenchard/Alamy Stock Photo; page 284, nito100/iStock.com; page 285, AP Photo/Ahn Young-joon; page 286, ©iStockphoto/Edward Westmacott; page 287, Gwengoat/iStock.com; page 290, PureRadiancePhoto/Shutterstock.com

CHAPTER 13
Page 296, Sonsedska Yuliia/Shutterstock.com; page 300, Rido/Shutterstock.com; page 301, Barone Firenze/Shutterstock.com; page 302, antoniodiaz/Shutterstock.com; page 304, AYA images/Shutterstock.com; page 308, © age fotostock/Alamy Stock Photo; page 309, Niall Carson/PA Wire URN:20068438, (Press Assocation via AP Images); page 312, Monkey Business Images/Shutterstock.com; page 314, Goran Bogicevic/123RF

CHAPTER 14
Page 319, Courtesy Rutgers University Center for Communication and Health Issues; page 320, kyletperry/iStock; page 322, lofti photography/Shutterstock.com; page 323, Halfbottle/Shutterstock.com; page 324, © marc macdonald/Alamy Stock Photo; page 326, RichLegg/iStock; page 330, LeeTorrens/iStock; page 333, LightFieldStudios/iStock; page 339, Photo by Andy Kropa/Invision/AP; page 341, Nastco/iStock

Author Index

Note: Page numbers with a *b* indicate boxes. Numbers in italics indicate pictures.

Abay, S. M., 32
Abd-Allah, F., 32
Abdela, J., 32
Abraham, S., 105
Abrams, M., 22
Abroms, L. C., 204
Abuda, U., *257*
Adaikan, P., 262, 298
Adams, J. R., 65
Adams, N., 41
Adams, R., 41, 124
Addington-Hall, J., 58
Adelman, M. B., 159
Adelman, S. A., 96
Adler, E. P., 140
Adler, N., 135
Adolfsen, F., 244
Afifi, W. A., 175*b*
Ahmad, N., 144, 146
Ahn, G., 300, 301
Ahn, S. J., 313
Ajzen, I., 323
Alam, R., 168
Albrecht, T. L., 159
Albright, K., 106, 115
Alden, D. L., 147–48
Aldrich, R. A., 148
Aldridge, A., 228
Alegría, M., 115
Aleo, G., 23
Alexander, G. C., 290–91
Ali, S., 281
Allen, K. A., 172
Allenbaugh, J., 81
Alperin, E., 117
Alston, S., 160
Alter, C., 252*b*
Altieri, L., 203
Altman, W., 122
Alvaro, E. M., 334*b*
Amadeo, K., 31
Amarasekara, S., 333
Ambuel, B., 142
Amelung, D., 219
Amori, G., 96
Anas, A. P., 125
Anderberg, L., 254
Anderson, B. J., 44
Anderson, D. M., 312
Anderson, J. O., 164, 168
Anderson, K. B., 288
Anderson, L. A., 181

Anderson, M., 128, 189
Anderson, P. M., 50
Anderson, R., 162
Anderson, W. B., 150
Andrews, *309*
Andrews, G. R., 159
Andrews, J. E., 67
Andrews, K. R., 323, 324
Andrews, N. F., 168
Andsager, J. L., 249
Angelini, J. R., 309
Angell, M., 247, 248
Anghelcev, G., 314
Anschütz, D., 253–54
Antoun, J., 142
Apker, J., 99
Apolloni, L., 50
Appenzeller, T., 286, 287
Arasaratnam, L. A., 309
Arendt, F., 115
Argentero, P., 93
Armour, K., 203
Armstrong, D. M., 24
Armstrong, J. L., 244
Armstrong, L., 331
Armstrong, S., 242
Arnetz, B. B., 50
Arnetz, J. E., 50
Arnold, S., 244
Arora, N., 4, 41
Arpey, N. C., 106
Artiga, S., 113
Ashley, B. M., 75
Ashraf, A. A., 15
Aslam, S., 253
Assendelft, W., 188
Atherly, A., 127
Atkin, C., 340
Atwood, L. E., 334*b*
Audrey, S., 315
Austin, E. W., 264, 265, 308
Ayers, D., 163
Azevedo, D., 99

Babazadeh, T., 323
Babrow, A. S., 167, 340
Bachman, J. G., 296
Bachner, Y. G., 127
Backer, T. E., 296
Bae, H.-S., 264
Baek, T. H., 245, 256, 257
Baglia, J., 146, 246*b*

Bagnasco, A., 23
Baier, M., 309
Baker, D. W., 109
Baker, K., 244
Baker, M., 256
Baker, R., 70
Balbale, S. N., 306
Balint, J., 47
Ball, J., 249
Ballard, D., 125
Ball-Rokeach, S. J., 106
Baltes, M., 127
Banas, J. A., 308
Bandeali, F., 32
Bandura, A., 162, 240
Banerjee, S. C., 265, 309
Banja, J. D., 93, 94, 96
Banks, L., 269
Bao, Y., 107
Barbarin, O. A., 164
Barclay, E., 241
Bar-David, G., 176
Baringer, D., 160
Barker, S. A., 172
Barlett, C., 260
Barlow, P., 272*b*
Barnes, A., 245
Barnes, D., 204
Barnes, L., 141
Barnes, M., 159
Barnes, M. K., 164
Barnes, R. K., 50
Barnett, G. V., 97
Barnlund, D., 8
Barrera, M., 168
Barry, C., 337
Bartholomew, K., 259
Bartholow, K., 260
Bartolo, D., 336
Baryeh, N. A. K., 106, 113
Basow, S. A., 254
Basu, A., 190, 192
Batalova, J., 117
Batra, N., 4
Bauer, G. R., 105
Baxter, L. A., 163
Beach, W. A., 171, 192
Beach Slatten, T., 143
Bealieu-Volk, D., 148
Beaudoin, C., 306
Beaudoin-Ryan, L., 189
Beavin, J. H., 9, 41

401

Bechara, A., 246*b*
Beck, A. M., 136
Bedford, T., 125
Beijer, L., 188
Bell, D. J., 86, 192
Bell, K., 272*b*
Bell, K. K., 153
Bellafante, G., 272*b*
Bender, P., 261
Benjamin, J. M., 50
Bennett, C., 271
Bennis, W., 215
Berger, P., 173
Berggren, V., 142
Bergstrom, M. J., 159
Berkman, N. D., 194
Berkowitz, E. N., 228
Berlin Ray, E., 123, 173
Bernard, P., 325
Bernhard, T., 164, 165
Bernhardt, B. A., 48
Bernhardt, J. M., 190
Bernheim, S. M., 106
Bernstein, S., 272*b*
Berry, J. A., 87
Berry, J. D., 160
Berry, L. L., 82, 98, 99, 206, 218, 221, 226, 227
Bertakis, A. F., 71
Bertolino, M. V., 246*b*
Berwick, D., 28
Berwick, D. M., 30
Best, A. L., 334
Bethea, L. S., 55
Betts, D., 4
Betts, K., 243
Beutel, S., 113
Bevan, J. L., 168
Bias, S., 140, *140*
Bibace, R., 123
Biddlecom, A. E., 189, 196
Billicic, W., 23
Billings, D., 334
Bilmes, A., 254
Bilotte Verhoff, C., 189
Bindler, R. C., 97
Binns, J., 146
Birkeland, S., 14
Birkholt, M., 92
Bissell, K., 228, 242
Bitner, M. J., 320
Blair, J., 120, 121
Blanc, N., 337
Blascovich, J., 172
Blaszczynski, A., 259
Bleustein, C., 71
Blevins, C. E., 44
Bliss, W. G., 226
Block, S., 179
Blumler, J., 198

Bochner, S., 41
Bock, B. C., 53
Boden, W. E., 249
Bodie, G. D., 192
Boer, H., 334*b*
Boerner, K., 159
Bohm, D., 137*b*, 329
Bohrer, G. G., 175*b*
Bokhour, B. G., 40
Bolt, D., 240
Bonaguro, E. W., 11
Bond, B., 260
Bonnefon, J.-F., 183
Bono, C., 260
Bonsteel, A., 147
Boodman, S., 96
Booms, B. H., 320
Booth-Butterfield, M., 162
Booth-Butterfield, S., 162
Borden, N. H., 320
Boris, C., 262
Borkhoff, C. M., 142
Borkman, T., 331
Borreani, C., 181
Borzekowski, D. L. G., 240
Bose, N., 245
Bosman, J., 245
Boswell, R., 242
Botan, C. H., 303
Botta, R. A., 160
Bouchard, G. M., 40
Boulet, J. R., 50
Boulton, J., 70
Bowleg, L., 105
Boyce, J., 338
Boyd, J. E., 140, 332
Boyland, E., 242
Boylstein, C., 162
Braddock, K., 336
Bradley, E. H., 106
Bradshaw, Y. S., 122
Brady, M. J., 59
Braga-Mele, R., 81
Braithwaite, D. O., 121, 164, 259
Branch, W. T., Jr., 54
Brann, M., 163
Brannon, L., 314
Branstetter, J. E., 81, 89
Brashers, D. E., 167
Braun, B., 334
Braun, K. L., 108
Braveman, P., 106
Brazda, M. A., 171
Breen, N., 72
Brehm, J. W., 308
Brendryen, H., 204
Brennan, P. F., 296
Brett, A. L., 81, 89
Brett, R., 174
Brick, C., 71

Brier, P., 119
Brigaud, E., 337
Bringman, J., 86
Briñol, P., 313
Britton, P. C., 53
Brock, T. C., 336
Broderick, J. S., 21, 304
Brohi, N. A., 220
Broom, A., 48, 154
Broome, B., 144, 292
Brosius, H., 315
Brosnan, P., 245
Broussard, D., 288
Brown, J., 58
Brown, J. D., 260
Brown, T., 72*b*
Brown, V. A., 192
Brown, Z., 254
Brüggemann, A. J., 46
Buchholz, B., 124
Buckley, L. M., 45
Budden, J. S., 224*b*
Budzi, D., 87
Buhrau, D., 241
Buijzen, M., 242
Bulik, B. S., 252*b*
Bull, S., 203
Burda, D., 95, 204
Burgoon, J., 72
Burgoon, M., 72, 334*b*
Burke, A., 195
Burke, C., 314
Burkhammer, S., 274
Burleson, B. R., 166, 181, 315
Burroughs, E. L., 6
Burton, *309*
Buscaglia, L., 157
Bush, A., 86
Bute, J., 161*b*
Butler, H. A., 334*b*
Butler, J., 111
Butler, R. N., 126
Byck, R., 135
Bylund, C. L., 151, 199

Caba, J., 139
Caburnay, C., 337
Cacioli, J., 253
Cacioppo, J. T., 160, 313
Caldroney, R., 96
Callister, M., 125
Cameron, K. A., 244, 334*b*
Campbell, R., 315
Campbell, R. G., 340
Campo, S., 334*b*
Candib, L., 104
Caplan, S. E., 181
Cappella, J., 245
Capriotti, T., 154
Carbaat, L., 253–54

Carcioppolo, N., 338
Carlisle, M., 245
Carlsson, M., 71
Carmel, S., 127
Carpiac-Claver, M., 166
Carrese, J., 48
Carroll, D., 14
Carroll, M., 242
Carroll, S. E., 122
Carter, J., 219
Casabé, A., 246b
Casper, M. F., 304, 334b
Cassedy, J. H., 80
Cassell, E., 147
Castle, D., 197
Castle Bell, G., 112
Catania, G., 23
Cates, R. J., 222, 226, 232
Catlin, A., 91
Cavallaro, F., 125
Caviness, C. M., 44
Cegala, D. J., 60
Cella, D., 59b
Chaffee, S. H., 313
Chaiken, S., 191
Chamberlain, M., 211
Chan, E. A., 87
Chan, P., 254
Chang, L., 137, 222
Chanthavongas, S., 269
Charchuk, M., 165–66
Charlton, C. R., 87
Charmaz, K., 70
Charon, R., 57, 58, 60b
Chee, Y. T. F., 125
Chen, G., 220–21
Chen, H.-Y., 152
Chen, R., 201
Chen, S., 106, 191, 289
Chen, Y.-C., 136, 265
Cheng, W. J., 243
Cheong, P. H., 305
Chesler, M. A., 164
Chesser, A., 189, 195, 196
Chetty, R., 21, 105
Cheung, O., 262, 298
Cheung, T. L., 300
Chewning, L., 257
Chia, H. L., 159
Chi-Chuan, W., 154
Child, J. T., 304
Chilkotas, N. E., 84
Cho, H., 324–25
Cho, J., 194–95
Cho, N., 334b
Cho, S., 251
Cho, S.-H., 152
Cho, Y., 245
Choi, J., 249
Chokski, D. A., 4

Chou, W.-Y., 67
Chow, M., 30
Chowdhury, N., 245
Christakis, N., 334b
Christensen, J., 195
Christiaens, M., 164
Christmas, C., 127
Chung, P. H., 83, 125
Chung, Y., 313
Cimiotti, J. P., 224b
Citroner, G., 283–84
Clark, M., 203
Clark, S., 25
Clarke, C., 249–50
Clarke, J. N., 146
Clarke, L., 125, 270
Clark-Hitt, R., 304
Clayton, M. F., 4, 41, 48
Clayton, R., 311
Clements, B., 74
Clinch, C. R., 60
Cline, R., 248, 249
Clinton, B., 76b
Coast, J., 176
Cobb, C., 245
Coeling, H., 163
Cohen, C., 231
Cohen, E., 325
Cohen, J., 250
Cohen, M., 265
Cohen, S., 159
Collins, J. C., 223, 226
Collins, S. R., 113
Conley, B. J., 181, 183
Conley, M., 252b
Conlin, L., 228, 242
Conner, K. R., 53
Connor, T., 249, 272b
Conrad, P., 83
Cook, E., 40
Cooper, R. S., 112
Cooper, S., 120
Copas, A. J., 305
Corbelli, J., 81
Córdova, D., 44
Cornwall, L., 224b
Cornwell, T. B., 241
Corriea, A. R., 253
Cortés, D. E., 75
Cortese, D., 82, 99
Costabile, R. A., 246b
Coughlin, S. S., 206
Coulson, G., 259
Coupland, J., 54, 126
Coupland, N., 54, 126
Cousin, G., 66
Covello, V. T., 284
Cowart, D., 182b
Cox, L., 260
Cozma, R., 25

Craft, N., 203
Crandall, S. J., 119–20
Cranley, L. A., 81, 89
Creagan, E., 172
Crenshaw, K. W., 105
Crosby, L., 228
Crowder, M. K., 143
Cruz, D., 272b
Cruz, G. G., 106
Cubanksi, J., 32
Cunningham, C. B., 183
Currie, D., 232
Cutrona, C. E., 165

Daalmans, S., 253–54
D'Agostino, N., 168
D'Agostino, T. A., 81
Dahlstrom, A., 252b
Dahm, M. R., 71
Da Leo, G., 206
Dalgliesh, J., 143
Dall, T., 224b
Damhewage, G., 281–82
D'Antonio, M., 53, 91b
Daratha, K., 97
Davey, R., 140
Davidoff, F., 47
da Vinci, L., 10
Davis, B., 122b
Davis, D., 140
Davis, F. D., 193
Davis, G. B., 193
Davis, J., 249
Davis, K., 32, 341
Davis, K. C., 295, 309, 341
Davis, L., 107, 257
Davis, S., 4, 119–20
Davison, W. P., 240
Dawson, K. S., 172
Deagle, G., 44
Dean, M., 88
Dearing, K. S., 87
Deary, I. J., 251
Deatrick, L. M., 308
De Bonis, W., 246b
DeBuono, B., 15, 109
de Charms, R., 224–25
de Droog, S. M., 242
Defenbaugh, N., 68, 84
DeFrank, J., 247, 248
Deinard, A., 137
De Laender, N., 107
Delgado, C., 332
DeLucia, M., 172
De Maeseneer, J. M., 107
DeMatteo, D., 244
De Meulenaer, S., 330
Demiris, G., 13
Demmel, R., 54
DeMonner, S., 144

Dempsey, A. F., 106, 115
Denham, B. E., 338
Dennis, M. R., 160
Dens, N., 330
Dentel, E., 200
De Pelsmacker, P., 330
De Ridder, D. T., 300
de Rijk, A., 164
Dervin, B., 51
de Souza, R., 6, 328
Desrochers, D. M., 241
Desroches, N. G., 44
Deveugele, M., 107
DeVries, R., 334b
DeWalt, D. A., 110
Dharmananda, S., 134
Diamond, G. A., 249
Dickson, H. G., 115
DiClemente, C. C., 324
DiCorcia, M., 257
Diekema, D., 43b
Diem, S., 256, 257
Dierckx de Casterl, B., 164
DiFranza, J. R., 261
Dilger, D., 108–9
Dill, M. J., 224b
Dillard, A. J., 338
Dillard, J., 336
Dillard, J. P., 240, 340
Dillon, J. M., 189, 193
Dillon, P. J., 48
Dillow, M. R., 163
DiMatteo, M. R., 139, 150
D'Innocenzo, L., 220
Dinwiddie, G. Y., 113
Dixon, G. N., 250
Dizon, Z. B., 44
Dluzewska, T., 88
Do, T.-P., 122
Dodd, V., 190
Doidge, K., 218, 220
Doles, B., 246b
Dolman, L., 112
Domschke, T., 159
Donahue, M. O., 222
Donceel, P., 164
Done, N., 33
Donelan, K., 219
Donohew, L., 308, 309
Donohue, G. A., 305
Donovan, E. E., 109
Donovan-Kicken, E., 161b
Dorsey, J. L., 28, 30
Dossaji, M., 40
Doty, M. M., 113
Douki, S., 142
Dozier, D. M., 229
Dragojevic, M., 330, 331
Drainoni, M.-L., 75
Drayson, M. T., 14

Dreisbach, S., 254
Dreyer, J., 53
Drucker, P., 97
D'Silva, M. U., 309
Dube, S. P., 85
Duck, S., 159, 164
Duewald, M., 254
Duggan, A., 89, 121, 122
Duggleby, W., 146
Duke, A., 145
Dumlao, R., 160
Duncan, J., 308
Duncan, T., 279, 281
Dunlop, S., 336
Dunwoody, S., 191
Duplaga, M., 193
du Pré, A., 125, 173, 174, 220, 222
Durà-Vilà, G., 135
Durkin, E., 271
Durso, S. C., 127
Dutta, M. J., 6, 132, 190, 192, 264, 315, 326, 328, 329, 332
Dutta-Bergman, M. J., 306, 326, 327, 328, 329
Dwyer, F. R., 228
Dyer, J., 181
Dykes, P. C., 222, 232
Dym, H., 16, 41
Dyrbye, L. N., 16

Ebener, D., 258
Eckert, S., 279
Edgar, T., 47, 48, 115, 123, 124, 306
Edwards, H., 171
Effertz, T., 308
Egbert, N., 163, 174
Egerton, J., 71
Eggly, S., 59b
Eisenberg, L., 134
Eisenman, D. P., 113
Elam-Evans, L. D., 272b
Elbert, S., 332
Ellard, J. H., 166
Ellingson, L. L., 92
Ellington, L., 4, 41
Ellis, B. H., 92
Elwyn, G., 65
Emanuel, E. J., 182
Emanuel, L. L., 182
Emed, J., 40
Emilsson, M., 73
Emme, C., 205
Endy, T. P., 288
Eneli, I. U., 324
Engelen, S., 332
Englehardt, C., 260
English, J., 161
Epstein, R. M., 4, 41, 81, 88
Erceg-Hurn, D., 312
Erdelyi, M. H., 262

Erdman, L., 181
Erickson, S., 95
Eriksson, M., 279
Eriksson, T., 40
Escarce, J. J., 107
Escudero, V., 9
Esmaeilzadeh, P., 209
Estrada, L. F., 4
Evans, B. C., 131
Evans, N., 106, 113
Evans, W. D., 341
Everett, M. W., 309
Ezeanochie, N., 203

Faden, R., 327b
Fadiman, A., 139
Fagioli, J., 135
Fahey, K. F., 52
Fallon, E. A., 254
Farahani, B., 197, 207
Farber, N. J., 45, 46
Fardouly, J., 254
Farrar, J., 286
Farrar, K. M., 260
Farrelly, M. C., 295, 298, 309, 341
Farsch, K., 54
Fathi, J., 209
Faulkner, S. L., 189
Fawcett, K., 257–58
Fearn-Banks, K., 231
Fellinghauer, B. G., 258
Fenton, J. J., 71
Ferguson, B., 110
Ferguson, E., 54
Fernandez, A., 135
Fernandez, S., 227
Ferraro, A. J., 14
Fertig, N., 245
Festinger, L., 241
Fiabane, E., 93
Fico, A. E., 70
Field, L., 41
Fincham, F. D., 259
Fine, L., 159
Fink, S. V., 296
Finkelstein, A., 127
Finney Rutten, L. J., 67
Fiscella, K., 50, 81
Fischer, P. M., 261
Fishbein, M., 193, 323
Fisher, C. L., 160
Fisher, J. A., 147
Fitzgerald, E., 265
Fitzpatrick, J. J., 222, 232
Fleming, M. D., 107
Flood-Grady, E., 141
Flora, J. A., 313, 320
Flower, L., 49
Floyd, K., 160
Flynn, J. J., 168

Flynn, T. N., 176
Folwell, A., 127
Forbes, G., 206, 254
Ford, D. E., 207
Ford, L. A., 167
Forman, J., 144
Forsythe, L. P., 165
Fossum, S., 244
Foster, E., 180–81
Fouad, A. M., 4
Fowkes, F. G. R., 251
Fowler, B. A., 107
Fowler, C., 125, 126, 127
Fowler, E. F., 251
Fowler, J., 334b
Fox, M., 249, 272b
Fox, R., 91
Fox, S., 189
Fox, S. A., 107
Frank, A., 237
Frank, L., 289, 290, 292
Frank, L. B., 106
Franke, M., 308
Frankel, R., 42
Frankel, R. M., 183
Frankl, V., 173
Franks, P., 71
Frates, J., 175b
Freed, G. L., 272b
Freeman, G., 70
Freimuth, V., 191, 274, 306
Fremonta, L. M., 46
Frenette, M., 51
Frey, L. R., 303
Freytag, J., 257
Fried, T. R., 83, 181
Friederichs, S. H., 314
Friedersdorf, C., 272b
Friedman, D. B., 6, 111, 251, 334
Friedman, H., 139, 150
Friedman, P. G., 303
Friedmann, E., 172
Frizell, S., 281
Frosch, D. L., 65
Fry, R. B., 162
Fryar, C., 242
Fryberg, S. A., 14
Fry-Johnson, Y., 208
Frymier, A. B., 160
Fuedtner, C., 43b
Fukuda, H., 73
Fullam, F., 40
Fuller, J., 133, 134
Fullman, N., 30, 32
Furber, L., 192

Gabrhelik, R., 204
Gade, C. J., 46, 60b
Gaglioti, A. H., 106
Gahbauer, S., 189

Galanti, G.-A., 132, 133, 134
Gallagher, S. S., 14, 15, 256
Galloway, M., 244
Gantz, W., 251
Gao, H., 132
Gardner, E., 123
Garfield, R., 33, 106
Garret, P. W., 115
Garza, M. A., 113
Gates, L., 58
Gaudet, H., 315
Geertz, C., 9
Geist, P., 53, 58, 122
Geist-Martin, P., 153, 164, 168
Geller, G., 48
Gelsema, T. I., 93
Gentile, D. A., 258, 261
George, A., 277
Gerbner, G., 240, 261
Gerrard, M., 334b
Gerritsen, M., 188
Getman, R., 195
Ghadlinge, M. S., 85
Ghafhari-Fam, S., 323
Gibbons, F. X., 334b
Giles, H., 54, 125, 126
Giles, L. C., 159
Gill, E. A., 167
Gill, J., 89
Gill, P., 120
Gillespie, R., 69
Gillespie, S. R., 73
Gillis, K., 208
Gillotti, C., 184
Gilman, S. L., 139
Gilmour, D., 304
Gilotra, N. A., 73
Gilstrap, C. M., 163
Giner-Sorolla, R., 191
Ginossar, T., 113
Giorgi, I., 93
Giuliani, R., 274
Gjorgievska, A., 260
Glass, R., 150
Glaysher, K., 120
Glik, D. C., 271
Glittenberg, J. E., 148
Glonek, G. F., 159
Go, E., 332
Goble, R., 117
Goffman, E., 68, 140
Goins, E. S., 111, 112
Golden, A., 298, 299b
Goldsmith, J., 178, 180
Goldstein, A. O., 261
Goldstein, K., 251
Good, B., 134
Goode, E. E., 137
Goodhart, F. W., 334
Goodyear, V., 203

Gordon, E. J., 73
Gordon, G. H., 91b
Gordon, R., 320
Gothe, N., 321, 322
Goyal Wasan, P., 320
Gozu, A., 127
Grady, M., 115
Grandpre, J. R., 334b
Granja, C., 197, 208, 210
Grant, J. A., 127
Graubard, B. I., 72
Gray, K., 197
Gray, S. W., 107
Green, C. E., 247
Green, E. C., 338
Green, K. C., 224b
Green, M. C., 336
Green, R., 174b, 175–76
Greene, K., 46, 47, 265
Griffin, M., 125
Griffin, M. Q., 232
Griffin, R. J., 191, 222
Grist-Gordon, V., 258
Grönroos, C., 320
Groopman, J., 56, 67, 115, 209
Gross, L., 240, 261
Grunig, J. E., 229
Grunig, L. A., 229
Guadagno, M., 109
Gualtieri, L., 15
Gubler, J., 261
Guidry, J., 279
Guiton, G., 116
Gunningberg, L., 71
Gunther, A. C., 240
Guntzviller, L. M., 107
Guo, H., 338
Gupta, V., 136
Gurevitch, M., 198
Gustafson, D. H., 169
Gustafsson, P. A., 73
Gustavo, S. A., 142
Guy, B., 228

Hagemeier, N. E., 84
Hagen, K. S., 84
Hägglund, D., 143
Hain, D., 151b
Haines, M. P., 334b
Hakoyama, M., 302
Halbesleben, J. R., 89
Halbreich, U., 142
Hales, C., 242
Halkowski, T., 58
Hall, H. T., 179
Hall, I. J., 72, 190, 334
Hall, J. A., 66
Hall, L. H., 89
Hall, S., 97
Haller, B., 258

Halpern-Felsher, B., 245
Hamdidouche, I., 73
Hammond, D., 245
Hammond, S. L., 306
Hample, D., 337
Hample, J. M., 337
Han, J. Y., 169
Handley, L., 201
Hankivsky, O., 104
Hanna, G., 50, 53
Happell, B., 90
Haque, F., 21
Hardy, Y., 85
Harkness, E. L., 259
Harmon, C., 88
Harres, A., 54
Harrington, N. G., 67
Harris, B. S., 254
Harrison, K., 241–42
Harrison, R., 120
Harrison, T. R., 175b, 257
Harter, L., 57–58, 121
Hartzband, P., 209
Harvey, J., 205
Harwood, J., 68–69
Haskard, K. B., 81
Haskell, H., 124
Haslett, B. J., 181
Haviland, M. L., 295, 341
Hawkins, R., 199
Hawkley, L. C., 160
Haynes, M. T., 160
He, X., 54
Healton, C. G., 295, 341
Heath, C., 64
Heboyan, V., 206
Hecht, M. L., 336
HeeKyung, C., 127
Hegedus, K., 178
Heifetz, M., 121
Heisler, M., 144
Heldman, C., 259
Heley, K., 337
Helft, L., 272b
Hellen, A., 246b
Helme, D. W., 309, 326, 332
Helms, S. W., 308
Helmstetter, K., 260
Henault, L. E., 75
Hendrich, A., 30
Hendriks, H., 338
Hendrix, K. S., 272b
Henley, S., 83
Hennessy, M., 260
Hergenrather, K. C., 111
Heritage, J., 44
Herman, D. S., 44
Hermann, J., 190
Herrick, S., 261
Herzberg, F., 225

Hess, R., Jr., 84, 319
Hesse, B. W., 67
Hesse, C., 160
Hessler, R. M., 80–81, 134
Hesson, A., 54
Hetsroni, A., 257
Heuer, C., 140
High, A., 195
Hildebrandt, C. A., 119–20
Hilgard, J., 260
Hill, D., 240
Hillier, D., 273, 283
Hills, R., 258–59
Himes, K. L., 163
Hines, S., 167, 244
Hinkelbein, J., 256
Hinojosa, R., 162
Hinton, L., 198, 199
Hirschmann, K., 83
Hitchman, S., 245
Hitti, E. A., 256
Ho, A. L., 81
Ho, C., 136
Ho, E. Y., 137, 151
Hodes, M., 135
Hofstede, G., 147
Hogan, H., 125, 175–76
Hoge, M. A., 89
Holden, W., 288, 289
Holland, E., 254
Holland, J. C., 139
Holland, J. J., 305
Hollenstein, T., 168
Holliday, J., 315
Hollister, L., 97
Holmes, M. E., 159
Holt, D. J., 241
Holtgrave, D. R., 324
Holton, A., 250
Hong, S. G., 190
Hooker, R., 87
Hooker, S. P., 6
Hoor, G., 338
Hoppe, R. B., 54
Horan, N. M., 85
Hornik, R. C., 107, 193, 198
Horosewski, M. L., 309
Horowitz, A., 106, 159
Horvath, K. J., 196
Horwath, C., 325
Hou, J., 169, 198
Houston, T., 207
Hovick, S. R., 107
Hoy, W., 221
Hrisanfow, E., 143
Hsiao, A.-F., 33
Huang, K. T., 81
Hubbell, A. P., 305
Hudson, A. P., 22, 23
Hudson, J., 331

Huebner, N., 232
Hufford, D. J., 150
Huhman, M., 306
Hullett, C. R., 338
Hummert, M. L., 45, 125
Hunt, J. M., 73
Hunt, S., 228–29
Hurley, R. J., 251
Hust, S. J. T., 244, 259, 260
Huston, L., 201
Hutch, R., 149
Hutchinson, A., 278
Hwang, S. S., 113
Hyun, J. H., 190

Iacob, E., 4, 41
Iles, I., 332
Imes, R., 199
Inbar, M., 309
Irungu, E., 284
Isaacson, J., 42
Itou, T., 86

Jackson, D. D., 9, 41
Jackson, K. T., 229–30
Jacobs, E., 135
Jacobs, J., 210
Jacobson, S. K., 40
Jadad, A. R., 71
James, J. T., 124
James, S. D., 246b
Jamieson, K., 251, 288
Jamieson, P. E., 261
Al-Janabi, H., 176
Jang, S. A., 334b
Jangland, E., 71
Janis, I., 99
Janssen, L., 338
Jaouad, S., 169–70, 170, 172
Jarrett, T., 246b
Jauhar, S., 76b, 83
Jenkins, H., 117
Jenkins, M., 324
Jenner, C., 260
Jensen, J. D., 107, 251, 333
Jeong, H. J., 162
Jerant, A. F., 71
Jerit, J., 250–51, 289
Jernigan, D. H., 244
Jha, A. K., 70
Jiang, J., 189
Jiang, S., 25, 40, 198, 207
Jimenez-Zambrano, A. M., 115
Jin, H. K., 81
Joa, 193
Jobes, M., 222
Johal, P., 87
Johnson, C., 333
Johnson, D., 274
Johnson, J., 89

Johnson, J. A., 302
Johnson, J. Q., 264
Johnson, K., 203
Johnson, L. J., 209
Johnson, M. J., 87
Johnson, P., 254
Johnson, R. A., 136
Johnson, S., 325
Johnson, T. P., 113–14
Johnston, L. D., 296
Jones, A., 87
Jones, C., 321
Jones, D., 120
Jones, J., 269
Jones, K. O., 338
Jones, R., 71, 189
Jones, R. K., 196
Joo, J. H., 81
Jordan, Z., 50
Juckett, G., 117
Judd, D., 81
Julliard, K., 45
Jung, J., 254
Junghans, A. F., 300

Kahled, DJ, 331
Kahlor, L., 107
Kaiser, K., 113–14
Kaiser, S., 244
Kakai, H., 43*b*
Kaldjian, L. C., 219
Kalenderian, E., 195
Kalkbrenner, M., 203
Kane, C., 208
Kane, R. L., 127
Kang, H., 244–45
Kang, S., 264
Kaplan, R., 49
Kaplan, S. A., 258
Kappel, S., 33
Karabenick, S. A., 143
Karadas, N., 115
Karcher, N., 203, 204
Kareklas, I., 330
Karlsson, M., 331
Kashima, Y., 336
Katz, E., 198
Katz, J., 42, 74
Kaufman, J. S., 112
Kaur, M., 140
Kawabata, H., 86
Kay, L. S., 324
Kealey, E., 194
Kean, J., 290
Kean, L. G., 242
Kean, S., 139
Kean, T. J., 191
Kearney, M., 149
Kearney, T., 164
Keddington, K., 259

Keeley, M., 179
Kees, *309*
Keller-Olaman, S., 161
Kelso, P. D., 338
Kemmelmeier, M., 143
Kennedy, J., 154
Kennedy-Hendricks, A., 337
Kenney, C., 86
Kessels, L., 332, 338
Kevorkian, J., 182*b*
Khawaja, M., 142
Khosravi, P., 206
Khullar, D., 4, 24–25
Khvitsko, T., 8
Kilbane, M., 54
Kilbourne, J., 252*b*
Killawi, A., 144
Kilonzo, N., 284
Kim, D. W., 190
Kim, E., 169, 336
Kim, H., 195
Kim, H. J., 333
Kim, H. Y., 336
Kim, J., 336
Kim, K., 189
Kim, M., 245
Kim, S., 256
Kim, S.-H., 310*b*
Kimppa, K. K., 190
King, 264
King, A. J., 107
King, W., 93–94
Kinsler, J., 260
Kipling, R., 336
Kiragu, M., 284
Kirby, D., 88
Kirch, M., 25
Kirkham, S. R., 132, 144
Kisa, K., 86
Klass, P., 83
Kleemans, M., 253–54
Klein, W. M. P., 338
Kleinman, A., 134
Klinken Whelan, A., 115
Klum, H., *339*
Knerr, W., 284
Knight, S. J., 33, 181
Knight-Agarwal, C. R., 140
Kober, H., 242
Koch, L., 163
Koch-Weser, S., 15, 189
Koczwara, A., 54
Kodish, E., 42
Kodjebacheva, G. D., 4
Koenig Kellas, J., 141
Koerner, C. D., 54
Kok, G., 338
Kolasa, M., 272*b*
Kolodner, K., 48
Komaroff, A. L., 135

Kopfman, J., 123
Koszalinski, R. S., 68
Kotler, P., 320
Koven, S., 111
Kowalewski, D., 260
Kowalski, K. M., 197
Krajewski, L. A., 143
Kramer, H., 178
Kramer, K., 178
Kramer, S., 260
Krantz-Kent, R., 239
Kravitz, R. L., 192
Krcmar, M., 260
Kreps, G. L., 4, 10, 11, 15, 92, 99, 149, 174, 303
Kreuter, M., 337
Krieger, J. L., 51
Krug, P., 182
Krumholz, H. M., 106
Kübler-Ross, E., 181
Kuijer, R., 338
Kulhánek, A., 204
Kulik, J. A., 336
Kulkarni, M. B., 85
Kumar, R., 143, 189, 199
Kundrat, A. L., 68, 121, 160
Kurinczuk, J. J., 198
Kwon, N., 189
Kyrrestad Strøm, H., 244
Kyrsko, M., 44

Lacks, H., 43, 74–75
Lafata, J., 206
Laframboise, D., 176
Lagoe, C., 70
Laine, C., 47
Laitman, L., 334
Lambert, B. L., 59*b*
Lane, D., 277
Lane, L. T., 308
Lang, A., 309, 313
Lansdale, D., 128
Lantos, J., 256
Lapinski, M. K., 334*b*
Lapowsky, I., 331
Larasi, I., 259
Larkin, M., 202
Larson, S., 207
Lau, J., 324
Lauer, C. S., 82
Lauricella, A., 189
Laux, J. P., 181
Lavoie, N. R., 296
Lazarsfeld, P., 315
Lederman, L. C., 319, 320, 334
Ledlow, G. R., 302
Lee, C., 107
Lee, E. L., 334*b*
Lee, F., 79, 221–22, 229
Lee, H. E., 194–95

Lee, J., 332
Lee, J.-S., 152
Lee, K., 249
Lee, M. J., 199, 244–45
Lee, P., 325
Lee, S., 194, 309, 313
Lee, S.-J., 265
Lee, T., 337
Lee, Y. J., 189, 193, 194, 198
Lefebvre, R. C., 307, 320
Légaré, F., 50, 65
Lehman, D. R., 166
L'Engle, K. L., 260
Leon, J. B., 73
Lepage, K., 40
Lesser, C. S., 50, 81
Levin, D., 252*b*
Levinsky, N., 114*b*
Levinson, W., 168–69
Levy, B. R., 125
Levy-Storms, L., 166
Lewis, C., 22
Lewis, L. S., 248
Lewis, N., 107
Lewis-Fernández, R., 134
Li, C.-C., 40, 41
Li, H. Z., 44
Li, J., 244
Li, N., 192
Li, Y., 85
Liang, A., 249
Liang, C., 315
Liang, M., 107
Liebhart, J. L., 240
Lief, H., 91
Lim, J. C. J., 137
Lim, R., 262, 298, 300, 311
Lin, F., 181
Lin, J., 189, 194, 198
Lin, S.-M., 222
Lindberg, D. A. B., 128
Lindley, L. L., 111
Ling, P., 245
Lipkin, M., Jr., 87
Lipkis, I., 333
Little, V., 134
Littlefield, R. S., 277
Liu, K., 73
Lo, M.-C. M., 67, 70
Lockwood, N. L., 160
Long, A., 113
Long, S. D., 175*b*
Longcope, W. T., 39
Longino, C., 12
Lordly, D., 83
Loustaunau, M. O., 136, 137, 142
Love, A., 187–88
Lovell, B., 14
Lowe, G., 246*b*
Lowman, S. G., 110

Lowrey, W., 150
Lozano, R., 32
Lu, J., 278
Lu, Z., 30
Luc Honore Petnji, Y., 199
Luciano, M. M., 220
Luckmann, T., 173
Ludtke, M., 253
Lui, X., 210
Lunsky, Y., 121
Lurie, S., 87
Lustria, M., 309, 313
Luszcz, M. A., 159
Lwin, M., 278, 279, 289, 324
Lyapustina, T., 290–91
Lyon, A., 248

Maathius, E., 45
Mabry, A., 109
MacDonald, M., 139
Macias, W., 128, 248
Macías-González, V. M., 143
Mackert, M., 109
Mackey, A., 168
MacLellan, D. L., 83
Madanikia, Y., 259
Maertens, J. A., 115
Maezawa, M., 86
Magee, M., 53, 91*b*
Magoffin, D., 125
Magsamen-Conrad, K., 189, 193–94, 198
Maher, D., 284
Mahler, H. I. M., 334*b*
Mahomed, N. N., 70
Maibach, E., 302
Maier, J. A., 258
Major, A. M., 334*b*
Makarem, S. C., 73
Makoul, G., 4, 41
Malani, P., 25
Malik, T. K., 54
Malis, R. S., 160
Mallon, M., 280*b*
Maloney, E., 245
Mammen, S., 334
Manfredi, C., 113–14
Mannix, M. E., 124
Manns, H., 160
Manolis, C., 199
Manzoor, M., 206
Marantz, P., 141
Margesson, R., 281
Margonelli, L., 75
Marin, A. J., 119–20
Maring, E., 334
Marion, G. S., 119–20
Marks, J., 160
Markus, H. R., 14
Marras, C., 205

Mars, R., 85
Marshall, E., 338
Marteinsdottir, I., 73
Martin, C., 91*b*
Martins, N., 161*b*
Martinussen, M., 244
Marwick, C., 134
Masi, C. M., 160
Maslach, C., 89
Mast, M. S., 66
Mastin, T., 249
Mata, A., *217*
Mata, K., *217*
Mathieu, J. E., 220
Matsaganis, M. D., 107, 298, 299*b*
Matthews, A. K., 40, 113–14
Matthews, J., 84
Mausner, B., 225
Maxmen, A., 268, 282, 283
May, N. B., 95
May, S. G., 65
Mayer, D., 124
Mayer, M., 245
Mayer, T. A., 222, 226, 232
Maynard, D. W., 183
Maynard, M. T., 220
Mazloff, D., 45
Mazur, A., 241, 242
McAlister, A. R., 241
McCague, J., 124
McCall, C., 47
McCann, R. M., 125
McCarley, P., 53
McCarthy, D., 279, 281
McCarthy, J., 272*b*
McCaul, K. D., 338
McComas, K., 271–72
McConatha, D., 128
McCormack, L., 341
McCormick, T. R., 181, 183
McCreaddie, M., 55
McCue, J. D., 178–79
McCune, S. K., 136
McDonald, P., 288, 289
McElligott, J., 205
McGinnis, T., 330
McGregor, D., 225
McIntyre, K. A., 304
McKeever, B. W., 250
McKinley, C. J., 50, 89
McKnight, L., 252*b*
McLean, S., 239
McMillan, S., 128
McPherson, E., 339*b*
McQueen, A., 337
McWhinney, I., 149
Mead, E. L., 135
Mead, G. H., 83
Meakin, R., 120
Medina, L., 24

Meerkerk, G.-J., 243–44
Mehrotra, A., 205
Meili, H. K., 264
Melki, J. P., 256
Meltzer, W., 272, 275b
Mendenhall, E., 135
Mendes, W. B., 172
Menegatos, L., 319
Meredith, L. S., 113
Merritt, A., 262
Merz, M. Y., 148
Messeri, P., 295, 341
Meterko, M., 40
Metts, S., 160
Micalizzi, D. A., 94
Michelson, L. D., 23
Miech, R. A., 296
Milika, R. M., 71
Miller, A., 265
Miller, C. H., 308, 334b
Miller, K., 171
Miller, K. I., 92
Miller, K. S., 142
Miller, L., 165, 166
Miller, M., 121
Miller, S., 221
Miller, W., 52
Miller-Day, M., 160, 336
Mills, A. B., 229
Mills, C. B., 172–73
Milne, C., 97
Minor, L., 200
Minton, L., 226
Miovic, M. K., 46
Mirren, H., 125, *126*
Mirzaeian, K., 323
Mishler, E. G., 65, 82
Mizobe, M., 73
Modahl, M., 209
Modave, F., 195
Modin, H., 209
Moffatt, L., 117
Moldogaziev, T., 227
Moldovan-Johnson, M., 198
Mollen, S., 332
Montague, H., 189
Montgomery, B. M., 163
Moonhee, Y., 264
Moore, G., 197, 198
Moore, J., 125
Moore, L., 315
Moore, L. G., 148
Moore, L. W., 121
Moradi, F., 323
Moran, M. B., 106, 306
Morgan, L. A., 171
Morgan, M., 240, 261
Morgan, R., 228–29
Morgan, S. E., 54, 175, 175b, 257
Moriarty, C. M., 251

Moritsugu, K., 281b, 291b
Morozov, S., 207
Morrell, B. L. M., 84
Morris, D., 84
Morris, J. L., 143
Morris, M. G., 193
Morrison, D., 331
Morse, 264
Mosavel, M., 305
Moser, R. P., 67
Moss, M., 14, 255b
Moulton, P., 224b
Mouton, A., 54
Moyse, E., 126
Mudambi, S. M., 73
Muehling, D., 330
Mufarrij, A. A., 256
Mugo, N., 284
Mulac, A., 126
Mullan, B. M., 259
Mullet, E., 184
Mungal, S. U., 85
Muralidharan, S., 336
Murgatroyd, C., 139
Murphy, E., 222
Murphy, S. T., 106
Murphy-Graham, E., 14
Murray, D., 95
Muskin, P. R., 171, 183
Mussap, A. J., 253

Nabi, R. L., 337, 340
Nacef, F., 142
Naeem, A. G., 139
Nagel, S., 289, 290, 292
Nan, X., 332
Napier, D., 132
Nass, C. I., 265
Nathanson, A. I., 265
Navrazhina, K., 125
Needleman, J., 224
Neihardt, J. G., 139
Neiman, A. B., 72
Nelkin, D., 139
Nemeth, S., 121
Nestle, M., 243
Netemeyer, 309
Netherton, T., 172
Neuwirth, K., 191
Newman, M., 137b
Ng, B. C., 125
Ng, R., 152
Ngure, K., 284
Nguyen, A.-M., 41, 195
Nicholas, D. B., 168
Nicksie, N., 245
Nicolai, J., 54
Nie, J., 73
Niederdeppe, J., 196, 251, 309, 336, 337

Nishimoto, N., 86
Noar, S. M., 309, 322
Nøhr, O. N., 50
Nolan, D., 292
Noller, P., 171
Noorani, T., 331
Norcross, J. C., 324
Nordby, H., 50
Norling, G. R., 67
Novack, D. H., 46, 88
Novák, D., 204
Nowak, K. L., 260
Nussbaum, J. F., 11, 68, 121, 123, 124, 125, 126, 127, 160
Nutt, K., 143
Nyhan, B., 272b
Nyström, L., 142

Obama, B., 281
O'Brien, M. K., 46
Occa, A., 54
O'Connell, N., 205
O'Connor, D. B., 89
October, T. W., 44
O'Daniel, M., 90
Oeldorf-Hirsch, A., 195, 203
O'Flynn, J., 239
Ogden, C. L., 242
Oghia, M. J., 256
Oh, S., 228
Ohnstrom, G., 73
O'Keefe, D. J., 333, 337
Okoror, T., 132
Okwerekwu, J. A., 115
Olien, C. N., 305
Oliver, D. P., 13
Olson, K. D., 89
Olufowote, J. O., 82
O'Malley, P. M., 296
O'Neil, K., 254
Ophir, Y., 251, 278, 288, 289
Orav, E. J., 70
O'Reilly, K. B., 110
Orgera, K., 33, 106, 113
O'Rourke, K. D., 75
Orrange, S., 192
Ortman, J. M., 125, 175–76
Ositelu, F., 80
Osler, W., 43
Østvang, T., 200
Otilingam, P. G., 140
Ots, P., 332
Overton, B. C., 125, 196, 197, 198, 205, 209, 210
Owens, J. E., 95
Owermohl, S., 245

Paasche-Orlow, M. K., 75
Pacey, A., 256
Padela, A., 144

Padon, A., 245
Paek, H.-J., 308
Paganini, N., 139
Page-Reeves, J., 105
Palmer, S., 204
Palmer-Wackerly, A. L., 51
Palmgreen, P., 308, 309
Palokangas, M., 197
Pan, R., 85
Pan, W., 254, 333
Pang, J. S., 243
Papi, A., 73
Paris, M., 89
Park, E., 127
Park, J., 194
Park, M., 81
Park, S., 332
Parker, P. A., 192
Parker, S., 4
Parker-Pope, T., 246*b*
Parker-Raley, J., 183
Parkes, C., 181
Parrott, R., 11, 124, 302, 306, 339
Pashupati, K., 248
Passalacqua, S. A., 160
Pasteur, L., 134
Pateet, J. R., 46
Patel, D. S., 270
Patel, S., 134
Patel, U., 244
Paterniti, D. A., 85
Patterson, E., 70
Patterson, F., 54
Patterson, J., 231
Patterson, J. D., 208
Payne, S., 55
Pearson, J. C., 304
Peate, I., 143
Pecchioni, L., 55, 125, 127
Pedala, M., 174*b*
Peeke, P., 263*b*
Pelto-Piri, V., 42
Peña, J., 254
Peñaranda, E., 195
Pendleton, D., 148
Pennic, J., 206
Pennycott, A., 258
Pepicello, J., 222
Peretti-Watel, P., 106
Perino, C., 89
Perrin, A., 128, 189, 199
Perrin, E., 242
Perry, B., 180
Peters, E., 337, 340
Peters, L., 228
Peters, T., 140
Peterson, B., 163
Peterson, C. C., 160
Petroff, A., 281
Petty, R. E., 313

Phillips, A. C., 14
Phillips, O. P., 86
Philogene, G., 159
Philpott, A., 284
Phua, J., 331
Piazza, I. M., 222
Pighin, S., 183
Pilling, V., 314
Pincus, C. R., 91
Pincus, H., 134
Piñeiro, B., 113
Pinkleton, B. E., 265
Piotrow, P. T., 262
Plante, C., 261
Platt, F. W., 91*b*, 168–69
Plews-Ogan, M., 95–96
Plotkin, I., 269
Polmear-Swendris, N., 241
Polonec, L. D., 306, 334*b*
Ponnet, K., 259
Popova, L., 245
Porter, R. E., 132
Porticella, N., 336
Potter, E., 176
Potter, J., 54, 111
Potts, K. A., 308
Pratt, M., 206
Prentice-Dunn, S., 162
Press, I., 221, 232
Presser, N., 203, 204
Pribble, J., 251
Price, K., 41
Price, R., 261
Prividera, L., 242
Prochaska, J. O., 324, 325
Puhl, R., 140
Purnell, L. D., 139
Pye, D., 111, 112

Qian, S., 337
Qiang, J. K., 205
Quant, C., 203
Quenqua, D., 253
Query, J. L., Jr., 11, 92
Quesada, A., 265
Quick, B. L., 296
Al-Qutob, R., 142

Ra, C., 240
Rabinowitz, F. E., 143
Rack, L., 81
Radesky, J., 240, 243
Raffel, M. W., 134
Raffel, N. K., 134
Ragan, S., 124, 125, 127, 178, 179, 180
Rains, S. A., 169, 305, 308
Ramanadhan, S., 162
Ramasubramanian, S., 257
Ramírez, A. S., 107
Rampell, C., 143

Rao, J. K., 181
Rapaport, L., 4
Rasmussen, P. W., 113
Rattigan, S. H., 122
Ratzan, S., 272, 275*b*, 281, 291*b*
Ravanbakht, S., 242
Real, K., 334*b*
Reblin, M., 4, 41
Recktenwald, D., 187–88
Redfern, J. S., 111, 112
Reed, K. P., 244
Reeds, K., 134
Reese, S., 207
Reid, J., 245
Reifler, J., 272*b*
Reilly, P., 84
Reinhardt, J. D., 258
Reinhardt, J. P., 159
Rendle, K. A. S., 65
Reno, J. E., 53
Renwick, R., 258
Reyes, J., 195
Reynolds, B., 287
Rheaume, C. E., 6
Rhiannon, 23
Rhoades, E., 244
Rhodes, H., 113
Rhodes, N. D., 51
Rhodes, S. D., 111
Richard, J. W., 261
Richards, A. S., 308
Richardson, B., 97
Richey, S., 272*b*
Richtel, M., 245
Rideout, V., 189
Rifkin, L., 292
Rimal, R., 162, 331, 334*b*
Rimon, J. G., II, 262
Rittman, M., 162
Rizo, C. A., 71
Roberto, A. J., 313
Roberts, D. F., 265
Roberts, J. A., 199
Robertson, T., 182
Robinson, A. J., 305
Robinson, J. D., 44, 159, 164, 207
Robinson, T., 125
Rocque, G. B., 23
Rodgers, R., 239
Rodgers, S., 259
Rodriguez, H. P., 81
Rodzwicz, S., *165*
Rodzwicz, V., *165*
Rogers, E. M., 296, 315, 331
Rogers, K. B., 244
Rogers, K. E., 168
Rogers, L. E., 9
Roggenkamp, S. D., 228
Rohde, J. A., 141
Rohrberg, T., 195

Rollnick, S., 52
Roloff, M. E., 122, 160
Romain, A. J., 325
Romer, D., 261
Rooney, B., 281
Rose, I. D., 111
Rosenbaum, M. E., 106
Rosenbaum, S., 15, 109
Rosenberg, A., 43*b*
Rosenstock, I. M., 276, 321
Rosenthal, L., 151
Roser, C., 313
Roskos-Ewoldsen, D. R., 264
Ross, J. S., 106
Ross, K. A., 112
Rossiter, C., 88, 135
Rosti, G., 40
Roter, D. L., 44, 66, 207
Rothman, A. J., 332
Rothman, L., 260
Rouder, S., 260
Routsong, T. R., 199
Ruben, M. A., 40
Rubenstein, A., 143
Rubio, D., 81
Rubyan-Ling, D., 279
Rucinski, D., 305
Rudolph, J., 87
Ruiter, R., 338
Ruppert, R. A., 176
Rushani, D., 112
Rushton, C. H., 48
Russ, T. L., 320
Russell, C. A., 241
Russell, L. D., 167
Rust, G., 208
Ryan, E. B., 125, 126
Ryan, G., 113
Ryan, L., 108
Ryan-Wenger, N., 123
Rydahl-Hansen, S., 168
Rynn, T., 229

Saadi, A., 115
Sabatino, A. A., 72
Sabee, C. M., 199
Sachdeva, N., 190
Sacks, R. J., 305
Saeed, N., 206
Saffitz, G., 262
Saha, S., 116
Salamon, J., 119
Salander, P., 183, 184
Salas, E., 99
Saleem, B. T., 85
Salmon, C., 315
Salmon, C. T., 243, 324–25, 340
Salovey, P., 332
Salsberg, E. S., 224*b*
Samovar, L. E., 132

Sanchez, R., 93–94
Sanchez-Reilly, S., 180
Sanders, L., 16*b*
Sanders-Jackson, A., 311, 312, 336
Sandman, P., 270, 271, 273, 288
Sands, D. Z., 207
Sandy, D., 151*b*
Sanford, A. A., 199
Santa Cruz, J., 255*b*
Sar, S., 314
Saraf, A., 195
Sarbazi, E., 323
Sasso, L., 23
Sastre, M. T. M., 184
Savage, M., 330
Scarpaci, J., 314
Schein, E. H., 86
Scherr, K. A., 71
Schillinger, D., 181
Schmaltz, H., 127
Schmid Mast, M., 48
Schnall, R., 134
Schneider, E., 22
Schneider, M.-J., 269
Schneiderman, G., 168
Schoen, C., 32
Schoenberg, N., 142
Scholl, J. C., 55
Schooler, C., 313
Schormans, A. F., 258
Schreiber, L., 152
Schulenberg, J. E., 296
Schulman, K. A., 114
Schulz, P., 278
Schur, L., 125
Schurr, P. H., 228
Schuyler, S., 217–18
Schwartz, L., 247, 248
Schwartz, M. P., 261
Schwartz, N., 309
Schwenk, N., 98
Schwingel, A., 306
Scott, A., 330
Scott, C., 92
Scott, J., 209
Scott, M., 298, 299*b*
Scruggs, S., 325
Seeger, M. W., 275*b*
Seervai, S., 107
Sefko, J., 337
Segert, I., 260
Segrin, C., 159, 160
Sehgal, A. R., 73
Seigel, B., 103
Seihamer, M. F., 125
Sellnow, T. L., 275*b*, 277
Sellnow-Richmond, D., 277, 281
Seltman, K. D., 82, 98, 99, 206, 218, 221, 226, 227

Seltzer, T., 229
Senge, P., 5, 86, 329
Sentell, T., 108
Seo, M., 107
Seymour, B., 195
Sezginis, N., 106, 113
Sguazzin, C., 93
El-Shaarawi, N., 305
Shah, A., 22
Shah, J., 66–67
Shah, T., 22
Shaner, J. L., 125
Shapiro, M. A., 336
Sharf, B., 160
Sharmeen Shommu, N., 23
Shaunfield, S., 13
Sheldenkar, A., 278
Shelton, W., 47
Shepard, D. S., 143
Shi, J., 315
Shih, C.-H., 222
Shim, M., 198
Shokar, N. K., 195
Shore, D., 258
Shortsleeve, C., 188
Shuler, L., *170*, 170–71
Shuler, S., *170*, 170–71
Siegel, J. T., 169
Signorielli, N., 240, 261
Silberner, J., 247
Silk, K. S., 322, 324
Silver, M., 75, 201
Silvester, J., 54
Simpson, J., 331
Sinclair, B., 111, 112
Singer, D., 25
Singer, D. G., 264, 265
Singer, J. L., 264
Singh, K., 87
Singh, S., 106, 113
Singleton, J. A., 272*b*
Sinha, S., 159
Sisk, B., 42
Sismondo, S., 248
Sitzman, K., 81
Skelton, J., 242
Skierczynski, B. A., 30
Skinner, A., 242
Skluth, M., 150–51
Skolnick, P., 290
Slack, P., 139
Slater, M. D., 326, 332
Smedema, S. M., 258
Smith, K. C., 329
Smith, L. F., 85
Smith, M. A., 127
Smith, M. F., 73
Smith, R., 4
Smith, R. A., 306
Smith, R. C., 54

Smith, S. G., 107
Smith, S. W., 304
Smith, T. M., 84
Smith-McLallen, A., 193
Snyderman, B. B., 225
Soares, J., 159
Sobo, E. J., 136, 137, 142
Solway, E., 25
Son, H., 332
Sopory, P., 334
Sorah, E. L., 84
Sorum, P. C., 184
Soule, K. P., 122
Spagnoletti, C., 81
Spalding, S., 86
Sparks, L., 68–69, 160, 168, 183
Speaker, A., 280b
Spear, S. F., 334b
Spencer, M., 334
Springston, J. K., 338
Stage, C., 92
Stange, K. C., 50, 81
Starks, H., 43b
Stavrositu, C. D., 336
Stein, J. A., 191
Stein, M. D., 44
Steinbinder, A., 222
Stephens, N. M., 14
Stephenson, M. T., 175b
Stepler, R., 41, 176
Stepner, M., 105
Stetler, C., 54
Stevens, W., 188, 210
Stewart, J., 206
Stewart, L. P., 319, 320, 334
Stiff, J. B., 92
Stivers, T., 50–51
St. John, W., 70
Stohl, C., 167
Stout, P. A., 109
Street, J. L., 4
Street, J. R. L., 41
Street, R., 88
Street, R. L., 25, 60
Stretcher, V. J., 276, 321
Strick, M., 338
Strothers, H., 208
Struble, C., 111
Stryker, J., 251
Studer, Q., 220, 227
Studts, C. T., 142
Suchman, A. L., 54
Suchwalko, J., 53
Sudore, R. L., 181
Sugai, W., 74
Sugg, C., 279
Suhr, J. A., 165
Sullivan, M., 281
Summers, S., 265
Sumner, P., 250

Sun, J., 85
Sun, T., 54, 286
Sun, Y., 337
Sundar, A. A., 195
Sundin, Ö., 159
Suomi, R., 190
Sussman, S., 306
Sutton, R. L., 223
Sutton, S., 68, 70
Swahnberg, K., 46
Swanson, A., 248
Swayze, P., 160
Swazey, J. P., 134
Swiderski, R. M., 147
Swinnen, W., 107
Sylvia, 264
Sypher, B. D., 208
Szabó, B., 178
Szanton, S., 113

Taha, H., 70, 142
Tai, Z., 286
Tan, A., 311
Tan, A. S. L., 198
Tan, M., 250–51, 289
Tangka, F. K. L., 72
Tanner, A. H., 251
Tar, J., 66, 66–67
Tarasenko, Y. Y., 142
Tardy, C. H., 161
Tarrant, C., 70
Tarter, C. J., 221
Tauber, M., 145
Taylor, J., 67
Taylor, K., 201
Teichert, T., 308
Tetteh, D., 193
Thabane, L., 152
Tham, D., 262, 298
Thang, C. K., 83
Thi, L. M., 148
Thomas, A. L., 192
Thomas, D., 175b
Thomas, K., 248
Thomas, S., 245
Thomas, S. A., 172
Thomas, S. J., 288
Thompson, D., 282
Thompson, L., 125
Thompson, T., 178, 184
Thompson, T. D., 72
Thompson, T. L., 11, 121
Thomsen, T., 168
Thomtén, J., 159
Thornton, B. C., 10, 15
Thorson, E., 306
Thrasher, J., 245
Thubron, R., 200
Tian, Y., 159, 256
Tichenor, P. J., 305

Tiedtke, C., 164
Tietbohl, C., 65
Tiggermann, M., 254
Tinsley, B. J., 324
Tirrell, M., 339
Topol, E., 200–201, 202b
Toppenberg-Pejcic, D., 276–77, 279, 284
Torres, J., 203
Torres-Ruiz, M., 314
Tough, E. A., 152
Tourangeau, A. E., 81, 89
Tovey, P., 154
Transue, E., 49, 82–83, 93
Travis, S. S., 55
Trimi, S., 190
Tripathi, G., 320
Trorey, G. M., 71
Trost, C., 251, 253
Troth, A., 160
Trujillo, A., 15, 85, 109
Trump, D., 245
Tsai, T. C., 70
Tsipa, A., 89
Tu, H. T., 136
Tucker, G., 41
Tuikka, A., 190
Tulsky, J., 256
Turner, A., 281
Turner, C., 105
Turner, J. W., 259
Turner, M. M., 308
Turpin, T. P., 105
Tustin, N., 192
Twaddle, A. C., 80–81, 134

Uba, L., 136
Ubel, P. A., 71
Uhrig, J., 341
Ulmer, R. R., 275b
Ume, E., 131
Ünal, S., 47
Unger, K., 117
Unguru, Y., 43b
Unsworth, C., 97
Updegraff, J. A., 333
Uscher-Pines, L., 205
Usta, J., 142
Utjtdehaage, S., 83
Uwujaren, J., 258

Valaitis, E., 71
Valkenburg, P. M., 242
Van Arsdale, P. W., 148
van den Putte, B., 332
van der Riet, P., 88
van der Sande, R., 188
Vangeest, J. B., 110
van Gemert-Pijnen, J., 198
Van Ouytsel, J., 259

Van Roen, J., 49
van Straaten, B., 243–44
van Zanten, M., 50
Vardeman-Winter, J., 106
Vardigan, B., 248
Vaughan, C., 230–31
Veatch, R. M., 148b
Velkoff, V. A., 125, 175–76
Venetis, M. K., 110, 164
Venkatesh, A. K., 113
Venkatesh, V., 193
Verhoff, C., 193
Verlinde, E., 107
Vermillion, M., 83
Vernon, J. A., 15, 109
Vespa, J., 24
Vest, J., 261
Viccellio, P., 210
Vickers, C., 117
Vidrine, A., 30
Vidrine, J., 30
Vilhauer, R. P., 171
Villagran, M. M., 183
Viswanath, K., 162
Vladzymyrsky, A., 207
Vogel, D. L., 258
Vollrath, M. W., 190
von Bertalanffy, L., 5
Vuckovich, M., 125

Wagner, C. V., 81, 89, 107
Wagner, L., 168
Wagner, P. D., 81
Wahl, H.-W., 127
Wahlström, R., 142
Waitzkin, H., 66
Wakefield, A. J., 239, 272b
Wakefield, M., 329, 336
Walker, B., 21
Walker, N., 269
Wallace, P., 120
Wallace, S., 203
Walrave, M., 259
Walsh, K., 47, 50
Walsh, M. E., 123
Walsh, S., 187
Walters, E., 202
Wang, B., 67
Wang, F., 193
Wang, G. E., 82
Wang, H., 81
Wang, X., 85
Wang, Z., 251
Wanzer, M. B., 75, 160
Ward, C., 219
Warnke, J. H., 143
Warren, A. M., 142
Warren-Jeanpiere, L., 142
Wartella, E., 189, 196
Washington, K., 13

Watson, A., 239
Watson, T. J., 41
Watt, I., 89
Watzlawick, P., 9, 41
Wax-Thibodeaux, E., 271
Weaver, J., 194, 195, 196, 199
Webb, T., 261
Weber, K., 163
Weber, T., 330
Wechsler, H., 334b
Weimann, G., 315
Wei-Na, L., 249
Weinberg, D., 86
Weiner, J. L., 192
Weiner, S. J., 110
Weir, K., 88
Weisman, E., 93
Weiss, C., 14
Weiss, G., 48
Welch, B., 205
Welch, G., 52
Welch, S. J., 110
Wernhart, A., 189, 194, 196, 197
West, C. P., 88
West, D. C., 85
West, T., 224b
Westhoff, Y., 334b
Weston, W. W., 87
Wetherell, M. A., 14
Wexler, D., 219
Whaley, B., 123, 124, 125, 127
Wheeler, M., 250–51, 289
White, A., 159
White, A. D., 139
White, A. R., 152
White, J., 203
White, Z. M., 163
Whiteman, M. C., 251
Whitten, P., 208
Wicks, R. J., 89, 92
Widdows, R., 194
Wijma, B., 46
Wikler, D., 310b
Wilcox, S., 6
Wilding, H., 197
Wilharm, A., 210
Wilkerson, L., 116
Wilkes, M., 82
Wilkinson, D. M., 305
Willems, S., 106, 107
Williams, C., 68
Williams, D. E., 262
Williams, D. R., 228
Williams, G. C., 53
Williams, L. T., 140
Williams, M., 106, 113
Williams, R., 145
Willing, R., 182
Willingham, E., 272b

Willis, L. A., 310b
Wills, T. A., 159
Wilson, D., 41
Wilson, E. O., 136
Wilson, K., 161
Wilson, W., 163
Wimmers, P. F., 116
Windridge, K., 70
Winfrey, O., 331
Winkelman, M., 131, 136
Winslow, C.-E. A., 269
Winsten, J., 300
Wise, K., 228
Witte, F. M., 67
Witte, K., 338
Witteman, H. O., 50
Wittenberg, E., 179
Wittenberg-Lyles, E., 13, 180
Wojtek, C., 306
Wolf, M. S., 107, 110
Woloshin, S., 247, 248
Wong, K., 87
Wong, M., 262
Wong, V. T., 152
Wood, D., 261
Wood, H., 203
Wood, J., 253
Woods, T., 72, 73
Woodyard, C., 146
Wordell, D., 97
Wortman, C. B., 166
Wright, K. B., 169
Wright Nunes, J. A., 70
Wu, C.-H., 154
Wynia, M., 43b

Xie, X., 73
Xu, J., 81
Xu, Z., 338

Yang, B., 243, 332
Yang, M.-S., 265
Yang, X., 315
Yankey, D., 272b
Yanovitzky, I., 334b
Yarsevich, J., 309
Yazdi, D., 201
Ye, J., 208
Yeanwood, N., 32
Yee, A., 324
Yee, L. J., 111
Yeon-Hwan, P., 127
Yie, K., 311
Yip, K.-C., 152
Yoo, J., 256
Yoshimura, S. M., 160
Young, A., 49
Young, A. M., 308
Young, H., 248, 249
Young, L., 115, 206

Zakrzewski, P. A., 81
Zaltman, G., 320
Zambrana, R. E., 113
Zana, Á., 178
Zaner, R., 58
Zanini, M., 23
Zeitz, H. J., 110
Zhang, L., 258
Zhang, L. H., 195
Zhang, Z.-J., 152
Zhao, X., 313, 332
Zhao, Y., 250–51, 289

Zhdanova, L., 50
Zheng, Y., 251
Zhong, E. H., 224*b*
Zhong, Z.-J., 73
Zhu, X., 85
Zhu, Y., 85
Ziebland, S., 198
Zikmund-Fisher, B. J., 50
Zimmerman, B., 134
Zimmerman, D., 134
Zimmerman, F. J., 243
Zimmerman, R. S., 309

Zineb, S. B., 142
Zisman-Ilani, Y., 50
Zittleman, L., 309
Zittoun, R., 139
Zizak, D. M., 262
Zook, E., 171
Zook, R., 46
Zoucha, R., 144
Zuckerman, M., 309
Zusman, E. E., 219
Zwerner, A. R., 99

Subject Index

Note: Page references followed by *t* indicates tables; *f* indicates figures; *b* indicates boxes. Numbers in all italics indicates pictures.

ACA. *See* Affordable Care Act
acceptance
    dialectics, 163
    medical mistakes, 95
accommodation, 59, 125–26
accountability, 222, 311
Accreditation Council on Graduate Medical Education (ACGME), 81
action-facilitating support, 165–66
activation model for information exposure, 308–9
activity level, advertising, 243
acupuncture, 151, *152*
addictions, 24
    opioid epidemic, 289–92, *290*
ADHD. *See* attention-deficit-hyperactivity-disorder
administrative fatigue, 89
adolescents
    alcohol, 243–44
    body image, 253–54
    eating disorders, 255
    e-cigarettes, 245
    media literacy, 265
    safer sex, 260
    smartphone apps, 203
    smoking, 295–96
    social support, 160
    steroids, 255–56
    video game violence, 261
advance-care directives, 167, 181–82
advertising
    activity level, 243
    alcohol, 243–45, *244*
    beauty, 256
    body image, 254, *254*
    children, 241–42
    cultivation theory, 240
    entertainment, 261–64
    nutrition, 241–43, *243*
    obesity, 241–43, *243*
    pharmaceuticals, 245–49, 246*b*
    communication skill builder, 249
    DTC, *247*, 247–49
    smoking, 245
    Viagra, 246*b*
Advertising Age, 296
affective moments, 168
Affordable Care Act (ACA), 34–35, 224*b*
Africa, 152.
    See also Ebola

HIV/AIDS, 24, *283*, 283–85
African Americans, 24, 135
    cancer, 114
    death, 113
    diabetes, 115
    DTC, 249
    gender identity, 111
    opioid epidemic, 292
    stroke, 112
    women, 105
    obesity, 242
    storytelling, 299*b*
age and aging, 24, 123–28, *126*.
    See also children; older adults
    eHealth, 193
ageism, 125, 127
AIDS. *See* HIV/AIDS
Al-Anon/Alateen, 169
alcohol
    advertising, 243–45, *244*
    health promotion campaigns, 297, 319–20, 334*b*
    mHealth, 202
    peer pressure, 334*b*
    SMS, 203
allopathic medicine, 153*b*
ALS. *See* amyotrophic lateral sclerosis
alternative medicine, 152
Alzheimer's disease, 176, 177*b*, 201
AMA. *See* American Medical Association
ambivalence, MI, 52
American College of Health Care Administrators, 11*b*
American College of Health Care Executives, 11*b*
American Medical Association (AMA), 109, 290
American Pain Society (APS), 290–91
American Psychological Association, 126
amyotrophic lateral sclerosis (ALS), *339*
analytic stage, media literacy, 265
anger (*coraje*), 135
AngiesList.com, 150
anguish of spirit, 149
animal companions, 172
anonymity, health promotion campaign questionnaires, 304
anti-vaxxers, 273
anxiety

Ebola, 272
immigrants, 24
SARS, 285
SMS, 203
apologizing
    coping, 172
    medical mistakes, 95
    service failures, 233
Appalachian culture, 142
Apple Watches, 187–88, *188*, 200, 201, 206
APS. *See* American Pain Society
arousal, health promotion campaign channels, 313
Asian Americans, 24, 116
Assassin's Creed Syndicate (video game), 253
assertions, 51
asthma, 21, 73
A-team players, 226
attention-deficit-hyperactivity-disorder (ADHD), 240
audience, health promotion campaigns, 298
    children, 308
    as person, 306
    segmentation, 302–11, *304*
    sensation-seekers, *308*, 308–11
    target, 305
    underinformed, 306
autism, MMR, 249, 272–73
avian flu (H5N1), *286*, 286–88
    vaccinations, 286, 287*b*
Ayurveda, 152, 153

bad news, 182–84
    eHealth, *192*
Barbie dolls, *252*, 252*b*
battle metaphor, 145–46
beauty, 125
    advertising, 256
    body image, 256
    media images, 238
The Beauty of Aging (documentary), 125
behavior change theories, 321–25
believers, 148–49.
    See also health belief model
Be My Eyes, 190, *190*
bereavement, 181
Better Business Bureau, 197
Be You. Be Bold, Be #Unapologetic, 252

415

The Biggest Loser (TV show), 263*b*
binge drinking, 244
biofeedback, 153
biomedical model, 12–13
biophilia hypothesis, 136
biopsychosocial care (model), 13–14, 85, 99, 121
biosensor patches, 206
bisexual. See LGBTQ+
blindness, eHealth, 190, *190*
blood donation, health promotion campaigns, 339*b*
body image, *241*
   Barbie dolls, *252*, 252*b*
   boy's toys, 255, *255*
   media, 253–56, *254*
   steroids, *255*, 255–56
   video games, *264*
body mass index, 241
boy's toys, 255, *255*
breast cancer, 141, 199, 333
   coping, 161
   health promotion campaigns, *324*
   Hispanic Americans, 305
   news coverage, 251
B-team players, 226
bubonic plague, 139
buffering hypothesis, social support, 159, 160
buffer zone, pandemics, 287
Building Reputational Capital (Jackson, K.), 229–30
bullying, 260
bureaucracy, 29–30, 98
burnout, 89–93, *92*
   conflict, 90–91
   emotions, 91–92
   empathy, 92
   family, 176
   health communication, 4
   patient-caregiver communication, 41

CAM. See complementary and alternative medicine
cancer, 64, 270, 271.
   See also breast cancer
   African Americans, 114
   holistic are, 154
   identity, *68*, 68–70
   informed consent, 74–75
   MI, 52
   social liability, 139
capacity, 8
   community, 329
capitation, 27, 28, 74
cardiopulmonary resuscitation (CPR), 202, 256
career opportunities
   caregivers, 80*b*

diversity, 120*b*
   health care administration, 217*b*
   health communication, 16
   health communication research, 41*b*
   health information technology, 211*b*
   health promotion campaigns, 297*b*, 331*b*
   health-related jobs, 3*b*
   holistic medicine, 154*b*
   managed care, 29
   mental health, 184*b*
   patient advocacy, 72*b*
   public health, 269*b*
   social services, 184*b*
caregivers.
   See also parents; patient-caregiver communication; *specific topics*
   career opportunities, 80*b*
   caring for, 176–77
   confidence, 88–89, 121
   eHealth, *197*, 197–98
   emotions, 87–88, *88*
   end-of-life experiences, 179
   family, 144, 174–77, *175*
   friends, 174–77
   identity, 83
   isolation, 82–83, 176
   mHealth, 203
   mindfulness, 88
   older adults, 127
   organizational culture, 85–86
   patient cooperation, 73–74
   perspectives, 79–99
   preparations, 80–85, *81*, *84*
   privileges, 83
   psychological influences, 87–89, *88*
   satisfaction, 89
   service excellence, 232
   SES, 107
   shortages, 224*b*
   socialization, 81–82, 176
   systems-level influences, 85–87
   telehealth, 207–11
   time constraints, 86–87, *87*
catastrophic cap, 26
#CATmageddon, 295, *296*
CDC. See Centers for Disease Control and Prevention
celiac disease, 56
cell phones. See smartphones
Center for eHealth Research and Disease Management, 197–98
Centers for Disease Control and Prevention (CDC), 11*b*, 269, 271
   CERC, 278
   Ebola, 281
   vaccinations, 272*b*
   Zika, 288–89
CERC. See Crisis and Emergency Risk Communication

channels (health promotion campaigns), 312–15, *314*
chief operating officers (COOs), 200
children, 123–24.
   See also adolescents
   ACA, 34
   advertising, 241–42
   cultivation theory, 240
   health insurance, 33
   health promotion campaign audience, 308
   obesity, 242, 255
   sleep deprivation, 243
   smoking, 243
   video game violence, 261
chiropractic medicine, 151, 152, 153
Christian Science Church, 149
chronic conditions, communication, 69–70
chronic fatigue syndrome, 135
chronic obstructive pulmonary disease (COPD), 204–5
CI. See collaborative interpretation
climate change, 24
closed-ended questions, 44, 56, 303
collaborative interpretation (CI), 48–49
collaborative medical communication
   CI, 48–49
   decision making, 50–51
   dentists, 55*b*
   dialogue, 53
   MI, *51*, 51–52
   narrative medicine, *56*, 56–59
   nonverbal encouragement, 53–54
   patient-caregiver communication, 47–51, *48*
   quality of life, 49–50
   verbal encouragement, 54–55
collaborative sense-making, 9
collective efficacy, 329
commercialism, entertainment, 261–64
commitment-trust theory of relationships, 228–29
Communicating at the End of Life (Foster), 180
communication.
   See also *specific types and topics*
   chronic conditions, 69–70
   collaborative sense-making, 9
   context and culture, 9–10
   coping, 15–16, 165–69
   defined, 8–9
   disabilities, 121–23
   Ebola, 282–83
   eHealth, 188
   health, *15*, 15–16
   health care, 23
   health care administration, 219

health promotion campaigns, 298–99
holistic care, 154
identity, 68, 69–70
managed care, 25–30
PI, 167
relational approach, 9
SARS, 285
satisfaction, 70–71
saving time and money, 16
SES, 106–7
social support, 161*b*
technology, 25
transactional model, 8–10
two-way symmetrical, 229, 230–31
communication accommodation theory, 125–26
Communication as Comfort (Ragan, Wittenberg-Lyles, Goldsmith, and Sanchez-Reilly), 180
communication skill builder, 6, 7*b*
bad news, 182–84
children, 124
coping with death, 181
difficult patients, 91*b*
disabilities, 122–23
emotional expression, 168–69
health literacy, 109–10
internet, 196–97
medical mistakes, 95–96
news coverage, 251–53
pharmaceutical advertising, 249
servant-leadership, 219–23, 220*f*, 222
social media, 230–31
supportive listening, 166–68
teams, 225–27
two-way symmetrical communication, 230–31
community capacity, 329
compassionate engagement, 57
complementary and alternative medicine (CAM), 152
concrete-logical conceptualization, 123
condoms, 259–60
confidence
caregivers, 88–89, 121
social media, 231
confidentiality, 46, 142
conflict, 90–91, 99, 160
consciousness, theoretical foundations, 137*b*
consent. *See* informed consent
consumerism, health care, 149–50
ConsumerReportsHealth, 150
containment zone, pandemics, 287–88
contingent personal identity, 69
control, sense of.
See also locus of control
communication, 71

coping, 161, 162–63
crisis, 164
theory of personal causation, 224, *225*
convergence, 54, 126
cooperation, patients, 72–74, *73*
COOs. *See* chief operating officers
copay, 27
COPD. *See* chronic obstructive pulmonary disease
coping
animal companions, 172
communication, 15–16, 165–69
control, sense of, 162–63
crisis, 163–64
with death, communication skill builder, 181
dialectics, 163, *163*
emotions, 168–69, 183
metaphors, illness, 145–46
normalcy, 164–65, *165*
social support, 161–62
coraje (anger), 135
coronavirus (COVID-19), 2, 24, 205, 268, 288
corporate identity, 230
Cosmopolitan (magazine), 242, 245
costs, 4
addictions, 290
consumerism, 150
eHealth, 197
health care administration, 219
HIV/AIDS drug, 284
managed care, 29
single-payer system, 33
support groups, 169
telehealth, 207, 208
coverage gap, 33
COVID-19 (coronavirus), 2, 24, 205, 268, 288
CPR. *See* cardiopulmonary resuscitation
crisis, 231, 290
coping, 163–64
Crisis and Emergency Risk Communication (CERC), 278
crisis communication
avian flu, *286*, 286–88
case studies, 279–92
Ebola, 279, 281–83
emotions, 274
fear, 272, 273–74, *274*
HIV/AIDS, *283*, 283–85
lessons, 291*b*
models and guidelines, 276–78
opioid epidemic, 289–92, *290*
panic myth, 270–71, *271*
public health, 268–93
risk communication, 270–74

risk management/communication framework, 275*b*
SARS, *285*, 285–86
social media, 278–79
Zika, 288–89
crisis management, 228, *231*, 231–32
critical-cultural approach, health promotion campaigns, *326*, 326–29
cultivation theory, media, 240
cultural appropriateness, 109, 146
cultural competence, 24
cultural sensitivity, 132, 133
culture, 24–25, *25*.
See also multiculturalism
believers, 148–49
communication, 9–10
coping metaphors, 145–46
emotions, 135–36
energy, 136–37
family, 143–44
health, 131–55
health care, adaptability, 133–34
health communication, 132–34, *133*
HIV/AIDS, 283
holistic care, 151–54, *152*
hot and cold, 136
illness, 131–55
nature, 136
patient-caregiver communication, 146–51, *147*
roles, 146–51, *147*
spiritualism, 135–36, 148–49
culture-centered, 132
curanderos, 149
cyberbullying, 260
cyberchondriacs, 248

DARE. *See* Drug Abuse Resistance Education
data collection, health promotion campaigns, 302–3
data security, mHealth, 204
DD-MM. *See* disclosure decision-making model
death.
See also end-of-life experiences
African Americans, 113
with dignity, 179–81
Ebola, 24
health care dramas, 257
HMOs, 29
right to, ethics, 182*b*
decisional balance, TTM, 325
decision making, 50–51, 127, 219, 221–22
CI, 49
dialectics, 163
informed consent, 75
MI, 52–53
deconstructing, media literacy, 265

deductible, 26, 27, 28
dentists, 55b
Department of Health and Human Services (HHS), 289
depersonalization, 89
depression, 24, 73, 134, 168, 256
 mHealth, 202
 SMS, 203
descriptive norm, peer pressure, 334b
detached concern, 91–92
diabetes, 73, 106, 115, 240, 270
 herbal remedies, 153
 mHealth, 203
 MI, 52–53
diagnosis-related groups (DRGs), 26–27
diagnostic centers, managed care, 28
dialectics, coping, 163, *163*
dialogue, collaborative medical communication, 53
dieticians, 60b, 97, 255
difficult patients, 91b
diffusion of innovations, 315
digital divide, 189, 193, 305
direct-effect model, social support, 159
direct-to-consumer advertising (DTC), *247*, 247–49
disabilities, 8, 120–23
 alcohol, 243, *244*
 communication, 121–23
 communication skill builders, 122–23
 entertainment, 258
 intersectionality theory, 105
 perspectives, 122b
disclosure decision-making model (DD-MM), 46–47
discrimination, 106, *168*
dispersed leadership, 227
distress markers, 54
distrust, 113, 228
 African American women, 299b
 eHealth, 211
 noncooperation, 73
 risk communication, 270
divergence, communication accommodation theory, 126–27
diversity.
 See also age and aging; culture; disabilities; language; race and ethnicity; sexual orientation; socioeconomic status
 career opportunities, 120b
 gender identity, 110–12, *111*
 health care, 104–28
 health literacy, 108–10, 109t, *110*
 intersectionality theory, 104–5
 language, *117*, 117–20
 social mobilization, 270
doctors. *See* physicians

DoctorScorecard.com, 150
doorknob disclosures, 44
double bind, 91
Down syndrome, 172–73
drain circlers, 84
DRGs. *See* diagnosis-related groups
Drug Abuse Resistance Education (DARE), 14
drug-resistant illnesses, 24
DTC. *See* direct-to-consumer advertising
dualism, 82

earthquakes, 271, 281
eating disorders, 160, 239, 254–55
Ebola
 anxiety, 272
 crisis communication, 279, 281–83
 deaths, 24
 empathic communication, *282*, 283
 fear, 281, 282–83
 IDEA model, 277
 news coverage, 250, 281
e-cigarettes (vaping), 245, 296, 311–12
ED. *See* erectile dysfunction
education
 entertainment-education programming, 262–64
 public health, 269
 SARS, 286
 SES, 106, 107
effectiveness study, 341
efficacy study, 341
eHealth, 25, 187–200, *188*
 advantages, 194–95
 age, 193
 bad news, *192*
 blindness, 190, *190*
 caregivers, *197*, 197–98
 conflicting information, 196
 defined, 188
 digital divide, 193
 disadvantages, *191*, 195–96
 health information acquisition model, 191
 health information efficacy, 190
 health literacy, 193–94
 HIV/AIDS, 196
 impact, 198–200
 integrative model of online health information seeking, 192–93
 interoperability, 198
 older adults, 189, 193, *195*
 participatory design, 197–98
 patient-caregiver communication, 199–200
 patients, 194–97
 privacy, 196
 social support, 194–95
 TMIM, 191–92, 194

 unreliability, 195–96
 usefulness, 194–98
 UTAUT, 193–94
EIC. *See* Entertainment Industries Council
elaboration likelihood model, 313
elderly. *See* older adults
electronic medical records (EMRs), 197, 209–10
emergency
 defined, 290
 public health, 270
emergency medicine/department
 language, 118b
 public health, 270
 service excellence, 233
emotional adjustment, coping, 161
emotional appeals, 337–40
emotional contagion, 171
emotional exhaustion, 89, 91
emotional preparedness, 87–88
emotional response, narrative messages, 336
emotions.
 See also feelings
 burnout, 91–92
 caregivers, 87–88, *88*
 coping, 168–69, 183
 crisis communication, 274
 culture, 135–36
 death, 181
 expression, allowing, communication skill builder, 168–69
 health literacy, 108–9
 Hispanic Americans, 135
 stress, 13–14
 suppression, depression, 168
empathic communication, 92, *282*, 283
empathic concern, 171
empathy, 71, 84, 340
 difficult patients, 91b
 overempathizing, 171
 support groups, 169
Empire (TV show), 260
empowerment, 58–59, 75, 91b, 220
endangered plants, holistic care, 154
end-of-life experiences, 49, 167, 178–81
enduring narratives, 58
energy, culture, 136–37
entertainment
 advertising, 261–64
 commercialism, 261–64
 disabilities, 258
 health care, 256–57
 health images, 263b
 mental illness, *257*, 257–58
 product placement, 261–62, *262*

safer sex, 259–60
sex, 258–60
sexual orientation, 260, *260*
violence, 260–61
entertainment-education programming, 262–64
Entertainment Industries Council (EIC), 262
entertainomercials, 261
environmental factors, social cognitive theory, 322
ePatients, 189
epidemics
　defined, 290
　opioids, 289–92, *290*
epilepsy, 139
EPPM. *See* extended parallel process model
e-quality theory of aging, 128
ER (TV show), 256
erectile dysfunction (ED), 246*b*
Essence (magazine), 242
esteem support, 166
ethics
　avian flu vaccinations, 287*b*
　entertainment and health images, 263*b*
　health care, 114*b*
　health care reform, 35*b*
　health communication, 16*b*
　health promoters, 327*b*
　health promotion campaigns, 303, 310*b*
　informed consent, 76*b*
　medical mistakes, 94
　paternalism, 148*b*
　physicians, 148*b*
　power differentials, 42, 47
　prevention, 310*b*
　right to die, 182*b*
　satisfaction, 72*b*
　truth, 43*b*
ethnic concordance, 115
ethnicity. *See* race and ethnicity
ethnocentrism, 132
euthanasia, 182
exemplification theory, 277
expectations
　dialectics, 163
　health promotion campaigns, 334
　medical mistakes, 96
　SES, 106
　UTAUT, 193
experiential stage, media literacy, 265
explicate order, 137*b*
extended parallel process model (EPPM), 338
external locus of control, 162, 256–57
extreme talkers, 127
eye contact, 54

Facebook, 230, 278, 279, 288
facework, 68–69
faith healers, 149
family
　burnout, 176
　caregivers, 174–77, *175*
　health communication, 143–44
　stress, 176
Family and Medical Leave Act of 1993, 176
fatalism, 162
FDA. *See* Food and Drug Administration
fear.
　See also anxiety
　appeals, 272
　crisis communication, 272, 273–74, *274*
　Ebola, 281, 282–83
Federal Trade Commission, 197
feedback
　health promotion campaigns, 340
　medical mistakes, 96
　verbal encouragement, 54
fee-for-service, 28
feelings, 148
　mindfulness, 88
　Voice of Lifeworld, 65–66
female identity, 142
The Field Guide to the Difficult Patient Interview (Platt and Gordon), 91*b*
Fifty Shades of Grey, 259
"fight for your life," 145–46
Fitbit, 206
fixed-alternative questions, health promotion campaign questionnaires, 303
flooding out, 171
focus groups, *304*, 304–5
folk medicine, 149
Food and Drug Administration (FDA), 153–54, 204
forgotten publics, 291*b*, 292
formal-logical conceptualization, 123
fracturing narratives, 58
friends
　caregivers, 174–77
　social support, 169–70, *170*
fright (*susto*), 135
fundraising, 228

gain-frame appeal, 332–33
gappiness, 51–52
gatekeepers, 340
gay. *See* LGBTQ+
gender.
　See also women
　health, 142
　identity, 110–12, *111*

Genetic Information Nondiscrimination Act of 2008 (GINA), 116
genetic profiling, 116*b*
germander, 154
germ theory, 134
gigantism, 139
G.I. Joe (toy), 255
GINA. *See* Genetic Information Nondiscrimination Act of 2008
global health, 24
globalization, public health, 281
Global Observatory, 211
glossolalia, 149
gomers, 84
got milk?, 330
Greedy for Life (documentary), 125
Grey's Anatomy (TV show), 256
groupthink, 99
The Guardian, 254, 292
Guideline on Communication Risk (WHO), 276–77
guilt appeals, 338

H5N1. *See* avian flu
hand-tremblers, 149
happy violence, 261
harmonic balance, 135
HDHPs. *See* high-deductible health plans
healer roles, 146–51
health.
　See also specific topics
　CI, 49
　collaborative medical communication, 48
　communication, *15*, 15–16
　culture, 131–55
　cyberchondriacs, 248
　defined, 7–8
　female identity, 142
　gender, 142
　harmonic balance, 135
　identity, *68*, 68–70
　inequities, 105–6
　male identity, 143, *143*
　MI, 52
　Native Americans, 139
　organic model, 134–35, *135*
　patients, *68*, 68–70
　sex, 142
　social asset, 139
　social liability, 139
　social support, 160
　universal coverage, 31
health apps. *See* smartphones
health belief model, 276, 321–22

health care.
See also specific topics
  access and disparities, 21–22
  communication, 23
  consumerism, 149–50
  culture, adaptability, 133–34
  current issues, 20–23
  distrust, 113
  diversity, 104–28
  entertainment, 256–57
  ethics, 114*b*
  evolution, 10
  multiculturalism, 24–25, *25*
  navigators, 22–23
  race and ethnicity, 24–25, *25*
  SES, 106
  staffing shortages, 224*b*
  system complexity, *22*, 22–23
  systems-level approach, *5*, 5–6
  world rankings, 32*t*
health care administration, *217*, 217–23, 220*f*, *222*
  career opportunities, 217*b*
  journals, 219*b*
health care interpreters, 117, *117*, 120
health care models
  biomedical model, 12–13
  biopsychosocial model, 13–14
  sociocultural model, 14–15
health care reform, 30–35, *34*
  ethics, 35*b*
  universal coverage, 30–34
health communication
  burnout, 4
  career opportunities, 16
  changing world, 23–24
  context, 1–36
  culture, 132–34, *133*
  defined, 10–11
  ethics, 16*b*
  family, 143–44
  history of, 11
  importance of, 2–6
  integrative health model, 59
  intercultural, 115–16
  landscape, 20–36
  narrative medicine, 58
  organizations, 11*b*
  patient-caregiver communication, 41
  perspectives, 8*b*
  preventive care, 21
  product placements, 262
  research, career opportunities, 41*b*
  technology, 4
  theoretical foundations, 10*b*
Health Communication (journal), 11, 49
health information.
See also health literacy
  communication, 71
  digital divide, 189
  narrative medicine, 58
  older adults, 127–28
  SES, 107
  technology, career opportunities, 211*b*
  telehealth, 208
  therapeutic privilege, 42–47
health information acquisition model, 33, 191
health information efficacy, eHealth, 190
health information scanning, 196
health information seeking, 196
health insurance.
See also Affordable Care Act
  health care access and disparities, 21
  holistic care, 152–53
  managed care, 26–27
  multi-payer system, 33
  older adults, 32
  SES, 106
  telehealth, 208–9
health literacy, 108–10, 109*t*, *110*
  eHealth, 189, 193–94
  informed consent, 75
health maintenance organizations (HMOs), 27, *27*, 29
health passport, 121, *121*
health promoters, 296
  accountability, 311
  ethics, 327*b*
  fear appeals, 273
health-promoting behaviors, 296
health promotion campaigns, 270, *270*, 295–317
  audience, 298
  children, 308
  as person, 306
  segmentation, 302–11, *304*
  sensation-seekers, *308*, 308–11
  target, 305
  underinformed, 306
  background, 297–300
  behavior change theories, 321–25
  benefits, 301
  blood donation, 339*b*
  breast cancer, *324*
  career opportunities, 297*b*, 331*b*
  channels, 312–15, *314*
  communication, 298–99
  critical-cultural approach, *326*, 326–29
  current situation, 301–2
  data collection, 302–3
  emotional appeals, 337–40
  ethics, 303, 310*b*
  evaluation and maintenance, *341*, 341–42
  exemplary campaigns, 298
  expectations, 334
  focus groups, *304*, 304–5
  goals, 300, 311–12
  healthy options, 300, *300*
  implementation, 340
  interviews, 303, *304*
  logical appeals, 337
  media, 312–15, *314*
  messages, 329–40, *330*, *333*, *339*
  Meth Project, 312, *312*
  motivating factors, 297–98, 302, *302*
  multimedia, 300
  narrative messages, 336–37
  piloting, 340
  questionnaires, 303–4, *304*
  scapegoating, 327*b*
  smoking, *309*
  spokesperson, 330–31
  stigma, 327*b*
  tailored, 313–15
  timing, 327*b*
  truth® campaigns, 295–96
  virtual reality headsets, *301*
health savings accounts (HSAs), 28
health self-efficacy, 162–63
hearing loss, 73
heart disease
  DTC, 249
  nonadherence, 73
  public health, 270
hepatitis C, 290
herbal therapies, 153, 154
heroin, 290
HHS. *See* Department of Health and Human Services
hidden curriculum, 82
high-deductible health plans (HDHPs), 28
highly scheduled interviews, 303
Hispanic Americans, 24
  diabetes, 106
  discrimination, *168*
  DTC, 249
  emotions, 135
  folk medicine, 149
  HPV vaccination, 115
  intersectionality theory, 105
  obesity, 242
  organic model of health, 135
  patient-caregiver communication, 44–45
  roles, 146
  social support, 169
  women, breast cancer, 305
HIV/AIDS
  in Africa, 24
  crisis communication, *283*, 283–85
  eHealth, 196

entertainment-education programming, 262–64
health promotion campaign, 298
herbal remedies, 153
LGBTQ+, 111
news coverage, 250, 251
opioid epidemic, 290
patient-caregiver communication, 45
preventive drug, 283–84, *284*
shocking messages, 339
social liability, 139
social support, 160
stigma, 140
victimization, 141
HMOs. *See* health maintenance organizations
holistic care (medicine), 151–54, *152*, 153*b*
career opportunities, 154*b*
homeopathic medicine, 153
hospice, 179–80
hospitals.
See also specific hospitals
managed care, 28
perspectives, 13*b*
hot and cold, 136
How Doctors Think (Groopman), 67
Hoy-Tarter Model of Shared Decision Making, 221
HPV. *See* human papillomavirus
HSAs. *See* health savings accounts
human papillomavirus (HPV), vaccination
health promotion campaigns, 305
Hispanic Americans, 115
MI, 53
TTM, 325
human resources, *223*
hiring, 226
organizational culture, 226
recruitment, 226–27
staffing shortages, 224*b*
theoretical foundations, 223–25
humor
burnout, 93
difficult patients, 91*b*
social support, as hurtful jests, *170*, 170–71
verbal encouragement, 55
Hurricane Dorian, 281
Hurricane Katrina, 271
hypertension
alcohol, 243
mHealth, 202, 203
patient cooperation, 73
hypnosis, 152

"I Am Not a Victim of Breast Cancer" (Barnes), 141
ICF. *See* International Classification

for Functioning, Disability, and Health
IDEA model (Internalization, Distribution, Explanation, Action), 277–78
identity
caregivers, 83
communication, 69–70
corporate, 230
facework, 68–69
female, 142
health, *68*, 68–70
male, 143, *143*
older adults, 125
patients, *68*, 68–70
illness (disease).
See also mental illness; prevention; *specific illnesses*
Christian Science Church, 149
coping metaphors, 145–46
culture, 131–55
curse, 139
drug-resistance, 281
stigma, *140*, 140–41
victimization, 141
Voice of Lifeworld, 66–67
illusions of vulnerability, 272
image.
See also body image; media images
marketing and public relations, 229–30, *231*
imaginary audience, 308
immigrants, 24, 105
immunizations. *See* vaccinations
impact, health promotion campaign channels, 313
implicate order, 137*b*
implicit bias, 106
indemnity, 26
individual mandate, 33, 34
Industrial Safety & Hygiene News, 274
information.
See also health information
activation model for information exposure, 308–9
overinforming, 171
SARS, 285–86
informational support, 165
informative stage, media literacy, 265
informed consent, 74, 74–75, 76*b*
Instagram, 253
institutional review board (IRB), 303
instrumental support, 165
insurance. *See* health insurance
insurance premium, 26
Integrated Theory of mHealth, 203
integrative health model, 59*b*
integrative medicine, 153
Integrative Model of Online Health Information Seeking, 192–93

intercultural competence, 24
intercultural health communication, 115–16
internal factors, social cognitive theory, 322
Internalization, Distribution, Explanation, Action (IDEA model), 277–78
internal locus of control, 162, 256–57
International Classification for Functioning, Disability, and Health (ICF), 7–8, 13, 120
internet.
See also specific topics
communication skill builder, 196–97
older adults, 128
quality of care, 150
SARS, 286
support groups, 169
uses and gratifications theory, *198*, 198–99
interoperability, eHealth, 198
interpersonal communication, 15
interpreters, health care, 117, *117*, 120
interprofessional education (IPE), 84
intersectionality theory, 104–5
interviews
difficult patients, 91*b*
health care models, 12
health promotion campaigns, 303, *304*
MI, *51*, 51–52
intimate-partner violence, 142–43
involvement, health promotion campaign channels, 313
IPE. *See* interprofessional education
IRB. *See* institutional review board
isolation
caregivers, 82–83, 176
eHealth, 199

Jawbone, 206
Journal of Health Communication, Communication & Medicine, 11
Journal of Life (radio show), 262–64
Journal of the American Medical Association, 256

karma, 136
knowledge gap hypothesis, 305

Lammily dolls, 252
The Lancet, 284
language, *117*, 117–20
development, media, 240
emergency medicine, 118*b*
health literacy, 108
informed consent, 75
opioid epidemic, 292
Latinos. *See* Hispanic Americans

leadership
  dispersed, 227
  servant, 219–23, 220f, 222
  social mobilization, 270
  training, 227
Leadership for Great Customer Service (Mayer and Cates), 232
LGBTQ+, 111
  entertainment, 260
liability, telehealth, 209
life at all costs, 178–79
LinkedIn, 252b
listening
  Ebola, 283
  HIV/AIDS, 284
  identity, 70
  marketing and public relations, 229
  MI, 52
  narrative medicine, 56, 57, 59
  power differentials, 44
  servant-leadership, 220–21
  supportive, communication skill builder, 166–68
  verbal encouragement, 54
literacy
  media, 15, 264–65
  patients, 110
liver damage, 243, 256
living wills, 182
locus of control (LOC), 162, 256–57
logical appeals, 337
loss-frame appeal, 332, 333

machines, culture, 147
mad cow disease, 270
MADD. *See* Mothers Against Drunk Driving
main-effect model, for social support, 159
malaria, 153
male identity, 143, *143*
malpractice, 41, 95
managed care
  advantages of, 28–29
  bureaucracy, 29–30
  career opportunities, 29
  communication, 25–30
  costs, 29
  disadvantages, 29–30, 30f
  HDHPs, 28
  health insurance, 26–27
  HMOs, 27, *27*, 29
  holistic care, 153
  PPOs, *27*, 27–28
  prevention, 29
  selection, 31b
  spokesperson, 29
  teamwork, 29
  wellness, 28
managed care organization, 26

managing meanings of embodied experiences (MMEE), 69
marketing, 227–31
  foundations, 228
  image, 229–30, *231*
  relationships, 228–29
  reputation, 229–30, *231*
massage, 152
mass communication, 239
mass media, 15
Master Settlement Agreement (MSA), 245
Mayo Clinic
  biosensor patches, 206
  teams, 225–26
  teamwork, 98
  telemonitoring, 206
mean world syndrome, 261
measles-mumps-rubella vaccine (MMR), 249, 272–73
The Meat Puppet, 67
mechanics, caregivers as, 147
media.
  See also advertising; entertainment; mass media; news coverage
  body image, 253–56, *254*
  consumption, *239*, 239–40
  crisis management, 232
  cultivation theory, 240
  eating disorders, 239
  gatekeepers, 340
  health promotion campaigns, 312–15, *314*
  images, *238*, 238–66
  news coverage, 249–53
  public relations, 228
  race and ethnicity, 305
  sleep deprivation, 243
  smoking, 243
  social comparison theory, 241, *241*
  social learning theory, 240–41
  theoretical foundations, 239–40
  third-person effect, 240
media images, *238*, 238–66.
  See also advertising; body image; entertainment; news coverage; television
  entertainment, 263b
media literacy, 15, 264–65
Medicaid, 33, 219
medical centers, managed care, 28
medical costs, 4
medical mistakes, *93*, 93–97
  communication skill builders, 95–96
  ethics, 94
  malpractice, 95
medical models
  biomedical, 12–13
  biopsychosocial, 13–14, 85
  disabilities, 121

  teamwork, 99
  integrative, 59b
  organic, 134–35, *135*
  sociocultural, 14–15
medical talk, *42*, 42–47
  knowledge and power, 42–43
  patronizing behavior, 45
  sensitive subjects, 44–45
  transgressions, *45*, 45–46
  who talks, who listens, 44
Medicare, 32, 152, 219
meditation, 146, 151, 152
mental health
  career opportunities, 184b
  SMS, 203
mental illness.
  See also specific conditions
  entertainment, *257*, 257–58
  social liability, 139
  stereotypes, *257*
  stigma, 140
Merck Pharmaceuticals, 248
mercy killing, 182
messages.
  See also health promotion campaigns
  SMS, 203–4
Meth Project, 312, *312*
mHealth, 188
  caregivers, 203
  disadvantages, 204
  smartphone apps, *200*, 200–204
MI. *See* motivational interviewing
mindfulness, 88
minority groups. *See* race and ethnicity
MMEE. *See* managing meanings of embodied experiences
MMR. *See* measles-mumps-rubella vaccine
MND. *See* motor neuron disease
mobile apps. *See* smartphones
moderately scheduled interviews, 303
Modern Family (TV show), 260
moments of truth, 232
monologue heavy communication, 44
Mossman-Pacey Paradox, 256
Mothers Against Drunk Driving (MADD), 310b
motivational interviewing (MI), *51*, 51–52
motivation-hygiene theory, 225
motor neuron disease (MND), 58
MSA. *See* Master Settlement Agreement
multichannel campaigns, 315
multiculturalism
  challenges, 132
  health care, 24–25, *25*
multimedia, health promotion campaigns, 300
multi-payer system, 33

narrative medicine, 56, 56–59
narrative messages, 336–37
National Cancer Institute (NCI), 11b, 164
National Health Service (NHS), 339, 339b
National Institute on Drug Abuse (NIDA), 289
National Institutes of Health (NIH), 152
Native Americans, 24, 113
 folk medicine, 149
 health, 139
 Navajo, 136, 150
nature, culture, 136
naturopathic medicine, 153
Navajo, 136, 150
NCI. See National Cancer Institute
negative-affect appeals, 338
never events, 95
news coverage
 accuracy and fairness, 250
 communication skill builder, 251–53
 Ebola, 281
 media, 249–53
 overgeneralizations, 250
 sensationalism, 250, 250–51
 Zika, 288–89
Newsweek (magazine), 250
New York Times, 30, 72b, 210, 273–74
New York Times Magazine, 250
NHS. See National Health Service
The Nicholas Effect (Green, R.), 174b
Nicholas Green Foundation, 174b
nicotine. See smoking
NIDA. See National Institute on Drug Abuse
NIH. See National Institutes of Health
9/11 terror attacks, 271
The No Asshole Rule, 223
NO MORE Excuses, 330
nonverbal encouragement, 53–54
normalcy, coping, 164–65, 165
nouning, 51
novel messages, 339, 339
NPs. See nurse practitioners
nudging, 300
nurse practitioners (NPs), 87
nurturing support, 166
nutrition
 advertising, 241–43, 243
 counseling, pharmacies, 4
 SES, 106
 television, 241–42

obesity
 advertising, 241–43, 243
 African American women, 242
 body image, 254–55

children, 242, 255
 Hispanic Americans, 242
 media, 240
 patient cooperation, 73
 stigma, 140, 140
offers, 51
Office of Alternative Medicine (NIH), 152
older adults, 124–25
 communication accommodation theory, 125–26
 communication patterns, 127
 communication technology, 25, 127–28
 eHealth, 189, 193, 195
 empathy loss, 84
 health care dramas, 257
 health insurance, 32
 increase, 24
 internet, 128
 intersectionality theory, 105
 Medicare, 32
 social support, 160, 160
On Call (Transue), 49
On Death and Dying (Kübler-Ross), 181
online support, health care navigation, 23
open-ended questions
 health promotion campaign questionnaires, 303
 narrative medicine, 59
opioid epidemic, 289–92, 290
optimistic biases, 272
Orange Is the New Black (TV show), 257, 260
organ donations, 174b
 Ebola, 283
 health care dramas, 257
organic health model, 134–35, 135
organizational culture
 caregivers, 85–86
 human resources, 226
 teamwork, 98
organizational processes, 86
osteopathic medicine, 153
overaccommodation, 126, 127
overempathizing, 171
overgeneralizations, 250
overhelping, 171
overinforming, 171
oversupport, 171
OxyContin, 290, 291

PACE. See present information, ask questions, check understanding, express concerns
pain
 cancer, 52
 MI, 52
 patient-caregiver communication, 41

palliative care, 180
PandemicFlu.gov, 288
pandemics, 24
 WHO, 287–88
panic myth, 270–71, 271
parental mediation, media literacy, 265
parents
 children's care role, 124
 vaccinations, 272b
participatory design/model
 eHealth, 197–98
 theory of personal causation, 225
PAs. See physician assistants
passivity, rhetoric of, 49
pasteurization, 134
paternalism, 147–48, 148b
pathologizing the human body, 253
patient-caregiver communication, 40–61.
 See also collaborative medical communication
 culture, 146–51, 147
 DTC, 247
 eHealth, 199–200
 medical talk, 42, 42–47
 patronizing behavior, 45
 power differentials, 42, 42–47
 sensitive subjects, 44–45
 telemedicine, 210–11
 tips, 60b
 transgressions, 45, 45–46
patient-centered care
 collaborative medical communication, 50
 decision-making, 51
 telehealth, 206–7
patient portals, 205–6
patients.
 See also specific topics
 cooperation, 72–74, 73
 difficult, 91b
 DTC, 248
 eHealth, 194–97
 health, 68, 68–70
 identity, 68, 68–70
 informed consent, 74, 74–75, 76b
 literacy, 110
 perspectives, 63–77
 satisfaction, 70–71, 71, 81
 consumerism, 150
 service excellence, 232
 socialization, 63–65, 65
 standardized
  disabilities, 121
 PBL, 85
 Voice of Lifeworld, 65–67, 66
The Patient's Playbook (Michelson), 23
patronizing behavior, 45
PBL. See problem-based learning

PCP. *See* principal care provider
peace metaphor, 146
Pebble Time, 206
peer pressure, 334*b*
People (magazine), 145
performance, 8
personal choice
    health communication, 11
    health promotion campaigns, 298, 308, 327*b*
    sociocultural perspective, 14
personal fable, 308
personal identity, 68
perspectives
    Alzheimer's disease, 177*b*
    Barbie doll, 252*b*
    boy's toys, 255, *255*
    caregivers, 79–99
    dentists, 55*b*
    disabilities, 122*b*
    health communication, 8*b*
    hospitals, 13*b*
    patients, 63–77
    physical therapy, 17*b*
    son's duty, 144*b*
    uncertainty, 64*b*
Pet Partners, 172
pharmaceuticals, advertising, 245–49, 246*b*
    communication skill builder, 249
    DTC, *247*, 247–49
pharmacies
    health hubs, 4, *4*
    nutrition counseling, 4
    vaccinations, 4
Photoshop, 253–54
physical therapy, perspectives, 17*b*
physician assistants (PAs), 87
physician-assisted suicide, 182
physicians.
    See also patient-caregiver communication
    DTC, 248
    ethics, 148*b*
    shortages, 224*b*
    spokesperson, 154
PI. *See* problematic integration
piloting, health promotion campaigns, 340
placebo, 149
plan-choose-act-take responsibility model, 224
The Pleasure Project, 284
Point-A-to-Point-B companies, 230
pokkuri shinu (popping like a bubble), 179, *180*
pollution, 24, 106
popping like a bubble (*pokkuri shinu*), 179, *180*
pornography, 259

positive-affect appeals, 337–38
posttraumatic stress disorder (PTSD), 142
power differentials (distance), *42*, 42–47, 147–48
PPOs. *See* preferred provider organizations
preexisting-conditions, ACA, 34
preexisting narrative frames, 167
preferred provider organizations (PPOs), *27*, 27–28
pregnancy
    smartphone apps, *203*
    Zika, 288
prelogical conceptualization, 123
premium, 26
PrEP, 283–84, *284*
present information, ask questions, check understanding, express concerns (PACE), 67
preserving narratives, 58
pretest-posttest design, health promotion campaigns, 341, *341*
prevention
    ACA, 34
    ethics, 310*b*
    health communication, 21
    HIV/AIDS, 283–84
    managed care, 29
    morality, 141
    Zika, 288
principal care provider (PCP), 23
"PR in the ER" (Seltzer), 229
prisoners of systems, 86
privacy
    eHealth, 196
    health communication, 17
    informed consent, 75
    invasions of, 71
    patient-caregiver communication, 47
    telehealth, 209, *209*, 211
privileges, caregivers, 83
problematic integration (PI), 167*b*
problem-based learning (PBI), 84–85
problem solving
    CI, 49
    coping, 161
    social support, 160
process of change, TTM, 325
product placement, 261–62, *262*
professional prejudice, 99
pronouncements, 51
proposals, 51
prospective payment structure, 26
PSAs. *See* public service announcements
psychological reactance, 308
PTSD. *See* posttraumatic stress disorder

public health
    avian flu, *286*, 286–88
    career opportunities, 269*b*
    crisis communication, 268–93
    defined, 269
    Ebola, 281–83
    emergency, 270
    "four-legged stool," 282
    globalization, 281
    health promotion campaigns, 270, *270*
    HIV/AIDS, *283*, 283–85
    lessons, 291*b*
    opioid epidemic, 289–92, *290*
    SARS, *285*, 285–86
    Zika, 288–89
public relations, *217*, 227–31
    crisis management, 232
    foundations, 228
    image, 229–30, *231*
    relationships, 228–29
    reputation, 229–30, *231*
public service announcements (PSAs), 270
    alcohol, 243
    e-cigarettes, 311–12
    gain-frame appeals, 332–33
Purdue Pharma, 290–91

Qi, 136, 137
Qualitative Health Research (journal), 11
quality of care, 117, 150, 210
quality of life
    aging, 123
    collaborative medical communication, 49–50
queer. *See* LGBTQ+
queer theory, 111
questionnaires, health promotion campaigns, 303–4, *304*
questions
    closed-ended, 44
    health promotion campaign questionnaires, 303
    narrative medicine, 56
    fixed-alternative, health promotion campaign questionnaires, 303
    MI, 52–53
    open-ended
        health promotion campaign questionnaires, 303
        narrative medicine, 59
        patients socialization, 65
        Voice of Lifeworld, 67
quicker and sicker, 92

race and ethnicity, 24–25, *25*, 112–16.

See also African Americans; Asian Americans; Hispanic Americans; Native Americans
media, 305
opioid epidemic, 292
racism, 112
rape culture, 259
reach, health promotion campaign channels, 313
reactive care, 21
reassurance, verbal encouragement, 54
reductionism, 12, 59
reflective negotiation model, 133, 134
reform. *See* health care reform
Reiki, 153
relational approach, communication, 9
relational bankruptcy, 229
Relational Health Communication Competence Model, 92–93
relationships.
See also patient-caregiver communication
commitment-trust theory of, 228–29
crisis communication, 274
crisis management, 232
marketing and public relations, 228–29
reputation, marketing and public relations, 229–30, *231*
reputation-based companies, 230
resiliency, integrative health model, 59
The Resilient Clinician (Wicks), 92
resistance, integrative health model, 59
resources.
See also career opportunities
health communication organizations, 11*b*
restored self, 69
rhetoric of passivity, 49
right to die, ethics, 182*b*
risk communication
crisis communication, 270–74
distrust, 270
perception management, 271–72
risk management/communication framework, 275*b*
rite of passage, 334*b*
Robert Wood Johnson Foundation, 113
roles
culture, 146–51, *147*
social, 141–44
Rolling Stone (magazine), 245
RU SURE, 319–20, 334*b*
The Rutledge Handbook of Health Communication (Thompson, Parrott, & Nussbaum), 11

safer sex, 160, 259–60, 284
salvaged self, 69

sampling, health promotion campaigns, 304
SARS. *See* severe acute respiratory syndrome
satisfaction
caregivers, 89
service excellence, 232
ethics, 72*b*
older adults, 127
patients, 70–71, *71*, 81
consumerism, 150
service excellence, 232
Scandal (TV show), 260
scapegoating, 327*b*
schizophrenia, 203
scientific method, 12
segmentation, audience, 302–11
self-blame, 94
self-concept, 8
self-disclosure, 54
self-doubt, 89, 95
self-efficacy, 127, 162–63, 191, 325
self-esteem, 89, 241, *241*
media image, 239, 253
social support, 159
stigma, 140
seniors. *See* older adults
sensationalism, *250*, 250–51
sensation-seekers, *308*, 308–11
sensitive subjects, 44–45
September 11, 2001 terrorist attacks, 271
sequence of noticings, 58
servant-leadership, 219–23, 220*f*, *222*
service excellence, 232–33
service failures, 233
service learning, 6, 7*b*
service recovery, 233
SES. *See* socioeconomic status
"17 Goals to Change Our World," of United Nations, 24
severe acute respiratory syndrome (SARS), *285*, 285–86
sex and sexual behavior.
See also safer sex
Africa, 283
alcohol, 244
entertainment, 258–60
health, 142
objectification, 259
SMS, 203
transgressions, 46
Zika, 288
The Sex Myth (Hills), 259
sexual assault, 244, 330
sexually transmitted infections, 73, 260, 284, 305
female identity, 142
syphilis, 74–75, 76*b*, 113
Zika, *250*, 251

sexual orientation, 110–12, 260, *260*
shamans, 149
shame-free environments, 110
shocking messages, 339
short message services (SMS), 203–4
short-term memory, 240
sick roles, 146–51
silence, nonverbal encouragement, 54
single-payer system, 32–33
sin taxes, 310*b*
sleep deprivation, 243
smallpox, 139, 279
smartphones, 4
apps, 25
eHealth, 190
mHealth, *200*, 200–204
pregnancy, *203*
WhatsApp, 279
smoking (tobacco)
advertising, 245
cessation, SMS, 203, 204
children, 243
entertainomercials, 261
health promotion campaigns, *309*, 334*b*
media, 243
MI, 53
peer pressure, 334*b*
product placements, 262
truth® campaigns, 295–96
SMS. *See* short message services
social capital, 306
social cognitive theory, 322–23
social comparison theory, 241, *241*
social identities, 68
socialization
caregivers, 81–82, 176
hidden curriculum, 82
patients, 63–65, *65*
social learning theory, 240–41
social marketing, 320–21
social media, 15, 195, 199.
See also specific sites
body image, 253–54
communication skill builder, 230–31
crisis communication, 277, 278–79
health promotion campaigns, 315
social mobilization, 270
social networks, 169, 298
social norms theory, 320, *320*, 321
social roles, 141–44
social support, 6, 8.
See also coping
action-facilitating, 165–66
adolescents, 160
buffering hypothesis, 159, 160
communication, 161*b*
coping, 161–62
defined, 159
eHealth, 194–95

social support (*continued*)
  excess of, 171
  folk medicine, 149
  friends, 169–70, *170*
  health, 160
  Hispanic Americans, 169
  HIV/AIDS, 160
  humor, as hurtful jests, *170*, 170–71
  main-effect model, 159
  nurturing, 166
  older adults, 160, *160*
  problems, 169–72, *170*
  transformative experiences, 172–74
sociocultural model, 14–15
socioeconomic status (SES), 105–7, *107*
  patient cooperation, 73
  poor health with, 4
  race and ethnicity, 113
son's duty, 144*b*
So Sexy So Soon (Levin and Kilbourne), 252
source homophily, 331
Spanish flu, 286
specificity, health promotion campaign channels, 313
The Spirit Catches You and You Fall Down (Fadiman), 139
spiritualism, 135–36, 148–49
spokesperson, 126, 164, 285
  Barbie doll, 252*b*
  crisis communication, 278, 279
  health promotion campaigns, 330–31
  managed care, 29
  physicians, 154
Sports Illustrated (magazine), 245
staffing shortages, 224*b*
stakeholders
  crisis management, 232
  pandemics, 288
  public relations, 228
  risk management/communication framework, 275*b*
standardized patients, 85, 121
Star Trek (TV show), 297
stealth ads, 261
stepping in, medical mistakes, 95–96
stereotypes, 107, 115, *257*
steroids, *255*, 255–56
stigma, *140*, 140–41, 258, 290, 327*b*
"Still a Privilege to Be a Doctor" (Rifkin), 292
St. Jude Children's Research Hospital, 13*b*
stoic orientation, 171
storytelling
  African American women, 299*b*
  narrative medicine, *56*, 56–59
  service excellence, 233

stress.
  See also burnout
  biopsychosocial model, 13–14
  emotions, 13–14
  family, 176
  patient-caregiver communication, 40
stroke, 112, 243
subliminal advertising, 261
substance use disorders.
  See also alcohol; opioid epidemic; smoking
  SMS, 203
suggestions, 51
suicide, 53, 182
superficially image-based companies, 230
supernormal identity, 69
support groups, 23, 169
supportive listening, 166–68
survivor supports, 70
sustaining narratives, 58
susto (fright), 135
syphilis, 74–75, 76*b*, 113
systems-level approach, health care, 5, 5–6

tailored messages, 313–15
Taoism, 136
TB. *See* tuberculosis
teach-back method, 110
teams and teamwork, 97–99
  communications skill builder, 225–27
  managed care, 29
  SARS, 285
  social mobilization, 270
  telehealth, 208
technology.
  See also specific types
  communication, 25
  health communication, 4
  health information, career opportunities, 211*b*
teenagers. *See* adolescents
telehealth, 188, 204–11
  caregivers, 207–11
  patient-centered care, 206–7
  patient portals, 205–6
  telemonitoring, 206
telemedicine, 25, 188, 204–5, *205*
  patient-caregiver communication, 210–11
  pros and cons, 202*b*
telemonitoring, 206
television, 198–99, 239, 240, 243, 260.
  See also specific shows
  health care dramas, 256–57
  news coverage, 251
  nutrition, 241–42
  pharmaceutical advertising, 248

temptation, TTM, 325
tertiary identity, 68–69
Text2Quit, 204
Thai customs, 144*b*
theory of health as expanded consciousness, 137*b*
Theory of Motivated Information Management (TMIM), 191–92, 194
theory of normative social behavior (TNSB), 321, 334*b*
theory of personal causation, 224–25, *225*
theory of planned behavior (TPB), *323*, 323–24
theory of problematic integration, 167*b*
theory of reasoned action (TRA), 323–24
Theory X, 224
Theory Y, 224
"The Patient as a Central Construct" (Kaplan, R.), 49
therapeutic action, mindfulness, 88
therapeutic privilege, 42–43
thimerosal, 272
third-party payer, 26, 27
third-person effect, 240
time constraints, 86–87, *87*, 127
TMIM. *See* Theory of Motivated Information Management
TNSB. *See* theory of normative social behavior
tobacco. *See* smoking
touch, nonverbal encouragement, 54
TPB. *See* theory of planned behavior
TRA. *See* theory of reasoned action
traditional Asian medicine, 153
traditional Chinese medicine, 134, 146
transactional communication, 8–10, 44
transcendent experiences, 173
transgressions, *45*, 45–46
transportation, narrative messages, 336
transsexual. *See* LGBTQ+
transtheoretical model (TTM), 324–25
treatment duplications, 219
trust.
  See also distrust
  commitment-trust theory of relationships, 228–29
  crisis communication, 277
  health communication, 17
  health literacy, 128
truth
  ethics, 43*b*
  moments of, 232
truth® campaigns, 295–96
TTM. *See* transtheoretical model
tuberculosis (TB), 139

tumors, 64
Tuskegee Syphilis Study, 74–75, 76b, 113
Twitter, 230, 252, 289
two-way symmetrical communication, 229, 230–31
tyranny of urgent, 47

uncertainty
  perspectives, 64b
  PI, 167
  Voice of Lifeworld, 67
underinformed audience, 306
Unified Theory of Acceptance and Use of Technology (UTAUT), 193–94
United Nations, 24
universal coverage, 30–34
  multi-payer system, 33
  single-payer system, 32–33
unscheduled interviews, 303
urinary tract infections, 205
uses and gratifications theory, 198, 198–99
UTAUT. See Unified Theory of Acceptance and Use of Technology

vaccinations, 24
  avian flu, 286
  ethics, 287b
  HPV
    health promotion campaigns, 305
    Hispanic Americans, 115
  MI, 53
  TTM, 325
  MMR, 249, 272–73
  parents, 272b
  pharmacies, 4

public health, 269
  smallpox, 139
vaping. See e-cigarettes
verbal encouragement, collaborative medical communication, 54–55
verbing, 51
Viagra, 246b
victimization, illness, 141
video games, 240, 253, 260, 261, 264
violence
  alcohol, 243
  entertainment, 260–61
  intimate partner, 142–43
  sexual assault, 244, 330
  social learning theory, 240
Vioxx, 248
virtual reality headset, 301
Voice of Lifeworld, 65–67, 66
Voice of Medicine, 65, 82

watch one, do one, teach one, 83
wearable devices, 4, 206. See also Apple Watches
webs of significance, 9–10
Weight Watchers (WW), 255
well-being, 40, 256, 268
wellness, 28, 34
WhatsApp, 279
WHO. See World Health Organization
Without Pity (documentary), 258
women
  African American, 105
  obesity, 242
  storytelling, 299b

eHealth, 199
female identity, 142
gender identity, 111
Hispanic American, 44–45
breast cancer, 305
physical fitness, 305–6
intersectionality theory, 105
magazines, 242
older adults, 125
sexual objectification, 259
workload
  burnout, 92
  eHealth, 197
World Health Organization (WHO), 21, 135, 204, 206, 211, 269
  disabilities, 120
  Ebola, 281–82
  Guideline on Communication Risk, 276–77
  health definition, 7–8
  ICF, 7–8, 13, 120
  pandemics, 287–99
  SARS, 285
World Health Report, 285
worried well, 232
WW. See Weight Watchers

X-Men (film), 258

yang, 136
yellow fever, 279
yin, 136
yoga, 146, 152
YouTube, 253

Zika, 250, 250–51, 279, 288–89